Clinical Oncology

Edited by

Geoffrey R. Weiss
Associate Professor of Medicine
The University of Texas Health Science Center at San Antonio

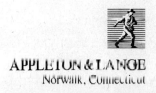
APPLETON & LANGE
Norwalk, Connecticut

0-8385-1325-5

93 94 95 96 97 / 10 9 8 7 6 5 4 3 2 1

Prentice Hall International (UK) Limited, *London*
Prentice Hall of Australia Pty. Limited, *Sydney*
Prentice Hall Canada, Inc., *Toronto*
Prentice Hall Hispanoamericana, S.A., *Mexico*
Prentice Hall of India Private Limited, *New Delhi*
Prentice Hall of Japan, Inc., *Tokyo*
Simon & Schuster Asia Pte. Ltd., *Singapore*
Editora Prentice Hall do Brasil Ltda., *Rio de Janeiro*
Prentice Hall, *Englewood Cliffs, New Jersey*

ISBN: 0-8385-1325-5
ISSN: 1068-6541

Acquisitions Editor: Shelley Reinhardt
Production Editor: Christine Langan
Designer: Kathy Hornyak

PRINTED IN THE UNITED STATES OF AMERICA

Table of Contents

Preface

The clinical and scientific disciplines that collectively contribute to the field of oncology span nearly all the disciplines of medicine and surgery. Few other areas of human endeavor draw from so many other knowledge bases and offer the opportunity for a fundamental understanding of mechanisms of disease and human biology. Perhaps it is for these reasons that those of us privileged to participate in the intellectual challenges of seeking the causes, prevention, and cure of cancer feel that this is where the action is. Indeed, the scope of the problem is so large that traditional divisions of clinical and scientific labor are giving way to new liaisons and collaborations. The concept of translational science, that is, the application of basic science discoveries to the clinical problems at the bedside, has become one of the imperatives of the oncologist.

In ten years of medical education, I have been struck by the dichotomy between the sense of scientific adventure offered to "students" of the oncologic disciplines and the sense of intimidation felt by physicians-in-training when confronted by problems related to cancer. The custodians of the knowledge related to the care of the cancer patient are viewed as individuals steeped in the problems of death, using poisonous drugs by their order alone, and sequestering their patients in special units with special rules understood only by the initiated. This new text seeks to reduce the mystery of this strange fraternity.

During the past decade, many excellent textbooks and handbooks devoted to the cancer problem and the care of its victims have emerged for use by the medical community. This text has been written to bridge some of the remaining gaps in communicating the cancer knowledge base, particularly for the physician-in-training, the graduate physician, the nonspecialist physician, and other health care professionals. We have assembled a distinguished group of authors to present a readable foundation in oncology for this audience. It is hoped that the effort will result in a tool useful in the clinic and as an introduction to more sophisticated areas of oncology. I welcome comments and criticisms, which I hope will lead to future editions even more useful and topical for readers of this work.

Geoffrey R. Weiss, MD
San Antonio, Texas
May 1993

Authors

Janna S. Blanchard, MD
Staff Anesthesiologist, Veterans Affairs Medical Center, Huntington, West Virginia

E. Randolph Broun, MD
Assistant Professor of Medicine, Division of Hematology/Oncology, Indiana University School of Medicine, Indianapolis

Thomas D. Brown, MD
Associate Professor of Medicine and Director, Gastrointestinal Oncology Program, Duke University Medical Center, Durham, North Carolina

Charles A. Coltman, Jr., MD
Professor of Medicine, Division of Medical Oncology, The University of Texas Health Science Center at San Antonio

Mary B. Daly, MD, PhD
Associate Director, Cancer Control Science Program, Fox Chase Cancer Center, Philadelphia

Calvin L. Day, Jr., MD
Clinical Professor of Medicine (Dermatology), The University of Texas Health Science Center at San Antonio

Creighton L. Edwards, MD
Professor of Gynecology, Ann Rife Cox Chair in Gynecology, The University of Texas M. D. Anderson Cancer Center, Houston

John J. Feldmeier, DO
Associate Professor of Radiation Oncology, Department of Radiation Oncology, Wayne State University Medical Center, Detroit

Suzanne M. Fields, PharmD
Director, Investigational Drug Section, Cancer Therapy and Research Center, San Antonio

Harold V. Gaskill III, MD
Associate Professor of Surgery, The University of Texas Health Science Center at San antonio

Philip D. Hall, PharmD
Assistant Professor, College of Pharmacy, Medical University of South Carolina, Charleston

Thomas C. Hardin, PharmD
Clinical Associate Professor of Pharmacology and Medicine, The University of Texas Health Science Center at San Antonio, and Clinical Pharmacy Coordinator, Audie L. Murphy Memorial Veterans Administration Hospital, San Antonio

Kathleen A. Havlin, MD
Assistant Professor of Medicine, Division of Hematology/Oncology, Duke University Medical Center, Durham, North Carolina

G. Richard Holt, MD, MPH
Clinical Professor of Otolaryngology—Head and Neck Surgery, The University of Texas Health Science Center at San Antonio

Rebecca Johnson Irvin, PharmD
Clinical Assistant Professor, College of Pharmacy, The University of Texas at Austin, and Clinical Assistant Professor, Department of Pharmacology, The University of Texas Health Science Center at San Antonio

Michael P. Kahky, MD
Junior Faculty Associate, The University of Texas M. D. Anderson Cancer Center, Houston

Steven P. Kalter, MD
Clinical Associate Professor of Medicine, Division of Medical Oncology, The University of Texas Health Science Center at San Antonio

John J. Kavanagh, MD
Associate Professor and Chief, Section of Gynecologic Medical Oncology, Department of Medical Oncology, The University of Texas M. D. Anderson Cancer Center, Houston

Jim M. Koeller, MS
Clinical Associate Professor, The University of Texas at Austin and Division of Medical Oncol-

ogy, The University of Texas Health Science Center at San Antonio

Andrzej P. Kudelka, MD
Assistant Professor, Departments of Gynecologic Medical Oncology and of Medical Oncology, The University of Texas M. D. Anderson Cancer Center, Houston

John J. Kuhn, PharmD
Professor, Department of Pharmacology/Clinical Pharmacy, The University of Texas at Austin and Division of Medical Oncology, The University of Texas Health Science Center at San Antonio

Milton V. Marshall, PhD
Director of Research and Development, Park One Research Laboratories, Sugar Land, Texas

T. Dwight McKinney, MD
Professor, Department of Medicine, and Director, Nephrology Section, Indiana University School of Medicine, Indianapolis

Frank L. Meyskens, Jr., MD
Professor of Medicine and Biological Chemistry, and Director, Clinical Cancer Center, The University of California at Irvine, Orange

Gregory R. Mundy, MD
Professor of Medicine and Chief, Division of Endocrinology and Metabolism, The University of Texas Health Science Center at San Antonio

Pamela Zyman New, MD
Assistant Professor of Medicine (Neurology), The University of Texas Health Science Center at San Antonio

Naziha F. Nuwayhid, PhD
Assistant Professor, Department of Internal Medicine, Texas Tech University Health Sciences Center at Amarillo, and Associate Director, Special Clinical Immunology Laboratory, Veterans Administration Medical Center, Amarillo, Texas

Timothy J. O'Rourke, MD
Chief, Hematology-Oncology, Brooke Army Medical Center, Fort Sam Houston, Texas

Carey P. Page, MD
Professor of Surgery, The University of Texas Health Science Center at San Antonio

Richard T. Parmley, MD
Professor of Pediatrics and Chief, Division of Pediatric Hematology/Oncology, The University of Texas Health Science Center at San Antonio

Jay Peters, MD
Associate Professor of Medicine and Director of Critical Care Medicine, The University of Texas Health Science Center at San Antonio

William P. Peters, MD, PhD
Associate Professor of Medicine and Director, Bone Marrow Transplant Program, Duke University Medical Center, Durham, North Carolina

Catherine A. Phillips, PhD
Associate Professor, Departments of Internal Medicine and of Biochemistry and Molecular Biology, Texas Tech University Health Sciences Center at Amarillo, and Director, Special Clinical Immunology Laboratory, Veterans Administration Medical Center, Amarillo, Texas

Marion P. Primomo, MD
Medical Director, Santa Rosa Hospice, San Antonio, and Associate Clinical Professor, Department of Family Practice, The University of Texas Health Science Center at San Antonio

Peter M. Ravdin, MD PhD
Assistant Professor of Medicine, Division of Medical Oncology, The University of Texas Health Science Center at San Antonio

Spencer W. Redding, DDS
Associate Dean for Advanced Education and Hospital Affairs and Associate Professor, Department of General Practice, The University of Texas Dental School at San Antonio

Michael F. Sarosdy, MD
Associate Professor and Chief, Division of Urology, The University of Texas Health Science Center at San Antonio

Jeffrey A. Scott, MD
Private Practice of Medical Oncology/Hematology, Atlanta

William W. Shockley, MD
Associate Professor of Surgery (Otolaryngology/Head and Neck Surgery), University of North Carolina Hospitals and the University of North Carolina School of Medicine, Chapel Hill

Theresa A. Shouse, MD
Private Practice of Pediatrics, Plano, Texas

Lon Shelby Smith, MD
Clinical Associate Professor of Medicine, Division of Medical Oncology, The University of Texas Health Science Center at San Antonio

Margaret C. Sunderland, MD
Private Practice of Medical Oncology/Hematology, Dallas

Daniel D. Von Hoff, MD
Professor of Medicine, Division of Medical Oncology, The University of Texas Health Science Center at San Antonio

Nicolas E. Walsh, MD
Professor and Chairman, Department of Rehabilitation Medicine, The University of Texas Health Science Center at San Antonio

Geoffrey R. Weiss, MD
Associate Professor of Medicine, The University of Texas Health Science Center at San Antonio

Arlene J. Zaloznik, MD
Internal Medical Consultant to the United States Army Surgeon General, Falls Church, Virginia

Section I.
Cancer Biology & Etiology

The Cancer Problem

1

Geoffrey R. Weiss, MD

Cancer remains a hugely expensive public health problem in the USA, both in economic terms and in terms of the amount of human suffering it produces. The past two decades have witnessed an explosion in the understanding of the molecular basis of malignant disease and in the rapid application of basic research concepts to the clinical arenas of diagnosis and treatment. Yet the excitement accompanying this new wisdom belies the stubbornness and tenacity with which cancer has resisted satisfactory control. Cancer has been the second leading cause of death in the USA for decades. Although heart disease leads cancer by more than 300,000 deaths per year, cardiovascular deaths are declining, a realization that has led some to project that cancer deaths will predominate by the turn of the century.

Cancer incidence exceeded 1 million cases for 1992. Of that number, one-half died. While half of cancer patients may expect to be cured, the sobering fact remains that the investment of billions of dollars in cancer research, particularly after passage of the National Cancer Act during the Nixon administration, has produced few discoveries having important impact on patient survival for the dominant cancers of the population. Can expenditure of this magnitude against such a daunting foe with so few tangible dividends be rationalized any longer? It may be instructive to examine the cancer problem in ways that elucidate its many facets and suggest that true advances have been made which are not easily measured in terms of cancer patient survival.

Cancer etiology intuitively represents a place to begin applying the resources necessary to solving the cancer problem. But the causes of cancer are multifold and may be viewed from perspectives spanning several orders of magnitude. For the epidemiologist, the problem is one of the human condition, reflecting the tension between environment and genetics. In Western industrialized nations, the impact of culture, habits, diet, and occupation may far exceed the effects of infection, sanitation, natural environment, and heredity that underlie the causes of cancers in less developed or Third World nations. The tasks for the cancer epidemiologist are the identification of those environment determinants of cancer and the alteration of behavior in favor of reducing cancer risk for the population of interest. The well-known determinants of cancer risk for Western or industrializing societies include tobacco consumption, diets high in fat and low in unrefined starches, and occupational exposure to radiation or toxic chemicals.

For the cancer biologist, the problem is viewed at the molecular level, biochemical level, chromosomal level, or cellular level in terms of perturbations of cell homeostasis that result in uncontrolled cell growth and division and the assumption of immortality by the cancer cell. The advances in these arenas have been real, exciting, and potentially prophetic for understanding not only cancer etiology but also normal cell growth and regulation. The discovery of oncogenes, tumor growth factors, chromosomal markers of disease, among others, as new foci for potentially arresting the development of the malignant cell has sparked the interest and imagination of basic scientists and clinicians alike. Conversion of a proto-oncogene to an oncogene may require only a single DNA base pair change coding for a single amino acid alteration in the gene product. Further, genes that suppress an otherwise universal ability of normal cells to assume malignant behavior may undergo mutation or loss under cellular or environmental mechanisms yet to be defined. Such events drive home the realization that all normal cells harbor the potential for becoming promptly malignant as a result of very limited and highly specific changes to the genome and cell machinery. Although the application of these concepts to the predicament of the cancer patient may seem at first far flung, it is becoming clear that many of these basic research techniques can be applied to clinical cancer management: detection of oncogenes in malignant tissues may be associated with poor prognosis for the afflicted host; specific chromosomal aberrations in malignant tissues may permit prediction of poor response to treatment among patients with the same types of leukemia or lymphoma. Now more than ever, advances in the understanding

1

of cancer biology may importantly contribute extraordinarily potent methods of altering the headlong progression of the malignant engine toward the destruction of the host.

For clinicians, the problem remains the struggle to avert the destruction of the patient by the unrelenting displacement of normal homeostasis accompanying malignant tumor growth, a struggle that all too often is fatal for the cancer patient. The clinical skills necessary to achieve the limited success possible in this era demand the use of destructive agents in a way that straddles the fine line between death of the malignant cell and preservation of the normal cell. The empiricism of the last 20 years in the use of anticancer drugs, radiation, and surgery is being displaced by a rationally based approach to therapeutics steeped in molecular and clinical pharmacology, biochemistry, high energy physics, computer modeling of therapeutic strategies, and other novel disciplines. The clinical problems faced by the oncologist include overcoming the inherent or acquired resistance of the malignant cell to therapy, ameliorating the toxicities of aggressively applied therapies, and exploiting the additive or synergistic potencies of radiation, drugs, and surgery to effect optimal anticancer results. Massive cooperative clinical treatment organizations have been created to explore the potencies of these strategies when offered to large populations of cancer patients in order to provide the most rapid plausible result to the treatment community.

The problem is massive in scope and multifaceted in its presentation to the observer. Its solution is unimaginable in terms of benefit to the human condition, both in the alleviation of the pain and suffering produced by malignant disease and in the understanding of the mechanism of cellular growth and senescence.

The Malignant State: The Molecular, Cytogenetic, & Immunologic Basis of Cancer

2

Catherine A. Phillips, PhD, & Naziha F. Nuwayhid, PhD

This chapter highlights areas of research, both clinical and basic, that give insight into the causes of cancer. It considers the genetic basis of cancer at the macro level—chromosomal abnormalities—and at the micro level—molecular biology of oncogenes. It also considers the role of the immune system in tumor development and progression.

GENETIC BASIS OF CANCER

The idea that cancer has a genetic basis is supported by clinical observations that certain tumors exhibit defined familial inheritance patterns and by observations that specific chromosomal abnormalities (eg, the Philadelphia chromosome translocation in chronic myelogenous leukemia) are associated with particular tumors. Evidence that specific genetic elements or alterations are involved in tumor formation was derived from studies of animal retroviruses that cause specific cancers.

In 1911, Rous described the induction of sarcomas in chickens using cell-free filtrates. The virus identified as the etiologic agent was called Rous sarcoma virus (RSV) and was the first retrovirus to be described. Its genome was characterized, and the gene responsible for oncogenesis was designated as *src*. Subsequently, a homologous gene was identified in normal chicken cells and in most vertebrates, including humans, using a complementary DNA probe. This work suggested that the viral oncogene evolved from a normal cellular gene.

To determine whether "transforming genes" in tumors were responsible for the malignant state, a series of transfection studies were performed by Weinberg and Cooper. These investigators demonstrated that DNA extracted from human tumors and introduced into normal cells via calcium phosphate precipitation could produce a transformed/malignant phenotype in nonmalignant cells. Their results suggested that such genes were present in tumor cells. (DNA derived from about 20% of all tumors can in-

duce transformation in some type of cultured cell lines.) Further characterization of this tumorigenic DNA has lead to the identification of altered cellular genes, mostly of the *ras* gene family. Specific oncogene families are discussed later in this section.

Mechanisms of Oncogene Activation

The mechanisms by which normal cellular genes acquire oncogenic activities are **mutation, chromosomal translocation, amplification, insertion,** and **deletion.**

A. Mutation: A cellular proto-oncogene can be converted to an oncogene via a single point mutation, causing a change of a single amino acid in the gene product. Genetic lesions of this type have been demonstrated to activate a number of the *ras* oncogenes; these single base changes result in the production of an altered p21 *ras* gene product. The normal *ras* gene product is a protein with a molecular weight of 21,000 referred to as p21. In the bladder carcinoma T24/EJ, a change from G to T in the p21 DNA coding sequence results in the incorporation of valine into the peptide chain instead of glycine at position 12. This small change is capable of changing the cell's phenotype. Chemical or environmental agents could induce transformation by generating mutations within these proto-oncogenes.

B. Chromosomal Translocation: Chromosomal rearrangements, particularly the transfer of a gene from its normal position on one chromosome to another chromosome, have been demonstrated in a number of tumors. Some translocations occur consistently in certain tumors. The consistent and specific appearance of particular rearrangements support the notion that they play a significant etiologic role in tumorigenesis. These rearrangements may lead to the activation of proto-oncogenes, as in Burkitt's lymphoma, or to the production of chimeric (fusion) proteins resulting from gene fusion, as in chronic myelogenous leukemia.

In Burkitt's lymphoma, reciprocal translocations between chromosome 8 at the c-*myc* locus and chromosomes 2, 14, or 22 at or near the immunoglobulin genes occur. The translocation of a segment of chromosome 8 to chromosome 14, t(8;14), puts c-myc into the immunoglobulin heavy chain alpha switch region. Reciprocal translocations [t(2:8) and t(8:22)] place the c-myc gene together with immunoglobulin enhancer or promoter elements. Because Burkitt's lymphoma cells with this rearrangement express increased levels of the c-myc gene, it has been inferred that the rearrangement has influenced the regulation of this gene.

In chronic myelogenous leukemia (CML), the c-abl gene on chromosome 9 is translocated to chromosome 22 at the bcr (break point cluster) locus. This results in the production of the c-abl-bcr transcript and the translation into a novel tumor-specific protein.

C. Amplification: Amplification is the increase in the number of copies of a particular gene or DNA sequence. The amplification of a gene may result in the overexpression of the product encoded by this gene. Many oncogenes have been shown to be amplified and their gene products overexpressed as the result of this change in copy number. For example, N-myc amplification has been demonstrated in both neuroblastoma and retinoblastoma, whereas a 16-fold amplification of c-myc has been shown in colon carcinoma and a 20- to 30-fold amplification in the human leukemia line HL60. The prognosis for individuals with certain tumors correlates with amplification or overexpression of particular oncogenes and their products, eg, the HER-2/neu oncogene in breast and ovarian cancers (see below).

D. Insertion: Insertion of endogenous cellular DNA regulatory sequences, either by direct transposition or by retroviruslike integration, can result in the activation of proto-oncogenes. The integration of regulatory sequences within viral long terminal repeats (LTRs) at a position near cellular proto-oncogenes can result in their activation. The insertion of an intracisternal–A particle genome near the proto-oncogene c-mos has been shown in mouse plasmacytoma. The activation of the c-mos has been shown to be the result of reinsertion of an endogenous intracisternal–A particle genome within the c-mos proto-oncogene. The exact mechanism of this insertion has not been determined.

E. Deletion: Deletion may involve the loss of a whole chromosome, a chromosomal segment, or a gene. Some deletions are tumor specific while others are common to tumors of diverse cellular origins. The loss of the retinoblastoma gene on chromosome 13 and the loss of a specific region (q13) on chromosome 11 are unique to retinoblastoma and Wilms' tumor, respectively. On the other hand, loss of a specific region on chromosome 3 is observed in small-cell carcinoma of the lung, renal cell carcinoma, and ovarian carcinoma.

Deletion often results in the loss of tumor suppressor genes (also referred to as antioncogenes or recessive oncogenes), which function as negative growth regulators, ie, they regulate uncontrolled cellular proliferation by inhibiting cell division or by enhancing differentiation. Therefore, the loss of these suppressor genes or a mutation that leads to the loss of their function results in tumorigenesis. Because of their recessive behavior, the involved mutation or loss should affect both gene copies on homologous chromosomes (see below).

RB1 is a tumor suppressor gene that encodes for a nuclear protein which is involved in transcriptional regulation and control of cell division. This protein exists in phosphorylated and unphosphorylated forms. The presence of phosphorylated RB1 protein correlates with the number of cells entering DNA synthesis phase (S) of the cell cycle. Dephosphorylation of RB1 takes place during growth phase (G_1) of the cell cycle and inhibits cell division. In addition, RB1 protein is inactivated by binding to transforming proteins encoded by DNA tumor viruses such as adenovirus and human papillomaviruses.

The p53 gene is another tumor suppressor gene that encodes for a nuclear phosphoprotein with DNA binding activity. Similar to RB1 gene product, p53 also binds to several proteins encoded by DNA tumor viruses. A wide variety of tumors exhibit mutations in RB1 and p53. Transformation of cell lines occurs when the products of either of these genes are lost or rendered nonfunctional by mutation.

Viral Oncogenesis

Much of what is known about the genetic etiology of cancer is based on studies of **retroviruses** (RNA viruses). A hallmark of these viruses is the incorporation of the viral sequences into the cellular genome via the formation of a DNA intermediate that is transcribed from the RNA viral genome by the structural viral protein reverse transcriptase. The viral genome consists of three main structural genes—gag, pol, env—encoding for internal viral proteins, the replicative enzyme reverse transcriptase, and the envelope protein, respectively. The oncogenic potential of these viruses is independent of the replicative genes. It has been determined that the oncogenic form of the virus cannot replicate and that one of the original three genes has been replaced by a "transforming" gene.

Examples of retroviruses that are important in the etiology of human disease states are HTLVs (human T cell lymphotropic viruses) involved in the production of T cell leukemias and lymphomas (HTLV-I), hairy cell leukemia (HTLV-II), and AIDS [acquired immunodeficiency syndrome; HIV-I (human immunodeficiency virus), formerly termed HTLV-III]. Studies on these viruses and their life cycles reveal that they behave similarly to transposons (or movable genetic elements). These elements are capable of moving or "jumping" around the genome and were discovered because of their ability to alter or modify the expression of genes by inserting into or near them.

In addition to retroviruses, **hepdnaviruses (hepatotropic DNA viruses)** and **papillomaviruses (DNA viruses)** are also capable of inserting themselves into the cellular genome and thereby altering gene expression.

Epidemiologic evidence that the hepdnavirus hepatitis B virus (HBV) is involved in the etiology of hepatocellular carcinoma (HCC) is striking. However, the molecular mechanisms that lead to HCC development are poorly understood. Data suggest that integration of the HBV into the host chromosome may lead to tumor induction either by direct activation of cellular oncogenes or by disrupting the function of tumor suppressor genes. In addition to integration, chronic inflammation and continuous regeneration of the infected liver contribute to increased mutational events and subsequent tumor development. This virus replicates through an RNA intermediate requiring reverse transcriptase and has been shown to integrate into the tumor cell genome. The hepatitis B viral DNA may be extensively rearranged and may cause chromosomal damage. DNA extracted from hepatocellular carcinomas can cause transformation in *in vitro* transfection studies. The exact mechanism of oncogenesis is unknown and probably involves more than simple integration of a viral retroelement.

Human papillomaviruses (HPV) have also been implicated as transforming viruses and have been associated with precancerous lesions and invasive cervical cancers. Additional factors may be required to produce cellular transformation. Like the hepdnaviruses, HPV 16 and HPV 18, which demonstrate high risk for malignant progression, have been shown to be integrated in the cellular genomes of invasive cancers; however, the HPV DNA is not integrated into the cellular genome in the precancerous lesions. These high-risk types are able to transform primary rat cells in cooperation with *ras* and immortalize primary human fibroblasts and keratinocytes. The transforming proteins of HPV 16 and HPV 18 bind pRB1 and p53, both of which have been shown to participate in tumor suppression. HPV-tumorigenesis is believed to be a complex multistage process. Understanding this process is important to the development of preventive, diagnostic, and curative strategies.

Temin (1989) suggested that all these viral types were derived from an ancient bacterial retron and that all these genetic elements be termed **retroelements.** This terminology suggests that the means by which the retroelements replicate and survive is related to their oncogenic potential.

Oncogenes & Their Products

Oncogenes can be classified by the relatedness of nucleic acid sequences, by the amino acid sequences

of gene products, or by the enzyme activity of these products. These products may be located in the cytoplasm, nucleus, or plasma membrane, and they are similar to growth factors, growth factor receptors, protein tyrosine kinases (PTKs), or guanosine triphosphate (GTP)–binding (signal transduction) proteins. They function as regulators of DNA replication, gene transcription, GTP binding, and protein phosphorylation. Uncoupling of these activities could result in uncontrolled growth and development of tumors. Three families of these genes are described below.

A. The *ras* Gene Family: The three genes of the *ras* family are H-*ras,* K-*ras,* and N-*ras.* These genes are activated owing to a single point mutation in codons 12, 13, 59, and 61 in their p21 coding region as previously described. The H-*ras* gene is the cellular homolog of the viral oncogene found in the Harvey strain of murine sarcoma virus and has been associated with bladder, mammary, and lung carcinomas. The single base changes that are found in these tumors are at codons 12 and 61; they result in single amino acid changes from glycine to valine or aspartic acid, or from glutamine to leucine, in the peptide sequence. The amino acid change in the transforming p21 results in a more rigid molecule rather than the flexible hinge that allows the amino terminus to fold into the core of the normal p21 molecule.

Normal p21 has GTP-binding GTPase activity and an amino acid sequence homologous to signal-transducing proteins coupled to specific cell surface receptors. Mutant p21 may not be able to hydrolyze GTP (GTPase activity) and hence not be able to modulate intracellular signal transduction; the mutation in codon 12 results in loss of the ability of p21 to bind GTP. Transfection of an estrogen-dependent breast carcinoma cell line with the mutant *ras* converts it into an estrogen-independent line.

B. The C-*myc* and *myc*-like Gene Family: C-*myc* is associated with progression of cells from a resting state to a dividing state, ie, progression from G_0 to G_1 and maintenance of the potentially proliferative state. Thus, it is associated with cell growth, division, and differentiation. The c-*myc* gene product is a nuclear protein with DNA binding activity. It is activated in Burkitt's lymphoma by the chromosome translocation t(8;22) as previously described. This translocation not only activates this gene but also results in the overexpression of its product, pp62 (a phosphoprotein of MW 62,000) located in the nucleus. It has been postulated that the rate of cellular proliferation is related to the turnover rate of pp62. The increased c-*myc* expression probably contributes to the high rate of proliferation observed in these tumors.

Another member of the *myc* gene family, N-*myc,* has been shown to be amplified 75- to 500-fold in some neuroblastoma lines. This gene is homologous to the c-*myc* gene on chromosome 8 but is located on chromosome 2. Amplification of this gene is most likely preceded by its translocation together with variable lengths of its flanking sequences. The degree of overexpression correlates with the gene copy number. C-*myc* is reported not to be expressed in tumors that express N-*myc*. In general, the greater the amplification, the shorter the time to relapse and hence the poorer the prognosis. Furthermore, it is overexpression of N-*myc* rather than simply amplification that correlates with the worst prognosis. As with c-*myc,* the N-*myc* gene product is associated with increased proliferation; proliferation of neuroblasts prevents their differentiation.

C. The HER-2/*neu* Gene: HER-2/neu (also called c-*erb* B2) was originally identified by transfecting DNA derived from chemically induced rat neuroglioblastomas into NIH/3T3 cells. It has partial sequence homology with, but can be distinguished from, the epidermal growth factor (EGF) receptor. Moreover, it has structural similarity to peptide hormone receptors, which consists of an extracellular encoding region, approximately 40% homologous to EGF receptor; a hydrophobic transmembrane domain, approximately 80% homologous to the EGF receptor; and a third (cytoplasmic) domain that contains sequences with protein tyrosine kinase activity.

This gene is amplified in 25–30% of all human primary breast tumors. Amplification and overexpression are clearly associated with stage of disease. Slamon et al (1989) assayed for gene amplification, mRNA levels, and expression of the *neu* gene product (a protein of MW 185,000; p185) in primary breast tumors by immunohistochemical staining and Western blotting. They confirmed that amplification of the gene correlates with time to relapse and survival. Overexpression is highly predictive of a poorer outcome in both node-negative and node-positive patients. It has also been shown to be associated with increased mitotic fraction. If either overexpression or amplification conclusively demonstrates an increased tumor growth fraction, then chemotherapeutic agents that are S phase–specific might be efficacious in the treatment of these cancers.

The normal HER-2/*neu* gene has been shown to induce transformation in in vitro transfection studies. Cells transformed in this way expressed the *neu* gene product at levels comparable to human breast and ovarian cancer cells. Evidence that a *neu* gene may play an etiologic role in the development of breast tumors also comes from studies in which the mutated HER-2/*neu* gene was introduced into mice. In these transgenic mice, adenocarcinomas developed in both males and females in a synchronous and polyclonal manner; no normal breast tissue could be found. This finding supports the notion that either the normal or mutant gene alone can induce the transformed state.

Data from several groups suggest that the activation of this gene results in the stimulation of the cytoplasmic receptor protein tyrosine kinase activity causing signal transduction into the cell that ultimately results in increased cell growth.

Brandt-Rauf et al have explained the mechanism by which changes in the preferred (or lower energy) three-dimensional conformation of p185 due to a single amino acid change (valine to glutamine, position 664) in the transmembrane region could cause transformation (Fig. 2–1). In the absence of p185-associated growth factor, the majority (91%) of non-transforming p185 molecules favor a three-dimensional conformation that has a "bend" in the transmembrane region which prevents receptor aggregation, signal transduction, and hence cell growth (Fig. 2–1A). In the presence of the growth factor, the normal p185 assumes an α-helical ("straight") conformation resulting in aggregation, signal transduction, and cell growth (Fig. 2–1B). The transforming mutant p185 molecules preferentially assume the "straight" conformation that permits aggregation, signal transduction, and cell growth in the absence of p185-binding growth factor, ie, growth factor–independent or autonomous cell growth (Fig. 2–1C).

How does the expression of the normal or nontransforming p185 cause transformation? A minority (9%) of the normal p185 molecules assume the higher energy or "straight" conformation of the mutant p185 (Fig. 2–1D). This small amount of the activated form of the receptor, while normally present, is insufficient to cause cell transformation. Overexpression of the normal p185 could increase the absolute number of the "straight" conformation causing autonomous cell growth. Overexpression of p185 has been described in human breast and ovarian cancers. Experimentally, 5- to 10-fold overexpression of the normal *neu* proto-oncogene causes transformation of (NIH/3T3) cells in culture, while lower levels (1- to 4-fold) do not. The conformational analyses provide a reasonable explanation for the mechanism whereby overexpression of a normal product causes cell transformation.

The use of both immunohistochemical and molecular biologic techniques for this gene and its product could be of great strategic importance in the diagnosis, treatment, and follow-up of breast and ovarian cancer.

Chromosomal Abnormalities in Cancer

Genetic rearrangement of genomic sequences is an important if not essential step in tumor development. Specific chromosomal alterations have been shown to be closely associated with various tumor types and cancer risk syndromes. For example, trisomy 21 and deletions of chromosomes 11 and 13 are associated with an increased risk of leukemia, Wilms' tumor, and retinoblastoma, respectively. The Philadelphia chromosome t(9;22) is commonly found in chronic myelogenous leukemia and the t(8;14) in Burkitt's lymphoma. (See the references at the end of this

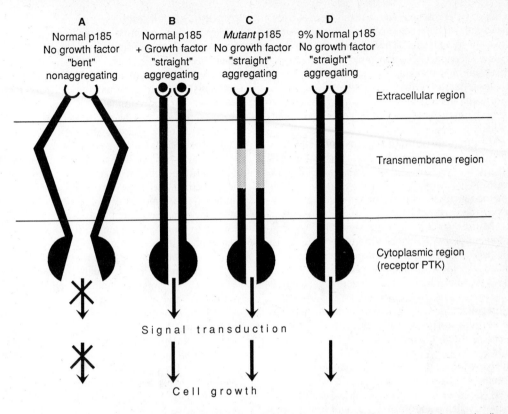

Figure 2–1. Alternative conformations of the *neu* oncogene product, p185, correlate with normal and abnormal cell growth states. **A:** 91% of normal (nontransforming) p185 molecules preferentially assume a conformation which has a bend in the transmembrane (TM) region that does not permit aggregation, signal transduction, and induction of cell growth. **B:** The interaction of normal "bent" p185 with its growth factor cause a conformational change in the TM region from "bent" to "straight" that permits aggregation, signaling, and induction of cell growth. **C:** Mutant (transforming) p185 molecules preferentially assume the "straight" conformation that leads to autonomous (non–growth factor–dependent) growth or transformation. **D:** 9% of normal p185 are found to assume the "higher energy requiring" or "straight" conformation and resemble the mutant p185 molecules in their ability to induce aggregation, signal transduction, and cell growth in the absence of growth factor. Overexpression of normal p185 causes an increase in the absolute number of the "straight" normal molecules to growth factor–independent (autonomous) cell growth or neoplasia if the critical mass of receptors is attained. PTK = Protein tyrosine kinase. (Modified and redrawn, with permission, from Brandt-Rauf PW, Rackovsky S, Pincus MR: Correlation of the structure of the transmembrane domain in the *neu* oncogene–encoded p185 protein with its function. *Proc Natl Acad Sci USA* 1990;**87**:8660.)

chapter for extensive reviews and cataloging of chromosomal aberrations.)

Virtually all adult solid tumors have abnormal heterogeneous karyotypes, in contrast to pediatric tumors and leukemias that have a few clonal chromosomal defects. However, the general mechanisms that operate in chromosomal rearrangements are **translocation, inversion, amplification, partial deletion, and abnormal segregation of chromosomes.** The break points are often associated with oncogene loci. As discussed above, a positional change of genetic material can alter a gene's regulatory environment (eg, c-*abl-bcr* sequence in Burkitt's lymphoma). Often, inheritable tumor types show abnormal segregation of chromosomes, resulting in either mono-

somy or duplication of a whole chromosome complement with or without structural rearrangements. In some cases, the tumor becomes hemizygous for part of the genome because of a deletion.

In neuroblastomas, amplification of the N-*myc* oncogene is cytologically evidenced by the appearance of double minute chromosomes or by homogeneous staining regions.

In retinoblastoma, tumor cells most commonly have the chromosomal deletion 13q14 (ie, band (14) of the long arm (q) of chromosome 13 is deleted). Additional rearrangements involving chromosomes 1 and 6 also occur. In Wilms' tumor, all or portions of the chromosome region 11q13 are deleted; however, chromosome 1 abnormalities are also common. Both these tumor types are believed to result from two separate and independent genetic events as proposed by the "two-hit hypothesis." They can be used to illustrate that secondary chromosomal rearrangements can result in the unmasking of an initial predisposing recessive mutation ("first hit") that leads to the homozygosity of this mutation. The mechanisms proposed by Nordenskjold and Cavenee (1988) are the following:

(1) Mitotic nondisjunction (failure of sister chromatids to migrate to opposite poles during mitosis) results in the loss of the wild-type chromosome. Hence, somatic hemizygosity will be attained at all loci on the remaining chromosome including the predisposing recessive mutation.

(2) Mitotic recombination (between chromosomal homologs with the break point between the tumor locus and the centromere) results in homozygosity at all loci most distal to the centromere, which includes the tumor locus, and in heterozygosity at all loci proximal to the centromere.

(3) Secondary events (**gene conversion, deletion, or point mutation**) may also occur in the affected region and lead to the unmasking of the initial genetic event.

The basic idea is that both chromosomes must bear the mutated RB1 (retinoblastoma) locus, *rb*. This homozygous state can be attained either by inheriting one recessive gene and having a second somatic mutation, or by having two somatic mutations occur as has been demonstrated in sporadic cases of retinoblastoma.

Wilms' tumor has several characteristics in common with retinoblastoma. Deletions in the chromosome region 11q13 constitute a predisposition to this disease but are not sufficient to cause it. This idea is supported by the fact that discrete tumor foci are seen against a background of normal kidney cells even in cases in which the 11q13 band of one chromosome is missing. A second postzygotic event is required before tumor development can occur. Wilms' cells lost their ability to form tumors in nude mice after having a normal chromosome 11 introduced into them. Such data support the idea that Wilms' tumor is the result of unmasking of a recessive mutation located on chromosome 11.

IMMUNOLOGIC BASIS OF CANCER

The host's immune response to a tumor is assumed to be beneficial and therefore desirable. It is the notion that the immune system surveils the body for aberrant changes, growths, or neoplasms and mobilizes armies of immune lymphocytes or killer cells to attack and subdue the invasive tumor, once recognized. Is this the only role that the immune system plays in tumor growth and progression? Could the immune system facilitate tumor growth?

Immune Surveillance

The theory of **immune surveillance** proposes that the immune system routinely recognizes and eliminates mutant cells that develop throughout an individual's life span. Potential tumor cells can be distinguished from "self" antigenically and therefore be recognized and eliminated. Several lines of evidence support this theory. Firstly, immunocompromised animals produced by treatment with antithymocyte serum, carcinogens, or viruses that attack the immune system and neonatal or old animals, have greater susceptibility to carcinogenesis or to enhancement of carcinogenesis. Moreover, the ability to form tumors in such animals can be inhibited by reconstituting the immune system with exogenous lymphoid cells or by immunostimulants. Secondly, there is an increased incidence of tumors in transplant patients who have been immunosuppressed to prevent organ graft rejection and in individuals who have either acquired or congenital immunodeficiency syndromes. This idea is the basis of the many immunotherapies that have been proposed or that are being tested. Other situations have caused this theory to be questioned. In the nude (congenital athymic) mouse, the incidence of spontaneous tumors is not increased as would have been predicted. However, these animals have high levels of natural killer (NK) cell activity that may partially compensate for their defective T cell immunity.

Immunofacilitation

Prehn et al have proposed a "flip side" or "dark side" of tumor immunity—immunostimulation or **immunofacilitation.** This hypothesis suggests that tumor growth and progression require or are dependent on a positive immune response, ie, the immune system encourages or fosters tumor growth and progression! Furthermore, this immunity is unique for each tumor, and the tumor adjusts its immunogenicity to a level that is most favorable to its growth. From this argument, it follows that *immunosuppression may be as good as or better than enhancement of the immune response for the treatment of malignancy.* The immunofacilitation hypothesis warrants further consideration because of its possible impact on the recently accelerated use and development of immunotherapies.

Data supporting the hypothesis of immunofacilitation are that **(1)** in immune restoration or titration experiments (by addition of varying numbers of lymphocytes), a level of immunity existed that favored the formation of 3-methylcholanthrene (MCA)–induced tumors; **(2)** the growth of tumors in vivo and in vitro could be inhibited or facilitated by varying the concentration of a specific antibody in the culture; and **(3)** MCA-induction of tumors in adult mice could be favorably influenced by the autoimmune state induced by 3-day neonatal thymectomy.

The immune system maintains the level of immunogenicity of a tumor by immunologic selection, establishing a level that is most conducive for growth and progression even after many experimental passages in animals. As a consequence of this selection, a change in the immunizing capacity of a tumor is compensated for by an opposing change in its sensitivity to the immune response, thereby preserving the tumor's overall immunogenicity. The tumor is constantly changing to adapt to its immune environment. It is important to note that adaptation cannot occur before there has been significant proliferation (generating heterogeneity) to permit selection. Thus, tumors that have undergone less progression are probably less malignant and more homogeneous and are better treated by immunotherapy regimens. However, after progression has been established, immunosuppression may be as beneficial an immunotherapy as enhancement of immune response.

Immunodeficiency Syndromes & Tumor Formation

Individuals with acquired and congenital immunodeficiency syndromes have been reported to have an increased incidence of certain malignancies relative to normal individuals. [For a review of immunodeficiency diseases, see Ammann (1991).] It has been postulated that the breakdown or absence of immune surveillance in these states permits formation and growth of tumors because of a ubiquitous environmental, microbial, or carcinogenic agent. In these patients, including immunosuppressed transplant recipients, tumors are restricted to a few types such as ultraviolet-induced skin cancers, tumors of the lymphoreticular system—lymphomas and leukemias—and Kaposi's sarcoma. In HIV-1–infected individuals, Kaposi's sarcoma is a common clinical feature. Previously this relatively rare form of skin cancer had been seen primarily in elderly males of Mediterranean origin. Other tumors associated with HIV-1–infected individuals are squamous cell carcinoma of the oral cavity, cloacogenic carcinoma of the rectum, non-Hodgkin's lymphoma, and acute and chronic leukemias. These tumors may result from the transformation of cells by viruses such as Epstein-Barr virus (EBV) and cytomegalovirus (CMV). Coupled with other events such as oncogene activation or overproduction of growth factors, these cells could attain a proliferative advantage and aid in tumor formation.

Two-thirds of X-linked lymphoproliferative syndrome–affected males develop infectious mononucleosis that is associated with high morbidity and mortality. These patients are specifically immunologically deficient in their ability to respond to EBV, and they develop extranodal non-Hodgkin's lymphoma of the Burkitt type or become hypogammaglobulinemic or both. Because of their specific inability to destroy the EBV-infected, transformed B cells, these cells continue to proliferate and invade virtually all organs; the activated but ineffective killer cells (T and NK) cause widespread damage to the organism owing to nonspecific cell-mediated cytotoxicity. The result is immune dysregulation and dysfunction.

Immune Surveillance Versus Immunofacilitation

Does an immunodeficiency state predispose an individual to develop cancer owing to the lack of immune responsiveness or because of it? What is the role of the immune system in growth and progression of tumors?

The picture that can be assembled from currently known data is that the tumor and the host are involved in a symbiotic relationship at least at the beginning of development; however, if conditions are conducive, the transformed cell begins to grow, and as growth progresses, immunoselection favors the growth of certain clones of transformed cells or eliminates others, by either cytostatic or cytotoxic mechanisms. If the immune response is effective early in this scenario, then the host's interests are served. On the other hand, if tumor growth continues and immunoselection prevails, then the tumor's interests are served, leading to tumor adaptation and progression. A balance is established between the tumor and its host. If the immune status of the host changes, then clones previously held in check may begin to grow because the new environment is conducive, while other clones will be eliminated.

Clearly, the relationship between the host and the tumor is neither simple nor fully understood. In designing immunotherapies it is important to consider the possible consequences of enhancing the host's immune responsiveness. For certain malignancies, immunosuppression may be preferable. Early detection is essential; the earlier a tumor is detected, the less chance there is for tumor heterogeneity to develop and therefore the best conditions exist for eliminating it.

REFERENCES

Oncogenes

Aaronson SA: Growth factors and cancer. *Science* 1991;**254**:1146.

Aaronson SA, Tronick SR: The role of oncogenes in human neoplasia. In *Important Advances in Oncol-*

ogy, 1985. DeVita VT, Hellman S, Rosenberg SA (editors). Lippincott, 1985.

Brandt-Rauf PW, Rackovsky S, Pincus, MR: Correlation of the structure of the transmembrane domain of the *new* oncogene-encoded p185 protein with its function. *Proc Natl Acad Sci USA* 1990;**87**:8660.

Korsmeyer SJ: Immunoglobulin and T-cell receptor genes reveal the clonality, lineage and translocations of lymphoid neoplasms. In: *Important Advances in Oncology, 1987.* DeVita VT, Hellman S, Rosenberg SA (editors). Lippincott, 1987.

Merkel DE, McGuire WL: Oncogenes and cancer prognosis. In: *Important Advances in Oncology, 1988.* DeVita VT, Hellman S, Rosenberg SA (editors). Lippincott, 1988.

Park M, Vande Woude GF: Principles of molecular cell biology of cancer: Oncogenes. In: *Cancer: Principles & Practice of Oncology,* 3rd ed. DeVita VT, Hellman S, Rosenberg SA (editors). Lippincott, 1989.

Slamon DJ et al: Studies of the HER-2/*neu* proto-oncogene in human breast and ovarian cancer. *Science* 1989;**244**:707.

Temin HM: Retrons in bacteria. *Nature* 1989;**339**:254.

Weinberg RA: The genetic origins of human cancer. *Cancer* 1988;**61**:1963.

Viral Oncogenesis

Beasley RP: Hepatitis B virus: The major etiology of hepatocellular carcinoma. *Ann Intern Med* 1988;**108**:390.

Gallo RC, Blattner WA: Human T-cell leukemia/lymphoma viruses: ATL and AIDS. In: *Important Advances in Oncology, 1985.* DeVita VT, Hellman S, Rosenberg SA (editors). Lippincott, 1985.

Werness BA, Munger K, Howley PM: Role of the human papillomavirus oncoproteins in transformation and carcinogenic progression. In: *Important Advances in Oncology, 1991.* DeVita VT, Hellman S, Rosenberg SA (editors). Lippincott, 1991.

Cytogenetics

Nordenskjold M, Cavenee WK: Genetics and the etiology of solid tumors. In: *Important Advances in Oncology, 1988.* DeVita VT, Hellman S, Rosenberg SA (editors). Lippincott, 1988.

Rowley JD: Principles of molecular cell biology of cancer: Chromosomal abnormalities. In: *Cancer: Principles & Practice of Oncology,* 3rd ed. DeVita VT, Hellman S, Rosenberg SA (editors). Lippincott, 1989.

Immunology

Ammann AJ: Immunodeficiency diseases. Chapters 23–27 in: *Basic & Clinical Immunology,* 7th ed. Stites DP, Terr AI (editors). Appleton & Lange, 1991.

Greenberg PD: Mechanisms of tumor immunology. In: *Basic & Clinical Immunology,* 7th ed. Stites DP, Terr AI (editors). Appleton & Lange, 1991.

Penn I: Cancers following cyclosporine therapy. *Transplantation* 1987;**43**:32.

Prehn RT: Tumor-specific antigens as altered growth receptors. *Cancer Res* 1989;**49**:2823.

Prehn RT, Bartlett GL: Surveillance, latency and the two levels of MCA-induced tumor immunogenicity. *Int J Cancer* 1987;**39**:106.

Prehn RT, Prehn LM: The autoimmune nature of cancer. *Cancer Res* 1987;**47**:927.

Prehn RT, Prehn LM: The flip side of tumor immunity. *Arch Surg* 1989;**124**:102.

Shearer WT, Parker CW: Antibody and compliment modulation of tumor cell growth in vitro and in vivo. *Fed Proc* 1978;**37**:2385.

Carcinogenesis

3

Milton V. Marshall, PhD

Carcinogenesis is the study of the origins of cancer. In a broad sense, epidemiologic studies are performed to corroborate clinical observations. Investigations in biologic systems can be performed to reproduce these observations to determine the steps involved in conversion of normal cells to malignant cells. One goal of this chapter is to classify diverse chemical and physical agents by known or suspected mechanisms of action. Once it is known how exposure to such diverse agents can lead to tumor formation, it will be easier to understand how to prevent their activities both by identifying susceptible individuals as well as by blocking or reversing the actions of such agents.

Although tumors have been observed in patients for centuries, the origins of the study of human cancer are generally attributed to physicians in the 18th century. A suspected link between tobacco use and cancer was reported by Hill. Shortly thereafter, a relationship between scrotal cancer and occupational exposure of chimney sweeps to coal tar and soot was established by Pott. It was not until 1917 that the first experimental documentation of coal tar as a carcinogen in animals was reported. In this study, tumors were observed on the ears of rabbits following application at that site. Several years later, fractionation of coal tar made possible the identification of a class of chemical carcinogens known as polycyclic aromatic hydrocarbons (PAHs). PAHs are formed during the incomplete combustion of organic material and are therefore present in the environment from numerous sources including automobile exhaust, burning tobacco products, municipal incineration facilities, and wood burning.

The observation that workers in the dye industry experienced an unusually high incidence of bladder cancer was reported by Rehn in 1895. Evidence that 2-naphthylamine, an aromatic amine to which dye workers were occupationally exposed, was carcinogenic was reported in 1938 by Hueper. In this study, bladder tumors were induced in dogs following exposure to 2-naphthylamine. Conversely, the carcinogenicity of bischloromethyl ether in animals resulted in epidemiologic studies that established a link between occupational exposure and tumors in humans. Dietary carcinogens such as aflatoxin B_1 and cycasin

were found to cause tumors in animals and were thus suspected of causing cancer in humans. In areas where liver cancer was endemic, a positive correlation was observed between the presence of aflatoxin in the diet and urine levels of aflatoxin metabolites covalently bound to nucleosides arising from the repair or degradation of DNA.

Viruses also cause tumors in animals. Rous first isolated an infectious agent that caused sarcomas in fowl. Isolation of a filtrable agent capable of causing mammary tumors in rodents led to the discovery of mouse mammary tumor virus. Until the identification of viruses associated with hepatitis and immune deficiencies, a direct role for viruses in human cancer had not been established. Viruses, notably the Epstein-Barr virus and its association with Burkitt's lymphoma, have been implicated in the etiology of several types of cancer in humans. Other associations between viruses and cancer include the Epstein-Barr virus and nasopharyngeal carcinoma, human papillomavirus and cervical cancer; hepatitis B virus has been associated with an increased risk for the development of liver tumors. Although viruses have been associated with these various malignancies, a causal relationship has not been directly established in humans. In some cases, other factors, such as predisposing diseases (eg, malaria), may also figure in the development of cancer associated with virus exposure.

IDENTIFICATION OF SUSCEPTIBLE INDIVIDUALS

Pharmacogenetics is the study of the heritable basis for idiosyncratic responses to xenobiotics, including clinically prescribed agents as well as other foreign substances. Several polymorphisms have been associated with malignancy in humans, three of which involve differences in expression of cytochrome P-450 genes. Cytochrome P-450 polymorphisms associated with lung cancer susceptibility include the *Ah* locus, which involves metabolism of aromatic hydrocarbons, the debrisoquine 4-hydroxylase gene, and the cytochrome P-450 2E1 gene (*CYP2E1*) that is involved in ethanol metabolism. An additional polymorphism is in the cytosolic N-acetyltransferase enzyme, which has been linked to susceptibility to bladder cancer. Animal polymorphisms exist to provide model systems for their human counterparts.

The most extensively studied genetic polymorphism in humans and rodents is the *Ah* polymorphism. In inbred strains of mice, it was observed that certain strains (ie, C57B1/6) were inducible for aryl hydrocarbon (benzo[a]pyrene) hydroxylase (AHH) activity, whereas other strains (ie, DBA/2) were not. The lack of AHH induction was autosomally recessive. It was subsequently found that a defect in the *Ah* receptor was responsible for the decreased AHH induction in DBA/2 mice. In *Ah*-responsive animals, the binding of compounds to the cytosolic receptor leads to internalization and translocation of the inducer-receptor complex to the nucleus, causing increased expression of several genes including cytochrome P-450 enzymes, uridine diphosphate glucuronyltransferase (UDPGT), glutathione S-transferase, and the multidrug resistance (MDR) gene. These enzyme systems act in a coordinated manner to detoxify lipophilic compounds. The MDR-1 gene product serves as an efflux pump for xenobiotics. Increased expression of cytochrome P-450 genes leads to increased metabolism (hydroxylation) of aromatic hydrocarbons such as benzo[a]pyrene. These compounds are more readily excreted, and they also serve as substrates for phase II (detoxification) enzymes such as UDPGT, sulfotransferase, and glutathione S-transferase.

In mice, the high AHH inducibility phenotype is associated with an increased risk for development of cancer following exposure to PAHs. In humans, an increased risk of bronchogenic carcinoma was reported for *Ah*-responsive smokers. Levels of a particular cytochrome P-450, CYP1A1, and inducible AHH activity are correlated in mitogen-stimulated lymphocytes following PAH exposure. Furthermore, polymorphism in this gene has been observed in patients with lung cancer.

The ability to 4-hydroxylate debrisoquine occurs at a 10- to 200-fold greater extent in extensive metabolizers compared to poor metabolizers, who account for up to 10% of the population of Great Britain. The poor metabolizer group is at greater risk for developing hypotension. In two separate studies, a greater proportion of extensive metabolizers of debrisoquine was observed in the cancer populations. It was subsequently reported that defects in mRNA splicing in poor metabolizers resulted in the lack of production of a functional cytochrome P-450 protein capable of metabolizing debrisoquine. Size variations in DNA fragments have been reported from DNA isolated from circulating lymphocytes of poor metabolizers of debrisoquine following digestion of DNA with restriction enzymes that cleave DNA only at certain sequences, which provides further evidence

for the synthesis of a defective protein in poor metabolizers. Nonhuman primates also exhibit a polymorphism for debrisoquine metabolism similar to that reported for humans. Controversy regarding the debrisoquine polymorphism in rodents may enable the debrisoquine polymorphism to be investigated in greater detail in nonhuman primates.

Epidemiologic evidence associates occupational exposure to arylamines which an increased incidence of bladder cancer. Bladder cancer incidence is increased in cigarette smokers, but there are conflicting reports about the contribution of aromatic amines present in cigarette smoke to the associated increase incidence of bladder cancer. The relative amounts of arylamine metabolites present depend primarily on the N-acetyltransferase and arylacetamide deacetylase enzyme systems. The hepatic N-acetyltransferase activity in humans is genetically regulated such that the slow acetylators are homozygous for an autosomal recessive gene for N-acetylation. There is a statistically significant association between slow acetylators and bladder cancer following exposure to aromatic amines. In contrast, high levels of N-acetyltransferase are present in the human colonic mucosa, and rapid acetylators may be at greater risk for development of colon cancer. The slow acetylator phenotype is not, however, associated with an increased incidence of lung carcinoma. When the results of eight different studies of bladder cancer and acetylator phenotype were analyzed (a total of 1672 subjects), 59% of the control population were found to be slow acetylators, whereas 65% of bladder cancer patients were slow acetylators. The observation that the slow acetylator phenotype predominated in a rural population that lacks industrial exposure to aromatic amines suggests that N-acetyltransferase also is of importance in bladder cancer within this population, although the causative agents are unknown. No association between poor and extensive metabolizers of debrisoquine and bladder cancer was observed.

CLASSIFICATION OF CARCINOGENS

Chemical carcinogens can be classified into two general categories based on the ability of compounds to bind to DNA. Compounds that bind to DNA are termed **genotoxic,** whereas compounds that are carcinogenic but have no evidence of DNA binding are termed **epigenetic.** Chemicals that bind to DNA are more readily detected. Short-term assays for detecting genotoxic agents are inexpensive and reliable indicators of the potential carcinogenicity of such compounds. The principle of such tests is the ability of this class of compounds to cause a mutation that can be detected by growth in a selective medium.

GENOTOXIC CARCINOGENS

Most genotoxic carcinogens (Table 3–1) are small molecules with a molecular weight less than 500. The ultimate reactive species are generally electrophilic, as postulated by Miller and Miller. Genotoxic carcinogens can be further categorized as **direct-acting** or as **procarcinogens** that require metabolic activation to ultimate reactive species. Direct-acting carcinogens are active at the site of application, whereas procarcinogens require metabolic activation. Procarcinogens may be metabolized by one organ and transported to a second site for the final step in activation. Also within the category of genotoxic carcinogens are inorganic compounds that do not directly bind to DNA but cause alterations in normal DNA replication.

Some compounds have a high degree of organ specificity in tumor formation, particularly nitrosamines. They are ubiquitous and may be found in tobacco products and tobacco smoke, in certain industrial settings, and in the diet. Of particular importance is the potential for in vivo formation from amines and nitrite, which has been demonstrated in humans for N-nitrosoproline. The in vivo formation of nitrosamines is of particular concern in bacterial infections of the bladder and may also be a factor in bladder cancer associated with *Schistosoma* infection.

Carcinogen Metabolism
A. Polycyclic Aromatic Hydrocarbons: The metabolism of PAHs is complex, but for some compounds such as benzo[a]pyrene, the details of metabolism have been determined. Benzo[a]pyrene serves as a prototype PAH owing to widespread distribution in the environment, ease of detection of the parent compound and metabolites, and ready availability of metabolite standards. The initial metabolism by the cytochrome P-450 1A1 enzyme system results in formation of epoxides that are converted to phenols nonenzymatically or that are conjugated with glutathione. The phenols can be conjugated with uridine diphosphoglucuronic acid (UDPGA) or sulfate. All these reactions represent detoxification reactions. Alternatively, the epoxides can be converted to dihydrodiols by epoxide hydrolase. The 7,8-dihydrodiol of benzo[a]pyrene also can be further metabolized to the ultimate carcinogenic metabolite of benzo[a]pyrene, the benzo[a]pyrene-7,8-dihydrodiol-9,10-epoxide. The benzo[a]pyrene-7,8-dihydrodiol-9,10-epoxide is extremely reactive and has a short half-life in aqueous solutions. Benzo[a]pyrene also can be metabolized by a one electron oxidation pathway, which may predominate in some tissues. During prostaglandin metabolism, peroxyl radicals can react with PAHs such as benzo[a]pyrene to catalyze formation of the benzo[a]pyrene-7,8-dihydrodiol-9,10-epoxide.

B. Aromatic Amines: In general, aromatic amines and amides are activated by N-hydroxylation and detoxified by ring-hydroxylation. The initial step in N-oxidation of arylamines can be catalyzed by the cytochrome P-450 monooxygenase system, flavin-containing monooxygenases, or peroxidases. Aromatic amides are N-hydroxylated only by the cytochrome P-450 monooxygenase system. One of the most widely studied aromatic amides is 2-acetylaminofluorene (AAF). Following N-hydroxyl-

Table 3–1. Genotoxic carcinogens.

Type	Mode of Action	Example	Structure
Direct-acting	Electrophile, interacts with DNA	Dimethyl Sulfate	$CH_3OSO_2OCH_3$
		Cytoxan	$ClCH_2CH_2$ O N-CH_2 >N-P< CH_2 $ClCH_2CH_2$ O-CH_2
Procarcinogen	Converted to direct-acting electrophile through metabolic activation	Benzo[a]pyrene	
		2-Acetylaminofluorene	
		Dimethylnitrosamine	
Inorganic	Alters DNA replication	Nickel	Ni_1S_3
		Chromium	Na_2CrO_1

ation, further metabolic activation steps to ultimate reactive metabolites include sulfate esterification, deacetylation, or acyl transfer.

These reactions are tissue dependent, resulting in target organ specificity for tumor formation. For example, hepatic tumors are formed in male rats via activation of AAF by N-hydroxylation followed by sulfate esterification. In female rats, liver tumors are rare owing to low levels of hepatic sulfotransferase, whereas mammary tumors can result from deacetylation of N-hydroxylated AAF and subsequent binding to DNA. Activation of aromatic amides and amines can occur in the urinary bladder mucosa. In both male and female rodents, urinary bladder tumors are found. The urinary bladder mucosa contains cytochrome P-450 monooxygenase enzymes that can metabolize arylamines and arylamides. The cooxidation of arylamines by prostaglandin endoperoxide synthetase during arachidonic acid metabolism is another pathway for metabolic activation of these carcinogens in the urinary bladder mucosa. Additionally, O-glucuronides that are present in the urine owing to transport from other organs are reactive electrophilic species that can bind to DNA under acidic conditions.

Thus, several metabolic activation routes exist for this class of chemical carcinogen in the urinary bladder. An important feature of both bladder and breast carcinogenesis by AAF is the initial activation to an arylhydroxamic acid and transport to the target tissue for the final activating steps and subsequent covalent binding to nucleic acids.

C. Nitrosamines: N-Nitrosamines are metabolized by cytochrome P-450 enzymes (CYP2E1, CYP2A3) different from those previously discussed that metabolize benzo[a]pyrene (IA1) or 2-acetylaminofluorene (CYP1A2). Both alkyl and cyclic nitrosamines are carcinogenic, and **organotropism** is a major characteristic of this class of compounds. A key step in the metabolic activation of this class of chemical carcinogens appears to be alpha hydroxylation. Nitrosamines derived from nicotine are found in tobacco and in tobacco combustion products. The ultimate reactive species of nitrosamines are alkylating agents. Tobacco usage thus probably represents the largest human exposure to alkylating agents. Evidence exists for induction of nitrosamine metabolizing enzymes by previous exposure to the tobacco-specific nitrosamines N'-nitrosonornicotine and 4-(methylnitrosamino)-1-(3-pyridyl)-1-butanone. In countries with high levels of gastric cancer, nitrosamines found in the diet (ie, smoked or cured foods) may be responsible for the increased levels of cancer observed. Further evidence for a dietary component (or components) being responsible for the increased incidence of gastric cancer comes from epidemiologic studies which indicate that the gastric cancer level of immigrants decreases when they relocate to a country with a lower gastric cancer incidence and their dietary habits reflect those of the new environment.

The in vivo formation of nitrosamines and subsequent tumor incidence can be reduced following administration of ascorbic acid. However, ascorbic acid does not significantly reduce tumor incidence in animals when administered concurrently with nitrosamines.

DNA Binding & Repair

A key step in the carcinogenic process is the covalent modification of DNA by genotoxic carcinogens. Most genotoxic carcinogens (or their active metabolites) are electrophilic and can bind to bases in DNA that have many nucleophilic sites. This covalent binding to DNA presents a unifying concept whereby structurally diverse chemicals share a common fate. Binding of compounds to DNA can result in decreased fidelity of DNA synthesis, leading to mutated protein products. Two examples of such an action are deletion of a base, leading to a frameshift mutation, and disruption of the normal hydrogen bonding between strands of DNA, which can lead to a base pair substitution. The consequences of a single point mutation are illustrated by the activation of a cellular transforming gene in T24 bladder cells. Arylamine binding to the C8 and N^2 position of guanine are predicted to result in guanine to thymidine or cytosine transversions, O^6 DNA adducts in guanine to adenine transitions, and C8- or N^6-substituted adenines in adenine to thymidine or cytosine transversions. Activation of *ras* cellular oncogenes can occur by single base pair transversions or transitions at specific codons, leading to a single amino acid change.

A DNA base that is covalently bound to a carcinogen can be removed by the DNA repair system, thus restoring the normal gene sequence. Several factors that determine the efficiency of DNA repair include the size of the compound that is covalently linked (a methyl group, compared to a fused ring structure), whether the covalent bond lies in a coding or control region, and the three-dimensional orientation of the carcinogen-DNA adduct. For example, formation of a covalent adduct perpendicular to the DNA backbone could be more easily recognized by a repair enzyme than by one oriented within the major groove of the DNA helix. DNA repair enzymes also may be more efficient in certain cell types, resulting in a lower probability of errors during transcription or translation of the DNA. Some examples of covalently modified DNA bases and the resulting effects on hydrogen bonding are shown in Figure 3–1.

EPIGENETIC CARCINOGENS

Carcinogens for which there is no evidence for genotoxicity are considered to be epigenetic. Possible mechanisms of action include chronic tissue injury,

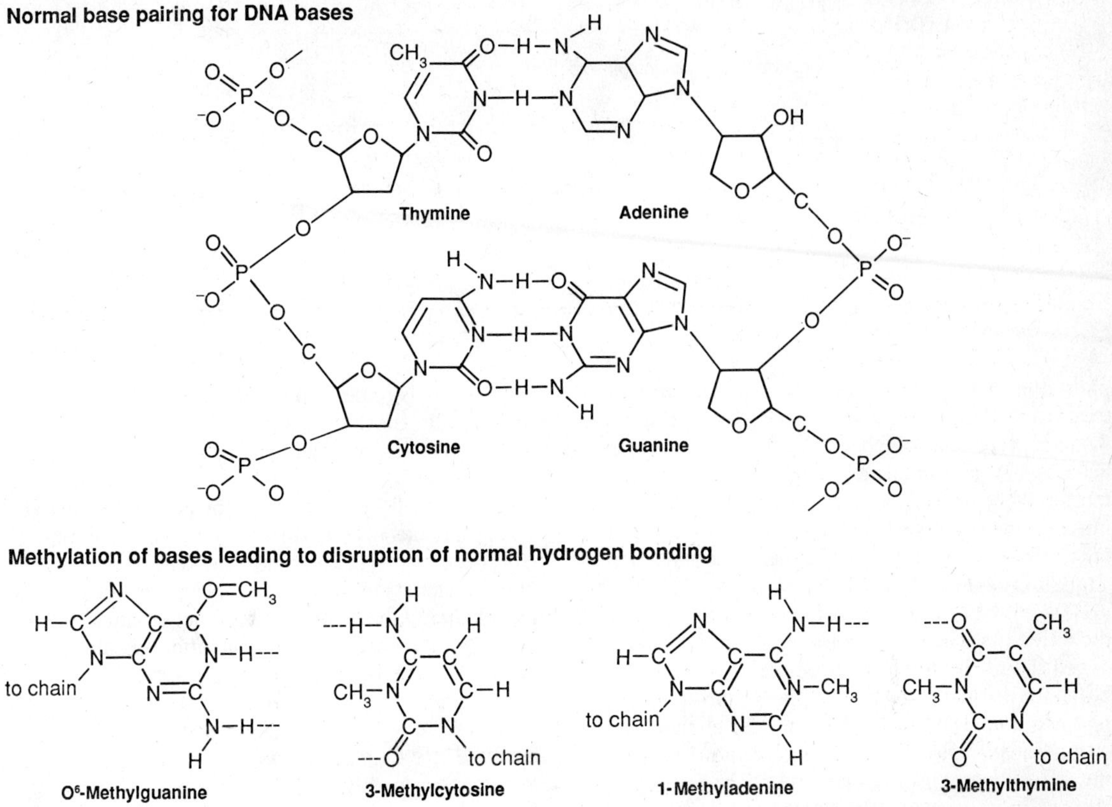

Normal base pairing for DNA bases

Methylation of bases leading to disruption of normal hydrogen bonding

O⁶-Methylguanine 3-Methylcytosine 1-Methyladenine 3-Methylthymine

Figure 3–1. Covalent binding of alkylating agents and effects on hydrogen binding in DNA.

alteration of immune system function, and hormonal alterations. For example, diethylstilbestrol and asbestos are carcinogenic, but a mechanism of action for these agents remains to be determined. Because these agents do not bind to DNA, they have been classified as epigenetic carcinogens. Genotoxic carcinogens also may have epigenetic effects. Compounds that enhance tumor incidence also fall into the epigenetic category. Two such examples are cocarcinogens and tumor promoters. Both classes of carcinogens have a similar end point, increasing the overall tumor yield of genotoxic carcinogens. Cocarcinogens are compounds that increase tumor yield when administered concurrently with compounds of known carcinogenic potential. Tumor promoters are compounds that increase the tumor yield when administered after a genotoxic agent. Tumor development can thus be divided into an initiation phase with exposure to known genotoxic agents, and a promotion phase that occurs following exposure to the initiator. Several characteristics of this phenomenon are illustrated in Figure 3–2.

Carcinogens that are encountered in the environment are generally not pure compounds but rather exist within complex mixtures that also contain anti-carcinogens, cocarcinogens, tumor initiators, and tumor promoters. A good example is cigarette smoke, the particulate fraction of which is reported to contain over 3800 compounds. Cigarette smoke consists of a gaseous and a particulate phase. A majority of the analytic studies with cigarette smoke have utilized the particulate phase, or cigarette tar. Cigarette tar contains chemical carcinogens from the following classes of chemical carcinogens: PAHs, nitrosamines, and aromatic amines. However, cigarette tar itself is weakly carcinogenic and requires multiple applications to obtain tumors in animals. An example of a cocarcinogenic effect is demonstrated by the association between cigarette smoking and asbestos exposure. From animal studies with benzo[a]pyrene and ferric oxide particles, the cocarcinogenic effect has been proposed as a result of increased residence time of the cigarette tar in the lungs, the primary target organ for tobacco-related carcinogenesis.

Tumor Promoters

Tumor promoters have been best characterized in a mouse skin painting model. Using this animal model, specific stages of tumor promotion have been identified. Phorbol esters, particularly 12-O-tetradecanoyl

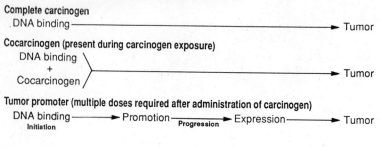

Figure 3–2. Types of carcinogens.

phorbol acetate (TPA), have been isolated from croton oil and identified as the primary tumor-promoting agent in croton oil, which was used for the early studies of tumor promotion. Another aspect of tumor promotion is the latency period between exposure to the initiator and promoter. In mouse skin, tumor promoters can be administered up to a year after exposure to a tumor initiator and still produce tumors. Tumor promoters have been identified in other organ systems, including lung, liver, and colon. In mice, urethane-induced lung tumors can be promoted by exposure to butylated hydroxytoluene. In liver, a promoting effect was observed by administration of phenobarbital or butylated hydroxytoluene. In the colon, a promoting effect was observed by administration of bile acids. Hormones can be classified as tumor promoters because they generally produce tumors in hormonally responsive target tissues, probably by interfering with the normal endocrine balance.

A mechanism of action for tumor promoters is not yet known but probably involves effects of tumor promoters on slowly replicating stem cells that have been previously damaged by initiating agents. Because hydrogen peroxide is a tumor promoting agent, it has been hypothesized that tumor promoters may act by producing reactive oxygen species to cause DNA damage. Within this framework, cytotoxic agents could also act as tumor promoters by causing lysis of cells with consequential damage to DNA in surrounding cells from lysosomal enzymes. If DNA damage occurs in germ-line cells, genetic defects can be transmitted to the offspring, thus maintaining the defect in subsequent generations. In a manner analogous to the alkylation of DNA bases by genotoxic carcinogens, the lack of methylation of control regions of DNA could lead to aberrant processing. In the former example, methylation of control regions also could lead to abnormal gene expression by protein transcription factors that recognize specific methylated or unmethylated sequences of DNA prior to interacting with RNA polymerases.

Cocarcinogens

Cocarcinogens differ from tumor promoters in that cocarcinogens act when present along with carcinogens, whereas tumor promoters act after tumor initiators (usually subcarcinogenic doses of known carcinogens) have already completed their damage (Figure 3–2). Examples of cocarcinogens are pyrene and catechol, both of which are present in tobacco smoke. Cocarcinogens may act by increasing the overall metabolism of a carcinogen, or by decreasing detoxification. In later stages of disease, cocarcinogens may act by enhancing the growth of carcinogen-altered cells. An example would be a cell that, after carcinogen exposure, requires specific growth factors for continued proliferation.

Solid-State Carcinogens

The most widely studied carcinogen in this category is asbestos. Although the mechanism of action of asbestos is unknown, several important considerations for the carcinogenicity of this inorganic material are known. The physical size and composition of the particles are important in determining the carcinogenic potential. Asbestos also can be considered a cocarcinogen when exposure is performed with cigarette smoke. In this example, asbestos may act by increasing the residence time of inhaled cigarette tar, which can bind to asbestos.

ONCOGENES

Two types of genetic alterations have been postulated to occur in tumor development. The first type involves the positive activation of genes termed cellular **proto-oncogenes** because of their relationship to the oncogenes identified in retroviruses. Activation can occur via a point mutation or a translocation as has been demonstrated with the *bcr/abl* fusion protein found in chronic myelogenous leukemia as a result of a chromosome translocation. An altered transcription factor has also been identified in some acute leukemias. Expression of proto-oncogenes following viral infection can lead to cellular transformation. The second type of alteration involves tumor suppressor genes, or **anti-oncogenes.** Loss of activity of this gene leads to tumor formation, which has been reported for retinoblastoma. The activation of cellu-

Table 3–2. Functional characterization of cellular proto-oncogenes.

Location of Protein Product	Proto-oncogene
Nucleus	*myc* family
	myb
	fos
	ski
Cytoplasm (membrane-bound protein kinases)	*erb*-B (EGF receptor)
	fms (CSF-1 receptor)
	src
	yes
	fes
	ros
	mos
	fps
	fms
	fgr
	raf
Cytoplasm (GTP-binding proteins)	*ras* family
Growth factor	*sis*
Others	*mcf*-3
	bcl-1
	bcl-2

lar proto-oncogenes or inactivation of tumor suppressor genes, which can occur by mechanisms described earlier in this chapter, is therefore the unifying concept whereby chemicals or viruses can cause cancer. Altered levels of cellular proto-oncogenes have frequently been described in tumors or in cell lines de-

rived from tumors. A list of common cellular proto-oncogenes, grouped by functionality, is presented in Table 3–2 (see also Chapter 2).

A model to explain the role of signal transduction systems in carcinogenesis has been proposed by Schuller. This concept provides evidence for the role of epigenetic agents in carcinogenesis, particularly peroxisome proliferators and hormonal agents that act via cellular receptors to regulate cell growth. This model also provides an explanation for the observed decreased risk for developing lung cancer associated with smoking cessation: removal of the chemicals that trigger cellular proliferative responses. Agents that cause proliferation can also work in conjunction with genotoxic agents to commit cells on a pathway toward uncontrolled growth.

Cellular protooncogenes can be activated by several different mechanisms including gene amplification, chromosomal translocation, and point mutations. Activation of specific proto-oncogenes is negatively correlated with survival in breast and lung cancer. Conversely, inactivation of anti-oncogenes is implicated in the etiology of diverse types of cancer. Although protein products from proto-oncogenes have been identified, the activities of these proteins are largely still unknown. A model that illustrates the pivotal role of oncogenes in carcinogenesis is shown in Figure 3–3.

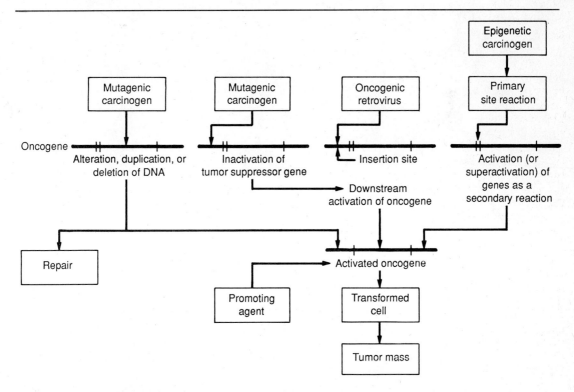

Figure 3–3. Hypothetical model for tumor production by genotoxic and epigenetic carcinogens.

REFERENCES

Adams JD et al: Toxic and carcinogenic agents in undiluted mainstream smoke and sidestream smoke of different types of cigarettes. *Carcinogenesis* 1987;**8**:729.

Caporaso N et al: Lung cancer risk, occupational exposure, and the debrisoquine metabolic phenotype. *Cancer Res* 1989;**49**:3675.

Cerutti PA: The role of active oxygen in tumor promotion. Page 167 in: *Biochemical and Molecular Epidemiology of Cancer*. CC Harris (editor). Liss, 1986.

Friend SH et al: Oncogenes and tumor-suppressing genes. *N Engl J Med* 1988;**318**:618.

Gonzalez FJ: The molecular biology of cytochrome P450s. *Pharmacol Rev* 1989;**40**:243.

Gottesman MM: Multidrug resistance during chemical carcinogenesis: A mechanism revealed? *J Natl Cancer Inst* 1988;**80**:1352.

Hajj C et al: DNA alterations at proto-oncogene loci and their clinical significance in operable non–small cell lung cancer. *Cancer* 1990;**66**:733.

Hayashi S-I et al: Genetic linkage of lung cancer–associated *Msp*I polymorphisms with amino acid replacement in the heme binding region of the human cytochrome P450IA1 gene. *J Biochem* 1991;**110**:407.

Hickman D, Sim E: *N*-Acetyltransferase polymorphism: Comparison of phenotype and genotype in humans. *Biochem Pharmacol* 1991;**42**:1007.

Law MR et al: Debrisoquine metabolism and genetic predisposition to lung cancer. *Br J Cancer* 1989;**59**:686.

Marnett LJ: Peroxyl free radicals: Potential mediators of tumor initiation and promotion. *Carcinogenesis* 1987;**8**:1365.

Miller EC, Miller JA: Mechanisms of chemical carcinogenesis. *Cancer* 1981;**47**:1055.

Mitsudomi T et al: *ras* Gene mutations in non–small cell lung cancers are associated with shortened survival irrespective of treatment intent. *Cancer Res* 1991;**51**: 4999.

Ohshima H, Bartsch H: Quantitative estimation of endogenous nitrosation in humans by monitoring N-nitrosoproline excreted in the urine. *Cancer Res* 1981;**41**:3658.

Puisieux A et al: Selective targeting of *p53* gene mutational hotspots in human cancers by etiologically defined carcinogens. *Cancer Res* 1991;**51**:6185.

Reddy EP et al: A point mutation is responsible for the acquisition of transforming properties by the T24 human bladder carcinoma oncogene. *Nature* 1982;**300**:149.

Schuller HM: The signal transduction model of carcinogenesis. *Biochem Pharmacol* 1991;**42**:1511.

Seidegard J et al: Isoenzyme(s) of glutathione transferase (class Mu) as a marker for the susceptibility to lung cancer: A follow-up study. *Carcinogenesis* 1990;**11**:33.

Selikoff IJ et al: Mortality effects of cigarette smoking among amosite asbestos factory workers. *J Natl Cancer Inst* 1980;**65**:507.

Skoda RC et al: Two mutant alleles of the human cytochrome P-450db1 gene (P450C2D1) associated with genetically deficient metabolism of debrisoquine and other drugs. *Proc Natl Acad Sci USA* 1988;**85**:5240.

Slaga TJ: Overview of tumor promotion in animals. *Environ Health Perspect* 1983;**50**:3.

Uematsu F et al: Association between restriction fragment length polymorphism of the human cytochrome P450IIE1 gene and susceptibility to lung cancer. *Jpn J Cancer Res* 1991;**82**:254.

Wong-Staal F, Gallo RC: Human T-lymphotrophic retroviruses. *Nature* 1985;**317**:395.

Epidemiology of Cancer

4

Mary B. Daly, MD, PhD

Epidemiology may be defined as the study of the distribution and determinants of disease in population groups. In speaking of the epidemiology of cancer, one must also speak of the preventability of cancer, for it is the role of the cancer epidemiologist to investigate the causes of cancer with a view toward developing preventive strategies. Cancer epidemiology is a dynamic discipline that continually seeks to monitor incidence and mortality statistics, to evaluate changes in time and geographic trends, and to identify both personal and environmental factors associated with cancer risk. Epidemiologic research is a progression from observation and correlations in populations, to studies in specially characterized subgroups, to experimental trials with manipulation of study conditions. Through the application of epidemiologic concepts and skills, the cancer epidemiologist hopes to gain an understanding of cancer etiology, to measure the magnitude of the problem in a given society, to evaluate interventional measures, and to develop strategies for cancer control.

Both descriptive and analytic sources of data are used by the epidemiologist to understand cancer causation. Descriptive data are those statistics which measure the frequency of cancer in human populations:

(1) Incidence: The number of new cases of cancer during a specified time period in a defined population. Incidence rates estimate the probability of developing a disease and provide valuable measures of temporal or geographic differences.

(2) Prevalence: The number of cancer cases, both old and new, present at a point in time in a defined population. Prevalence rates provide an estimate of the burden of disease in a population.

(3) Mortality: The number of deaths attributed to cancer during a specified time period in a defined population.

(4) Case-fatality: The number of persons among all those who have a form of cancer who die of it during a specified period of time. This provides a measure of the aggressiveness of a cancer or of the success of medical intervention.

Much of this information is derived from vital statistics, national and international cancer surveys, and tumor registries. In a more experimental fashion, the epidemiologist conducts studies in specific subgroups of the population in either a prospective or retrospective manner. The **prospective, or cohort, study** identifies members of a defined population by their exposure or risk factor status and then follows them over time to quantify their incidence of disease, thereby allowing causal relationships to be defined. Because a prospective study starts before development of a disease, it is better able to demonstrate that cause precedes effect. In a **retrospective study,** on the other hand, the population is first identified by disease status and then investigated for a history of exposure to certain risk factors. Because a retrospective study starts after development of a disease, its ability to demonstrate cause and effect may be weakened by recall errors. To summarize, the retrospective study looks backward from disease to prior risks, while the prospective study starts with the risk factors and monitors subsequent disease occurrence.

Epidemiologic analyses are concerned with defining etiologic relationships and rely on certain qualities of the data to strengthen causal inferences:

(1) Strength: Often defined as relative risk; a measure of the importance of a certain risk factor for the etiology of a disease.

(2) Consistency: The repeated observation of an association in different population groups at different times.

(3) Specificity: The production of a single effect by a causal agent.

(4) Temporality: The demonstration that the risk factor precedes the disease in time.

(5) Biologic gradient: The demonstration of a dose-response relationship between the risk factor and the subsequent disease.

(6) Plausibility: The coherence of the demonstrated relationship with known scientific facts.

In addition, the cancer epidemiologist uses statistical tools to distinguish true causal relationships from those due to chance, errors of data collection, or other confounding variables.

Cancer represents the second largest cause of morbidity and mortality in the USA and is the principal health concern of the nation. Cancer epidemiology, with its emphasis on defining the progression of the disease in the population and its goal of optimizing cancer control through prevention, is assuming an expanding role in the fight against cancer.

CAUSES OF CANCER

Cancer accounts for approximately 500,000 deaths per year in the USA and 4,000,000 deaths worldwide. Research data currently available support the position that close to 90% of all cancer is related to life-style and environmental factors (Table 4–1). This discussion of the epidemiology of cancer focuses on these major determinants of cancer, their association with specific tumor types, and the use of this information for cancer control strategies.

Tobacco

The use of cigarettes and other tobacco products accounts for over 30% of cancer deaths. Cigarette smoking is responsible for 80–85% of lung and laryngeal cancers, is a major cause of oral and esophageal cancer, and plays a causative role in development of cancers of bladder, kidney, pancreas, and cervix. Pipe and cigar smokers are also at increased risk for oral and pulmonary cancers, and the use of smokeless tobacco is related to cancers of the mouth.

The role of cigarette smoking in the etiology of lung cancer has been well documented in retrospective and prospective studies. In 1950, Wynder and Graham published the results of a case-control study performed among 684 new cases of bronchogenic carcinoma and 780 hospital controls that demonstrated a highly significant difference in the number of smokers in the two groups as well as in the duration of smoking and number of cigarettes smoked. The first cohort study was begun in 1950 by Hammond and Horn, who obtained smoking histories on 189,854 men aged 50–69 years and then followed these men for several years to obtain data on incidence of and mortality from lung cancer. They were able to demonstrate an increased risk for lung cancer

among smokers, with a strong dose-response relationship. Doll and Peto subsequently quantified the relative risk for smokers versus nonsmokers as 14 (25 for heavy smokers) in a prospective study of British physicians begun in 1951. They also documented a drop in risk over time for those smokers who stopped smoking. Animal studies in the mid and late 1950s demonstrated the carcinogenicity of components of both tar and cigarette smoke. A number of well-known carcinogens, including benzo[a]pyrene, nitrosamines, and dibenzanthracenes have since been isolated from tobacco products. By 1964, cigarettes were identified by the Surgeon General of the USA as a health hazard. While the exact pathophysiologic mechanism of cancer initiation and promotion is still not known, the magnitude of data identifying tobacco as a cause of lung cancer is incontrovertible. Recently, studies in the USA and Japan found an increased risk for cancers of the lung and paranasal sinus among passive smokers.

The epidemiologic evidence implicating tobacco as a cause of lung cancer fulfills many of the criteria for causal association. The data are consistent throughout multiple studies. There is a strong and specific relationship between cigarettes and lung cancer, a clear-cut temporal sequence between exposure and disease, and a strong dose-response relationship.

The epidemiologic evidence supporting a causal relationship between tobacco use and incidence of laryngeal cancer also is strong and consistent across many studies, with risks for smokers of 10–30 times that for nonsmokers. Pipe and cigar smokers share a similar risk, and approximately 75–80% of laryngeal cancer can be attributed to tobacco products.

Oral carcinomas, which account for approximately 2% of cancer deaths, are related to all forms of tobacco products including smokeless tobacco, with risks for smokers ranging from 2 to 12 times higher than those for nonsmokers. Additionally, a synergistic relationship between tobacco and alcohol has been demonstrated in the etiology of oral carcinoma and increases the risk by a factor of 2.5 over their additive effects. Similarly, the synergistic effects of tobacco and alcohol account for over 85% of esophageal cancer seen in the USA, with a strong dose-response relationship.

Cigarette smoking appears to be a contributory factor in cancers of the bladder, pancreas, and kidney. Risk for these malignancies in smokers is 2–5 times that for nonsmokers and is related to duration of use. While the pathophysiologic mechanisms are unknown, there is some evidence that the polynuclear aromatic hydrocarbons derived from tar can act as bladder carcinogens.

Cigarette smoking is a major risk factor in development of cancer of the uterine cervix. The relative risk when other known risk factors are controlled for is approximately 2.5. It is speculated that a carcinogen derived from tobacco products is secreted into

Table 4–1. Causes of cancer mortality.[1]

Factor or Factor Class	All Cancer Deaths (%)	
	Best Estimate	Range of Acceptable Estimates
Tobacco	30	25–40
Alcohol	3	2–4
Diet	35	10–70
Reproductive and sexual behavior	7	1–13
Occupation	4	2–8
Pollution	2	1–5
Industrial products	1	1–2
Medicines and medical procedures	1	0.5–3
Geophysical factors	3	2–4

[1]Data from: *Cancer Control Objectives for the Nation: 1985–2000.* NCI Monograph No. 2. US Public Health Service, 1986.

the cervical epithelium, where it acts as a promoter or cocarcinogen.

Many studies have documented a gradual reduction in cancer risk for those individuals who quit smoking. The percentage of adults quitting smoking has increased steadily since cigarettes were first identified as a major health hazard in early 1960. The rate of decline is higher for males than for females, and rates have actually risen over the last two decades in certain subgroups of the population, such as teenaged girls, blacks, and Hispanics. Achievement of the goal of the former Surgeon General of the USA of a smokeless society by the year 2000 would result in the elimination of 30% of all cancer deaths.

Diet

While there is a voluminous and constantly growing body of literature linking dietary elements to different forms of cancer, many data are observational or retrospective and therefore lack the experimental precision needed to determine truly causal relationships. Correlations of food consumption, which in most studies is in fact a measure of food disappearance in a defined population, with disease incidence have been used to implicate dietary fat as a cause of several cancers, including colorectal, breast, uterine, prostate, and ovarian (Figure 4–1). These observations are based on crude measurements, are ecologic in nature, and therefore refer only to population

groups, not individuals. The associations discovered through these types of analysis may be indirect. Fat consumption may be indirectly related to some other variable that is the true causal factor.

Difficulties are also encountered in interpretation of case-control data when relative risk is used as the measure of association. The level of exposure to various constituents of the diet among cases and controls is based on dietary recall, which can be fraught with inaccuracies. Finally, truly experimental studies, prospective in nature, are extremely difficult to perform in the area of nutrition, since they require assignment of large groups of individuals to certain dietary manipulations and long periods of follow-up. Problems of long-term dietary compliance and cost severely restrict initiation of such studies.

Theories of dietary carcinogenesis include the following potential mechanisms of action:

(1) Direct ingestion of carcinogens or their precursors, eg, aflatoxin, a hepatic carcinogen derived from *Aspergillus flavus,* a fungal contaminant of ground nuts.

(2) Production of carcinogens by cooking processes, eg, production of nitrosamines by the charring of meat.

(3) Facilitation of endogenous carcinogen formation by provision of substrates or induction of enzymatic activation of substrates.

(4) Alteration of delivery of carcinogens to their

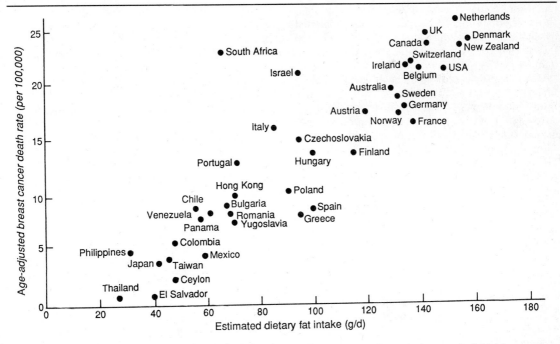

Figure 4–1. Correlation between age-adjusted death rate from breast cancer and estimated per capita fat intake among a number of countries. (Reproduced, with permission, from Wynder E et al: *Nutrition and metabolic epidemiology of cancers of the oral cavity, esophagus, colon, breast, prostate, and stomach.* In: *Nutrition and Cancer: Etiology and Treatment.* Newell G, Ellison NM [editors]. Raven Press, 1981.)

site of action at the cellular level by altering membrane permeability, or at the organ level by controlling contact time of a carcinogen with its target tissue.

(5) Inhibition of cellular protective mechanisms both at the biochemical level, eg, production of superoxide radicals, and at the immune system level, eg, suppression of cellular immunity.

Conversely, certain dietary factors may play a protective role against cancer development by promoting cellular differentiation or by trapping or metabolizing other carcinogens. The food groups stimulating the most interest in terms of association with cancer risk are fat and fiber, vitamins, and alcohol.

A. Fats and Fiber: No other dietary hypothesis has received more attention than the proposed relationships between dietary fat and fiber to the incidence of colorectal carcinoma. Brukitt was the first to use international comparisons to demonstrate an inverse relationship between colorectal cancer and the proportion of nonabsorbable fiber in the diet. He pointed out the clustering of colorectal cancer with other intestinal diseases such as polyps and diverticular disease, all of which are seen more commonly in economically developed populations consuming "westernized" diets, which are relatively low in fiber. He suggested a mechanism whereby dietary fiber might alter the interaction of potentially carcinogenic bile acids and gut flora through the dilution of stool contents, the binding of carcinogenic chemicals such as bile acids in the feces, and the reduction of contact time with intestinal mucosa through more rapid transit of fecal material. This hypothesis was supported by animal models in which high-fiber diets decreased the incidence of carcinogen-induced intestinal tumors.

Other investigators have pointed out that dietary fiber is inversely correlated with dietary fat, which is in itself a promoter of carcinogenesis by way of increasing bile acid excretion. The action of bacterial enzymes in the large intestine on these bile acids to form carcinogens or cocarcinogens is thus seen as the primary event. Animal studies in which diets high in polyunsaturated fats increase the incidence of spontaneous or induced intestinal tumors support this hypothesis.

A number of observational and case-control studies support an association between westernized diets, high in fat and low in fiber, and risk for colorectal cancer. Further support is supplied by studies of Japanese who have emigrated from Japan to Hawaii and California. Their risk for colorectal cancer gradually rises from the low rates prevailing in Japan to the high rates found among white populations in the USA.

Dietary fat has also been associated with several other cancers, especially those with a component of hormone stimulation, namely, cancers of the breast, uterus, ovary, and prostate. The large international variation observed in rates of breast cancer is positively correlated with per capita intake of both meat and total fat. A natural experiment that occurred in Great Britain during the Second World War revealed a 13% decrease in breast cancer rates coincident with the meat restrictions imposed by the war. Following the war, fat consumption gradually rose by 25%, followed by a 14% rise in breast cancer mortality. Migrant studies and studies among special population groups that adhere to vegetarian diets are also consistent with an association between diets high in animal fat and excess risk of cancer of the breast, uterus, ovary, and prostate.

Several case-control studies report an increased relative risk for breast and uterine cancer with increased dietary fat intake and also with body weight. It is hypothesized that the amount of fat included in the diet can alter the production or metabolism of endogenous hormones and thereby alter cancer risk.

A large-scale prospective study of diet and subsequent cancer incidence among 88,751 women aged 34–59 years has recently provided evidence of a positive association between fat intake and risk for colon cancer. No association was seen for breast cancer risk. Finally, a meta-analysis of the epidemiologic evidence concerning dietary fiber and colon cancer risk provides support for a protective effect associated with fiber-rich diets.

The National Research Council in the USA holds the opinion that the combined evidence of animal research and population-based studies is of sufficient strength to suggest a causal relationship between fat intake and cancer occurrence, particularly for cancers of the breast and gastrointestinal tract.

B. Vitamins: It has long been observed that vitamin deficiencies can result in altered growth patterns and differentiation of tissues. It is natural then to investigate the role that vitamins or vitamin deficiencies may play in the deranged growth characteristics of cancer cells.

1. Vitamin A–Vitamin A is a fat-soluble vitamin present both as plant-derived carotenes and animal-derived retinol and retinal. Its biologic activities include roles in vision, reproduction, and control of epithelial growth and differentiation. Vitamin A deficiency leads to alteration of epithelial tissue to a more keratinizing form. In animal models, vitamin A deficiency results in premalignant epithelial changes and enhanced susceptibility to the induction of experimental tumors. Pretreatment of the animals with retinoids, on the other hand, inhibits experimental induction of carcinogenesis. Both case-control and prospective dietary recall studies support an association between increased intake of vitamin A and protection from cancers of the lung, oropharynx, larynx, bladder, and colon. Prospective studies in which serum levels of retinol were measured in groups that were then followed for cancer occurrence found an inverse relationship between serum retinol levels and risk for lung cancer. Trials are under way to assess the role of vitamin A in the prevention of cancer among high-risk groups.

2. Vitamin C–Vitamin C, a water-soluble vitamin, is known to block the production of nitrosamine compounds from their nitrogen-containing precursors. Several case-control studies have linked low intake of vitamin C with cancers of the gastrointestinal tract, especially esophagus and stomach, but the associations found are modest and interpretation of findings is limited by the confounding effects of other nutrients.

3. Others–Vitamin E, an intracellular antioxidant, selenium, a natural element with antiperoxide activity, and riboflavin, which participates in hepatic demethylation reactions, have been proposed as having a role in human carcinogenesis, but to date no consistent data support these proposals.

C. Alcohol: A synergistic relationship between alcohol and tobacco smoke has been documented for cancers of the mouth, pharynx, larynx, and esophagus. Several mechanisms have been proposed for the role of alcohol as a cocarcinogen, including alteration of membrane permeability through solvent action, alteration of hepatic metabolism through decreased mitochondrial function, or indirectly by causation of nutritional deficiencies associated with alcohol abuse. Hepatic cirrhosis, whether alcohol- or virus-induced is a precursor lesion for hepatocellular carcinoma, one of the most prevalent cancers worldwide. Most recently, a growing body of both cohort and case-control studies support an association between moderate alcohol consumption and elevation in breast cancer risk, with a consistent dose-response relationship.

Dietary recommendations of the Committee on Diet, Nutrition, and Cancer of the National Research Council are based more on balanced principles of nutrition than on precise scientific data. They include the following:

(1) Decrease fat intake from 40% to 30% of total calories.

(2) Include fruits, vegetables, and whole grain cereals.

(3) Minimize the consumption of food preserved by smoking or salt-curing.

(4) Minimize the intake of food additives.

(5) Minimize alcohol consumption.

Chemicals—Occupational, Environmental, & Pharmaceutical

More than 4 million known chemicals, both natural and synthetic, are present in the environment today. More than 60,000 of them are in widespread use, and 1000 new chemicals enter the environment in significant quantities each year. Chemical carcinogens are usually identified by in vitro mutagenicity tests or by in vivo rodent bioassay tests for chromosomal damage. The International Agency for Research in Cancer (IARC) has established a list of industrial processes and chemicals known to be carcinogenic to humans (Table 4–2). Occupational carcinogens are thought to account for 4–6% of cancer deaths in industrialized nations, with much higher risks in specific groups with heavy exposures. The most significant contributors to cancer risk through chemical exposure are thought to be asbestos and benzene products, mainly because of their widespread use in many industries. Additionally, substances encountered in the workplace in high concentrations by relatively few individuals may also contaminate the environment through air, soil, and water pollution and thus reach the general public. Attempts to implicate air pollution as a major cause of lung cancer have been largely unsuccessful, although a synergistic relationship between certain particles in the air and smoking has been suggested.

What have clearly emerged as carcinogenic risks are specific pharmaceutical agents used to treat a variety of medical conditions. Arsenicals, prescribed for over 2000 years for the treatment of a host of conditions, including skin diseases, are causally associated with the development of squamous and basal cell carcinomas of the skin. In the occupational setting, arsenic has also been associated with lung cancer. Diethylstilbestrol (DES), a synthetic nonsteroidal estrogen given to pregnant women in high doses in the 1940s and 1950s to prevent miscarriage, is linked with adenocarcinoma of the vagina and cervix in their female offspring. Estrogen supplements used commonly for treatment of menopausal symptoms have been associated with an increased risk of uterine cancer. Unopposed estrogen stimulation, whether exoge-

Table 4–2. Industrial processes and chemicals carcinogenic for humans as determined by the IARC.[1]

Industrial processes and occupations
Auramine manufacture
Isopropyl alcohol manufacture (strong-acid process)
Nickel refining
Underground hematite mining (with exposure to radon)
Chemicals and groups of chemicals
4-Aminobiphenyl
Arsenic and arsenic compounds
Asbestos
Benzene
Benzidine
N,N-bis(2-Chloroethyl)-2-naphthylamine(chlornaphazine)
Bis(chloromethyl) ether and technical-grade chloromethyl methyl ether
Chromium and certain chromium compounds
Diethylstilbestrol
Melphalan
Mustard gas
2-Naphthylamine
Soots, tars, and oils
Vinyl chloride

[1]Data from: Cancer Control Objectives for the Nation; 1985–2000. NCI Monographs No. 2, US Public Health Service, 1986.

nous or endogenous, results in endometrial hyperplasia, a condition thought to be precancerous. The risk of endometrial cancer in women taking exogenous estrogens is dependent on both dose and duration of use and ranges from 1.7 to 8.

Oral contraceptives, particularly when used for long duration, have been linked to development of hepatic adenomas. Several case-control studies, however, have failed to document any appreciable risk for breast cancer associated with their use. In the case of ovarian cancer, oral contraceptive use appears to offer a protective advantage, possibly by the suppression of ovulation. An increased risk of liver tumors is associated with androgen therapy. Antineoplastic drugs, particularly alkylating agents, have been shown to increase the subsequent risk for acute myelocytic leukemia, especially when combined with radiation therapy. Immunosuppressive agents, used to treat a wide variety of disorders, are associated with an increased risk of lymphoma and Kaposi's sarcoma.

Habitual users of analgesic preparations containing phenacetin are at increased risk of papillary necrosis of the kidney and interstitial nephritis. An additional association of phenacetin with transitional cell carcinomas of the renal pelvis has been confirmed in a rat animal model.

Methoxsalen, a photosensitizing drug taken in conjunction with ultraviolet radiation exposure (psoralen plus ultraviolet A; PUVA) has become over the past 15 years a popular form of treatment for psoriasis. In mice, PUVA therapy results in increased incidence of dermal and epidermal tumors, and a number of case reports now suggest an association between PUVA therapy and increased risk of skin cancer in humans.

While exposure to chemicals and drugs in the environment accounts for a minority of cancer deaths, it represents an especially important cause of morbidity and mortality because of its potential for prevention. Through continual research, monitoring of the environment, and application of existing knowledge, some of these associated cancers may be avoided.

Radiation

Ionizing radiation is well documented as a human carcinogen and is associated with increased risks for leukemias and lymphomas as well as solid tumors. Although radiation accounts for less than 3% of all cancer deaths, it has been extensively studied and is a topic of great public concern.

The greatest source of radiation exposure is natural, eg, cosmic rays, terrestrial deposits, and internal radionucleotides. Most of the remaining contribution is from medical diagnostic and therapeutic applications. Less than 1% is related to nuclear energy, nuclear weapons, occupational exposure, and radioactive waste.

A. Natural Sources: Perhaps one of the most important causal associations to be described, in terms of both prevalence and increased incidence over time is that of skin cancer and exposure to ultraviolet radiation from the sun. All forms of skin cancer—squamous cell, basal cell, and malignant melanoma—appear to be related at least in part to sun exposure. They are more common in sun-exposed areas of the skin and occur more frequently in light-skinned people and those living closer to the equator. Changes in personal behavior and dress styles are correlated with the alarming increase in incidence of malignant melanoma, a disease which is relatively rare in dark-skinned peoples and which has a high case-fatality rate when diagnosed in later stages.

Recent evidence associates radon and radon daughters, decay products of trace elements in the soil that emit alpha particles of high energy and mass, with an increased risk of lung cancers, particularly among miners who exposure is high.

B. Medical Sources: Several retrospective studies have documented an increased risk of approximately 40% for leukemia and other cancers among children exposed to diagnostic radiation in utero, although the causal nature of this relationship is difficult to prove. Before the hazards of irradiation were appreciated, the use of relatively high doses to treat a variety of nonmalignant conditions was fairly common. Several surveys have documented an increased risk of cancer of the thyroid in patients treated with local irradiation to the head and neck for enlarged thymus glands, ringworm of the scalp, and acne. Long term follow-up of over 14,000 patients given radiation therapy to the spine for ankylosing spondylitis documents increased mortality from leukemia, aplastic anemia, and solid tumors in this group.

Women undergoing frequent fluoroscopy of the lung after treatment by pneumothorax for tuberculosis experienced an increased risk for breast cancer beginning 10 years postradiation. Another group at increased risk for breast cancer were those women treated with low doses of radiation for postpartum mastitis. The risk appears to inversely correlate with age.

C. Nuclear Energy, Nuclear Weapons, and Occupational Exposure: One of the most important sources of information of the carcinogenic effects of ionizing radiation comes from long-term follow-up of survivors of the atomic bomb explosions in Hiroshima and Nagasaki. Although data on individual dose estimates are crude, the Atomic Bomb Casualty Commission estimates that 530 deaths, or 0.8% of all deaths among the 283,000 survivors, are attributable to radiation exposure. What emerges from this exhaustive study is that a simple linear dose-response relationship will not explain the pattern of carcinogenesis, that the leukemogenic effect of radiation occurs earlier than the induction of solid tumors, and that age at exposure is a critical fact, with highest risks for those at the two extremes of age. There is at this point, however, no evidence that the low-level monitored emissions from nuclear energy facilities pose any risk to residents or workers in the vicinity of these plants. Radiologists represent an occupational group who experienced high levels of radiation exposure in the early years of the profession before the potential hazards were appreciated. Those who practiced radiology before 1920 have subsequently experienced excessive rates of leukemia, skin cancers, and cancers of the lung and pancreas.

D. Electromagnetic Fields: A vast amount of epidemiologic data has accumulated on the potential risks of electric power and electromagnetic fields (EMF). Limitations in the research methodology and inconsistencies in the findings to date preclude definitive conclusions, although weak associations between residential EMF exposure and childhood leukemia and between occupational EMF exposure and a variety of cancers warrant further study.

Endogenous Hormones

Hormone-related cancers, namely, cancers of the breast, ovary, uterus, and prostate, account for a large proportion of all cancer deaths in westernized societies and are thought to be related to a variety of lifestyle factors. While it is an oversimplification to suggest that increased hormonal stimulation of a target organ leads to neoplastic growth, some function of the hormonal milieu clearly affects cancer risk for these malignancies.

There is overwhelming evidence in the case of breast cancer that ovarian function plays a role in the initiation, promotion, or both, of the disease. The mitotic activity of breast epithelium varies greatly during the menstrual cycle and is under the control of cyclic fluctuations of estrogen, progesterone, and prolactin. Many epidemiologic variables associated with breast cancer may be explained in terms of their relationship to the hormonally driven cell kinetics of breast tissue. The increased risk associated with early menarche, late menopause, and nulliparity, as well as the decreased risk associated with early artificial menopause, may be explained in terms of the duration and intensity of ovarian activity. The protective effect of bearing a first child at an early age may be mediated by the early commitment of breast epithelial cells to differentiation, thereby decreasing the proportion of cells susceptible to mitotic activity. The increased risks associated with race, socioeconomic status, obesity, and westernized diets high in total fat content may all be related to increased conversion of androstenedione to estrone in peripheral adipose tissue. There is even some evidence that the increased risk among family members of a breast cancer patient may be partly related to inherited patterns of hormone production.

Hypotheses relating risk of endometrial cancer to the endothelial proliferation induced by high levels of unopposed estrogen are supported by the increased risk associated with obesity and that seen in women treated with replacement estrogens for menopausal symptoms. A protective role for progesterone, which exerts antiestrogenic effects on endometrial tissue, is supported by the findings that both increased parity and use of oral contraceptives that inhibit ovulation are protective.

Theories regarding the etiology of ovarian carcinoma propose a correlation between risk and the number of ovulatory cycles and the amount of gonadotropin secretion. The prediction that decreased stimulation of the ovary would offer protection from ovarian carcinoma is supported by the findings that both increased parity and use of oral contraceptives that inhibit ovulation are protective.

Epidemiologic data to support an "androgen excess" theory for prostate cancer are sparse but supportive. Cancer of the prostate is not seen in men who have been castrated. Likewise, rates are low in men with cirrhosis of the liver, in whom levels of testosterone are reduced. Even stronger evidence comes from the development of an animal model in which testosterone alone can cause prostate cancer in rats.

Similar lines of evidence linking hormonal stimuli to the development of cancer are being developed to explore the relationship between maternal estrogen levels and the risk of testicular cancer in male offspring, the role of thyroid-stimulating hormone in the induction of thyroid cancer, and the relationship between growth hormone levels and the risk of osteosarcoma in adolescents.

Infectious Agents

Although the theory of cancer causation by contagion has long been pursued, in very few instances has an infectious agent been identified as a cause of cancer. A notable exception is the association of Epstein-Barr virus (EBV) with Burkitt's lymphoma in Africa. The accumulated evidence includes the correlation of serologic evidence of EBV infection with incidence of disease, demonstration of the genome in tumor cells, and experimental transmission of the disease in an animal model. EBV is estimated to be involved in the pathogenesis of over 95% of endemic Burkitt's lymphoma in Africa and in 15–25% of sporadic Burkitt's lymphoma in nonendemic areas. EBV has also been associated with nasopharyngeal carcinoma and with carcinoma of the thymus.

Hepatitis B virus is most certainly responsible for development of a large proportion of cases of hepatocellular carcinoma, a major cause of cancer morbidity and mortality worldwide. Other chronic liver infections, particularly liver flukes, are associated with an increased risk of cholangiocarcinoma. *Schistosoma haematobium,* a parasite endemic to certain parts of Africa, is thought to increase the risk for bladder cancer through chronic fibrosis and granulomatous proliferation of bladder epithelium leading to metaplastic and neoplastic changes.

The epidemiologic features associated with cancer

of the cervix in women, ie, low socioeconomic status, early age at first intercourse, and multiple sex partners, point to a venereal pattern of etiology. Current information suggests the coexistence of two viruses, herpes simplex type 2 and papillomavirus, as necessary for the induction of malignant transformation. Evidence of papillomavirus infection is also beginning to be documented among men who develop penile cancer.

A retrovirus, the human T cell lymphotropic virus (HTLV), has been linked to an aggressive T cell leukemia endemic to the southwestern coast of Japan. The same disease has also been described among American blacks from the southeastern USA and immigrants from the West Indies. In addition to a high correlation of antiviral antibodies to incidence of the disease, proviral segments have been isolated from the leukemic cells, which strongly supports a causal relationship.

There are a number of cancers (Hodgkin's disease is the prime example) whose natural history and epidemiologic patterns strongly suggest an infectious etiology but for which no organism has been conclusively identified.

Genetics

While aggregation of cancer in families may be the result of a variety of factors ranging from the inheritance of single-gene syndromes to the sharing of common environments, the concept of familial predisposition to cancer is an area of great public interest. A large number of known genetically inherited disorders, both autosomal and sex-linked, are associated with increased risk for cancer.

A. Autosomal Recessive Disorders: Ataxia-telangiectasia, which involves a translocation of genetic material to chromosome 14, is associated with increased risks for leukemia, lymphoma, gastric cancer, liver cancer, and ovarian cancer. A defect in DNA repair is thought to be involved. Furthermore, heterozygotes, who comprise approximately 1% of white populations in the USA, are at increased risk for cancer, especially breast cancer in women carriers, who appear to have a heightened sensitivity to diagnostic and occupational radiation. Other syndromes such as Fanconi's anemia, Bloom's syndrome, and immunodeficiency syndromes produce an increased risk of leukemia and lymphomas. Xeroderma pigmentosum, which involves a defect in DNA repair of ultraviolet light–induced skin damage, is highly associated with skin cancer.

B. Autosomal Dominant Disorders: Neurofibromatosis is associated with an increased risk of neurofibrosarcoma, a tumor of nerve sheath origin, as well as with acute myelocytic leukemia. Familial polyposis; its variant, Gardner's syndrome; and Peutz-Jeghers syndrome all share a strong association with intestinal neoplasms. The use of molecular genetics has contributed to the development of a model of colon tumorigenesis which describes a series of mutational events in at least four to five genes and which may serve as a prototype for other common malignancies, such as familial breast and ovarian cancers. Of retinoblastomas, 20–30% are familial and inherited in an autosomal dominant fashion. The dysplastic nevus syndrome, with its associated risk for malignant melanoma, also appears to be inherited in an autosomal dominant pattern.

C. X-linked Recessive Disorders: Wiskott-Aldrich and other sex-linked immunodeficiency syndromes are associated with an increased risk of leukemia and lymphoma. Dyskeratosis congenita, in addition to its common association with aplastic anemia, is also linked to cancer of the mucous membranes.

By far more common than those single gene mutations is the familial aggregation of cancers where no single genetic defect can be identified. The "cancer family syndrome" consists of the development of excess numbers of single or multiple primary cancers in successive generations, with a frequency higher and age of onset earlier than in the general population. Often the cancers appearing in these families are hormone-related cancers or cancers of gastrointestinal tract. Presumably some poorly understood genetic determinant predisposes to the physiologic events leading to malignant transformation.

REFERENCES

Bal D, Foerster S: Changing the American diet. *Cancer* 1991;**67**:2671.

Bourke G: *The Epidemiology of Cancer.* The Charles Press, 1983.

Cannon-Albright L et al: Genetic predisposition to cancer. In: *Important Advances in Oncology.* DeVita R, Hellman S, Rosenberg S (editors). Lippincott, 1991.

Fearon E, Vogelstein B: A genetic model for colorectal tumorigenesis. *Cell* 1990;**61**:759.

Greene M. The dysplastic nevus syndrome: Precursors of hereditary and nonfamilial cutaneous melanoma. In: *Important Advances in Oncology.* DeVita R, Hellman S, Rosenberg S (editors). Lippincott, 1986.

Greenwald P, Sondih E: Cancer control objectives for the nation: 1985–2000. NCI Monographs No. 2, 1986.

Harley N, Harley J: Potential lung cancer risk from indoor radon exposure. *CA* 1990;**40**:265.

Holbrook J: Tobacco and health. *CA* 1987;**37**:49.

Longnecker M et al: A meta-analysis of alcohol consumption in relation to risk of breast cancer. *JAMA* 1988;**260**:652.

Novotny T et al: Trends in smoking by age and sex, United States, 1974–1987: The implications for disease impact. *Prev Med* 1990;**19**:552.

Riegelman R, Povar G: *Putting Prevention into Practice.* Little, Brown, 1987.

Saracci R: The interactions of tobacco smoking and other agents in cancer etiology. *Epidemiol Rev* 1987;**9**:175.

Schatzkin A et al: Alcohol consumption and breast cancer in the epidemiologic follow-up study of the first national health and nutrition examination survey. *N Engl J Med* 1987;**316**:1169.

Schottenfeld D et al: *Cancer Epidemiology and Prevention.* Saunders, 1982.

Severson R, Davis S: Are there cancer risks associated with electrical power lines? *Cancer Prevention* (April) 1991; p. 1.

Shopland D et al: Smoking-attributable cancer mortality in 1991: Is lung cancer now the leading cause of death among smokers in the United States? *JNCI* 1991;**83**:1142.

Smith P: Radiation. In: *Cancer Risks and Prevention.* Vessey MP, Gray M (editors). Oxford Univ Press, 1987.

Swift M et al: Incidence of cancer in 161 families affected by ataxia-telangiectasia. *N Engl J Med* 1991;**325**:1831.

Trock B: Dietary fiber, vegetables, and colon cancer. Critical review and meta-analyses of the epidemiologic evidence. *JNCI* 1990;**82**:650.

Willett W, MacMahon B: Diet and cancer: An overview (2 parts). *N Engl J Med* 1984;**310**:633,697.

Willett W et al: Relation of meat, fat, and fiber intake to the risk of colon cancer in a prospective study among women. *N Engl J Med* 1990;**323**:1664.

Section II.
Approach to the Cancer Patient

Diagnosis & Management of Early & Advanced Cancer

5

Geoffrey R. Weiss, MD

The ability of the practitioner caring for the cancer patient to bring order to the understanding and management of this chaotic disease has been a skill in evolution for centuries. It has been a product largely of the early and middle parts of this century that application of knowledge based on careful clinical observations, high-resolution diagnostic technology, and clinical trials methodology has permitted therapeutic interventions to produce improvement in the survival of cancer patients. This improvement in survival has plateaued for many of the commonest cancers as the benefits of aggressive surgical, radiation, and chemotherapeutic approaches to cancer management are enjoyed by that fixed fraction of the population most likely to respond. In the last quarter century, survival gains have been made in relatively uncommon cancers (testis cancer, leukemia, lymphoma, gestational tumors, and childhood cancers). It is likely that impact upon the control of the common and treatment-resistant cancers will require advances drawn from the newer disciplines in cancer research: molecular biology, cytogenetics, cell biology, radiation biology, carcinogenesis, immunology, and clinical pharmacology. In addition, increasing emphasis is being placed on prevention of cancer as it becomes more widely realized that most malignancies of Western industrialized societies are a product of lifestyles and occupation.

Until the time that cancer is better controlled by the utilization of as yet unrealized advances in diagnosis and treatment and by widespread application of preventive maneuvers, the most effective manner of offering the cancer patient the best opportunity for survival improvement and protection from disability is to practice state-of-the-art medical care in aggressive and timely fashion. Guidelines for recognizing and exploiting these opportunities are provided in this chapter.

PRINCIPLES OF CANCER DIAGNOSIS

The biologic and clinical hallmark of cancer is a disturbance of tissue growth in the host, most often distinguished by expansion of the aberrant tissue, invasion into local tissues, dissemination to distant sites, and ultimately death of the host as a consequence of the perturbations of normal organ function. Although this behavior seems chaotic and uncontrolled, uniform progress of malignant growth through these stages seems shared by most of the phenomena characterized as "cancer." It is the uniformity of behavior which directs the diagnostic and therapeutic approach to the cancer patient and which is reflected in the following principles.

Obtain Histopathologic Evidence of Malignancy

As stated frequently in this book, histopathologic confirmation of the presence of cancer is a principle that should remain inviolate. The diagnosis of cancer is such a stigmatizing fact that its presence should be unequivocally assured. At moments of diagnostic doubt, seeking additional opinions from recognized experts is a common and frequently useful pursuit. Additionally, when potentially disabling, disfiguring, or life-threatening treatment is envisioned for the patient, the diagnosis of malignant disease should be assured before treatment commences.

Corollary: The initial diagnosis of cancer should only rarely be based exclusively upon fine needle aspirate cytologic evidence.

Again, ensurance of the correct diagnosis is improved by the ability of the examining pathologist in reviewing adequate tissue. It may be fairly stated that the diagnosis of lymphoma and its subtypes cannot satisfactorily be made on less than whole nodal tissue; aspiration material is entirely inadequate. The use of needle-aspirated material may be only rarely condoned when evidence of malignancy without more specific characterization is sought (eg, the terminally ill patient or the patient too medically infirm to tolerate more invasive evaluation).

A further caveat demands that special attention be paid to histopathologic diagnoses of "poorly differentiated carcinoma," "poorly differentiated adenocarcinoma," "poorly differentiated spindle cell tumors," and "poorly differentiated small cell tumors." The ominous ring of such diagnoses may stifle the clinician's enthusiasm that a treatable or curable malignancy is being dealt with. However, in such circumstances, the scrutiny of the patient's tumor and clinical condition may provide evidence of treatable cancers that mimic diseases carrying a poor prognosis. For example, germ cell tumors, poorly differentiated lymphomas, and the more treatable carcinomas (breast cancer, small cell lung cancer) may emerge from more intense diagnostic evaluation of ill-described malignancies.

Obtain Histopathologic Evidence of Recurrence of Cancer for Disease Previously in Remission

The rationale for assuring the presence of recurrent malignant disease is similar to that for diagnosing primary malignant disease. In addition, a new site of malignancy must be demonstrated not to represent a new primary cancer, particularly when the neoplasm arises at a time distant from the original cancer. The occurrence of two or more primary cancers in a single individual is extraordinarily common, particularly since many cancers share common risk factors. In addition, nonmalignant conditions may mimic cancer. Despite the consistency of the clinical presentation of a lesion with the behavior of advanced cancer, the safest route to accept is biopsy of the lesion for confirmation of the clinical suspicion.

Make Use of Clinical Leads Likely to Provide the Highest Dividends

If an abnormal and suspect lesion is detected by physical examination, radiologic examination, or other technique, useful diagnostic evidence may be obtained by a direct approach to the suspect lesion. For example, if a rectal mass is palpated, slight liver enlargement is present, and the patient complains of dysphagia, diagnostic efforts should be devoted to the rectal mass as the most likely source of useful material; evaluation of the liver and dysphagia by other studies may await the characterization of the more obvious lesion. Furthermore, if the existing data suggest multiple possible sources of malignancy, pursue those possibilities suggested by the patient's symptoms or signs.

Review Previous Biopsy Slides of Resected Malignant or Nonmalignant Tissues

If the clinical behavior of a patient's malignant or nonmalignant condition is atypical or brings into doubt the initial diagnosis, review of the original tissue in light of the clinical perspective may provide new insight and revision of the histopathologic diagnosis. For example, a patient thought to be afflicted with an aggressive lymphoma who fails to enter a durable remission and suffers from recurrent lymphoma over a long period of time despite multiple aggressive therapeutic attempts may be found to have an incurable indolent lymphoma upon review of the original pathologic material.

Obtain a Second Opinion

Many malignancies provide the examining pathologist diagnostic challenges that may be resolved in the hands of individuals experienced in the evaluation of large numbers of rare diseases or of critical differential diagnostic subtleties. Obtaining a second opinion is a fact of life in all disciplines of medicine and should not be resisted when sought. If the diagnosis is not straightforward and requires increasingly sophisticated techniques (special stains, electron microscopy, etc), or if tissue for analysis is extremely limited, additional input should be sought from individuals with experience in the review of difficult diagnostic dilemmas.

CANCER STAGING

Once the histopathologic diagnosis of cancer has been completed, the process of cancer staging may be commenced. Cancer staging is an extremely important endeavor that contributes to a better understanding of cancer behavior in the following settings:

Prognosis

Staging provides information to the clinician and patient that permits estimation of prognosis of the disease. Most major cancers have been studied for decades and manifest patterns of spread that permit prediction of the likelihood and duration of survival, whether or not some therapeutic maneuver is applied to the care of the patient.

Treatment

Cancer staging provides the clinician an estimate of the likelihood of success of some therapeutic intervention against the cancer. Staging information assists the physician in planning treatment. Most modern cancer clinical trials are carried out with considerable effort in the population sample treated to ensure reproducibility and comparability of results in individuals with the same cancer. These staging efforts then permit an understanding of the appropriateness of a therapy for all stages of a cancer. For example, radiation therapy may be entirely appropriate alone for curative treatment of early-stage Hodgkin's disease but entirely inappropriate alone as curative therapy for Hodgkin's disease with visceral involvement.

Vital Statistics

Cancer staging ensures the comparability of treatment results in cancer clinical trials, tumor registry data, quality assurance of treatment programs, and demographic data for city, state, and federal health organizations. Cancer staging data are extremely important in monitoring the vital statistics of various populations in order to identify changes in incidence, prevalence, and death trends. Accuracy of cancer staging is virtually the only way the effects of a therapy can be certified as effective or ineffective, by comparison with an identically staged control group.

Staging

Cancer staging codifies the description of cancer states to enhance communication of cancer data between institutions, practitioners, and monitoring or treatment organizations. The most commonly accepted staging methods reflect a cancer biology dogma that is well entrenched, namely, an untreated primary cancer increases in size progressively, eventually manifests dissemination to lymph nodes, and ultimately manifests metastatic spread to distant anatomic sites. Both the American Joint Committee on Cancer (AJCC) and the Union International Contre le Cancer (UICC) have proposed the **TNM staging system** for universal application. Tumor growth (T), spread to primary or regional lymph nodes (N), and metastatic dissemination (M) are the events in the natural history of a cancer that this system seeks to define. Once classified, a malignancy may be grouped with classes of the disease with similar behavior or prognosis (stage classification). This process of staging may utilize only clinically derived parameters (physical examination, radiologic procedures, blood and serum data) or surgically/pathologically derived parameters (histopathologic examination of surgically resected tissues). Occasionally, the grade of a tumor (its differentiation or "degree of malignancy") is utilized in the further stage grouping of a cancer.

In following chapters it will be seen that cancer staging is fundamental to management of the disease.

APPROACH TO EARLY CANCER

The patient who presents to a physician promptly after detection of early evidence of cancer is the patient most likely to reap the benefits of early, aggressive, and intelligent application of modern cancer diagnosis and care. For most cancers, particularly those having a finite period of clinically detectable localized disease, the moment of first detection is the best and often only opportunity for cure. The primary physician or cancer specialist caring for the new cancer patient must proceed through a number of deliberate and well-defined steps to ensure the patient the chance for eradication of this disease (Table 5–1).

Obtain Histopathologic Evidence of Cancer

This step is critical to the primary management of cancer. Although the first evidence of cancer often occurs at its site of origin (the primary site), such an assumption is not a dependable one. Yet the assumption that a clinical sign of malignant disease is sufficient to proceed with further diagnostic or therapeutic procedures in the absence of confirming histopathologic evidence is hazardous; such procedures may carry a risk of disability, deformity, or death that can be rationalized only if cancer is unequivocally documented. Consequently, the safest approach to take is direct biopsy of the suspected site or origin. Once tissue documentation of malignancy is assured, further evaluation may proceed.

The clinician seeking retrieval of tissue for diagnosis of cancer should be prepared to glean as much diagnostic information from the sample as possible. Therefore, the clinician and pathologist must be alerted to the special requirements of tissue handling in certain circumstances. So many newly developed histochemical, immunologic, and molecular techniques applicable to diagnosis in resected human tissues are available that preparatory handling of tissues is far from routine. It may be necessary to divide resected tissue for placement in formalin, in glutaraldehyde for electron microscopy, in saline or tissue culture medium for later growth of cells in tissue culture, or in liquid nitrogen to snap-freeze for special techniques requiring vital cells (cell surface marker expression, tissue receptors for hormones or other agents).

Although fine-needle aspiration biopsy may serve simply to certify the presence of malignancy, biopsy of larger tissue specimens may provide important additional diagnostic information with therapeutic and prognostic impact. One of the most important derivatives of the definitive surgical removal of the primary cancer is the provision of additional material for diagnosis.

Table 5–1. Approach to early cancer.

Obtain histopathologic evidence of cancer.
Establish extent of primary cancer.
Evaluate nodal and distant sites for evidence of metastases consistent with natural history of cancer.
Obtain multidisciplinary evaluation for definitive primary management of cancer.
Apply primary therapy aggressively.
Evaluate patient's need for additional treatment (adjuvant) following primary therapy.
Develop apppropriate follow-up examination schedule based on patient's risk of recurrence.

Establish Extent of the Primary Cancer

The extent of the primary cancer (its size, its location, the extent to which it locally invades other structures) is of prognostic importance and is a determinant of the type of primary therapy appropriate to the disease. These are two of the functions of cancer staging. This information is drawn from careful physical examination (direct palpation of the tumor), radiologic procedures (standard plain x-rays, computed tomographic [CT] scans, magnetic resonance imaging [MRI], sonography, radionuclide imaging), endoscopic evaluation (bronchoscopy, endoscopy of the gastrointestinal tract or genitourinary tract, etc), collection of blood for tumor markers (carcinoembryonic antigen [CEA], α-fetoprotein, beta subunit of human chorionic gonadotropin [β-hCG], CA-125 for ovarian cancer, prostate-specific antigen, acid phosphatase, among others). Compilation of these data will permit the specialist to design the appropriate surgical or radiotherapeutic approach to the cancer, to estimate the likelihood that the approach will encompass the entire extent of the disease, and to offer some prediction of the likelihood of primary treatment failure and cancer relapse. Table 5–2 lists those cancers for which primary surgical or radiotherapeutic management offers the best chance of cure of localized cancers.

Evaluate Nodal and Distant Sites

Implicit in the evaluation of the extent of the primary cancer is the evaluation for evidence of metastatic cancer. This evaluation is addressed in the next section (Approach to Advanced Cancer), but it is noteworthy that aggressive treatment for cure of the primary cancer is futile in most cases if even a single deposit of metastatic cancer remains. The search for metastatic cancer should not elicit a wholesale diagnostic screen of the patient. The metastatic screen should be tailored to the known natural history of the disease, to its more likely sites of dissemination, and to the likely interventions applied to the patient's care.

Critical information is provided in the effort to detect malignant disease in regional lymph nodes. For selected cancers, the primary surgical management includes evaluation of the regional lymph nodes, the resultant data directing subsequent therapy and establishing reliable prognostic information (Table 5–3).

The detection of metastatic cancer carries uniformly grave prognostic meaning in all but a few cancers curable in the advanced state. The observation that spread of cancer is well beyond the confines of the primary tumor may spare the patient a major surgical or radiotherapeutic undertaking unlikely to have important impact on the natural history of the disease.

Obtain Multidisciplinary Evaluation

The major evolutionary advance made in the management of cancer in the last 20 years has been the multidisciplinary treatment approach. The limitations of surgery, radiation therapy, or chemotherapy alone are well known. Although surgery remains the dominant method for achieving arrest of still-localized cancer, the frequent postoperative relapse of cancer at local or metastatic sites remains tangible evidence of the limitations of this macroscopic modality alone for the control of a microscopically active disease. For the common solid tumors of Western society, it is believed that the initial emergence of cancer may have preceded its clinical detection by 5–15 years, ample opportunity for metastatic spread.

The simultaneous or rapid sequential administration of two or more anticancer maneuvers may be rewarded by objective improvement in time-to-relapse, disease-free survival, and overall survival, the common measures of therapeutic effect in cancer treatment. The term "adjuvant" has long been applied to those treatments which follow surgical management of a primary cancer. The concept of adjuvant therapy is one which recognizes that certain patients harbor a risk of relapsing cancer unaddressed by state-of-the-art surgery. Adjuvant radiation therapy or chemotherapy seeks to eradicate that undetectable residue of cancer inadequately retrieved by surgery, either local advancement of the cancer unencompassed by the surgical procedure or micrometastatic cancer requiring systemic treatment. Cancers for which such "adjuvant" therapy has had definite effect on survival outcome are listed in Table 5–4.

Apply Primary Therapy Aggressively

It cannot be overemphasized that the primary management of a cancer when first detected is the best

Table 5–2. Cancers cured by surgery or radiation therapy.

Cancers frequently cured by primary surgery
  Cancers of the head and neck region
  Skin cancers, including malignant melanoma
  Bronchogenic lung cancer (not small cell)
  Breast cancer
  Cancers of the hollow viscera of the gastrointestinal tract
  Cancers of the male and female genitourinary tract
  Soft tissue sarcomas
Cancers frequently cured by primary radiation therapy
  Hodgkin's disease
  Testicular seminoma
  Skin cancers other than melanoma

Table 5–3. Cancers for which regional nodal involvement by metastases is strongly prognostic.

Breast cancer
Non–small-cell lung cancer
Malignant melanoma
Cancers of the head and neck
Gastrointestinal cancers
Female and male genitourinary cancers

Table 5–4. Cancers for which adjuvant therapy has improved survival.

Breast cancer
Osteogenic sarcoma
Colorectal carcinoma

and may be the only opportunity for cure. The treating clinician should not seek reasons for ameliorating the toxicity of therapy or suspending the need for its application. The clinician should attempt to apply the elected therapy at full potency, only rarely reducing its full application when attendant medical conditions warrant. Most cancers are extremely sensitive to small changes in "dosage," responding beneficially to maximum treatment effects but manifesting disappointing therapeutic outcome following minor attenuation of treatment aggressiveness. It is worthwhile keeping in mind that the alternative to toxicity of therapy, no matter how debilitating, disfiguring, or risky, is death. This same tenet applies to the scheduling of cancer treatments. The interval between courses of treatment or between different modalities of treatment should be kept as tight as possible.

Evaluate Need for Adjuvant Therapy

The rationale for follow-up therapy after primary management of a cancer has been alluded to. The intent of such therapy is to attempt eradication of residual tumor soiling the resected or irradiated primary site, or to destroy microscopic lymphatic or blood-borne deposits of cancer at sites distant from the primary tumor. Clues that such adjuvant therapy may be necessary derive from staging information obtained during the initial noninvasive workup of the patient or during the primary surgery. Risks of recurrent or metastatic cancer may be inferred from tumor size, the presence of regional lymph node metastases in the resected specimen, histopathologic differentiation of the cancer, symptoms, or elevation of blood-borne tumor markers. Many individuals with very early cancers may have sufficiently favorable results from primary treatment that the risk of relapse is extremely low and the value of adjuvant therapy is negligible. The benefits of adjuvant therapy are often extremely subtle and may be detected only by large-scale randomized controlled clinical trials. Adjuvant therapy should be applied when the following two qualifications are met: (1) the risk of relapse exceeds the risk of death or permanent disability of the adjuvant therapy, and (2) the adjuvant therapy has been unequivocally shown by clinical trial to enhance the survival of the patient with disease of the appropriate stage of advancement and risk of recurrence.

Base Follow-up on Patient's Risk of Recurrence

Clinical data gleaned from the primary management of a patient's cancer will provide a strong indi-

cation of the likelihood of its recurrence. Previous published experience will suggest how rapidly this recurrence may occur. Because the prompt detection of newly recurrent cancer may yet permit occasional curative as well as survival-prolonging interventions, the interval between follow-up visits and surveillance should reflect the growth potential of the recurrent disease. A disease whose ability to double in size requires only the passage of weeks may require patient follow-up monthly; alternatively, the more indolent disease whose doubling time is measured in months or years may safely be monitored at more extended intervals (3–6 months). Furthermore, the natural history of most common malignancies is well established, and the duration of time that relapse remains a risk in patients is usually a consistent characteristic of the disease. In some cases, the risk of relapse never plateaus, and continued death of patients from cancer is an uninterrupted continuum to the last patient.

Follow-up of the cancer patient requires judicious application of the most useful and the most sensitive methods available. The approach is summarized below.

(1) History and physical examination are the foundation of the follow-up of all treated cancer patients.

(2) Known sites of cancer involvement prior to definitive treatment should be continuously monitored for relapse.

(3) Choice of follow-up diagnostic studies should reflect the known common sites of relapse for the disease.

(4) The least expensive high-resolution diagnostic methods should be selected for long-term sequential follow-up.

(5) The duration of the most intense follow-up based on the known interval of highest risk of relapse for that disease should be decided on; follow-up frequency and intensity should be adjusted at the passage of the planned initial follow-up period.

APPROACH TO ADVANCED CANCER

Advanced cancer may become a component of the cancer patient's condition at any time. The condition of advanced cancer generally reflects disease that is incurable and may lead to death. However, this realization should not paralyze the patient's or the clinician's commitment to aggressive management of the disease. The rationale for maintaining an aggressive and upbeat approach to advanced disease includes the following:

(1) A few cancers are curable in the advanced or metastatic state (testis cancer, gestational trophoblastic cancers, osteogenic sarcoma, Hodgkin's disease, intermediate- and high-grade non-Hodgkin's lymphoma).

(2) Although published reports of the treatment outcome or natural history of advanced cancers sug-

gest disturbingly short median, mean, or 2- to 5-year survival, survival distributions may have very long tails. Not all patients with a given advanced cancer may experience prompt disability or demise. Such patients may enjoy long holidays from active treatment or durable asymptomatic periods during disease stability.

(**3**) Although treatment statistics may suggest discouragingly low response rates for a treatment regimen, very brief response duration, or survival advantages no different from those of minimal or no treatment, the opportunity for any response, no matter how small, may be accepted easily by the advanced cancer patient. In the view of many patients, should they be fortunate enough to respond, the benefit is 100% for them. Indeed, the occasional patient may enjoy dramatic response or prolonged control of cancer upon receipt of a treatment regimen of low published activity.

(**4**) Despite evidence of advanced or metastatic cancer at the time of diagnosis of the primary disease, exploiting opportunities to remove relatively limited advanced disease may rarely be accompanied by cure of the disease, durable remission, or enhanced freedom from onset of cancer-induced symptoms.

The approach to the advanced cancer patient is summarized in Table 5–5. Adherence to this approach may enhance the patient's likelihood of prolonged survival and freedom from symptoms.

Obtain Histopathologic Evidence of First Recurrence

Chance clearly favors the prepared mind. Although most recurrences of malignant disease are strongly suspected by their manner of presentation on physical examination or noninvasive diagnostic evaluation, it must be remembered that other diseases are quite common, including additional de novo cancers. Indeed, cancer is a risk factor for other cancers. Consequently, obtaining biopsy material of a suspected recurrent cancer will rarely be met by argument from the patient or operator. The biopsied material may confirm a new cancer that may restore curative potential to the situation. In addition, patients treated for advanced malignancies who demonstrate residual evidence of disease at the conclusion of therapy deserve consideration for biopsy if the disease (1) has responded and then plateaued or stabilized in response, (2) shows little evidence of persistence by other criteria (eg, normalization of blood tumor markers), and (3) is creating no disability or symptomatology in the patient. In such cases, the evidence of residual disease may be scar tissue or fibrosis that has little capacity to resolve.

Table 5–5. Approach to advanced cancer.

Obtain histopathologic confirmation of first recurrence of cancer and any recurrences widely separated in time.

In the newly recurrent cancer patient, restage noninvasively all symptomatic sites and all sites commonly known to harbor metastases.

Actively treat advanced cancer no matter how dismal the treatment statistics. Corollary: Obtain second opinions about treatment for advanced cancer.

In Newly Recurrent Cancer, Restage Noninvasively All Symptomatic Sites and All Sites Commonly Known to Harbor Metastases

The aggressive management of advanced cancer requires a comprehensive understanding of the magnitude of the problem. Such knowledge is necessary in order to judiciously choose among local or systemic cancer therapies to ensure the most prompt and therapeutically parsimonious control of disease advancement and symptom control. For example, although a weight-bearing bone may be at risk of fracture from a large metastasis of breast cancer, the metastasis may also be a hallmark of bone dissemination of disease. Irradiation of the threatened bone may be warranted, but further thought should be given to performing a bone scan and treating the patient with chemotherapy or a hormonal modality if disseminated bone disease is detected.

Actively Treat Advanced Cancer

It is the rare patient who elects to forgo active treatment for advanced cancer no matter how dismal the treatment statistics. Although the prospect for survival in a patient with advanced cancer may be grim, the clinician should avoid an attitude of hopelessness and should not convey opinions suggesting complete futility of treatment. Patients may be prepared to accept the news that their cancer represents an immediate threat to life, but this threat is infrequently a stimulus for inaction. Indeed, the more limited the options for successful treatment, the more difficult are the decisions for appropriate treatment (particularly among marginally active treatment regimens) and the more likely that a patient will seek additional opinions about more controversial, less well-proved, or investigational forms of therapy. Requests for second opinions should be routinely honored unless the therapy sought is blatantly dangerous or without scientific or ethical merit. In addition, the patient with terminally advanced and treatment-resistant cancer may be a candidate for investigational therapy. In the absence of reliably effective therapy for the patient's disease, every effort should be exerted to permit the patient's participation in a legitimate clinical trial of cancer therapy.

Cancer Screening

6

Mary B. Daly, MD, PhD

The ultimate control of cancer will be the result of a combination of cancer prevention, risk reduction, and early detection. Efforts at primary prevention seek to forestall the biologic onset of malignancy by altering host susceptibility or by removing etiologic agents from contact with the host. Secondary prevention, or screening, on the other hand, seeks to detect the disease at a preclinical stage in the asymptomatic host, at a time when it is presumably most treatable (Figure 6–1).

Widespread application of a screening test requires demonstration of benefit from early detection, and certain criteria must be fulfilled to identify those cancers which are suitable for screening. The burden of suffering associated with a particular cancer must be sufficient, in terms both of prevalence and of morbidity and mortality, to warrant the risks and costs associated with a screening program. Furthermore, the cancer must have a treatment which, when applied during the preclinical stage of disease, is more effective than treatment applied after symptoms have developed. Effective treatment for early-stage disease should ultimately translate into decreased mortality from the disease. The screening test itself must fulfill certain standards. For widespread application in a population, a test must be safe, convenient, acceptable to the public, and relatively low in cost. In addition to being feasible, it must be accurate and reliable.

Accuracy refers to the sensitivity and specificity of a test, ie, its ability to detect the maximum number of true cases without falsely labeling others with positive tests. **Reliability** is the capacity of a test to give the same results on repeat examinations. To optimize the results of a screening program, efforts should be targeted at those persons who are identified by known risk factors to be at highest risk for a particular cancer. A program must attempt to achieve a high compliance rate and to define both the proper screening interval as well as the most appropriate follow-up of positive tests. Finally, the health care system in general must have the resources to cope with the screening efforts themselves, as well as with the consequences of identifying preclinical disease.

Some hazards associated with screening programs for cancer, in addition to cost, include the unnecessary morbidity of those with falsely positive tests, the potential overtreatment of borderline lesions, and the false reassurance offered to those with falsely negative tests.

Ideally, the effectiveness of a screening test is first demonstrated by one or more randomized trials which take into account the biases inherent in early screening for cancer. These biases include lead-time bias, length bias, and self-selection bias.

Lead-Time Bias

One goal of screening for cancer is to gain lead time, ie, to identify the cancer earlier. However, simply moving forward in time the date of diagnosis by early detection, without subsequently also delaying the time of death by successful intervention, creates a spurious increase in the duration of survival, and this is called lead-time bias. The magnitude of lead-time bias is determined by the sensitivity of the test, the testing interval, and the duration of the preclinical stage.

Length Bias

Length bias can occur because slow-growing cancers with presumably more favorable prognoses will have longer preclinical stages than fast-growing, aggressive tumors with worsened prognoses. Therefore, the more favorable cases are more likely to be detected in the preclinical stage by a screening effort. The improved survival observed in the screened population therefore derives at least in part from the growth properties of the tumor rather than from the benefits of the screening program.

Self-Selection Bias

Those persons who agree to participate in a voluntary screening effort may vary in terms of social and physical characteristics from those who decline participation. Depending on the relationship of these characteristics to disease outcome, a bias may be created, interfering with comparisons of survival between the screened and unscreened group.

Screening programs for some of the most common forms of cancer have been developed, tested, and subjected to scientific evaluation. The following discussion concentrates on the role of screening for cancer of the cervix, breast, colon and rectum, and lung, which represent the leading causes of cancer death in the Western world today.

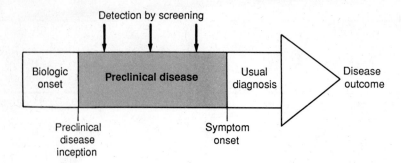

Figure 6–1. Goals of screening: Find cancers at an earlier stage; improve the chances of cure.

CANCER OF THE CERVIX

Although no randomized, controlled trials for cervical cytologic screening for cancer of the cervix have ever been performed, a large body of evidence clearly links the dramatic decline in incidence and mortality of this disease over the past 30 years with the introduction of the Papanicolaou smear and its routine use as a screening tool (Figure 6–2). The natural history of the disease suggests a long preclinical stage, progressing from dysplastic changes to carcinoma in situ and finally to frank malignancy over 12–20 years. This pattern and the success of treatment in the early stages makes cancer of the cervix an ideal candidate for secondary prevention by screening. The

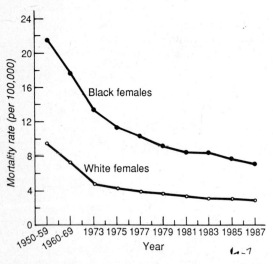

Figure 6–2. Mortality rate of cancer of the cervix per 100,000 population. [Data from: Gloeckler Ries L, Hankey B, Edwards B (editors): *Cancer Statistics Review, 1973–1987.* US Department of Health and Human Services, NIH Publication No. 90-2789, 1990; and Riggan W et al: *US Cancer Mortality* Rates and Trends, 1950–1979. National Cancer Institute (September) 1983.]

bulk of evidence supporting a role for screening with the Papanicolaou smear derives both from case control studies and from retrospective analyses of mortality rates in areas before and after the introduction of screening.

Gellman et al surveyed the incidence and mortality rates for cancer of the cervix in the provinces of Canada between 1960 and 1970. They report a negative correlation between mortality rates and intensity of screening with Papanicolaou smears over that decade.

A cervical cancer screening program was introduced in Toledo, Ohio, in 1947, and by 1954 it was estimated that over 90% of all adult females had received at least one Papanicolaou smear. The age-adjusted incidence rates for invasive squamous cell cancer of the cervix declined by 66% over that same time period. Similarly, a review of cancer mortality rates in Iceland shows a sharp decline for cancer of the cervix starting in 1969, approximately 5 years after the initiation of a mass cervical cancer screening program. At the same time, a shift from stage II and higher tumors to early stage I disease was observed.

Data from the Second and Third National Cancer surveys revealed a 35–60% decline in the incidence of cervical cancer in the USA between 1950 and 1970 and a strong correlation on a state-wide basis between rate of decline in rates and rate of screening with Papanicolaou smears.

Dunn and Schweitzer used data from the California Tumor Registry and household interviews in Alameda County to evaluate the impact of cervical cytologic screening on the occurrence of cervical cancer. Between 1960 and 1975, the number of women reporting having had at least one Papanicolaou test rose from 50% to 90%. At the same time, both incidence and mortality rates declined by 33% and 36%, respectively.

A case-control study conducted in Toronto between 1973 and 1976 matched all newly diagnosed cervical cancer patients by age with five neighborhood controls. Through interviews with both groups, twice as many controls as cases were found to have received Papanicolaou smears in the prior 5 years. The calculated relative risk was 2.7, and the negative relationship between Papanicolaou smear and incidence of disease persisted when all other known risk factors were controlled.

It is unlikely that a prospective randomized trial will ever be performed. In fact, on the basis of the weight of evidence accumulated to date, development and implementation of cytologic screening programs for cervical cancer have been recommended for all women over age 18 by both the American Cancer Society (ASC) and the American College of Obstetricians and Gynecologists. The recommended screening interval is at least every 3 years after three consecutive yearly negative tests. It is estimated that uniform compliance with these recommendations will lead to a 70–95% reduction in cervical cancer mortality.

BREAST CANCER

Breast cancer is the second leading cause of cancer death in women in the USA. More than 175,000 new cases are diagnosed each year, and in 1991 approximately 45,000 American women died of breast cancer. Breast cancer incidence has been rising at the rate of 3% per year since 1980. There is a clear relationship between stage at diagnosis and disease-free survival for breast cancer. Most breast cancer detected by routine clinical practice is stage II or greater. Therefore, a screening tool that can detect stage I or earlier breast cancer is likely to have an impact on survival. The screening techniques currently in use include breast self-examination, clinical breast examination by a health care provider, and mammography.

The value of breast self-examination (BSE) as a screening tool is controversial. Several studies have demonstrated an increase in earlier stage at diagnosis and a subsequent reduction in mortality among women who were regular BSE performers, while other studies fail to show such a relationship. A meta-analysis of 12 studies (total of 8118 patients) found evidence of a significant decrease in lymph node involvement and a significant reduction in tumor size for women who practiced regular BSE prior to their diagnosis. Randomized controlled trials are under way to determine the true benefit of regular BSE as a component of a breast screening program.

The efficacy of clinical breast examination and screening mammography, on the other hand, has been clearly demonstrated by several studies. In 1963–1967, the Health Insurance Plan (HIP) of New York enrolled 62,000 women aged 40–64 in a mass breast cancer screening program. The women were randomized into either a study group, which was offered annual physical examination and mammography for 4 years, or into a control group, which received "usual care." One-third of the cancers in the study group

were detected by mammography alone. Over 75% of the tumors found by screening, either through mammography or physical examination, were stage I tumors, compared to 45% stage I tumors in the control group. More importantly, the early detection afforded by the screening program has translated into a 23% reduction in mortality for all women in the screened group (25% for women aged 40–49 and 20% for women aged 50 or above), which has persisted beyond 18 years of follow-up.

A similar randomized, controlled trial of 162,981 women in Sweden, using mammography as the only screening technique, also documented a 24% overall reduction in mortality from breast cancer in the screened group.

The Breast Cancer Detection Demonstration Project (BCDDP), begun in 1973 and founded jointly by the American Cancer Society and the National Cancer Institute, was designed to test the acceptability and feasibility of a large-scale nonrandomized population-based breast cancer screening project. Twenty-nine centers were invited to enroll 10,000 women each, for mammograms, physical examination, and education on breast self-examination, for a total of five annual examinations. Over 280,000 women participated, with 51.7% attending all five screenings. In the interval between the HIP and the BCDDP studies, improvements in the quality of mammography involving both the hardware and the image receptors resulted in improved sensitivity of the examination as well as decreased dose of radiation to a negligible level to the patient. In fact, mammography played a significantly greater role in the diagnosis of breast cancer in the BCDDP than in the HIP study. Mammography alone revealed 48% of all detected cancers among women with negative physical examinations. Even among women aged 40–49, mammography alone was responsible for detecting 45% of cancers. Less than 20% of the cancers detected by BCDDP were node positive. Unfortunately, the collection of mortality data was not included in the design of this study. If, however, the distribution of stage at diagnosis found in the BCDPP was duplicated in the general population, the estimated in mortality would be 50% in women aged 40–49 years and 58% in women aged 50 years and older.

Current American Cancer Society recommendations for the early detection of breast cancer include the following:

(1) Breast self-examination monthly for all women beyond the starting age of 20.

(2) Breast physical examination by a health care provider once every 3 years for women aged 20–40, and yearly thereafter.

(3) A baseline mammogram between 35 and 40 years, and every 2–3 years for women aged 40–50 years and yearly thereafter.

The number of women reporting ever having had a mammogram has risen sharply to over 60% in the last decade in the USA. This is coincident with a greater than threefold increase in the percentage of physicians who recommend screening mammography to their patients. However, significant barriers to full utilization continue to exist, including socioeconomic and cultural factors, problems of access to care, and knowledge and attitudinal barriers. The full implementation of these guidelines will require continued educational efforts aimed at the population at risk and their health care providers, and a firm commitment to preventive health services on the part of both public and private insurers.

COLORECTAL CANCER

The annual incidence of colorectal cancer is second only to lung cancer and accounts for 60,500 deaths per year. Five-year survival rates are best correlated with anatomic spread at the time of resection, implying that early detection and resection will result in improved survival. Additionally, there appears to be a relationship between the presence of adenomatous polyps and the subsequent development of colon cancer. Early identification and removal of polyps through screening may therefore actually contribute to the prevention of colon cancer in certain individuals.

The anticipated detection of large bowel cancer by digital rectal examination is less than 10% owing to the more proximal location of most of these tumors. However, approximately half of colorectal carcinomas and adenomas occur in the anatomic region that is accessible by proctosigmoidoscopy. A 10-year study conducted at the Preventive Medicine Institute–Strang Clinic in New York entailed 47,091 proctosigmoid examinations on 26,126 patients. A 15-year survival rate of 90% was demonstrated among the 58 patients diagnosed with colorectal carcinoma through this screening effort. A randomized trial performed at Kaiser-Permamente Hospital in California reports a statistically significant reduction in mortality at 10 years in a study group that underwent annual proctosigmoidoscopy. The University of Minnesota followed 18,000 patients who had undergone rigid proctosigmoidoscopy annually for approximately 25 years. All polyps found on examination were routinely removed. During the entire period of follow-up, only 13 colorectal carcinomas, or 15% of the expected number, were found, suggesting a role of primary prevention by polypectomy.

The potential benefit in terms of reduction in mortality from regular screening with proctosigmoidoscopy has not been realized in the USA because of underutilization by physicians and poor compliance by patients. The flexible sigmoidoscope offers the promise of increased comfort for the patient but requires additional training for physicians and will in-

crease costs. Its use has not been adopted on a wide scale for screening purposes.

Widespread screening with the use of the Hemoccult card, on the other hand, offers a potentially more feasible alternative. The Hemoccult card is impregnated with guaiac, which stains hemoglobin in feces by an oxidation reaction when a drop of hydrogen peroxide is added.

Screening by both proctosigmoidoscopy and occult blood slides has undergone extensive testing in several population groups. Several uncontrolled community trials of stool guaiac testing using Hemoccult slides have yielded these consistent findings:

(1) Compliance ranges from 15% to 70% and can be increased by the use of multimedia public education campaigns.

(2) Slide positivity in an unselected population is between 2% and 6%.

(3) Further evaluation of persons with positive slides is variable and often inadequate.

(4) Approximately 5% of persons with positive slides are eventually diagnosed with colon cancer.

(5) Dukes' staging of detected cases compares favorably with that of cancers detected in symptomatic persons, with most studies reporting a 70–80% distribution of Dukes' A and B stages.

Five randomized controlled trials are under way to address the effectiveness of the stool guaiac test as a screening tool. Between 1975 and 1979, the Memorial Sloan Kettering Cancer Center randomized 21,756 individuals over the age of 40, who were presenting for their annual physical examination, to either the control arm, which included rigid proctosigmoidoscopy as part of the routine evaluation, or the study group, which additionally was offered a stool guaiac test. Of the 59 cancers detected in the study group, over 60% were found by slide alone. Even more significant is the finding that twice as many Dukes' early-stage cancers were found in the study group (65% stages A and B versus 33% in the control group). While mortality from other causes was equivalent in both groups at 10 years, there was a 43% reduction in mortality from colorectal cancer, which persisted for all age groups. On the other hand, 25% of the carcinomas and 75% of the polyps actually seen on sigmoidoscopy in the study group were missed by Hemoccult testing.

The University of Minnesota randomly assigned 48,000 individuals aged 50–80 years, to one of three groups: **(1)** testing with Hemoccult slides every year for 5 years, **(2)** testing with Hemoccult slides every other year for 5 years, or **(3)** the control group. Of those undergoing Hemoccult testing, 2.4% had positive slides. One hundred cancers were detected through the screening, 78% of which were Dukes' stage A or B at detection.

A study in Nottingham, England, randomly allocated 20,525 individuals aged 45–74 to either screening with Hemoccult cards three times or to a control group. Of the study group 38.5% responded, and 2.1% of these had positive slides. Work-up of these 201 individuals detected 56 adenomas and 17 colorectal carcinomas. Ninety percent of the cancers were Dukes' stage A or B, compared with 47% of those diagnosed by usual means.

A fourth controlled trial was initiated in Goteborg, Sweden, in 1982, in which all residents of the city aged 60–64 years were randomized to either two serial Hemoccult screens or to a no-contact control group. Compliance was 66% for the first screening and 58% for the second. Sixty-five percent of the colon cancers diagnosed by Hemoccult were stage A or B, compared with 33% in the control group. No long-term data are available.

Finally, a fifth large population based trial in Denmark is randomizing 62,000 individuals, aged 50–74 years, to stool blood testing every other year or to a control group. Initial compliance in the study group is 66%, with a 1% rate of slide positivity.

Mortality statistics are pending in most of the above-mentioned studies, but earlier detection is expected to result in prolonged survival. None of these studies fully addressed the cost-benefit aspects of widespread screening for colorectal carcinoma. Furthermore, significant areas of both patient and physician uncertainty regarding the risks and benefits of screening for colorectal cancer have been identified. While a high level interest for mass screening has been expressed by various health organizations, there are conflicting guidelines for its use. The American Cancer Society has issued the following recommendations:

(1) Digital rectal examination yearly after age 40.

(2) Sigmoidoscopic examination after age 50 every 3–5 years after two initial negative examinations, 1 year apart.

(3) Stool occult blood test yearly after age 50.

Individuals at high risk for colon cancer by virtue of prior colon cancer, ulcerative colitis, familial polyposis, or the cancer family syndrome require a particularly aggressive approach. Colonoscopy may be the screening tool of choice, and screening efforts must begin at a younger age.

LUNG CANCER

The dramatic increase in the incidence of lung cancer over the past 30–50 years has resulted in its prominence as the leading cause of cancer deaths for both men and women in the USA. Lung cancer typically presents in an advanced stage when successful treatment is not possible. Furthermore, screening efforts to detect early lung cancer have uniformly failed to demonstrate a significant impact on survival. Regardless of the screening modality used, there has been no appreciable change in mortality rates (Table 6–1).

Starting in 1951, the Philadelphia Pulmonary Neoplasm Research Project screened 6136 men, aged 45 years and older, in a nonrandom design with a chest x-ray and health questionnaire every 6 months. The 5-year survival rate for lung cancer patients detected through this program was 8%, which is no different from figures derived from national statistics.

The Veterans Administration screened 14,607 residents of Virginia nursing homes with a chest x-ray and sputum cytologic test every 6 months for 3 years. Of the 200 lung cancers detected, only 26 were resectable, and only three patients survived 3 years.

In the late 1960s, the Kaiser Foundation initiated a randomized trial comparing annual chest x-rays and spirometry to "routine care." After 11 years of follow-up, there was no difference in mortality due to lung cancer between the two groups.

The Mayo Clinic Lung Project compared screening with an annual chest x-ray and sputum cytologic test to testing every 4 months in a group of 11,000 male smokers aged 45 years and older. Although cases found in the more intensively screened group were more likely to be resectable (46% versus 32%), there was no difference in mortality between the two groups.

Finally, both Memorial Sloan-Kettering and Johns Hopkins evaluated the addition of quarterly sputum cytologic testing to annual chest x-ray in male smokers and found no benefit in terms of stage of tumor at diagnosis, 5-year survival, or overall mortality rates.

Thus, the screening tools currently available for detection of lung cancer, namely, chest x-ray, spi-

Table 6–1. Age-adjusted lung cancer mortality rates in screened group versus control group.

Study Group/Screening Effort	Mortality Rate	
	Screen	Control
Mayo Clinic Lung Project Annual chest x-ray plus quarterly cytologic examination versus "standard care"	3.2/1000 person-years	3.0/1000 person-years
Memorial Sloan-Kettering study Annual chest x-ray plus quarterly cytologic examination versus annual chest x-ray only	3.8/1000 person-years	3.8/1000 person-years
Johns Hopkins study Annual chest x-ray plus quarterly cytologic examination versus annual chest x-ray only	3.4/1000 person-years	3.8/1000 person-years

rometry, and sputum cytology, apparently do not detect cancers early enough to affect survival. An additional consideration is the substantial risk and cost associated with the evaluation of a false-positive screening test by bronchoscopy, biopsy, and in some cases thoracotomy. Because lung cancer lends itself so well to primary prevention by the avoidance of tobacco products and other known causes, it seems more appropriate at this time to devote the energies of the health care system to achieving a "smoke-free society."

OTHER CAUSES

Recommendations can be found for a variety of screening endeavors for other cancers, usually in the absence of data to substantiate their use. Digital rectal examination for the detection of prostate cancer has been included in the recommendation of the American Cancer Society for men aged 40 and above. No randomized trials have been conducted to determine the effectiveness of this approach. Periodic self-examination and medical examinations of the skin are recommended by some for persons at high risk for melanoma by virtue of skin type, dysplastic nevus syndrome, or family history. Lack of controlled trials leave the value of these screening activities unverified. The value of monthly self-examinations for testicular cancer in males is likewise unknown. The search for sensitive and specific bioassays to detect early cancer cells has to date been unsuccessful, although research in this area continues.

The goal of screening for cancer control is improved survival through early detection, with minimum risk to the screened population and with acceptable costs to the health care system. The criteria initially outlined for a successful screening program must be carefully maintained, and efforts to refine screening techniques must continue to be sought.

REFERENCES

Cadman D et al: Assessing the effectiveness of community screening programs. *JAMA* 1984;**251**:1580.

Clark E, Anderson T: Does screening by PAP smears help prevent cervical cancers? *Lancet* 1979;**2**:1.

Cole P, Morrison A: Basic issues in population screening for cancer. *JNCI* 1980;**64**:1263.

Coleman E: Practice and effectiveness of breast self examination: A selective review of the literature (1977–1989). *J Cancer Educ* 1991;**6**:83.

Cramer D: The role of cervical cytology in the declining morbidity and mortality of cervical cancer. *Cancer* 1974;**34**:2018.

Dunn J, Schweitzer V: The relationship of cervical cytology to the incidence of invasive cervical cancer and mortality in Alameda County, California, 1960–1974. *Am J Obstet Gynecol* 1981;**139**:868.

Eddy D: Screening for breast cancer. *Ann Intern Med* 1989;**111**:389.

Eddy D: Screening for lung cancer. *Ann Intern Med* 1989;**111**:232.

Gellman D: Cervical cancer screening program. *Can Med Assoc J* 1976;**114**:1003.

Johannesson G, Giersson G, Day N: The effect of mass screening in Iceland, 1965–74, on the incidence and mortality of cervical carcinoma. *Int J Cancer* 1978;**21**:418.

Kim K et al: The changing trends of uterine cancer and cytology. *Cancer* 1978;**42**:2439.

Simon J: Occult blood screening for colorectal carcinoma: A critical review. *Gastroenterology* 1985;**88**:820.

Smart C: The role of mammography in the prevention of mortality from breast cancer. *Cancer Prevention* (June) 1990:1.

Stone A, Kallenberg G: Screening for colorectal cancer. In: *Putting Prevention into Practice.* Riegelman R, Povar G (editors). Little, Brown, 1988.

Taylor W et al: Some results of screening for early lung cancer. *Cancer* 1981;**47**:1114.

Winawer SJ, Schottenfeld D, Flehinger BJ: Colorectal cancer screening. *JNCI* 1991;**83**:243.

Cancer Prevention

7

Frank L. Meyskens, Jr., MD

The best and most effective treatment for cancer is its prevention. Most of the major human diseases of humankind have been controlled not through aggressive treatment approaches but rather by the application of basic science discoveries in support of preventive or public health strategies (Table 7–1). Pellagra and scurvy, once common and poorly understood diseases, have been essentially eliminated by assuring adequate intakes of nicotinamide and ascorbic acid. Infectious diseases have been particularly well controlled by preventive interventions. Syphilis and tuberculosis have yielded to the powerful combination of basic understanding of the disease process, design of targeted pharmacologic interventions, and application through medical and public health measures. Prevention is currently the only effective approach to controlling the acquired immunodeficiency syndrome (AIDS). Since more patients with AIDS are developing malignancies as they live longer, prevention of AIDS in subjects at risk for tumors also has a role in controlling the overall morbidity and mortality from cancer.

Although prevention reduces morbidity and mortality due to a number of nutrition-based and acute and chronic infectious diseases, whether preventive approaches can reduce morbidity and mortality in patients with chronic diseases, such as heart disease or cancer, is still unknown. Experience with cardiovascular diseases during the past two decades indicates that application of a few simple measures impacts on their outcome. Lowering of blood pressure and cholesterol and cessation of smoking significantly reduces mortality from heart disease and stroke. Both the incidence of and the morbidity and mortality due to cardiovascular disease have fallen in the USA during the past decade. This favorable change almost certainly reflects secular trends in adjustments in lifestyle (changing diet, decreased smoking) and application of simple medical strategies (dieting advice, control of hypertension).

In our understanding of risk factors for cancer and the use of prevention strategies to alter its natural history, we are about 15 years behind the science for cardiovascular disease prevention. Table 7–2 lists those risk factors which unequivocally contribute in a major way to the development of cancer. Reduction

of these risk factors should lead to a rapid fall in the incidence of certain cancers. Table 7–3 lists those factors for which there is considerable reason to make an association with cancer development. However, more confirmatory data are needed before strong preventive recommendations can be made. This chapter focuses on the scientific basis for cancer prevention, old and new intervention strategies, the role of the physician in participating in prevention strategies, and prospects for future development.

BIOLOGIC BASIS

Successful application of prevention strategies depends on general and detailed knowledge of the biologic basis of cancer causation and early transformation events. Over the past 30 years, a large number of laboratory studies have sought to reveal the mechanistic basis of cancer formation (carcinogenesis). The general schema of our current understanding of the process of carcinogenesis is presented in Figure 7–1. Tumor development can be divided into three major stages of each phase: initiation, promotion, and progression. The essential elements are outlined in Table 7–4.

Initiation

Three key steps have been identified: **conversion** of the agent to an active carcinogen, **interaction** of the carcinogen with the DNA to produce a lesion in the genetic material, and **fixation** of that damage. Not all carcinogens require activation, but among those which do the liver or kidney is the usual site of metabolism, and the event is rapid. Interaction of the carcinogen with DNA may be direct or indirect. Many initiators produce lipid-activated (oxidized) species that act secondarily to produce genetic damage. This step is generally regarded as rapid although ongoing damage to DNA from oxidized lipid species may occur over long periods of time. After nucleotides in the DNA are altered, the cell attempts to correct the damage. Under certain conditions, particularly when accompanied by cellular quiescence, the alterations can be corrected. Several agents can serve

Table 7–1. Control of major diseases using prevention strategies.

Disease	Role Laboratory	Role Epidemiology	Intervention
Plague	–	+	Sewer control
Rabies	+	+	Animal control, vaccination
Smallpox	+	+	Vaccination
Poliomyelitis	+++	+++	Vaccination
Scurvy	–	+	Vitamin C
Pellagra	+	+	Niacin
Vehicular trauma	+++	+++	Seat belts
Chronic diseases			
Cardiovascular	+++	+++	Lowering of blood pressure and cholesterol
Cancer	+++	+++	Smoking cessation, ? dietary changes

Table 7–3. Suspected major associations with cancer formation in humans.

Factor	Associated Cancer	Proposed Prevention Strategy
Viruses		
Sexually transmitted		
AIDS-related	Kaposi's sarcoma, lymphomas	Abstinence, condom
Papilloma	Cervix	Abstinence, condom
Endemic		
Hepatitis	Liver	Vaccination
Epstein-Barr	Burkitt's lymphoma, nasopharyngeal	?
Diet		
Fat	Endometrium, breast, prostate, colon	Decreased intake
Fiber	Colon, breast	Increased intake
Vitamins	Skin, liver, oropharynx, cervix, colon	Increased intake

as initiators, including viruses, physical agents, and chemicals.

A. Viruses: In animals, viruses are a causative agent for many cancers. In humans, viruses suspected to have etiologic roles for cancer include T cell lymphotropic virus, Epstein-Barr virus, human papillomavirus (HPV), and hepatitis virus. Associations, respectively, with T cell lymphoma and nasopharyngeal, cervical, and liver cancers have been convincingly demonstrated.

The cultural epidemiology of T cell lymphotropic virus and Epstein-Barr virus has not been sufficiently worked out that preventive intervention strategies can be proposed. In contrast, HPV subtypes 6, 8, 16, and 18 appear strongly associated with risk for cervical cancer, and this malignancy clearly belongs in the

Table 7–2. Major confirmed and avoidable risk factors for cancer formation in humans.

Factor	Associated Cancers	Prevention Strategy
Tobacco		
Cigarette	Lung, oropharyngeal, bladder, cervix	Abstention, cessation
Smokeless	Oral	Abstention, cessation
Radiation		
Ionizing	Lung, leukemia	Shielding
Nonionizing	Skin	Sun screens, "sun sense"
Chemicals		
Dyes	Bladder	Reduced exposure in workplace
Asbestos	Lung, mesothelium	Avoidance of contact, use of alternative building materials

realm of sexually transmitted diseases. Appropriate barrier contraception (condom) as a preventive strategy for prevention of cervical cancer is likely to block transmission of HPV, but direct proof for this assertion does not currently exist. Hepatitis virus presents a more complex problem, since the biologic agent is endemic in some societies (eg, Taiwanese, South African blacks) and is also transmissible through both sexual contact and intravenous routes. Additionally, aflatoxin B, a potent chemical mutagen that has a predilection for the liver, is found in fungi which contaminate foodstuffs. This potent carcinogen is thought to play a major cofactor role by damaging hepatocytes, which results in enhanced cellular proliferation and subsequent fixation of genetic damage caused by the virus. Several preventive strategies therefore appear relevant to control of liver cancer: a virus vaccine (being tested), altered cultural habits (barrier contraception, abstinence from shared needles, reduction of aflatoxin B in foodstuffs), and testing of blood products.

B. Radiation: A second major group of cancer-causing agents important in initiation include physical disturbances such as ionizing (x-rays) and non-ionizing (ultraviolet) radiation. Exposure to ultraviolet (UV) light largely occurs via outdoor contact with sunshine and is confined to the skin. Nevertheless, at high doses sunlight produces a generalized immunosuppression. The incidence of both non-melanoma and melanoma skin cancer worldwide has doubled in each of the last three decades and has risen more rapidly in sunny climates. Cutaneous malignant melanoma is in incidence the second fastest increasing cancer in the USA, where its rise is sharpest in the Southwest and West. The reasons for this change

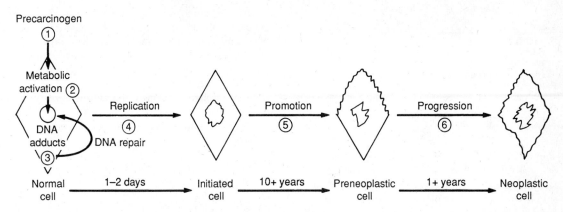

Figure 7–1. Steps in the induction of cancer. Loci for intervention. (Adapted, with permission, from Bertram JS, Kolonel LN, Meyskens FL Jr: Rationale and strategies for chemoprevention of cancer in humans. *Cancer Res* 1987;**47:**3012.)

probably are changing cultural habits and increased exposure to sunlight.

The UV light spectrum of sunlight is divided by length of waves into three major regions: UV-A (320–400 nm), UV-B (290–320 nm), and UV-C (<290 nm). UV-C is germicidal and highly mutagenic, but these shorter wavelengths of light are effectively filtered out by the ozone layer in the upper stratosphere. Although the role of ozone in blocking UV-C has been appreciated for some time, only recently has it been understood that manufactured fluorocarbons released to the atmosphere inactivate ozone via a simple chemical reaction. This depletion has been of sufficient magnitude to bring the ozone layer to dangerously low levels. Since the danger has been recognized, nearly all countries have agreed to stop the manufacture of these compounds. However, because fluorocarbons are integral to plastic manufacture and a phase-out period is required, the incidence of skin cancer is likely to rise at least until the year 2005. In addition, UV-B wavelengths are not completely filtered out by ozone, and exposure of the skin integument results in sunburn and tanning. The role of UV-A in producing skin damage and cancer is not completely clear, but these wavelengths probably

contribute to overall skin damage and cancer risk as well.

Prevention strategies that can be used to decrease overall exposure to sunlight are listed in Table 7–5. Gradual exposure to sunlight over short time periods and the use of sunscreens and sunblocks can help lower the incidence of skin cancers. These acculturations, however, involve long-term personal, cultural, and societal changes, and maintenance of these habits is difficult.

Significant exposure to ionizing radiation was until recently thought to be confined to diagnostic medical procedures, radiation accidents, and nuclear warfare. The amount of radiation exposure in diagnostic procedures has steadily fallen and is of minor concern if appropriate safeguards are followed. Radiation exposure in the medical workplace also has decreased markedly with appropriate shielding and precautions and improvement in equipment. The one group for which special vigilance is warranted is the pregnant female, since low exposure of the fetus to ionizing radiation results in a demonstrable increase in leukemia during childhood.

A recent issue of significance has been the identification of radon gas in many homes and its relation-

Table 7–4. Stages of tumor development (carcinogenesis).[1]

Stage	Time Duration	Genotype (DNA)	Phenotype	Common Examples	Reversibility
Initiation	Minutes	Abnormal	Normal	Cigarette smoke	?Molecular manipulations
Fixation	Days	Fixes damage	Normal	Necrosis with increased proliferation	?Delay proliferation
Promotion	Years	Abnormal	Abnormal, biochemical, histologic	Hormones, fats	Antipromoters
Progression	Months	Abnormal	Preneoplastic	?Viruses	Antipromoters/anti-proliferatives
Neoplasia	Weeks/months	Abnormal	Malignant		?Early differentiation or maturation agents

[1]Reproduced, with permission, from Meyskens FL Jr: Cancer prevention. In: *Current Therapy in Hematology-Oncology 3*. Brain MC, Carbone PP (editors). Decker, 1988.

Table 7–5. Methods for prevention of sunlight-induced cancers.

Reduce exposure
Cover up
Wear hat
Limit exposure between 10 AM and 3 PM
Prevent exposure
Use sunscreens
Use sunblocks

ship to lung cancer. Radioactive materials are found in most rocks, and without foundation shielding the level of radon gas in a home may rise to 100 times safe levels. Radon may offer an etiologic explanation for up to 20,000 cases yearly of lung cancer not associated with cigarette smoking, and it may also lower the carcinogenic threshold for tobacco. The control of residential radon has profound legal, economic, and public health implications, and effective strategies for managing the quality of indoor air have not been yet established.

C. Chemicals: The list of chemicals that have been associated with causation of various cancers is long. However, only a few of these compounds have a major role (Table 7–6), and most of these substances probably have their effect at the initiation stage of carcinogenesis. Aflatoxin, as a food contaminant, plays a major role in the development of liver cancer. Although uncommon in the USA, hepatoma is the second leading cause of death from cancer in the world. Aromatic amines have been directly linked to bladder cancer and account for at least half of the 50,000 cases diagnosed annually in the USA. Likewise, asbestos is an important carcinogen, contributing 10% of the risk for lung cancer and greater than 90% of the risk for mesothelioma, of which there were 3000 cases in the USA in 1988. Other chemicals that have been linked to cancer causation include benzene (bone marrow) and vinyl chloride (liver).

Promotion

After initiation and fixation of nucleotide changes in DNA have occurred, damage to the cell is generally regarded as irreversible. Whether future advances in genetic technology will allow correction of lesions in situ remains to be seen. The next major step in carcinogenesis is promotion. Cellular and tissue changes take years to unfold, and in experimental systems early and late stages have been identified. A progressive accumulation of phenotypic alterations occurs although generally no further genotypic changes are evident. Several common exogenous factors unequivocally play a role as promotion enhancers (Table 7–7). Less certain is the role of specific natural dietary factors (Table 7–3).

Established promoters of human cancer formation include alcohol, hormones, and drugs. Alcohol alone does not produce cancers in animal models, nor has an association been identified by epidemiologic investigations. However, alcohol is a potent cocarcinogen and markedly enhances cancer risk in the oropharyngeal cavity, larynx, and esophagus in association with smoking, and in the liver when associated with primary liver damage resulting from almost any cause.

Hormones are also potent promoters of cancer in individuals at risk. One of the most dramatic instances of promoter-enhanced cancers in humans was the "epidemic" of endometrial cancer that occurred in the late 1950s. It was traced to the use of unopposed estrogen (diethylstilbestrol, DES) in women for the management of osteoporosis. The incidence of this cancer promptly fell after this practice decreased. Older high-dose oral contraceptives produced benign liver tumors with fair regularity as well. Current contraceptives use lower doses of estrogen combined with progesterone, producing a more physiologic effect. Both these properties should obviate tumor development. Most worrisome is the currently popular use of anabolic steroids by athletes, since hepatomas

Table 7–6. Chemicals that are established major carcinogens in humans.

Agent	Exposure	Cancer
Aflatoxin	Foodstuffs (eg, cotton, milk)	Liver (hepatoma)
Aromatic amines (eg, benzidine)	Workplace (dyes)	Bladder (transitional cell carcinoma)
Asbestos	Workplace, buildings	Lung (squamous), pleura (mesothelioma)
Benzene	Workplace	Bone marrow (aplasia, leukemia)
Vinyl chloride	Workplace (plastics)	Liver (angiosarcoma)

Table 7–7. Established promoters of human cancer formation.

Agent	Exposure	Cancer
Alcohol	Social	Esophagus, larynx, oropharynx, liver
Estrogens	Medical	Endometrium, vagina[1]
Immunosuppressive drugs	Medical	All sites (especially marrow)
Overnutrition	Social	Breast, endometrium, gallbladder
Reproductive history[2]	Physiologic	Breast, ovary
Parasites	Environmental	
Clonorchis sinensis		Liver (cholangioma)
Schistosoma haematobium		Bladder (squamous carcinoma)
Steroids	Medical, cultural	
Anabolic		Liver
Contraceptive		Liver (benign hamartoma)

[1]Transplacental DES.
[2]Breast: late age at first pregnancy; ovary: zero or low parity.

are one of the many undesirable side effects of these drugs.

The role of dietary substances as modulators of cancer risk has been intensively discussed over the past few decades. A substantial number of epidemiologic studies support the notion that fat, fiber, vitamins, and micronutrients play a role in the expression of cancer risk. Likewise, laboratory investigations have shown that these substances can affect carcinogenesis.

The role of dietary fat intake remains hotly debated, and whether the effect is due to "calories" or fat has not been determined. Nevertheless, increased fat intake has been associated with increased risk for breast, colon, endometrial, and prostate cancers.

Ingestion of fiber is protective against colon cancer, although the type of fiber appears important. This protection probably is afforded through a combination of decreased transit time of stool, complexing with bile acids (potential mutagens), and absorption of harmful fat and lipid substances.

Vitamins A and C, β-carotene, and selenium probably have a strong protective effect against certain malignancies, particularly in combination.

Preneoplasia & Progression

Conventionally the premalignant state is regarded as synonymous with histologic alterations identified at the clinical or light microscopic level. With newer understanding of the process of carcinogenesis, this point of transition has become more nebulous. Nevertheless, changes that are clinically and microscopically identifiable and result in measurable lesions provide a useful point of reference for study. In most human tissues, a preneoplastic precursor has been identified. Some of the better known conditions include actinic keratoses (skin), leukoplakia (oropharyngeal cavity), dysplasia (cervix), and polyps (colon). Little is known about what changes occur as preneoplastic tissue progresses to neoplasia, nor are the factors that enhance this transition well understood. Good model systems are unavailable, and

there has been a lack of interest among investigators in this important step in tumor formation.

The observations about progression of preneoplasia that have been made in animal model systems include the following: (1) many of the same factors affect initiation, (2) new genetic changes occur and accumulate, (3) spontaneous regressions occur, and (4) progression is infrequent. Clinical study of preneoplastic conditions has been recorded for quite some time.

Two major themes emanate from these clinical observations. (1) The process by which different tissues evolve from normal to neoplastic varies among organs. An examination of this process in the gastrointestinal tract is instructive (Figure 7–2). (2) The process of preneoplastic evolution and the factors that affect progression are complex. Cervical dysplasia provides an excellent example (Figure 7–3).

The evolution from normal to neoplastic tissue in the gastrointestinal tract seems to occur via several different pathways although a common end pathway is followed. The initial damage in the esophagus occurs from reflux of acid from the stomach with inflammation being a prominent early change. In the stomach, the initial damage also appears to be inflammation, but before further progression an atrophic state frequently occurs.

Subsequently in the esophagus in some cases, the stratified squamous epithelium undergoes transition (or metaplasia) to a columnar epithelium. In contrast, the stomach uniformly evolves to precursor lesions via the native columnar epithelial pathway. Early events in the colon appear quite different from those in the esophagus and stomach, since hyperplasia or polyps are the initial abnormality.

These three pathways (stomach, colon, esophagus) likely represent fundamentally different strategies in the early event of preneoplastic lesions. In contrast, metaplasia in the esophagus, abnormal stomach columnar epithelium, and polyps in the colon all seem to later evolve through a dysplastic step before frank carcinoma appears.

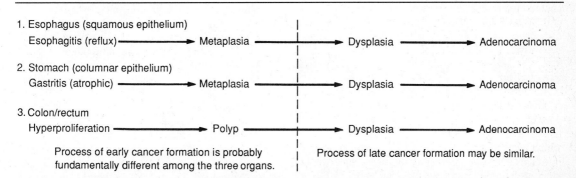

Figure 7–2. Evolution of preneoplastic lesions of the gastrointestinal tract into cancer.

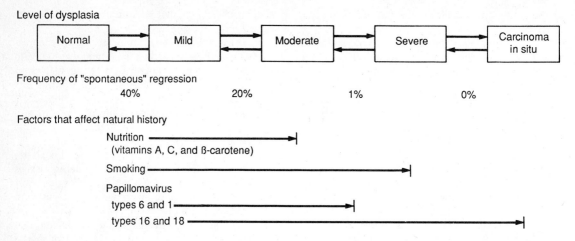

Figure 7–3. The natural history of cervical dysplasia, and factors affecting this process. Progression is complex, eg, in the cervix the transition from mild to moderate to severe dysplasia is not inevitable and a real spontaneous remission rate is evident, which decreases in frequency as the lesion progresses. Both human papillomavirus and mutagenic products from tobacco (eg, cigarette smoking) play a role in progression. Inflammation, other viruses, and nutrition are likely also involved. (Reproduced, with permission, from Meyskens FL Jr: Strategies for prevention of cancer in humans. *Oncology* 1992;**6(2 Suppl):**1.)

Early Neoplasia

The exact point at which a preneoplastic lesion becomes neoplastic is hard to define. Nevertheless, preneoplastic tissue becomes functionally neoplastic when cells are locally invasive or produce metastatic deposits. This transition stage is accompanied by a series of changes in which the tumor cells become less responsive to both host immunologic and tissue and cell regulation. Additionally, the cells gradually accumulate genetic alterations and acquire an independent biologic mandate.

INTERVENTION STRATEGIES

An understanding of cancer etiology and its biologic evolution into progressively more malignant states provides a rational approach to prevention. The management of cancer spans the therapeutic continuum from simple applied prevention to aggressive chemotherapy. For the most part, the major medical emphasis to date has been on the treatment of late cancer, and the early management of cancer has not been systematically approached.

Prevention

A. Primary: Advances in molecular biology have clearly identified deletions of genetic material as important in the initiation of cancer. The best studied of these conditions is hereditary retinoblastoma, in which a portion of chromosome 13p is constitutively lost. This deletion abnormality has been corrected in vitro by the delivery of the gene via retroviral vectors. Since deletions are being identified as a critical

early change in many common cancers (eg, colon cancer), refinement of delivery technology of genes for in vivo use is an important goal. This type of approach will probably play a major role in the control of cancer in the future.

Whether subtle constitutive changes exist in individual nucleotides of certain genes in individuals at high risk for a cancer will be important to determine. With the identification of specific genes closely related to various cancers, exploration of this goal will be both important and attainable. For example, if constitutive changes are known to exist in an individual's genes that raise the risk considerably for a particular type of cancer, screening and early detection as well as health promotion advice could be directed toward that organ in that individual.

The application of conventional primary prevention strategies can have an enormous impact on cancer incidence. Most prominent among these are elimination of smoking and use of sunscreens. The effect of inhibitors of initiation (anti-initiators) is being actively investigated as well. Examples include β-carotene, vitamin E, selenium, soybean extract (protease inhibitors), and a wide range of antioxidants.

B. Secondary: Once genetic change has occurred and been fixed, a cell is irreversibly initiated. Secondary prevention management is therefore directed toward decreasing exposure to promoters (eg, aniline dyes, hormones, and fat), providing substances (eg, fiber) that reduce exposure to promoters, and improving the milieu in which the tissue is found so that proliferation is suppressed or differentiation enhanced (eg, ensure adequate vitamin intake).

C. Tertiary: Once phenotypic alterations have re-

Table 7–8. The therapeutic continuum and cancer prevention.[1]

Type of Management	State of Cell	Strategy	Example	Intervention
Prevention				
Primary	Constitutive abnormality Normal	Correct genetic defect Prevent exposure to carcinogen	Retinoblastoma	Molecular correction by gene replacement
		Proscriptive	Lung cancer Oral cancer	Elimination of tobacco products Sunscreens
		Prescriptive	Skin cancer (melanoma, non-melanoma)	Anti-initiators (eg, β-carotene, protease inhibitors)
Secondary	Genotypic damage (initiated)	Prevent phenotypic changes Remove promoters		
		Chemical	Bladder cancer	Removal of aniline dyes
		Hormones	Endometrial cancer	No use of DES
		Nutrients	Breast cancer	Less fat in diet
		Improve host milieu	Skin, lung, cervix, stomach cancer	Adequate intake of vitamins A, C, E Selenium intake
			Colon cancer	Fiber supplements
Tertiary	Phenotypic changes (preneoplasia)	Reverse or suppress preneoplasia	Oral or cervical leukoplakia	Retinoids, β-carotene
Treatment				
Early	Neoplasia			
	Host	Improve immune status	Colon cancer	Levamisole
	Tumor cell	Differentiate or mature the cancer	Neuroblastoma Melanoma	Retinoids, polyamine synthesis inhibitors
Late	Cancer	Kill tumor	Most cancers	Chemotherapy, biologic therapy, radiation

[1]Reproduced, with permission, from Meyskens FL Jr: Cancer prevention. In: *Current Therapy in Hematology-Oncology 3.* Brain MC, Carbone PP (editors). Decker, 1988.

sulted in histologic changes, clinical lesions can be identified and followed. Some common preneoplastic lesions and their management are outlined in Table 7–8. Surgery or ablation has been used most frequently for the management of these conditions. These approaches are not always feasible, and lesions frequently recur even after removal. Secondary intervention such as improving the nutritional environment should also play a beneficial role. Investigations are being performed to determine whether active intervention with antiproliferative or differentiating agents can reverse preneoplasia or inhibit preneoplastic progression to malignancy.

Cells and tissue making the transition from preneoplastic to neoplastic status should be an active target for intervention. This stage has been little studied, but advances in understanding of host-tumor interactions should allow rapid progress in this area. Likewise, certain malignancies in vitro and in animals appear peculiarly sensitive to differentiating agents. For example, human neuroblastoma cells in vitro terminally differentiate and mature in the presence of retinoic acid. Whether this change will occur in vivo has not yet been tested. Further understanding of such phenomena may allow highly targeted and benign therapy of certain cancers.

Behavioral Modification

A major limitation to the application of prevention strategies is that many of the interventions involve changes in personal, cultural, or social prerogatives. Effecting changes in diet, recreational alternatives, or sexual practices has not been in general part of medical education or practice. Nevertheless, the physician will need to be increasingly familiar with these issues as the practice of medicine becomes broader in its participation in the concerns of society. As leader of

Table 7–9. Smoking cessation for the busy clinician.[1]

1. Act as a role model by not smoking.
2. Use clinical opportunities to talk about smoking (eg, symptoms: cough, sputum production); tests: pulmonary function test, blood lipids; diagnosis of disease: chronic bronchitis, coronary heart disease).
3. Provide information on risks associated with smoking and reduction of risk if the patient stops.
4. Encourage abstinence by direct advice and suggestions.
5. Follow up on use of specific cessation and maintenance strategies (ie, treat smoking as a medical problem and cessation as the prescribed treatment).

[1]A complete guide is available in NIH Publication No. 86-2178: Clinical opportunities for smoking intervention: A guide for the busy physician (1986).

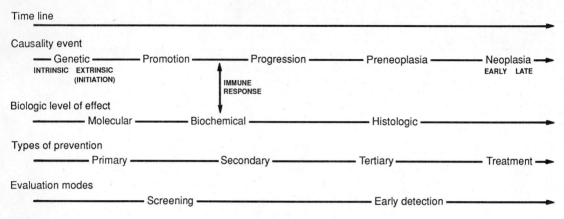

Figure 7–4. Cancer causality and the prevention of early cancer. (Reproduced, with permission, from Meyskens FL Jr: Thinking about cancer causality and chemoprevention. *JNCI* 1988;**80**:1278.)

the health care team, the physician will be increasingly called upon as a role model.

An area in which the physician should be highly knowledgeable is that of smoking prevention and cessation. Although the application of strategies to prevent smoking largely lie in the political arena, the techniques necessary to implement smoking cessation in patients (and their families) is a proper (and should be an integral) part of the physician's repertoire. Essential elements of a smoking cessation program are outlined in Table 7–9.

Avoidable Mortality

Most morbidity and mortality due to cancer is preventable (Tables 7–1 and 7–2). Conservative estimates are that cessation of cigarette smoking would decrease incidence of the following cancers: lung (75%), oropharyngeal (50%), bladder (25%), cervix (20%). Overall, cessation of cigarette smoking would lead to a 30% decrease (about 200,000 deaths) in mortality from cancer in the USA. Other large contributors to cancer incidence and mortality include radon (10–20% of lung cancers), aniline dyes (50% of bladder cancers), and asbestos (10% of lung cancers, 90% of mesotheliomas). Exposure to sunlight is a habit that can be modified and produce perhaps a

50% decrease in melanoma incidence and mortality. Virus exposure potentially represents a preventable cause of cancer, particularly for cervix and liver cancers.

The role of dietary modification in cancer prevention may be significant. An examination of incidence data of various cancers in different countries and comparison with dietary intake suggests that 30–50% of cancer risk is closely associated to diet. In particular, dietary intake seems to play an important contributory role in breast, colon, and prostate cancer development. Perhaps as much as 50% of the risk for these diseases can be explained by dietary interactions.

Synthetic Approach

Prevention is a strategy used to block the development of cancer. Necessarily, the approach draws its rationale from a multitude of disciplines. Figure 7–4 relates different aspects of early cancer development and proposed management. The process can be viewed at four levels: causal event, biologic effect, type of prevention, and evaluation mode. As our understanding of the genetics of cancer increases, individuals at high risk for common cancers will be identified. Such knowledge should lead to intervention and prevention of cancers.

REFERENCES

Atiba JO, Meyskens FL Jr: Chemoprevention of breast cancer. *Semin Oncol,* 1992;**19**:220.

Baquet CR et al: Socioeconomic factors and cancer incidence among blacks and whites. *JNCI* 1991;**83**:551.

Bertram JS, Kolonel LN, Meyskens FL Jr: Rationale and strategies for chemoprevention of cancer in humans. *Cancer Res* 1987;**47**:3012.

Clinical opportunities for smoking intervention: A guide for the busy physician. NIH Publication No. 86-2178,1986.

Doll R: The causes of cancer. *JNCI* 1981;**66**:1197.

Greenwald P: The new emphasis in cancer control. *JNCI* 1985;**74**:543.

Greenwald P, Cullen JW, Weed D: Cancer prevention and control. *Semin Oncol* 1990;**17**:383.

Lippman SM, Bassford TL, Meyskens FL Jr: A quantitatively scored cancer-risk assessment tool: Its development and use. *J Cancer Ed* 1992;**7**:15.

Lippman SM, Kessler J, Meyskens FL Jr: Retinoids as preventive and therapeutic anticancer agents. *Cancer Treat Rep* 1987;**71**:391.

Lippman SM et al: Biomarkers as intermediate endpoints in chemoprevention trials. *JNCI* 1990;**82**:555.

Meyskens FL Jr: Cancer causality and the prevention of early cancer: Thinking about cancer causality and chemoprevention. *JNCI* 1988;**80**:1278.

Meyskens FL Jr: Strategies for prevention of cancer in humans. *Oncology* 1992;**6(2 Suppl)**:1.

Trock B, Lanza E, Greenwald P: Dietary fiber, vegetables, and colon cancer: Critical review and meta-analyses of the epidemiologic evidence. *JNCI* 1990;**82**:650.

Wattenberg LW: Chemoprevention of cancer. *Cancer Res* 1985;**45**:1.

Wattenberg LW: Inhibition of carcinogenesis by minor dietary constituents. *Cancer Res* 1992;**52(7 Suppl)**:2085s.

8

Nutritional Care

Thomas C. Hardin, PharmD, & Carey P. Page, MD

Over the past decade, an interest in the relationship between nutrition and cancer has led to a significant body of information. There is little doubt that the presence of cancer and the treatment of cancer can adversely affect nutritional status. In addition, malnutrition has been implicated as adversely affecting response to therapy and quality of life of the cancer patient. Faced with this cycle of cancer-associated malnutrition, the clinician often turns to aggressive nutritional care of the cancer patient in hope of reversing the malnutrition and improving the patient's clinical status. This chapter reviews current understanding of cancer cachexia, the process of nutritional assessment, the delivery of enteral and parenteral nutrition support to cancer patients, and the evidence to support such therapy.

WEIGHT LOSS & CANCER CACHEXIA

Weight loss is a common finding among cancer patients. The frequency and extent of weight loss are variable and considered to be dependent on the type of malignancy and stage of the disease. For example, significant weight loss (>10% in the previous 6 months) has been reported at diagnosis in 25–30% of patients with gastric or pancreatic carcinoma and in only 5–10% of patients with breast cancer or leukemia. Pretreatment weight loss has been associated with a poorer response to chemotherapy in patients with breast cancer and a shorter survival in patients with colon cancer, prostate cancer, and non-Hodgkin's lymphoma. While the mechanisms responsible for these observed relationships are unclear, depletion of visceral and somatic proteins that are important for the maintenance of immunocompetence has been proposed. Moreover, malnutrition can contribute to delayed wound healing, increased infections, reduced tolerance to chemotherapy, increased postoperative complications, and prolonged hospitalization in some patients.

Cancer cachexia refers to a complex syndrome consisting of anorexia, asthenia, tissue wasting, biochemical abnormalities, and impaired organ function. The incidence and severity of cancer cachexia do not clearly correlate with the size, site, extent, stage, or cell type of the malignancy. Cancer cachexia may be directly related to the malignancy, since reversal has been described in animal models and in patients following tumor removal. A number of mediators of cancer cachexia, such as cachectin (tumor necrosis factor, TNF), have been suggested, but the mechanism of the syndrome remains uncertain. Table 8–1 lists several factors that may contribute to weight loss and malnutrition in cancer patients.

Decreased appetite and nutrient intake are frequent observations. Cancers that involve the cephalad portion of the gastrointestinal tract (oral cavity, neck, esophagus, stomach) may mechanically impair the patient's ability to eat. Depression and hopelessness associated with either a confirmed or a suspected diagnosis of cancer may result in the loss of appetite. Alterations in taste perception, such as a decreased threshold for salty and sour flavors, an increased threshold for sweets, and an aversion to meat proteins have been reported. In addition to problems of inadequate nutrient intake, observed alterations in the host metabolism of carbohydrates, lipids, and proteins are considered to be major factors in the development of cancer cachexia (Table 8–2).

NUTRIENT REQUIREMENTS

In general, the provision of appropriate amounts of energy, nitrogen, and micronutrients is essential for efficacious nutrition support. Nutritional care of the oncology patient requires an understanding of each patient's needs as altered by both the cancer and other disease processes.

Energy
The degree of weight loss and malnutrition seen in cancer patients is frequently greater than can be explained on the basis of a reduction in nutrient intake alone. This observation may indicate that the presence of a malignancy leads to increased energy requirements. Using the technique of indirect calorimetry, several investigators have assessed energy expenditure in patients with a variety of malignant conditions. Most hospitalized cancer patients usually manifest either normal or low resting energy require-

Table 8–1. Factors that may contribute to malnutrition in patients with cancer.

Mechanical impairment of nutrient ingestion
Aversion to food
Taste abnormalities
Altered visceral sensing (eg, early satiety)
Metabolic and hormonal abnormalities
Surgical therapy or procedures
Chemotherapy
Radiation therapy
Nutritional demands of the tumor
Paraneoplastic syndromes

ments, but the range of requirements is broad. Indeed, the resting energy expenditures measured in cancer patients vary from 50% to 175% of that predicted by formulas based on body surface area (Table 8–3). In addition, the energy requirements for patients with cancer are dynamic and reflect changes in the disease, treatment modalities, and associated morbidity (fever, sepsis, surgery). For these reasons, measurement of resting energy expenditures (REE) by indirect calorimetry is desirable to identify the patient's energy (caloric) requirements. When indirect calorimetry is unavailable, the Harris-Benedict equation can be used to estimate basal energy expenditure (BEE):

Males: BEE = 66 + (13.7 × wt) + (5 × ht) – (6.8 × age)
Females: BEE = 655 + (9.6 × wt) + (1.7 × ht) – (4.7 × age)
(where wt = weight (kg), ht = height (cm), age is expressed in years.)

REE is then estimated by adding a "factor" for the disease process.

If nutritional maintenance is the goal, 110–130%

Table 8–2. Abnormal host metabolism in cancer cachexia.[1]

Carbohydrate metabolism
  Glucose intolerance
  Insulin resistance
  Reduced insulin secretion
  Hepatic gluconeogenesis
  Aerobic glycolysis
  Increased glucose turnover
Lipid metabolism
  Hyperlipidemia
  Depletion of lipid stores
  Increased free fatty acids, glycerol turnover
  Increased lipolysis
  Decreased lipogenesis
  Decreased serum lipoprotein lipase activity
Protein metabolism
  Increased protein turnover
  Elevated rates of protein mobilization
  Decrease in peripheral protein synthesis
  Increase in muscle protein breakdown
  Increase in hepatic protein synthesis

[1]Adapted, with permission, from Kern KA, Norton JA: Cancer cachexia. *JPEN* 1988;**12**:286.

of the estimated or measured REE should be provided. If nutritional repletion is desired, up to 150% of the REE is appropriate. An alternative to the above guidelines is the provision of 25–40 kcal/kg/d, based on the patient's clinical status, activity level, and the goal of nutritional therapy. A patient rarely will require greater than 40 kcal/kg/d to meet energy needs.

Protein

Protein requirements for cancer patients are difficult to determine. In addition, concern regarding possible stimulatory or inhibitory effects of dietary protein on tumor growth has been raised. Nevertheless, at this time there appears to be no reason to limit the amount of protein (nitrogen) administered to cancer patients. On the other hand, many believe that more aggressive delivery of nitrogen substrates to cancer patients is appropriate based on the frequent findings of stress, sepsis, and hypoalbuminemia in these patients. Current accepted recommendations are for cancer patients requiring nutritional support to receive 1.5–2 g of protein/kg/d (0.25–0.35 g of nitrogen/kg/d). When evaluated on the basis of the NPC:N ratio (nonprotein calories to grams of nitrogen), a range of 100–150:1 is often recommended.

Vitamins, Minerals, & Trace Elements

While the nutritional value of vitamins, minerals, and trace elements is widely recognized, the optimal daily dose required to preserve nutritional status in cancer patients is unknown. In the absence of specific data defining the micronutrient needs of cancer patients, the clinician must apply the general recommendations for normal adults. Table 8–4 outlines the recommended daily dietary allowances (RDA) for vitamins, minerals and trace elements for adult men and women. These recommendations are based on maintenance of nutritional status, and any known deficits should be replaced in addition to these quantities. The cancer patient also may be at risk for potential drug-nutrient interactions resulting from chemotherapy or supportive adjunct drug therapy (Table 8–5).

NUTRITIONAL ASSESSMENT

Traditionally, the nutritional assessment process has incorporated information obtained through patient histories (medical, drug, dietary), physical examination, anthropometric measurements (weight, triceps skinfold thickness, mid-arm muscle circumference, creatinine-height index), laboratory tests (albumin, transferrin, nitrogen balance), and assessment of immunocompetence. Most of these techniques lack appropriate sensitivity and specificity and have not been shown to be superior to a careful clinical evaluation. In fact, a subjective global assessment (SGA) (Table 8–6) has been reported to be a better

Table 8–3. Metabolic status of selected cancer patients (percentage).[1]

Tumor Type	n	Hypometabolic (REE[2] < 90% PEE[3])	Normometabolic (REE = 90–110% PEE)	Hypermetabolic (REE > 110% PEE)
Colorectal	73	27	51	22
Other gastrointestinal	100	42	35	23
Lung	31	0	100	0
Mixed	200	33	41	26

[1]Adapted, with permission, from Dempsey DT, Mullen JL: Macronutrient requirements in the malnourished cancer patient: How much of what and why? *Cancer* 1985;**55**:290.
[2]REE = Resting energy expenditure as determined by indirect calorimetry.
[3]PEE = Predicted energy expenditure as estimated using Harris-Benedict equation.

predictor of patients at risk for nutrition-associated postoperative complications than traditional nutritional assessment methods and the prognostic nutritional index developed for surgical patients. While the SGA has not been evaluated in cancer patients for predictive value, it does offer an easy, economical, and valid means of assessing nutritional status clinically, especially when combined with an assessment of the patient's serum albumin concentration. Relying on information obtained from a thorough history and physical examination, the clinician subjectively classifies the patient's nutritional status as one of three general levels. Those patients determined to be severely malnourished are considered to be in greatest need of aggressive nutritional support.

Table 8–4. Recommended dietary allowances (RDA) for micronutrients.[1]

	Adult Males	Adult Females
Vitamins		
A (retinol)	1000 µg	800 µg
B$_1$ (thiamin)	1.4 mg	1.1 mg
B$_2$ (riboflavin)	1.6 mg	1.3 mg
B$_6$ (pyridoxine)	2.2 mg	2.0 mg
B$_{12}$ (cyanocobalamin)	3 µg	3 µg
C (ascorbic acid)	60 mg	60 mg
D (cholecalciferol)	200 IU	200 IU
E (alpha-tocopherol)	10 mg	8 mg
K (phylloquinone)	70–140 µg	70–140 µg
Biotin	100–200 µg	100–200 µg
Folic acid	400 µg	400 µg
Niacin	18 mg	13 mg
Pantothenic acid	4–7 mg	4–7 mg
Minerals		
Calcium	800 mg	800 mg
Iron	10 mg	18 mg
Magnesium	350 mg	300 mg
Phosphorus	800 mg	800 mg
Trace elements		
Chromium	0.05–0.2 mg	0.05–0.2 mg
Copper	2–3 mg	2–3 mg
Iodine	150 µg	150 µg
Manganese	2.5–5.0 mg	2.5–5.0 mg
Molybdenum	0.15–0.50 mg	0.15–0.50 mg
Selenium	0.05–0.2 mg	0.05–0.2 mg
Zinc	15 mg	15 mg

[1]Adapted from *Recommended Dietary Allowances,* 9th ed. Food and Nutrition Board, National Research Council, National Academy of Sciences, 1980.

CLINICAL APPROACHES TO NUTRITIONAL CARE

The physician should make a deliberate decision regarding the nutritional care to be prescribed for each cancer patient. Occasionally, the decision is easy because the patient is not initially malnourished and is able to eat. Frequently, however, the patient manifests preexisting malnutrition, a nonfunctional gastrointestinal tract, or both. In these circumstances, the clinical approach must meet the patient's individual needs. Figure 8–1 provides a proposed algorithmic guide to assist in selecting the patient's nutritional management.

Oral Nutrition

Many factors can lead to a reduction in oral nutrient intake with resulting weight loss (Table 8–1). Careful consideration in diet planning paid to any taste changes or preferences, unusual cravings, or aversions to certain foods along with creative assistance from dietary support services can improve oral nutrient intake in some patients. Others may require the use of adjunctive medications. Tricyclic antidepressants can reduce anorexia caused by depression, cyproheptadine is an appetite stimulant in some patients, and megestrol acetate has been reported to cause weight gain and appetite enhancement when given in high doses. Radiation therapy or chemotherapy may result in difficulty with chewing or painful swallowing secondary to stomatitis, mucositis, or associated fungal infections (thrush). Use of topical agents, such as antacids, diphenhydramine elixir,

Table 8–5. Potential drug-nutrient interactions in oncology patients.

Prolonged antibiotic therapy	Depletion to vitamin K–producing intestinal flora
Sulfonamides, methotrexate (other antifolate compounds)	Interference with folate metabolism
Fluorouracil	Thiamin deficiency
Cisplatin	Enhanced renal loss of magnesium
Amphotericin B	Enhanced renal loss of potassium and magnesium

Table 8–6. Components of the subjective global assessment (SGA).[1]

History
  Weight change over time
  Change in dietary intake relative to normal
  Presence of gastrointestinal symptoms for over 2 weeks
  Change in functional capacity
  Concurrent diseases or stress
Physical examination
  Evidence of loss of subcutaneous fat stores
  Evidence of muscle wasting
  Presence of ascites
  Presence of ankle or sacral edema
Diagnostic categories
  Well nourished
  Minimally malnourished
  Severely malnourished

[1]Abstracted, with permission, from Detsky AS et al: What is subjective global assessment of nutritional status? *JPEN* 1987;**11**:8.

clotrimazole, or nystatin, may improve these conditions. When food alone is insufficient to meet the patient's nutrient requirements, commercially available oral supplements may be used.

Enteral Tube Feedings

When the patient is unwilling or unable to eat or drink a nutritionally adequate diet and the gastrointestinal tract is functional, the clinician should consider enteral tube feedings. Small-bore feeding catheters have significantly reduced the high incidence of nasopharyngeal irritation and gastroesophageal reflux formerly associated with the use of larger tubes. In addition, longer tubes with a weighted end may allow for delivery of feeding formula via the small bowel rather than the stomach, further reducing the risk of aspiration. For long-term enteral feedings, consider a feeding gastrostomy or jejunostomy. The gastrostomy should ideally be by the Janeway (mucosa-lined tube) technique. Jejunostomy is particularly valuable when performed as an adjunct to a major abdominal operation.

The spectrum and number of acceptable, commercially available enteral feeding formulas make the choice between these products more often a function of formulary restrictions or financial concern than of which is "best." In general, the **monomeric** (elemental) formulations are characterized by being lactose-free and low-residue, and the nutrients are readily available with little or no digestion. Nitrogen is provided as dipeptides and tripeptides or crystalline amino acids; carbohydrate as glucose oligosaccharides, maltodextrins, or cornstarch; and fat as safflower or sunflower oil (for essential fatty acid requirements) and medium-chain triglycerides (MCT) (for energy). Many of these products are hyperosmolar and unpalatable. They are most often used as tube feedings. The **polymeric** liquid formula diets are of variable residue, and most are lactose-free. Intact pro-

tein derived from protein hydrolysates is the nitrogen source. Fat is from vegetable oil or MCT oil and represents a larger percent of calories, while the carbohydrate sources are complex sugars and starches. The higher fat content and more complex protein and carbohydrate components render these products more nearly isotonic. Many have added sucrose or fructose to make them taste sweeter and, therefore, are useful as oral supplements as well as tube feedings. Tables 8–7 and 8–8 provide a summary overview of selected products.

When the feeding formula is to be delivered into the stomach, concern about the osmolality of the product is rarely important and dilution is unnecessary unless it is to provide additional hydration to the patient. Initiation at a continuous rate of 25 mL/h with gradual titration to the desired flow rate to deliver the patient's nutrient needs over the next 24–48 hours is suggested. An alternative is periodic bolus administration of not more than 400 mL of formula with careful assessment of gastric residuals before further administration. Greater than 100 mL of residual gastric contents may signify problems with gastric emptying.

When the feeding is to be delivered into the intestines via a weighted feeding tube or invasively placed enterostomy, osmolality of the product becomes more important. While it is often unnecessary to dilute formulas with osmolalities of less than 450 mosm/kg H_2O, initial dilution of these products may be helpful in some cases. For intestinal delivery, the rate of administration becomes a more important concern. Initiation of the feeding at 25 mL/h with gradual increases in the administration rate as tolerated by the patient is recommended. Once the desired flow rate is achieved, the formula concentration can be increased to full strength if necessary. At times the intolerance to enteral feedings is associated with the content of the formula. A change to a more elemental formula or one with a lower content of fat or one characterized by the presence of dipeptides and tripeptides may lead to improved tolerance. If these efforts fail to improve tolerance and reduce diarrhea, the use of antidiarrheals (eg, loperamide, diphenoxylate/atropine, tincture of opium, psyllium) may be necessary.

Parenteral Nutrition

When the cancer patient is unable to rely on the gastrointestinal tract to meet nutritional needs, parenteral nutritional support should be considered, especially if the patient has preexisting nutritional deficits or if the gut will not be functional for 10–14 days in the normally nourished patient. The decision either to use peripheral vein access or to place a central venous catheter is based on several factors: availability of peripheral veins, expected duration of parenteral nutritional support, goals of nutritional care, and consideration of potential associated complications. If parenteral nutrition is expected to be prolonged (>2

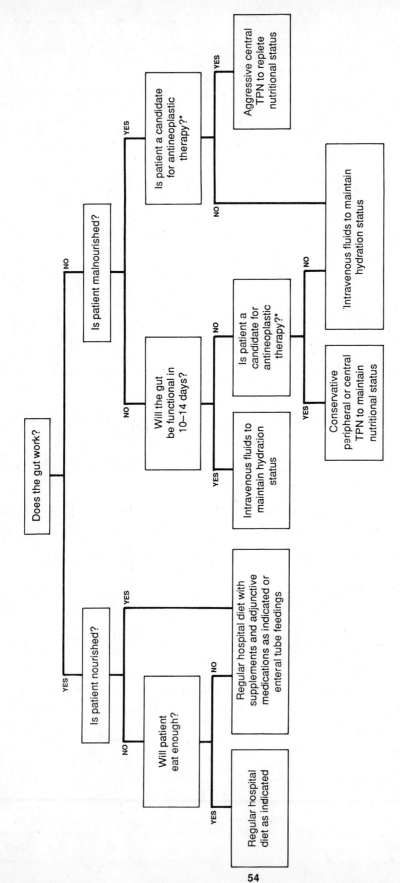

Figure 8–1. Algorithmic guide for nutritional support. *Is effective chemotherapy, surgery, or radiation therapy available?

Does the gut work?

YES — Is patient nourished?
NO — Is patient malnourished?

Is patient nourished?
- NO — Will patient eat enough?
- YES — Regular hospital diet with supplements and adjunctive medications as indicated or enteral tube feedings

Will patient eat enough?
- YES — Regular hospital diet as indicated
- NO — Regular hospital diet with supplements and adjunctive medications as indicated or enteral tube feedings

Is patient malnourished?
- NO — Will the gut be functional in 10–14 days?
- YES — Is patient a candidate for antineoplastic therapy?*

Will the gut be functional in 10–14 days?
- YES — Intravenous fluids to maintain hydration status
- NO — Is patient a candidate for antineoplastic therapy?*

Is patient a candidate for antineoplastic therapy?* (middle)
- YES — Conservative peripheral or central TPN to maintain nutritional status
- NO — Intravenous fluids to maintain hydration status

Is patient a candidate for antineoplastic therapy?* (right)
- YES — Aggressive central TPN to replete nutritional status
- NO — Intravenous fluids to maintain hydration status

Table 8–7. Selected monomeric (elemental) defined-formula feeding products.

Product (Manufacturer)	Caloric Density	Protein (% kcal)	Carbohydrate (% kcal)	Fat (% kcal)	mosm/kg	NPC:N Ratio	Carbohydrate Source	Fat Source	Protein Source
Vivonex TEN Powder (Norwich Eaton)	1.0	15	82	2.5	630	149:1	Maltodextrins	Safflower oil	L-Amino acids (33% BCAA)
Vital High Nitrogen Powder (Ross)	1.0	17	74	9	460	125:1	Sucrose and hydrolyzed cornstarch	45% MCT oil and 55% safflower oil	Protein hydrolysates and amino acids
Criticare HN Liquid (Mead-Johnson Nutritionals)	1.1	14	83	3	650	149:1	Maltodextrins, cornstarch	Safflower oil	Casein hydrolysates, peptides, and amino acids
Travasorb HN Powder (Clintec Nutrition)	1.0	18	70	12	560	114:1	Glucose oligosaccharides	40% MCT oil and 60% sunflower oil	Lactalbumin
Alitraq (Ross)	1.0	21	66	13	575	95:1	Cornstarch, sucrose	MCT oil, safflower oil	Amino acids, peptides

Table 8–8. Selected polymeric defined-formula feeding products.

Product (Manufacturer)	Caloric Density	Protein (% kcal)	Carbohydrate (% kcal)	Fat (% kcal)	mosm/kg	NPC:N Ratio	Carbohydrate Source	Fat Source	Protein Source
Osmolite Liquid (Ross)	1.1	14	55	31	300	153:1	Hydrolyzed cornstarch	50% MCT oil and 50% corn and soy oil	Caseinate salts and soy protein
Isocal Liquid (Mead Johnson Nutritionals)	1.1	13	50	37	300	167:1	Maltodextrin	20% MCT oil and 80% soy oil	Caseinate salts and soy protein
Precision LR Diet Powder (Sandoz Nutrition)	1.1	10	89	1	530	239:1	Maltodextrin and sucrose	Soy oil	Egg albumin
Ensure Plus Liquid (Ross)	1.5	15	53	32	600	146:1	Corn syrup and sucrose	Corn oil	Caseinate salts
Sustacal HC Liquid (Mead Johnson Nutritionals)	1.5	16	50	34	640	134:1	Corn syrup and sucrose	Soy oil	Caseinate salts
Magnacal Liquid (Sherwood)	2.0	14	50	36	590	154:1	Maltodextrin and sucrose	Soy oil	Caseinate salts
Enrich Liquid with fiber (Ross)	1.1	14.5	55	30.5	480	148:1	Hydrolyzed cornstarch, sucrose, and soy polysaccharide	Corn oil	Caseinate salts and soy protein (fiber-enriched)
Impact (Sandoz)	1.0	22	53	25	375	71:1	Hydrolyzed cornstarch	Structured lipid and refined menhaden oil	Caseinate salts, dietary nucleotides and arginine

weeks), if repletion of significant nutritional deficits is necessary, or if the patient has poor peripheral vein status, the technique of central total parenteral nutrition (TPN) is desirable.

Peripheral administration of nutrients necessary to meet the needs of most patients became possible with the introduction of lipid emulsions suitable for intravenous use. Since these products are isotonic, combination with crystalline amino acids and limited amounts of dextrose yielded admixtures with osmolalities near 900 mosm/kg (depending on electrolyte content) (Table 8–9). These formulations do not require a central venous route of administration. Rotation of the peripheral intravenous site every 48–72 hours is recommended to avoid associated phlebitis.

The choice to use central venous access for parenteral nutritional support is often based on availability of central venous access, desire to use carbohydrate (dextrose) as the primary nonprotein caloric source, necessity to limit the volume administered to the patient (a higher caloric density can be achieved by use of dextrose as the primary caloric source), or lack of suitable peripheral vein access. Traditionally, central TPN utilized hypertonic dextrose and crystalline amino acid solutions to deliver sufficient calories and nitrogen to meet the estimated patient requirements. Often, the amount of dextrose administered exceeded the oxidative capacity of the patient (5–7 mg dextrose/kg/min), thus leading to storage of these "extra" calories in such organs as the liver (hepatic steatosis). Moreover, glucose intolerance was occasionally observed, suggesting that administration of large quantities of dextrose was suboptimal. The last 5 years have seen acceptance of the daily use of lipid emulsions as a caloric source in patients receiving central TPN. By providing a more balanced nonprotein caloric profile (20–50% of total calories as lipid), some problems of cancer-associated glucose intolerance and insulin resistance may be avoided. Most cancer patients tolerate these admixtures well. However, limitation of lipid calories to no more than 500 kcal/d is recommended in patients with concurrent sepsis, based on the potential alterations in immune function with high dosages of lipid emulsions.

Regardless of route of parenteral nutrition delivery, micronutrient additives such as electrolytes, vitamins, minerals, and trace elements must be included in amounts to meet the patient's needs and replace deficits. Table 8–10 outlines a method for estimating electrolyte requirements.

Monitoring & Consultation

Appropriate monitoring and consultation help ensure both nutritional adequacy and safety of the nutrition support regimen selected for the patient. Consultation with the clinical dietitian may provide valuable insight into optimum and maximum use of both oral diets and tube feedings. Similarly, advice from the nutrition support team is valuable for all patients from the aspects of both assessment and therapy. Placement of elective central venous access should be performed and supervised only by those qualified by experience both to provide the access and to recognize and treat complications associated with the access (surgeons).

Monitoring the patient for response to whatever nutritional therapy is given is important. Periodic weight measurements and calorie counts are important in all cancer patients, even those on a "regular" diet. Monitoring is extended to include measurements of daily fluid balance, substrate tolerance, and chemical profiles in patients subjected to specialized enteral and parenteral feeding. Equally important, and frequently overlooked, is the monitoring technique of frequent patient interview and abdominal examination in patients receiving specialized enteral feeding.

All monitoring techniques have three aims: assessment of response, avoidance of complications, and early detection and treatment of the complications that occur in spite of appropriate monitoring. Complications fall into three categories: mechanical, metabolic, and infectious. Mechanical complications include problems associated with catheter placement (eg, pneumothorax, hemothorax), catheter malposition or migration, and admixture containers, tubing, or delivery (eg, malfunctioning pump). Metabolic complications can be detected through routine assessment of serum electrolytes, blood and urine glucose,

Table 8–10. Electrolyte requirements in total parenteral nutrition.[1]

Electrolyte	Amount/100 mL Volume Infused	Amount/1000 Carbohydrate kcal
Na+ (meq)	2–3	5–10
K+ (meq)	1.5–2	20–30
Cl- (meq)	2–3	10–15
Ca^{2+} (meq)		5
Mg^{2+} (meq)		8
P (mM)		10–15

[1]Basal daily electrolyte needs are equal to sum of amounts estimated based on volume infused and carbohydrate kcal. If there are abnormal loses (eg, due to nasogastric suction), additional electrolytes should be added as needed to replace loses.

Table 8–9. Example of peripheral parenteral nutritional solution.[1]

	Volume	Calories	mosm/kg
Lipid emulsion (20%)	500 mL	1000 kcal	300
Dextrose (20%)	1000 mL	689 kcal	1010
Crystalline amino acids (8.5%) with electrolytes	1000 mL	340 kcal	1160
Total admixture	2500 mL	2020 kcal	928

[1]This admixture yields a solution that is 8% dextrose, 4% lipid, and 3.4% crystalline amino acids; the NPC:N ratio is 120:1.

and acid-base status. In addition, daily weights are useful in assessing hydration status in the face of absent or incomplete recordings of input and output. Fever is often the sign of an infectious complication, although infections may be detected earlier by observations of new-onset glucose intolerance (glucosemia, hyperglycemia) in some patients. When catheter sepsis is suspected, the clinician may replace the intravenous catheter over a J wire, carefully culturing the catheter tip quantifiably. If the catheter tip demonstrates greater than 15 colony-forming units on culture, the new catheter should be removed and another site for access established.

EFFICACY OF NUTRITIONAL SUPPORT

Nutritional support is widely accepted to play an important role in the management of cancer patients. However, to date the data are confusing concerning the value of aggressive nutritional care in this population. Numerous controlled trials of parenteral nutrition in cancer patients undergoing surgical procedures, radiation therapy, and chemotherapy have been performed without producing clear evidence of improved outcome. Nevertheless, nutritional support can lead to weight gain, improved serum albumin, enhanced quality of life, and restoration of depleted fat stores and lean body mass in cancer patients. In addition to the general adjunctive role of nutritional support in cancer patients, work by several investigators regarding the importance of maintaining the gut mucosal barrier may be especially applicable. The gut mucosa is the most rapidly dividing cell mass in the body and functions not only as a digestive and absorptive surface but also serves as a critical barrier between the contaminated luminal contents of the bowel and the sterile tissue compartments. Antineoplastic therapy, particularly chemotherapy, often adversely affects the gut mucosa (mucositis, enteritis, colitis) because it is directed at rapidly dividing cell populations. Defects in this barrier may result in the translocation of bacteria, endotoxins, and toxic metabolic products. This translocation may result in activation of inflammatory mediators including the complement cascade, portal bacteremia and endotoxemia, and systemic sepsis.

The prime oxidative fuels for the gastrointestinal tract mucosa appear to be glutamine and ketone bodies (short-chain fatty acids). These fuels are provided in abundance in unperturbed simple starvation if body cell mass and fat stores are adequate. Intervention with TPN and some liquid formula diets, however, effectively eliminates these fuels. The amino acid admixtures used for TPN do not contain glutamine, and TPN suppresses ketosis as a result of the glucose administered. Thus, TPN administration results in gut atrophy.

Studies of enteral and parenteral glutamine administration suggest potential benefit from administering gut-specific fuels. Hwang et al reported better maintenance of the gut of experimental animals fed a TPN formulation enriched with 2% glutamine. Fox et al showed improved maintenance of the gut, less negative nitrogen balance, and a lower incidence of bacteremia in a rat methotrexate-induced enteritis model fed a glutamine-enriched liquid formula diet. The clinical utility of such intervention remains to be determined.

REFERENCES

Cancer Cachexia
Daly JM, Thon AK: Neoplastic diseases. Chapter 31 in: *Nutrition and Metabolism in Patient Care.* Kinney JM et al (editors). Saunders, 1988.
DeWys WD: Management of cancer cachexia. Semin Oncol 1985;**12**:452.
DeWys WD et al: Prognostic effect of weight loss prior to chemotherapy in cancer patients. *Am J Med* 1980; **69**:491.
Kern KA, Norton JA: Cancer cachexia. *JPEN* 1988;**12**:286.

Nutrient Requirements
Dempsey DT, Mullen JL: Macronutrient requirements in the malnourished cancer patient: How much of what and why? *Cancer* 1985;**55**:290.
Hansell DT et al: The relationship between resting energy expenditure and weight loss in benign and malignant disease. *Ann Surg* 1986;**203**:240.
Hoffman FA: Micronutrient requirements of cancer patients. *Cancer* 1985;**55**:295.

Merrick HW et al: Energy requirements for cancer patients and the effect of total parenteral nutrition. *JPEN* 1988;**12**:8.

Nutritional Assessment
Detsky AS et al: Evaluating the accuracy of nutritional assessment techniques applied to hospitalized patients: Methodology and comparisons. *JPEN* 1984;**8**:153.
Detsky AS et al: What is subjective global assessment of nutritional status? *JPEN* 1987;**11**:8.
Shizgal HM: Body composition of patients with malnutrition and cancer: Summary of methods of assessment. *Cancer* 1985;**55**:250.
Smale BF et al: The efficacy of nutritional assessment and support in cancer surgery. *Cancer* 1981;**47**:2375.

Clinical Approaches
Fleming CR, Nelson J: Nutrition options. Chapter 43 in: *Nutrition and Metabolism in Patient Care.* Kinney JM et al (editors). Saunders, 1988.

Klein GL, Rivera D: Adverse metabolic consequences of total parenteral nutrition. *Cancer* 1985;**55**:305.

Louie N, Niemiec PW: Parenteral nutrition solutions. Chapter 14 in: *Parenteral Nutrition.* Rombeau JL, Caldwell MD (editors). Saunders, 1986.

Efficacy of Nutritional Support

American College of Physicians: Parenteral nutrition in patients receiving cancer chemotherapy. *Ann Intern Med* 1989;**110**:734.

Fox AD et al: Effect of glutamine-supplemented enteral diet on methotrexate-induced enterocolitis. *JPEN* 1988;**12**:325.

Hwang TL et al: Preservation of small bowel mucosa using glutamine-enriched parenteral nutrition. *Surgical Forum* 1986;**37**:56.

Koretz RL: Parenteral nutrition: Is it oncologically logical? J Clin Oncol 1984;**2**:534.

McGeer AJ et al: Parenteral nutrition in cancer patients undergoing chemotherapy: A meta-analysis. *Nutrition* 1990;**6**:233.

Shike M, Brennan MF: Supportive care of the cancer patient. 1. Nutritional support. Chapter 59 in: *Cancer: Principles and Practice of Oncology,* 3rd ed. DeVita VT, Hellman S, Rosenberg SA (editors). Lippincott, 1989.

Hospice Care

9

Marion P. Primomo, MD

The National Hospice Organization (NHO) defines hospice as follows: "A hospice is a centrally administered program of palliative and supportive services which provides physical, psychological, social, and spiritual care for dying persons and their families. Services are provided by a medically supervised interdisciplinary team of professionals and volunteers. Hospice services are available in both the home and the inpatient setting. Home care is provided on a part-time, intermittent, regularly scheduled, and round-the-clock on-call basis. Bereavement services are available to the family. Admission to a hospice program of care is on the basis of patient and family need."

As early as 1858 the origins of hospice can be read in the words of Bigelow: "A physician's duties are to diagnose, to initiate treatment, to offer relief of symptoms, and to provide safe passage." "Safe passage" means competent control of pain and other symptoms, being with family and friends in familiar surroundings, being able to communicate with caregivers openly, and being involved in decision making. "Safe passage" asks for help in coming to terms with the fear, loneliness, and anguish of dying, being free from unwanted technical interventions that may prolong only suffering and not quality of life, and supporting grieving family and friends in their bereavement.

The Hospice Concept

The rapid development of the hospice concept of care in the past 20 years grew from a desire on the part of professionals and volunteers to address the needs of the dying and relieve the inadequacies of a health care system perceived as responding poorly to the needs of the terminally ill. Originating in "grass-roots" volunteer enthusiasm, the hospice movement is now firmly established within the health care system with its own policies, regulations, and paid employees.

Hospice is not a *place* but rather a *philosophy of care* that aims to help persons live until they die, free of pain and other distressing symptoms, able to share their feelings with loved ones and to find some sense of meaning even in their dying. Death is accepted as a natural part of life, and the final stages of life are viewed as important as or more important than other periods. The hospice approach rests on the belief that even when death cannot be avoided there are ways to render its approach less traumatic and even provide opportunities for growth.

Historical Perspectives

"Hospice," a medieval French word denoting a place of rest for pilgrims journeying to the Holy Land, found application in the 1960s to British programs of care for persons on life's last journey. In 1967, St. Christopher's Hospice was established in London by Dame Cicely Saunders, a social worker, nurse, and physician. She was the first to promote the multidisciplinary approach to palliative care for the dying and to recognize the importance of the patient/family unit. Today, St. Christopher's remains the model hospice in patient care, in the development of successful new approaches to pain and symptom control in terminal disease, in the education of professionals in this work, and in research to establish a valid scientific base for the rapidly growing new discipline.

In 1963 a lecture by Saunders at Yale University sparked the hospice effort in North America, and in 1974 the Hospice of Connecticut was established in New Haven. Aided by nationwide trends in death awareness and open communication and inspired by the popularity of Kubler-Ross's pioneer treatise, *on death and dying,* the hospice movement spread rapidly until today there exist an estimated 1700 programs in the USA.

Standards

Guidelines for the growing number of hospice programs were established in 1979 by the National Hospice Organization (NHO). A voluntary accreditation process was developed through the cooperative efforts of the NHO, the Joint Commission on the Accreditation of Hospitals (now the Joint Commission on the Accreditation of Healthcare Organizations), and other organizations (Table 9–1). From the 46 programs initially certified, the number has grown to over a thousand. Some states require licensure of hospice care.

Table 9–1. Requirements for hospice accreditation by the Joint Commission on the Accreditation of Healthcare Organizations.

Patient and family members are the unit of care.
Medical, nursing, social work, spiritual, volunteer, and bereavement services are available to patients and families in the inpatient and home settings.
Objectives of care are the management of physical and psychosocial needs.
Hospice services are available 24 hours a day, 7 days a week.

Types of Hospice Services

(1) "Free-standing" hospices containing all the elements of hospice care such as home care, inpatient care, respite care, and consultation services.

(2) Home care–based hospices with back-up inpatient hospital, residential, or nursing home beds.

(3) Hospital- or nursing home–based units.

(4) Hospital-based hospice teams—"floating" teams visiting patients throughout the hospital or in a designated area.

Hospice in the USA Today

According to a 1991 survey conducted by the NHO, an estimated 206,684 patients and families received hospice services in 1990. Of the patients, 84% had a diagnosis of cancer, 4% had AIDS, and 3% died of cardiovascular disease. The American Cancer Society reports that one of three persons dying of cancer in 1990 was served by a hospice program.

Forty percent of hospices were independent and community based, 30% were owned by hospitals, 24% were owned by home health agencies, and 7% operated as coalition or nursing home services.

The Medicare hospice benefit paid for 53% of hospice patients, private insurance provided 22% of patient support, and 4% were paid for by Medicaid.

Today, for the most part, hospice in the USA focuses on care in the home with inpatient or residential care as back-up, in contrast to that in Canada and England, where hospital-based programs predominate.

Reimbursement

Early hospice efforts were characterized by a sense of high idealism—the intent was to serve all dying patients whether funded or not, and to this end donations and volunteers were essential. Funding sources consisted of grants, memorials, donations, philanthropy, and support from religious groups. It soon became apparent that if hospice were to continue to grow, plans must include development of a firm financial structure to ensure continuity of professional staffs and organizations. Fortunately, as the public demand for hospice services increased, the major insurance companies, industry, and trade unions began to endorse hospice care.

Medicare Hospice Benefit in the USA

On November 1, 1983, hospice services were included under the Medicare benefit (Tables 9–2 and 9–3). The enabling legislation, part of the Tax Equity and Fiscal Responsibility Act passed by Congress in August 1982, has dramatically affected the growth of hospice in the USA.

Under the benefit, hospice programs are reimbursed by Medicare at a fixed daily rate for up to 210 days in each of four categories: basic home care, continuous nursing care, respite inpatient care, and hospital inpatient care. The patient relinquishes Medicare reimbursement for any other services related to the terminal illness except the services of the attending physician but may return to traditional treatment service at any time during the two 90-day and one 30-day certification periods. If the patient should live beyond the 210-day benefit period, the hospice may be reimbursed by Medicare under the terms of the Medicare Catastrophic Coverage Act of 1988. Medicaid provides almost identical coverage, and 33 states have adopted these benefits in their social welfare programs.

INTERDISCIPLINARY TEAM

The heart of hospice, the link between technology and personal caring, is the hospice care team. No one person can handle all the needs of the dying patient. The skills of many people working together in harmony, focusing on helping a patient and family prepare for a comfortable death, are required (Table 9–4).

The care team must be carefully selected, have a suitable work environment, and meet on a regular basis. In an atmosphere of open communication, close cooperation, and mutual trust and respect for one another, team members can form deeply satisfying relationships leading to a high degree of effectiveness, reducing unhealthy stresses, and promoting personal growth. The hospice that provides a warm, caring environment for its patients and families must

Table 9–2. Admission criteria for medicare hospice program.

Patient eligible for Medicare benefits
Terminal illness with a life expectancy of less than 6 months as certified by two physicians
Consent and cooperation of patient, family, and attending physician
Care focused on pain and symptoms of the illness, palliative in nature
Care provided by an interdisciplinary team including nurses, physicians, social workers, clergy, and specially trained volunteers
Care available 24 hours a day, 7 days a week
Patient cared for primarily at home, with family to participate in care

Table 9–3. Specific hospice services under medicare.

Nursing care
Physician's services
Medical social services
Physical, occupational, and speech therapy
Home health care by trained aide
Homemaker services
Medical supplies, including drugs and biologicals
Short-term inpatient care
Short-term respite care
Counseling, including bereavement counseling
Volunteer services

also nourish the people who work within it, from administrator to volunteer.

Because the hospice program attempts to meet a wide variety of needs of the dying person, other help may be called for, eg, a nutrition expert, an enterostomal therapist, a speech therapist, art and music therapists, a lawyer, even a funeral director. The growth and development of a good hospice team require time, a continuing commitment to the hospice concept, the acquisition of new skills and broader education, and a belief that one's input is important in program development and policy making.

Physicians

Physician leadership and involvement have obtained for hospice a respected position in the medical system. The newly formed Academy of Hospice Physicians now numbers almost 1000 and includes doctors from 49 states in the USA and 16 other countries. It has become a leading forum for physician education with emphasis on hospice academic and research activities.

The **hospice physician** who oversees the medical aspects of the hospice program and serves as consultant must have clinical competence, the ability to work with a team, and a good relationship with the medical community. In most hospice programs in the USA, the **attending physician** remains in charge of the patient's care and becomes as involved with hospice as desired. Attending physicians soon become familiar with hospice principles and learn that this is a useful and valued option for their dying patients.

Both hospice and attending physicians certify as to

Table 9–4. Five essential qualities required for hospice staff (after Zimmerman et al).

A high level of professional competence.
Sensitivity—caring not only for patients but also for each other and themselves.
Flexibility—willingness to improvise and accept change, being creative and imaginative.
Maturity—self-confidence rooted in a secure philosophy of life and a deep feeling of responsibility.
Spirituality—a sense that one is content to leave events in the hands of someone greater than oneself—faith in "letting go."

the patient's terminal condition, are responsible for hospice care plans, serve as role models, and give direction and support to the team, patient, and family. By means of this continued involvement, not only is the physician's care of the dying patient likely to be improved but discomfort in the face of death is alleviated. Increasing confidence in managing the dying event can also facilitate the often difficult ethical decisions that must be made.

House officers must be educated in matters of pain and symptom control and have a basic orientation to the principles of hospice. The undergraduate courses available in medical schools on topics of dying and death have been helpful, but there is scanty reference in the standard medical curriculum to the concepts of palliative care.

Nurses

Good nursing care is the foundation of good hospice care. Not only must nurses be skilled in patient assessment and evaluation but they also must be able to help meet the psychosocial needs of patients and families. Hospice nurses maintain symptom control, are knowledgeable about drugs for the relief of pain, and are able to tailor doses to the needs of the patient according to orders from the physician. Hospice nurses, frequently highly motivated and dedicated to their work, must have a sound understanding of hospice philosophy, principles, and practice and have achieved confidence and comfort in the face of death.

Coordination of the hospice team around the needs of patient and family is often orchestrated by the nurse who supervises nonprofessional workers such as volunteers. Much of the nurse's time is spent teaching patients about the disease, about medication, and about comfort techniques to relieve distressing symptoms. Preparing patient and family for the unexpected is an important part of the nurse's work and contributes greatly to the security of patient and caregivers at home. The peaceful outcome of a home death is frequently due in large part to the expertise of the nurse. Unfortunately, only a few university schools in the USA have recognized the need for graduate education to prepare nurses for advanced practice and research in palliative care.

Nurse's aides and homemakers must know hospice principles and be motivated by a sincere desire to help dying persons. Their moments of close physical contact with their patients may provide the "breakthrough" a patient requires to begin open communication.

Social Workers

Social workers in a hospice program by virtue of their training and interest are often keenly attuned to assisting others in matters of dying and death. They are well qualified to help patients and families deal with the social and personal problems of illness, disability, and death. They must work well with other members of the interdisciplinary team, be involved in supportive and bereavement counseling, and have thorough knowledge of community resources. Together with the nurse, they often participate in the initial contact with the patient and family and help set the tone for a successful hospice experience.

Pharmacists

Pharmacists are useful members of the hospice team because of the need for staff and patient/family education in the management of the drug regimen and monitoring of medication in the patient care plan.

Physical & Occupational Therapists

Physical and occupational therapists assist in maintaining patient comfort and maximizing patient capability as long as possible. They must be comfortable with the goal of diminishment rather than that of rehabilitation.

Counselors

Traditional psychiatric help is seldom needed by dying patients, and psychological counseling usually is provided by members of the hospice care team. However, psychologists and psychiatrists have been helpful to hospice staff in expanding their understanding of psychological events and family dynamics, and affording emotional support for staff members.

Spiritual/Pastoral Care

Providing spiritual care as needed is the task of all who engage in the work of palliative care. By listening and by being empathetic, a caregiver accompanies the patient in the struggle for growth and understanding. However, a trained person is frequently needed to address philosophic and theologic questions that arise and to celebrate the rites and rituals of a patient's religious preference. Palliative care chaplains, by acting in liaison with the dying person's own clergyman, are able to bring together the resources of spirituality, pastoral care, and religion in the service of the patient.

Volunteers

Volunteers have been fundamental to hospice since its earliest days. A well-functioning volunteer program requires proper selection, training, and supervision of volunteers who are active in patient care and administrative, clerical, and fund-raising activities. Volunteers interpret hospice to the community. Though they may incorporate their own area of expertise in their work, they often relate to patients and families on a nonprofessional level. Volunteers are often able to help a patient attain their "last wishes." Of the estimated 83,500 hospice workers in the USA in 1990, 64,000 were volunteers.

GOALS OF HOSPICE CARE

Good hospice care means creation of an environment in which a person can live up to the limit of his or her potential, physically, emotionally, socially, and spiritually. When a person, even in dying, can grow in a final search for meaning, then death can come peacefully. Family members, too, with the support of competent, compassionate caregivers can achieve a level of understanding and acceptance that is satisfying to them.

Physical Goals

A. Pain Relief: Unrelieved pain and physical distress are the foremost concerns of the dying patient. Pain control is key to hospice philosophy. No patient should want to die because of pain. Ideally, when a person arrives at hospice, the disease has been as carefully controlled as good medical and surgical care can achieve and the best efforts of medicine have been directed toward cure or palliation. Hospice medicine demands a thorough knowledge of the disease process and a high degree of clinical expertise. By means of meticulous attention to detail and competent assessment, hospice medicine focuses on each symptom as a problem and uses appropriate measures to obtain relief.

Terminal pain is different in character and meaning from pain encountered in acute care settings. It requires different methods of relief and has other standards of comfort.

Evidence that the pain of terminal disease was treated poorly prompted Saunders and Twycross to begin their work in England with an approach that included the whole person. "Total pain," as they called it, could be physical, emotional, interpersonal, spiritual, and even financial and required not only drug therapy but often environmental, social, physical, and spiritual therapies. Pain, they said, was a somatopsychic experience with its origin as much in the depression, anguish, and fear of death as in somatic sensation.

Central to their work was the oral use of opioids, regularly, around the clock, in a manner intended to prevent pain and not merely relieve it. Heroin, the first drug used, gave way to morphine as the drug of choice in England, Canada, and the USA. With further experience it became apparent to clinicians that terminally ill persons did not become addicted to the opioids, they developed tolerance very slowly, and respiratory depression was not a significant problem. The bioavailability of the oral opioids, previously thought to be low, and the presence of long-lasting metabolites became the most important factors in effecting a steady serum drug level that controlled pain evenly and prevented the erratic, fluctuating levels seen in parenteral use. Thus, controlling the patient's pain at home became not only effective but also simple for patient and family.

Chapter 17 deals with the specifics of analgesic drug therapy in the cancer patient. A few points are summarized here to clarify the unique application of such drug therapy to the control of pain in the patient who is dying.

(1) Pain must be treated as a problem in its own right and frequently reassessed.

(2) Pain can be relieved by an understanding of its source, an explanation to the patient regarding its meaning, and a successful demonstration that it can be controlled.

(3) Analgesics should be chosen appropriately according to the level of pain and half-life of the drug. When used properly for the control of pain, opioids do not cause addiction, tolerance, or respiratory depression.

(4) Regular administration of the selected analgesic at fixed time intervals is essential in the prevention of pain.

(5) The dosage of analgesics should be titrated so that the mental awareness of the patient is preserved.

(6) The oral use of morphine and other opioids can control pain effectively in most patients.

(7) The side effects of opioids, with the exception of constipation, generally subside within a short period of time.

(8) The use of adjuvant drugs, eg, nonsteroidal anti-inflammatory agents, antianxiety preparations, and antidepressants can improve the therapy of neuropathic pain, bone pain, and smooth and voluntary muscle pain and relieve concomitant insomnia and anxiety.

Not all pain control depends on the use of drugs. Important to palliative care are the skillful use of surgical measures, chemotherapy, and radiotherapy as well as neurolytic blocks and procedures and the wide array of physical therapy modalities. Worthy of mention are techniques that employ guided imagery, biofeedback, relaxation, acupuncture, and hypnosis as well as the soothing power of music, meditation, prayer, therapeutic touch, and spiritual healing. These methods are said to operate in a somatopsychic manner by releasing the body's own analgesic endorphins and, it is theorized, facilitating a person's connection with the inner self.

B. Other Symptoms: Symptoms other than pain may distress the dying patient, and good palliative care demands that they be relieved. We are indebted to pioneer clinicians on both sides of the Atlantic (Saunders and Twycross in England, Ajemian and Mount in Canada) as well as to hospice workers in the USA for their meticulous work in the alleviation of nausea, vomiting, dyspnea, weakness, dry mouth, cough, itching, bedsores, and confusion. For example, the medical management of malignant bowel obstruction designed by Baines for patients whose extensive disease, previous surgery, and severe illness make surgical intervention undesirable, enables a patient to be at home in relative comfort.

Often a small intervention can result in great comfort, eg, use of antifungal lozenges for candidiasis, and relieving terminal noisy secretions ("death rattle") by means of the scopolamine disk.

Finally, good hospice care mandates not only optimal techniques for managing pain and symptoms but doing so in a warm, secure, cheerful atmosphere where the patient's self-esteem is honored and the family's care is welcomed. Anxiety, loneliness, guilt, and fear all increase pain, but a sympathetic regard for the comfort of patient and family with attention to not only physical but also psychosocial and spiritual needs can make the difference between merely adequate and excellent control of pain and other symptoms.

Psychosocial Goals

A. Psychological Goals: Dying patients experience a multitude of emotions. Fear of pain, of abandonment, of the unknown, and of extinction as well as anxiety and anger may greatly intensify physical distress. The feelings of patient and family that impact the dying process were identified and described by Kubler-Ross. However, the "stages" of denial, anger, bargaining, depression, and acceptance are today more correctly seen as "process" rather than "stage." Kubler-Ross herself has pointed out their misuse in serving as guidelines for what a patient should experience, as some overly zealous caregivers once believed and taught. Certainly denial may be a useful way for patient and family to cope in the face of overwhelming disaster and for some may remain the major response. However, when a patient enters a hospice program, the inevitable progression of the disease with evidence of decline and deterioration have usually become apparent. Denial becomes increasingly difficult to maintain, and there is a growing awareness that the time together is short and that the focus must be on comfort. The process of acceptance may range from bitter resignation on the one hand to joyful acceptance on the other, but this goal is reached whenever the patient dies a death that is appropriate, for that patient.

B. Home Care: Caring for a patient with advanced cancer at home can be a satisfying experience for patient and family if medical, social, financial, and emotional support are available. Hospice nurses visit patients as often as necessary, and hospice physicians make house calls. Hospices can arrange for aide and homemaker help around the patient, organize friends and neighbors into helpful networks, and obtain hospital beds, wheelchairs, oxygen, and a wide variety of equipment for use in the home. Hospices can often supply drugs and biologicals required to control pain and symptoms. Hospice volunteers alleviate the boredom of tedious days by efforts at diversion, and by their presence enable family members to spend time away from the sick room. Spiritual comfort is brought to the patient by the hospice chaplain, who may provide the patient with a religious "reconnection" by means of ritual. Should the family's fatigue or stress become excessive, the patient can be admitted to a hospital for a short period of respite. Return to the hospital is also possible in order to achieve better control of pain or other distressing symptoms that cannot be managed adequately at home.

However, hospice care is not for everyone. Not every dying patient wishes to be at home; some feel more secure surrounded by hospital technology, and many children, during repeated hospital admissions, come to regard medical and nursing staff as "family" and the hospital as a secure home. Despite the best intentions of patient and caregiver, it is not always possible to manage successfully all stresses of the dying situation in the home. However, the caregiver is well supported by hospice at all times, the physical care of a dying person can help to relieve old feelings of guilt and remorse, can heal past emotional injuries, and can be a source of personal fulfillment. Gonda and Ruark in *Dying Dignified* reflect the feelings of hospice caregivers: " . . . we have often marveled at the courage and dignity with which certain patients and families manage to face the most horrifying situations. In many cases, we are profoundly uplifted by the essential nobility of the human spirit that we have been privileged to witness. It is thoughts such as these which sustain us through the moments of depression and despair that are inevitable for those involved in the care of the terminally ill."

C. Communication: Next to pain the greatest source of distress for the dying patient is loneliness. If a person is to live maximally until death there must be some shared awareness of the true situation. The hospice program tries to provide a framework in which patient, family, and friends can express their thoughts, fears, and fantasies about illness and death in an atmosphere where such discussions are openly accepted and communicated.

The anguish, fear, and pain of death can be eased most successfully by sharing the precious moments of life with another. Sadly, many couples who have shared years together in a good marriage often cannot acknowledge their feelings about death to one another, each trying to protect the other against the overwhelming grief. However, when feelings can be openly expressed and shared, patients and families often experience immense relief and freedom.

Shared meaning is rightly appreciated as one of the highest values in human life. However, clear communication may be blocked by deceit and game playing. Well-intentioned family and friends must be helped to realize that their efforts to shield the patient from the truth often only increase loneliness, anxiety, and suffering.

How a person dies has a profound effect on the survivors. A disturbing death creates uneasiness, guilt, and more intense grieving in the survivors. If there is

meaningful communication and reconciliation in the final days, long-standing quarrels and conflicts can be resolved and the family gains new strength, has less remorse, and experiences a healthier bereavement.

In her arguments against euthanasia, Saunders says, "the potential for personal and family growth at this stage is one of the strongest objections hospice workers feel for the legislation of a deliberately hastened death."

The patient should be informed of the illness and its extent in a responsible manner. Patients and families can tolerate bad news without losing hope if the truth is told gradually and gently with assurance that caregivers will continue to help them get the most out of living, will continue to be available to them, and will stay with them until the very end. Conversely, deceit creates distrust and arouses fear in the patient. Patients in whom unrealistic hopes of cure have been encouraged become anxious and fearful and unable to gain the peace that can come from an acceptance of the inevitable. Feeling that they are expected to continue the fight but knowing that they are becoming weaker, they tend to lose faith in themselves and their caregivers. Seravalli says, "The dying person needs to feel that he or she has not lost meaning for those who are close, one of whom is inevitably the doctor who has tried so hard to cure the patient."

D. Decision Making: Good communication facilitates decision making. When a patient's disease becomes terminal, the primary aim of treatment is to make the life remaining as comfortable and meaningful as possible. The focus shifts from "live as long as possible" to "live as well as possible." The use of total parenteral nutrition, dialysis, feeding tubes, antibiotics, assisted ventilation, and cardiopulmonary resuscitation may prolong only suffering. More importantly, if the patient goes home to die, the emphasis on the care of tubes and machines may stress patient and family so much that relationships are hindered and the critical saying of goodbyes, asking forgiveness, and giving of instructions may never be accomplished.

For most hospice patients, intensive efforts to improve nutrition and hydration are not appropriate unless improvement is foreseen. The role of hospice is to help family be comfortable with the decision and advise them that patients within a few days of death do not suffer hunger pangs and that thirst can best be relieved by good mouth care.

All therapy must be considered from the standpoint of whether or not it adds to the patient's comfort. A physician is not morally, legally, or ethically bound to prolong life at all costs. There is no obligation to employ useless or futile therapy. To support a lingering, painful death may even be immoral. Awareness of and comfort with the hospice philosophy of allowing death to come naturally may help doctors feel more at ease with letting go and not prolonging suffering out of a need for control or out of a sense of failure. Typical of the physician's dilemma is the remark made by a surgeon at the bedside of a dying patient: "I can stand for him to die of cancer, but I won't let him die of sepsis."

It is easier to forgo inappropriate measures to sustain life when the patient is at home or in a hospice, whereas in the setting of the acute care hospital it seems incongruous not to continue with high-technology efforts to sustain life.

Ideal resolution of ethical conflict can occur when patient, family, and physician can speak comfortably and openly with one another. McCormick says, "Decision making in health care, if it is to remain truly human, must be controlled primarily within the patient-doctor-family relationship, and these decisions must be tailor-made to individual cases and circumstances."

Existential & Spiritual Goals

When, comfortable and free of pain, secure in their environment and in their relationships, hospice patients become more aware of the emotional and spiritual changes that accompany dying, they are then free to ponder and search for those things in life that hold the deepest meaning for them. Some are overcome by fear, anger, and anguish; some die having missed the reason for living. However, many are able to confront this task and to use suffering as an opportunity for growth, as a chance to discover wholeness, and as the hope of finding meaning in life.

Existential and spiritual questions raised by a patient confronting death are many, and hospice workers try to help find answers as they seek new understanding. Hospice caregivers, by careful listening in genuine person-to-person contact, by their nonjudgmental attitude, and by their compassion and respect, encourage the personal search for meaning in their patients. In a practical way, patients are helped by gaining control of their situation. By enlisting the cooperation of family and friends and teaching them proper skills, the hospice worker helps them to meet challenges and find their own way through the situation. In this way, they regain a sense of worth, self-esteem, and mastery, enabling them to cope with crisis. Reviewing the past and completing any unfinished emotional business is part of the process of bringing order to the patient's life. This, in turn, contributes to the individual's finding meaning in dying and in each day of living until the end.

Many dying persons and their loved ones have said that the weeks or months before dying were the best of all. Time spent in shared preparation and completed relationships helped sweep away grief and remorse in a surge of tenderness. Often there occurred a deepened awareness of small joys and an intensified appreciation of love and human relationships. Proper care of the terminally ill patient offers an opportunity for patient and family to review, reconcile, explore, celebrate, and grow in the final search for meaning.

Hope must always be maintained even in the face of death—not unrealistic hope for cure but for more limited goals—a good day, another Christmas, the birth of a grandchild, a reconciliation. Often these hopes can be realized.

Most important is the hope of finding meaning in life. This search for meaning is the most basic quest and becomes of paramount importance as death approaches. Sometimes it is only under the pressure of impending death that a person learns life's lessons for the first time. In facing death, a person may achieve a degree of growth never before experienced and be able to complete his life with a sense of personal worth. Frankl acknowledged this when he said, "One can rise above oneself, one can grow beyond oneself, literally, up to one's last breath."

Creating an atmosphere that encourages personal fulfillment is not spiritual manipulation. Religious belief may or may not be a part of a dying person's experience. The thought of afterlife, reincarnation, or transcendent belief sustains some, but the belief of others that life ends with the end of the body also is worthy of respect. Peaceful, accepting deaths are not confined to patients with religious connections. All hospice patients are equally valued.

Byock speaks of the end of life as an opportunity for positive achievement and a process of "terminal growth." When relationships are mended, worldly affairs concluded, and goodbyes said, a person can focus on inner rather than outer concerns and make the connection to a larger reality. Thus, a person can be reconciled to the prospect of death and die without distress having achieved a completeness of being at the present moment. To provide a climate for growth, an opportunity for completion is a major task of hospice care for patients and caregivers.

HOSPICE FOR CHILDREN

Of the 1700 hospice programs in the USA, over 400 care for dying children and 14 are specifically designed for them. The American Academy of Pediatrics supports the concept of hospice care. Children's Hospice International (CHI), a nonprofit advocacy group established in 1983, is dedicated to the area that children with life-threatening conditions and their families have unique needs and deserve the option of hospice care in any setting. Soon to be available is a computerized, international network of services for seriously ill children based on the work of CHI in the USA and 18 other countries.

Various support groups such as Candlelighters and Make Today Count attempt to meet the needs of dying children and their families. Ronald McDonald houses play an important role in helping seriously ill patients with cancer and their families.

Home care, if the environment is suitable, is highly desirable for the dying child because it gives patient and family some sense of control. The focus in the home should not be on the death event but on making everyday life as normal as possible. When child and family can be home together, siblings and fathers are able to participate more fully than is possible in the institutional environment. Parents of children dying at home report less guilt and less anger. There are fewer negative effects on the marriage and an earlier return to work and social activities during bereavement.

Children with terminal cancer make up an estimated 1% of hospice-appropriate cases. The American Cancer Society reports that in the USA in 1988, 1638 children aged 1–14 died of cancer; conditions such as congenital anomalies, benign neoplasms, and HIV infection accounted for 1667 deaths. The hospice approach has been helpful for patients with severe congenital anomalies for whom cure is not possible but whose parents relish each day of life. Good hospice team support can lighten the burdens they carry, help them come to terms with the inevitable, and sometimes, despite their great sadness and distress, make the final journey together a rewarding spiritual event. Bereavement support after the child's death is an important ongoing hospice activity.

The increasing number of children with HIV infection will challenge hospice care in the future and require not only a broadening of admission criteria but also planning for adequate inpatient facilities devoted exclusively to their special needs.

HOSPICE FOR THE ELDERLY

Terminal care is an important aspect of geriatrics and increasingly recognized as worthy of attention. However, many disorders of the aged are characterized by long-term illness, such as Alzheimer's disease, and do not fit into the hospice criterion of a 6-month prognosis as to life. However, these patients too require a hospice type approach with emphasis on the family unit, relief of pain and symptoms, interdisciplinary planning, continuity of care, and attention to psychosocial and spiritual needs.

In England, the need for this approach has been clearly recognized since the beginning of the hospice movement. At St. Christopher's Hospice, 10–15% of patients are frail elderly, many with motor neuron disease, who often remain at the facility for years.

In the USA, hospice type care has been explored as a realistic option in the care of the elderly in different settings, especially in Veterans Administration hospitals and nursing homes. One such program is for patients with Alzheimer's disease headed by Volicir at the Veterans Administration hospital in Bedford, Massachusetts. This health care service emphasizes compassionate care for patients with Alzheimer's

disease and for their relatives and assists in decision making.

Hospice is interested in the alleviation of distressing symptoms and concerned with caring when cure is no longer a reasonable expectation. Hospice care should not be limited to the dying but should be offered to all those who need more personal care without the technology of the acute care setting. Such an approach is particularly well suited to the elderly so that maximum quality of living can still occur even at the end of life.

HOSPICE & AIDS

The admission of patients with acquired immunodeficiency syndrome (AIDS) to a hospice program poses new challenges. Most patients with this disease are young, have a protracted course of illness, and require and want curative, aggressive type therapy until the very end of life. However, the terminal stages of AIDS are not well defined. The introduction of new drugs has resulted in better control of the disease and prolongation of life although without affecting the ultimate outcome.

Caregivers must be protected against infection with the AIDS virus, and the patient, who is immunocompromised, must be protected against a host of infections possibly carried by the caregiver.

Problems associated with social status, emotional states, family dynamics, and finances are routinely encountered in patients suffering from AIDS and may be severe. Recognition of the special needs of these patients prompted Saunders to recommend that new hospice teams be developed with special expertise in the care of patients with AIDS.

Support groups have arisen in many cities in the USA. Many groups are closely allied with hospice programs and share in the expertise and caring of both organizations to form an AIDS care network. In many communities, such cooperation has become the nucleus for successful programs on AIDS education. Noteworthy is the RISE program, a health education program organized in California in 1987 to provide support for HIV-positive individuals. It has since spread to other Western states and Canada and has provided help for thousands of persons coping with HIV disease and other serious and chronic illnesses.

HOSPICE & EUTHANASIA

Hospice is not a method for euthanasia. Hospice care exists neither to hasten nor to unduly prolong death but to help patient and family accept it as part of life with as much comfort and peace as can be managed. When a person's pain and loneliness are relieved, when he or she feels welcome and not a burden and loved and understood by caregivers, the cry for euthanasia disappears.

Simpson points out that by listening carefully to a person who says "I don't want to live" we may really hear "I don't want to live like this." With today's advances in techniques of palliative care it is always possible to improve life and render it more acceptable to the patient and sometimes possible to make it a source of growth for both patient and family. Hospice is the alternative to euthanasia.

REFERENCES

Academy of Hospice Physicians: *Objectives*. 8800 49th Street North, Suite 102, Pinellas Park, FL 34666.

Billings JA: *Outpatient Management of Advanced Cancer.* Lippincott, 1985.

Buckman R: *I Don't Know What to Say: How to Help and Support Someone Who Is Dying.* Key Porter Books, 1988.

Corr CA, Corr DM (editors): *Hospice Approaches to Pediatric Care.* Springer, 1985.

Frankl V: *Man's Search for Meaning.* Simon & Schuster, 1962.

Gonda TA, Ruark JE: *Dying Dignified: The Health Professional's Guide to Care.* Addison-Wesley, 1984.

Howell DA, Martinson IM: Management of the terminally ill child. In: *Pediatric Oncology.* Pizzo PA (editor). Lippincott, 1989.

Johanson GA: *Physicians Handbook of Symptom Relief in Terminal Care.* Home Hospice of Sonoma County, Santa Rosa, CA, 1989.

Joint Commission on Accreditation of Healthcare Organizations: *Hospice Standards Manual.* Chicago, 1987.

Jonsen AR, Siegler M, Winslade WJ: *Clinical Ethics,* 2nd ed. Macmillan, 1986.

Kaye P: *Symptom Control in Hospice and Palliative Care.* Hospice Education Institute, 1989.

Kilburn LH: *Hospice Operations Manual.* National Hospice Organization, Arlington, VA, 1988.

Kubler-Ross E: *On Death and Dying.* Macmillan, 1981.

McCann BA: Hospice care in the United States: The struggle for definition and survival. *Palliative Care* 1988;**4**:16.

Milch RA, Freeman A, Clark E: *Palliative Pain and Symptom Management for Children and Adolescents.* Children's Hospice International, Alexandria, VA, 1985.

Mor V, Masterson-Allen S: *Hospice Care Systems: Structures, Process, Costs and Outcome.* Springer, 1987.

Paradis LF (editor): *Hospice Handbook: A Guide for Managers and Planners.* Aspen, 1985.

President's Commission for the Study of Ethical Problems in Medicine and Biomedical and Behavioral Research: *Making Health Care Decisions,* US Government Printing Office. 1982. *Deciding to Forego Life-Sustaining Treatment,* 1983.

Saunders C (editor): *The Management of Terminal Malignant Disease,* 2nd ed. Edward Arnold, 1984.

Simpson MA: Therapeutic uses of truth. In: *The Dying Patient.* Wilkes E (editor). Bogden, 1982.

Stedeford A: *Facing Death: Patients, Families, and Professionals.* Heinemann, 1985.

Stoddard S: *The Hospice Movement.* Stein & Day, 1978.

Torrens PR (editor): *Hospice Programs and Public Policy.* American Hospital Publishing, 1985.

Twycross RG, Lack SA: *Therapeutics in Terminal Cancer,* 2nd ed. Churchill Livingstone, 1990.

Walsh TD (editor): *Symptom Control.* Yearbook, 1988.

Zimmerman JM: *Hospice: Complete Care for the Terminally Ill,* 2nd ed. Urban and Schwarzenburg, 1986.

Section III.
Treatment Disciplines

Surgical Oncology

10

Harold V. Gaskill III, MD, Michael P. Kahky, MD, & Carey P. Page, MD

Before the 20th century, surgery was the only form of therapy available to the cancer patient. Accordingly, many important milestones in our understanding of the pathophysiology of cancer were made by observant surgeons. There is ample evidence that such basic principles of surgical oncology as wide local excision of malignant tumors were well known even to the surgeons of ancient Greece. In the 17th century, Hunter described the importance of the lymphatic system in the progression of cancer and discouraged operation in the presence of fixed regional lymph nodes. During the latter portion of the 19th century, advancement of operative technique made possible resectional therapy of malignant disease by surgeons such as Billroth (stomach, esophagus, larynx), Kocher (thyroid), and Halsted (breast). During the first half of the 20th century, surgical skills were refined to the point where it was technically possible to remove malignant tissue from virtually any organ. In addition, radiotherapy, chemotherapy, hormonal therapy, and immunotherapy were introduced. The need to integrate technically complex surgical procedures with these newer modalities led to the evolution of the surgical oncologist. The surgical oncologist is a surgeon who commits to the care of patients with cancer as an active participant in a multidisciplinary approach.

Screening & Physical Diagnosis

Screening for common cancers, such as cancer of the breast, and their diagnosis by physical examination is central to the successful treatment of cancer. Accordingly, the surgical oncologist is adept at physical examination of such critical areas as the oral cavity, neck, breast, abdomen, rectum, prostate, and regional lymph nodes. In cases when physical examination is the only way to establish the diagnosis early in the course of the disease, the special experience and skill of the surgical oncologist are critical.

Diagnostic Biopsy

Establishing the pathologic diagnosis is the first step to successful management of the patient with malignant disease. A variety of techniques are available for obtaining tissue.

A. Needle Aspiration Biopsy: The least invasive is the needle aspiration biopsy. This technique is performed by passing a 22-gauge needle percutaneously into the suspected tumor. The needle may be guided by direct palpation of the mass. For deeper lesions, the needle may be guided by ultrasound, CT scan, or other imaging techniques. The needle is then passed through the mass 4–6 times while aspirating continuously. Any material obtained is immediately expressed onto a microscope slide and fixed for cytologic examination. Depending on the type of tumor involved, the diagnostic accuracy of this technique can be greater than 90%, and a false-positive diagnosis of malignancy is rare. This same technique may yield enough material for Chromosomal analysis by flow cytometry and for immunoperoxidase staining for special markers. Needle aspiration biopsy is most useful for solid, epithelial neoplasms. Its utility is limited for many sarcomas. Its role in patients with lymphoid malignancies is restricted to differentiating the process from an epithelial neoplasm.

B. Needle Biopsy: Needle aspiration yields only enough tissue for diagnosis by cytologic techniques. If a histologic diagnosis is required, additional tissue may be obtained by the technique of needle biopsy. A specially designed needle (eg, Vim-Silverman, Trucut) is passed into the mass as described above. The needle is designed to remove a core of solid tissue from the lesion. This core of tissue is then frozen or fixed and submitted for standard histologic analysis. In contrast to needle aspiration cytology, needle biopsy may result in adverse complications such as bleeding or clinically significant perforation of the viscera or thorax. Seeding of malignant tissue across tissue planes is also possible.

C. Excisional Biopsy: A commonly employed technique for establishing a tissue diagnosis is the excisional biopsy. It involves complete excision of the lesion in question. This technique is ideally suited to cutaneous lesions less than 1 cm in diameter and small breast masses. In most cases, excisional biopsy is intended only to establish a definitive diagnosis;

thus, although it constitutes adequate therapy for most benign lesions, malignant lesions likely will require additional therapy. An advantage of the excisional biopsy is avoidance of the need for more extensive procedures when the diagnosis is uncertain. In addition, it may form the initial component of effective local therapy when combined with radiotherapy. Excisional biopsy is the method of choice for obtaining diagnostic nodal tissue from patients with lymphoma or leukemia. In these settings, examination of the architecture of the entire node is critical to definitive diagnosis.

D. Incisional Biopsy: To establish a tissue diagnosis before definitive resection, particularly when preoperative chemotherapy or radiotherapy is being considered, an incisional biopsy is useful. Careful planning should place the incision in a location that permits its excision as a part of a more extensive operation. In addition, careful hemostasis avoids dissemination of cancer cells along tissue planes by postbiopsy bleeding. This technique is useful for approaching large neoplasms and is the standard diagnostic technique for sarcomas.

Curative Resection

For many patients with solid neoplasms, surgical resection alone is curative. The success of this mechanical procedure is dependent on the size and location of the primary tumor, the presence of metastatic lesions, and the biologic behavior of both. The diagnosis of malignancy, however, does not give a license to perform the most extensive resection that is technically possible. The boundaries of the curative resection are determined with two objectives in mind. First, enough tissue is removed so that the patient is likely to be cured in the absence of clinically significant systemic disease. In the thyroid, this may represent the entire gland and no lymphatic tissue. By contrast, curative resection of a gastric antral cancer should include only enough stomach to assure margin-free removal of the cancer but all regional lymphatic tissue.

The second boundary of the potentially curative resection is established by the need to ascertain the likelihood of systemic disease. Thus, axillary dissection is an essential component of a curative resection for breast cancer, since the presence of metastatic cancer in axillary lymph nodes establishes a rationale for further systemic therapy. It does not, however, increase the number of patients cured by local resection alone.

Palliative Resection

Palliative therapy should be considered for a patient with evidence of widespread malignancy and no hope of cure by resectional therapy. For example, more than 25% of patients with gastric cancer present with advanced disease manifested by a palpable abdominal mass. Before a palliative resection is undertaken, several points should be considered. First, the patient must be truly symptomatic. Resection of the primary lesion in the asymptomatic patient with widespread metastatic disease is not palliative. Second, the surgeon must be thoroughly familiar with the symptoms to be palliated. For example, pain caused by invasion of retroperitoneal structures will not be alleviated by resection of the gastric primary. Third, the patient with advanced cancer is a poor operative candidate, and less invasive surgical procedures such as endoscopic laser therapy, stent placement, or radiotherapy should be considered.

Operative Debulking

In some cases, a patient presents with an extensive lesion such as a retroperitoneal sarcoma that is not amenable to curative resection. Although this patient is relatively asymptomatic, it may be advisable to recommend a debulking procedure. The procedure is designed to remove the greatest amount of tissue consistent with a safe operation and rapid postoperative recovery. This strategy facilitates further therapy with radiation or chemotherapy. There are several reasons for this phenomenon. First, the cells in the central portion of the tumor are the least metabolically active and the most resistant to both radiotherapy and chemotherapy. Second, debulking reduces the number of malignant cells in the body by one or two orders of magnitude before initiation of cytotoxic chemotherapy.

Staging

Pathologic staging of malignant disease is an important role. Most often, staging is incorporated into surgical management of the primary lesion. Thus, axillary node dissection is integral to surgical management of carcinoma of the breast. Similarly, resection of primary lesions of the head and neck as well as the gastrointestinal tract incorporates regional lymph node dissection. The presence or absence of lymphatic metastasis then serves as a guide to further regional or systemic therapy.

In some cases, such as Hodgkin's disease, the staging procedure is not related to any therapeutic operation. Stage I or stage II Hodgkin's disease may be treated with radiotherapy alone. Stage III patients may be treated with either radiotherapy or chemotherapy, or a combination of both, in the presence of bulky pelvic disease. Stage IV disease requires systemic chemotherapy. Accurate pathologic staging is a prerequisite to effective treatment. Fully one-third of patients with Hodgkin's disease are misstaged based on clinical findings alone. Addition of lymphangiography, radionuclide scans, and CT scans estimate but do not definitively diagnose intra-abdominal or systemic disease. Accordingly, the staging laparotomy has become integral to the management of patients with Hodgkin's disease. Patients with satisfactory cardiopulmonary function and no other contraindication to operation should be considered for staging laparotomy. This operation consists of a thorough exploration of the abdominal contents through a long midline incision, liver biopsy, splenectomy, and sampling of periaortic lymphoid tissue. Evaluation of this tissue guides the need for further radiotherapy and chemotherapy. The mortality rate for staging laparotomy should be less than 1%.

Second-Look Procedures

The second-look procedure was proposed by Wangensteen in 1951. Patients undergoing potentially curative resections or gastrointestinal malignancy were reexplored 6 months after their primary operation to test the theory that this strategy would result in early diagnosis and resection of intra-abdominal metastases. A few patients were rendered disease-free by second-look operations. However, the majority either underwent a negative exploration or were found to have unresectable disease at the time of the second look.

More recently, several authors have advocated second-look procedures after potentially curative resections for colon cancer based on an elevation of carcinoembryonic antigen (CEA). Again, some patients have probably been rendered disease-free by these operations, but most have disclosed either irresectable disease or no cancer at all. The advisability of recommending second-look procedures for all such patients remains controversial. Similar debate surrounds second-look operations for ovarian cancer.

Resection of Metastasis

In the past, presence of metastatic disease was considered evidence of incurability. More recently, resection of lesions metastatic to the central nervous system, lungs, and liver has become common. Although the most favorable results are associated with resection of a solitary metastatic lesion, resection of small numbers of multiple metastases is becoming more common. These operations are recommended most often when the patient is symptomatic, when further regional or systemic chemotherapy is planned, or when resection may render the patient disease-free. Resection of pulmonary and hepatic metastases from colorectal cancer should be performed, in appropriate patients, when there is a chance of achieving a "margin-free" resection and there is no other evidence of disease. Resection of pulmonary metastases from sarcoma prolongs survival in patients with a tumor-doubling time of more than 40 days. Axillary or femoral nodal metastases from melanoma should be removed to avoid breakdown of the overlying skin or to reduce tumor burden for chemotherapy or immunotherapy. Similarly, resection of isolated metastases for renal cell carcinoma may be an important adjunct to immunotherapy or curative in its own right.

Management of Complications of Therapies

Ideally, the surgical oncologist is included in the planning of aggressive medical management of malignant disease. Such a relationship facilitates the early and expeditious diagnosis and treatment of the complications inevitably associated with aggressive cancer therapy. These complications may be relatively minor, such as cutaneous burns after radiotherapy or extravasation of cytotoxic agents. Patients undergoing intensive therapy also suffer more serious complications such as gastrointestinal bleeding or perforation during treatment of tumors involving the gastrointestinal tract.

Management of these complications in the immunocompromised patient or the patient with widespread metastatic disease may differ markedly from that recommended for other groups of patients. For example, placement of gastrostomy of jejunostomy tubes should be avoided in immunocompromised patients. Similarly, operations involving division and reanastomosis of the bowel are avoided whenever possible. These patients require particular attention to preoperative and postoperative care. Correction of coagulation and platelet deficits preoperatively is essential. Postoperatively, meticulous attention to electrolyte balance, hydration, and nutritional support is essential.

Specialized Procedures

Among the surgical procedures unique to the field of surgical oncology is **isolated limb perfusion,** most commonly employed as an adjunct to the treatment of extremity melanoma. For example, a melanoma of the lower extremity is treated by cannulating the femoral artery and femoral vein. Cannulas leading from these vessels are then connected to a roller pump, an oxygenator, and a heating unit. Next, the limb is isolated by placing a tourniquet around the vessels separating the cannulas from the systemic circulation. Oxygenation and circulation is provided to the limb by the roller pump and oxygenator. The limb is then perfused with super-normal doses of cytotoxic agents, usually at elevated temperature. This form of therapy may be more effective than conventional systemic therapy for the treatment of metastatic melanoma confined to one region. Randomized trials are in progress.

Other forms of regional therapy include arterial perfusion of selected primary or metastatic cancers via an implantable pumping device. Such forms of treatment may be conducted by the surgical oncology service or in conjunction with the medical oncologist.

Vascular Access

Effective vascular access is an absolute prerequisite to effective systemic chemotherapy. Most cytotoxic agents are highly irritating to peripheral veins, and extravasation can cause necrosis and ulceration of surrounding tissues. Accordingly, access to the central venous system is required for most patients. The choice of technique depends on the individual requirements of the patient and the treatment regimen.

A. Percutaneous Catheters: Basic central venous access can be provided by a single-lumen 16- or 20-gauge polyurethane catheter passed percutaneously into the subclavian vein. These catheters may be safely placed under local anesthesia while the patient lies on a stretcher or hospital bed. The most common complications are pneumothorax and inadvertent puncture of the subclavian artery. These catheters are ideal for continuous infusions or very frequent intermittent use (ie, daily). They are easily removed upon completion of therapy or to diagnose or treat catheter infection. Their main disadvantage is that they provide only one lumen for vascular access. Percutaneous polyurethane triple-lumen catheters, like the single-lumen catheter, can be placed under local anesthesia outside of the operating room. They have the same advantages as the single-lumen catheter and are used in the same setting. They are selected when one lumen is inadequate to provide for the patient's intravenous needs. Their disadvantage is a higher incidence of infection related to more frequent access.

Routine maintenance for both single- and triple-lumen percutaneous catheters includes three-times-weekly aseptic cleansing of the skin entry site and application of a fresh sterile dressing. Each limb of the catheter is flushed with 1 mL of sterile heparin solution. The patient must be carefully taught to avoid inadvertent contamination of the catheter or a possible air embolus during the heparin flush. On completion of therapy, these catheters are easily removed.

B. Indwelling Cuffed Catheters: When continuous therapy for longer than 3 months is anticipated, an indwelling cuffed silicone catheter may be indicated. Single-, double-, and triple-lumen varieties are available. These catheters are usually placed in the operating room under local or general anesthesia. They require creation of a subcutaneous tunnel 15–20 cm in length and introduction of the catheter into the subclavian vein either directly using a sheath type introducer or via the cephalic vein. These catheters incorporate a porous Teflon or Dacron cuff placed 1–2 cm below the level of the skin. Ingrowth of tissue to this cuff provides secure anchoring. The role of the cuff in mitigating ascending infection from skin microorganisms is questionable. Maintenance includes a sterile dressing at the entry site and daily or weekly flushing of the catheter lumen with heparinized saline. Because these catheters are constructed of soft silicone material, they may develop leaks following abuse or long use. In many instances, leaks may be repaired by a variety of techniques. After tissue ingrowth of the cuff has occurred, removal of these catheters requires freeing the cuff from the subcutaneous tissue. However, it is often possible to remove these catheters under local anesthesia on an outpatient basis.

C. Implantable Infusion Ports: Yet another alternative for vascular access is provided by the totally implantable vascular access port. These devices contain a single- or multiple-lumen silicone catheter. Rather than extend through the skin, this device is connected to a subcutaneous port incorporating a compressed silicone septum. After introduction of the silicone catheter into the subclavian vein, the port body is placed in a subcutaneous pocket created below the clavicle. After the wound has healed, access to the port is achieved by carefully preparing the skin over the port with a bactericidal solution and passing a noncoring needle through the skin, through the compressed silicone septum, and into the lumen of the port body. Fluid may be introduced into the central venous system or blood may be aspirated from the central venous system without difficulty. Access is completed by flushing the port with heparinized saline. The noncoring needle is then withdrawn from the patient. The great advantage is that these ports are entirely subcutaneous and no parts protrude from the skin. Thus, patients with these ports are free to swim or engage in other activities without the obvious intrusion of a vascular access. Their main disadvantage is that they must be inserted and removed in the operating room. They are best suited for patients for whom access is required intermittently and for brief periods. All advantages are lost if an indwelling percutaneous needle is left in place for extended periods. They become occluded more frequently when used for blood sampling and for administration of drugs.

REFERENCES

Bailar JC III: Mammography: A contrary view. *Ann Intern Med* 1976;**84**:77.

Brinton LA, Hoover R, Fraumeni JF: Epidemiology of minimal breast cancer. *JAMA* 1983;**249**:483.

Cady B: Changing patterns of breast cancer. *Arch Surg* 1972;**104**:266.

Cady B: New diagnostic, staging, and therapeutic aspects of early breast cancer. *Cancer* 1990;**65**:634.

Feig S: Radiation risk from mammography: Is it clinically significant? *AJR* 1984;**143**:469.

Frank JW, Mai V: Breast self-examination: More harm than good? *Lancet* 1985;**2**:654.

Gallager HS: Pathogenesis of early breast cancer. Pages 14–19 in: *Early Breast Cancer.* Zander J, Baltzer J (editors). Springer-Verlag, 1985.

Henson DE, Ries LA: Progress in early breast cancer detection. *Cancer* 1990;**65:**2155.

Lundgren B, Helleberg A: Single oblique-view mammography for periodic screening for breast cancer in women. *JNCI* 1982;**68:**351.

Miller AB: Early detection of breast cancer. Pages 215–228 in: *Breast Diseases.* Harris JR et al (editors). Lippincott, 1991.

Pochin EE: Why be quantitative about radiation risk estimates? (Lecture 2, Lauriston S. Taylor lecture series in radiation protection and measurements.) National Council on Radiation Protection and Measurements, Washington DC, 1978.

Shapiro S: Evidence on screening for breast cancer from a randomized trial. *Cancer* 1977;**(Suppl 6):**2772.

Shapiro S et al: Ten to fourteen year effect of screening on breast cancer mortality. *JNCI* 1982;**69:**349.

Silverstein MJ et al: Hooked-wire directed breast biopsy and over-penetrated mammography. *Cancer* 1987;**59:**715.

Skrabanek P: Screening for disease: False premises and false promises of breast cancer screening. *Lancet* 1985;**2:**316.

Strax P, Venet L, Shapiro S: Value of mammography in reduction of mortality from breast cancer in mass screening. *Am J Roentgenol Radium Ther Nucl Med* 1973;**117:**686.

Tabar L et al: What is the optimum interval between mammographic screening examinations? An analysis based on the latest results of the Swedish two-country breast cancer screening trial. *Br J Cancer* 1987;**55:**547.

11

Radiation Oncology

John J. Feldmeier, DO

The first application of external radiation to treat a patient with a malignancy was reported in 1896, and by 1899 the first successful curative treatment of a patient with a malignant tumor by radiation had been accomplished. In the early 20th century, the therapeutic application of radiation made steady though uneven progress and was advanced mostly through empiric means. By 1934, Coutard had described a protracted fractionated course of therapeutic radiation that has become the cornerstone of clinical radiation oncology. Until the 1950s, the advance of radiation therapy was primarily limited by the shortcomings of the equipment. The introduction of cobalt units in the early 1950s made possible the reliable delivery of radiation doses to deep-seated tumors. Linear accelerators brought further improvements in radiation dosage at depths in the early 1960s.

A clinician practicing radiation oncology today has a wide range of available equipment. Low-energy x-rays produced by orthovoltage units are used to treat skin tumors or other superficial conditions. High-energy megavoltage photons are available from cobalt units, and even higher energy photons and electrons are produced by linear accelerators. These units have the capability of treating deep-seated tumors without overdosing the skin and superficial tissues. Today's radiation oncologist can also select the radioactive isotope with the optimal physical characteristics for a permanent or temporary interstitial or intracavitary radiation implant. The radiation oncologist making clinical decisions does so with a wealth of supporting knowledge from radiation physics and biology. He or she must be well versed in all aspects of oncology to provide optimal treatment and integrate radiation into an overall management plan that is likely to include a combined approach with surgery, chemotherapy, or both.

Just over one million new cases of invasive cancer are diagnosed annually in the USA, and nearly one-half of these patients will ultimately die as a result of their cancer. Fifty percent to 60% of those patients who are newly diagnosed to have cancer will undergo radiation therapy in the management of their disease. Annually, about 150,000 patients will receive radiation therapy for persistent or recurrent disease. In some cases, therapeutic radiation will be utilized with curative intent as the only modality of treatment. In other cases, radiation will be combined with surgery or chemotherapy in curative fashion. In still other cases, radiation will be delivered as palliative treatment with the intention of relieving pain or preserving or restoring function of a vital structure or organ.

Radiation oncology is a clinical specialty. As a practitioner, the radiation oncologist must master the disciplines of clinical oncology as well as the principles of radiation physics and biology that are unique to this specialty.

RADIATION PHYSICS

A clinician practicing the specialty of radiation oncology must have a command of the basic physical principles necessary to produce and quantify a therapeutic dose of radiation. The advancement and discovery of the tenets constituting radiation physics have been an integral part of radiation oncology since its inception. This chapter presents a brief overview of this complex subject. The reader is referred to other texts for a more thorough treatment.

Definitions

A. Dose: Radiation dose is the amount of radiation energy absorbed per unit mass of tissue irradiated. The current unit of radiation dose is the gray (Gy), and it is equal to 1 joule per kilogram. Usually the dose is prescribed or reported in centigrays (cGy) ($\frac{1}{100}$th of a gray). A centigray is mathematically identical to the rad, which is the older unit. One centigray (or rad) equals 1 erg per gram of tissue.

B. Energy: Radiation beams are characterized by their energy (usually peak energy). One keV (kilo-electron volt) is equivalent to the energy imparted to an electron by accelerating it through 1000 volts. An MeV (million electron volts) is the energy imparted by accelerating an electron through one million electron volts. Typical energies for therapeutic external radiation range from about 100 keV to about 25 MeV. Photon energies are often characterized in units of kVP (kilovolt potential) or MV (megavolts).

C. Skin Sparing: For low-energy orthovoltage

74

beams, the highest dose of radiation occurs at the skin, with a rapid decrease in relative dose as the depth increases. For higher energy beams, after entering tissue the radiation dose undergoes a buildup to maximum level and then decreases with depth beyond this maximum. The depth at which the maximum dose occurs is termed D_{max}. D_{max} increases with increasing energy. A cobalt beam has a D_{max} of about 0.5 cm, while a 10-MeV beam has a D_{max} of about 2.5 cm. D_{max} is characteristic for a given energy beam. Since the maximum dose for modern high-energy equipment does not occur until its characteristic depth is achieved, the dose to the skin is reduced relative to the tumor dose, and these high-energy machines are said to have a skin-sparing effect. Figure 11–1 compares D_{max} for various energy beams.

D. Depth Dose: The deposition of dose as a beam traverses a path in tissue varies with depth of penetration into tissue. Once D_{max} is achieved, the dose falls off with increasing depth. High-energy beams have a slower decrease with increasing depth, while lower energies are rapidly attenuated as they pass through tissue. For convenience, the dose at a given depth is compared to the dose at D_{max} as a percentage. When these percentages are plotted against the depth in tissue at which they occur, a depth-dose curve is plotted that is characteristic of a particular type or energy of radiation. A comparison of depth-dose characteristics of several photon energies is shown in Figure 11–1.

E. Free Radical: A free radical is a short lived but highly reactive chemical species that owes its highly reactive nature to the fact that it contains an unpaired electron.

F. Ionizing Radiation: Ionizing radiation has sufficient energy to eject one or more orbital electrons from an atom or molecule.

G. Excitation: Excitation is the process by which an orbital electron is moved to a higher energy level without being ejected from the atom.

Nature of Therapeutic Radiation

Therapeutic radiation is ionizing radiation. The interaction of ionizing radiation with the patient's tissues must result in the production of ions or charged particles. This ionization is caused by the ejection of electrons from their orbits in the atoms of the target tissues. The production of charged particles within tissues requires a larger amount of energy than that produced by nonionizing types of radiation such as microwaves, visible light, or radio waves. This large amount of energy is ultimately available to break chemical bonds and effect other biochemical changes required to destroy malignant cells.

Therapeutic ionizing radiation is highly efficient in its biologic impact. A whole-body dose of 400 cGy to human subjects would result in death to approximately half of those individuals so irradiated. If a physically equivalent amount of energy were delivered as heat to an individual, his or her body temperature would increase by less than 0.002 °C.

It is helpful to conceptualize and characterize ther-

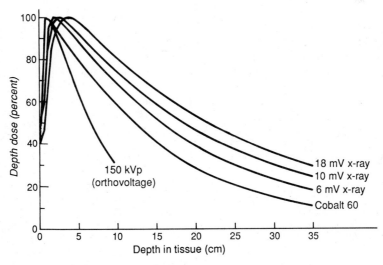

Figure 11–1. D_{max} and percentage depth dose curves for orthovoltage x-rays, cobalt gamma rays, 10-mV x-rays, and 18-mV x-rays. Orthovoltage x-rays have their maximum dose at the surface, with a rapid decrease as depth increases. Cobalt gamma rays have a maximum dose at 0.5 cm below the surface, with a fairly gradual fall-off with increasing depth thereafter. 10-mV x-rays from a high-energy linear accelerator have a D_{max} of 2.5 cm, with a very gradual decrease in percentage of D_{max} as depth of penetration into tissues increases. 18-mV x-rays exhibit their D_{max} at 3.5 cm and have an even more gradual decrease with depth.

apeutic radiation as bundles or packets of electro-magnetic energy (photons) or particles (electrons, protons, neutrons, and alpha particles). Photons are further described as either gamma rays or x-rays. Gamma rays are produced intranuclearly by the decay of a radioactive isotope. X-rays are produced outside the nucleus. Gamma rays and x-rays of the same energy are identical in their physical properties and differ only in their origins.

The interaction of ionizing radiation with its target of biologic material takes one of three forms:

A. Photoelectric Effect: The first phenomenon is called the photoelectric effect and occurs primarily at lower photon energies. It is this property that is utilized in the production of x-ray images. In this case, incident radiation interacts with an electron in one of the inner orbital positions of the atoms of the absorbing material. This electron is ejected from its orbit. The empty orbital position is filled by a "cascading" inward movement of electrons from the outer shell positions. As this inward movement occurs, additional energy is released. The photoelectric effect increases with the atomic number, Z, of the absorbing material. In fact, it increases in proportion to Z^3. Therefore, it follows that bone, which is composed of high Z materials, attenuates radiation much more readily than water, which is composed of low Z materials, in the energy ranges dominated by the photoelectric effect. This gradient of attenuation of the radiation beam by materials of varied Z produces the radiographic image as variable amounts of radiation penetrate the target material to expose the x-ray plate.

For several reasons, the photoelectric effect is not usually useful for radiation oncology. First, the low energies at which it occurs do not penetrate in adequate amounts to affect deeply located tumors. Furthermore, radiation that interacts primarily with matter through the photoelectric effect is preferentially absorbed by high Z materials. Such preferential absorption leads to an inhomogeneous distribution. If a tumor were to extend from soft tissue to bone, as much as two times as much radiation would be absorbed in bone as in the soft tissue component of the tumor.

B. Compton Effect: The interaction of radiation with matter that is of primary importance to radiation oncology is termed the Compton effect. In this case, incident radiation interacts with the atoms of the absorbing material to eject an outer shell electron. This outer shell electron acquires kinetic energy from the incident photon and either directly or indirectly through an intermediate reaction with a water molecule causes chemical bond breaks that can ultimately lead to cell death in the absorbing material.

This Compton reaction is primarily important to therapeutic radiology because it predominates at the energies commonly used for therapeutic purposes. Radiation at these energies is more penetrating and can impact on deeply seated tumors. Fortunately, it is also essentially independent from the atomic numbers of the radiated material. Thus, a tumor extending to involve both soft tissues and bone composed of atoms with varied Z's will receive a homogeneous dose of radiation.

C. Pair Production: This process is the third type of interaction of incident radiation with its target material. Pair production requires an energy of at least 1.02 MeV. It becomes more frequent at energies higher than 10 MeV. It therefore is not important to diagnostic radiology and occurs only with the highest energy therapy units.

When an incident photon of at least 1.02 MeV interacts with the *nucleus* of the absorbing material, the photon's energy can be converted into matter with the production of a pair of particles: a negatively charged electron and a positively charged positron. This energized pair of particles goes on to react with other atoms in the tissues to cause ionization and excitation. Ultimately the positron reacts with an electron in the tissues, resulting in the annihilation of both and the release of energy as two photons that can cause additional ionizations.

RADIATION BIOLOGY

General Principles

When ionizing radiation, either electromagnetic or particulate, is incident on tissues, a complex series of events is initiated that, if successful, leads to destruction of tumor cells and ultimately eradication of the tumor. The critical cellular target is believed to be the nucleus and its concentration of DNA.

The so-called **direct effect** occurs when an energetic electron resulting from a Compton reaction interacts directly with the target nucleus, and chemical changes (mostly breakage of chemical bonds) result within the DNA substance. The **indirect effect** occurs when the Compton electron reacts with a water molecule within the tissues, and a highly reactive free radical results. This free radical, usually a hydroxyl molecule, then reacts with DNA in the nucleus of a target cell to effect chemical bond breakage and set in action those changes which will lead to cellular death.

For either the direct or the indirect effect to be successful, the damage inflicted must not be repaired by the target cell's chemical reparative mechanisms and must be of sufficient severity to result in cell death. Some damage is termed **single-strand DNA breaks.** As its name implies, this damage is done to only one strand of the paired DNA chains. Most of these breaks are thought to be successfully repaired. It is also believed that **double-strand DNA breaks** occur in which both paired DNA chains sustain breaks in chemical bonds in close proximity to each other. This type of cellular damage is believed to be irreparable.

Cellular death due to radiation is characterized as

either **interphase death** or **reproductive death.** Interphase death occurs promptly and usually requires very high doses of radiation exposure. In the range of doses used in therapeutic radiation, it probably occurs consistently only in the case of lymphocytes and germ cells, which are unusually radiosensitive. The mechanism by which interphase death occurs is unknown.

Induction of reproductive death is the primary mechanism by which ionizing radiation has a therapeutic impact on tumors. Reproductive death occurs only in cells that are mitotically active or can be recruited to become active. For an individual cell to sustain a reproductive death, it must suffer such severe damage to the DNA composing its chromosomes that it cannot successfully replicate and no viable daughter cells can be generated. In reality an occasional cell may undergo one or two successful mitoses before succumbing to lethal radiation damage. Cells suffering reproductive death lose their ability to go on reproducing indefinitely. Such cells are said to be no longer clonogenic.

Relative Biologic Effectiveness (RBE)

Just as no two drugs will have the same biologic impact milligram for milligram, two different types or two different energies of radiation will not have the same biologic effect centigray for centigray. By convention, 250-kVP x-rays are the standard to which other types of radiation are compared. For the type of radiation in question, the dose required to produce the same biologic effect as a given dose of 250-kVP x-rays is compared mathematically:

$$RBE = \frac{\text{Dose of 250 kVP x-rays}}{\text{Dose of radiation in question}}$$

If the RBE is greater than 1, a lower dose of the type of radiation in question will cause the same biologic effects as the dose of 250-kVP x-rays. Likewise, if the RBE is less than 1, a dose greater than the dose of 250-kVP x-rays will be required to effect the same biologic changes.

Linear Energy Transfer (LET)

Not all incident radiation deposits its energy with the same linear density along the pathway it traverses in tissues. LET is the quantity used to describe these differences in the density of deposited energy. LET is equal to the amount of energy absorbed per unit length of penetration into the absorbing material. Typically x-rays and gamma rays are sparsely ionizing and have LETs on the order of one keV/μm (thousand electron volts per micrometer). Particulate radiation has typically higher LETs. For particulate radiation, LETs generally increase with increasing mass and charge. Neutrons have LETs on the order of 10 keV/μm, and alpha particles have LETs typically

around 100 keV/μm. Typically, radiation possessing a high LET also has a high RBE.

Cell Cycle & Radiosensitivity

Five distinct stages or positions of cells within the cell cycle (Figure 11–2) have been described: **M** represents mitosis, **S** is the DNA synthetic phase, **G_1** is a resting phase between M and S, **G_2** is another apparent resting phase between S and M, and **G_0** is also a resting phase. It occurs in cells that are not actively reproducing. Cells can rejoin the active phases of the cell cycle from G_0. Several investigators have shown that cells are most sensitive to radiation damage in M and G_2 and most resistant in late S. Cells in G_1 and early S are intermediate in their radiosensitivity.

Oxygen Effect

Hypoxic cells are not as sensitive to radiation damage as are well-oxygenated cells. It is generally accepted that the resistance of certain tumors, especially tumors that have grown to a large size, is at least in part due to the tendency of tumors "to outgrow their blood supply." Such large tumors often develop a necrotic core of hypoxic but viable cells.

A factor termed the oxygen enhancement ratio has been described to quantify the magnitude of the effect of oxygen tensions on the sensitivity of cells to radiation. Well-oxygenated cells are as much as 2.5–3 times as sensitive to radiation as are hypoxic cells. Most of this increased sensitization occurs as oxygen tensions increase to about 20 mm Hg, with only a gradual increase in sensitivity beyond 20 mm Hg.

Oxygen is the most potent radiosensitizer known. In the 1960s, trials were conducted in which radiation was delivered to patients in hyperbaric chambers. These chambers were usually compressed to 3 atm

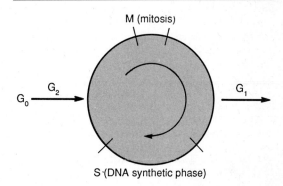

Figure 11–2. The cell cycle varies from 1 to 5 days for most human tumors. This value should not be confused with clinical volume doubling time, since it does not include cell loss factors or an allowance for growth factor. Growth factor is that percentage of cells that are actively proceeding through the cell cycle and averages only about 30%. Cell loss factor includes exfoliation and cell death due to necrosis and random effects.

absolute pressure, at which the patients breathed 100% oxygen. These studies for the most part demonstrated improved local tumor control. Unfortunately, there was also an attendant higher incidence of complications. Since such treatments were cumbersome and failed to show a selective sensitization of the tumor relative to normal tissue, the use of hyperbaric oxygen as a clinical radiation sensitizer has been largely abandoned.

Cell Survival Curve

Figure 11–3 shows an idealized plot of radiation dose versus proportion of cells surviving after radia-

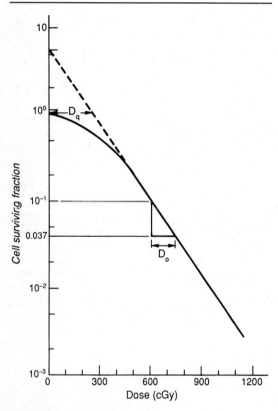

Figure 11–3. Idealized cell survival curve for photon radiation. Plot shows a logarithmic increase in cell kill as dose increases linearly. Certain parameters defined on the cell survival curve are characteristic for a given cell line. D_o is the dose that reduces the number of surviving cells to 37% of the original number. For mammalian cells, D_o generally varies from 100 to 200 cGy. D_q is obtained by extending the straight line portion of the plot upward and determining the dose at which this extension crosses the 100% value of the y axis plot. This value is termed the quasi–threshold dose. If the straight line portion of the plot is extended further until it intersects the y axis, the extrapolation number N is obtained. D_q typically varies from 300 to 700 cGy, and N typically varies from 2 to 20. Both D_q and N define the initial curved portion of the curve. This "shoulder" represents an accumulation of sublethal damage further modified by reparative efforts of the radiated cells.

tion exposure. Initially, the plot has a curved shoulder. This portion of the plot is commonly believed to demonstrate the accumulation of sublethal damage and effects of the simultaneous repair of some of this sublethal damage. A straight line plot follows the initial curved shoulder. On this semilogarithmic plot, a straight line is indicative of a logarithmic relationship of cell kill to a linear increase in dose. Several variables (as defined in the figure legend) can be quantitated for a given cell line to delineate its individual radiosensitivity. Not only will such plots vary from cell type to cell type, but for a given cell line, they can be shown to vary according to nutritional state, oxygen tension, or proportion of cells within a given phase of the cell cycle.

Hyperthermia

In the late 19th century, Coley reported dramatic but anecdotal tumor responses in patients in whom hyperthermia was induced by injection with bacterial toxins. Since that time intermittent attempts have been made to utilize hyperthermia as a treatment for malignancies either as a single modality or in combination with other modalities, especially radiation. Over the past 20 years, renewal of interest in hyperthermia has taken place. Both laboratory and clinical studies have shown promise especially when hyperthermia is used as a radiosensitizer.

As a single modality hyperthermia appears to have very limited application. There does appear to be a potentially useful synergism between certain cytotoxic chemotherapeutic agents and hyperthermia; however, the clinical experience combining chemotherapy with hyperthermia is limited so far.

Hyperthermia can be administered locally, regionally, or systemically. Most of the clinical experience to date has been with locally delivered hyperthermia. Local and regional heating is most frequently accomplished by microwave, ultrasound, or radiofrequency applicators. With external applicators, the delivery of a thermal dose is limited to a useful penetration of about 3 cm for microwaves and up to about 6 cm under optimal conditions for ultrasound. Improved delivery to larger tumors can be achieved with implanted microwave or radiofrequency probes. Such implanted hyperthermia devices combine especially well with interstitial radiotherapy, since the same implanted catheters can serve to carry the hyperthermia apparatus or the radioactive isotopes.

Regional hyperthermia has been less well investigated, but assemblies for regional heating consisting of several yoked microwave or ultrasound applicators are now commercially available. Such an apparatus has the multiple applicators arranged in a circular fashion with the patient positioned at the center of the circle. In this manner, the heat energy can be focused within a deep-seated tumor. A significant problem, however, exists for temperature monitoring. As yet there is no reliable technique for noninvasive thermometry, and thermometric probes must be invasively inserted into the tumor to ensure delivery of an appropriate thermal dose.

Systemic hyperthermia has also been attempted with techniques such as application of hot wax baths, use of thermal blankets, and use of radiant coil heating chambers. A unique system that creates hyperthermia with radiant heating while cooling the skin with convective currents is commercially available. Its primary advantage is the addition of skin cooling, which substantially reduces the systemic toxicity often seen with whole-body hyperthermia.

Several characteristics of hyperthermia make it especially well suited for combination with radiation for a synergistic effect. S phase cells (which are most resistant to radiation) are most sensitive to the effects of hyperthermia. Hyperthermia also selectively sensitizes other cells that are inherently radioresistant, ie, hypoxic cells and cells in a low pH environment. Finally, owing to the immature and disorganized nature of tumor vascularity, tumors appear to be preferentially heated. This selective heating of the tumor is due to the apparent inability of its blood vessels to vasodilate and carry off applied heat by convection.

A common hyperthermia treatment regimen for local or regional application is to heat the target volume to a temperature of 42.5–43 °C for 60 minutes. For whole-body hyperthermia, the maximum temperature appears to be limited to 42 °C owing to liver and central nervous system toxicity. An average whole-body hyperthermia treatment lasts about 2 hours. When combined with radiation, a typical course of hyperthermia varies from two to 10 total treatments. Hyperthermia treatments to any one site should be separated by at least 72 hours to allow for dissipation of the phenomenon of thermal tolerance. Studies have shown that cells develop increased tolerance to thermal effects with repeated applications; however, most of the original thermal sensitivity is restored if at least 72 hours transpires between thermal applications. Some experts advocate even longer intervals between treatments to further reduce the effect of thermal tolerance.

When used as a radiosensitizer, the heat treatment must also be timed with reference to the radiation treatment. The highest degree of radiation sensitization occurs when heat and radiation are simultaneously delivered. Clinically this arrangement is cumbersome. Significant sensitization occurs if the radiation is given within a time window extending from about 20 minutes before to 20 minutes after the heat treatment. Typically, the patient will be radiated first and the hyperthermia given just after the radiation. The radiation dose fractionation schemes used with hyperthermia have been variable. Both hypofractionated courses of 400 cGy twice weekly as well as conventional fractionation schemes of 180–200 cGy daily 5 days a week have been combined with one or two hyperthermia treatments per week. In pre-

viously irradiated tissues, standard-dose fractionation is considered preferable by this author.

The most frequent clinical application of hyperthermia to date has been in combination with radiation in the re-treatment of chest wall recurrences of breast cancer. A second nearly fall course of radiation therapy utilizing an electron beam generally can be safely tolerated when combined with hyperthermia. Many other tumor sites and histologic types have shown good response to hyperthermia and radiation. Perhaps the most potentially fruitful use of hyperthermia as a radiosensitizer will be with melanomas and sarcomas, which usually are resistant to radiation alone.

The toxicity of local hyperthermia is directly related to the thermal effect. Problems have been limited to pain during treatment, thermal blisters, and ulceration. The incidence of serious burns (beyond first degree) has been reported in only about 5–10% of cases.

Although hyperthermia appears to be a promising modality, for it to gain wide application, many technical problems must be resolved to permit the delivery of a thermal dose to a deep-seated tumor with adequate, reliable, and preferably noninvasive thermometry.

Other Radiation Sensitizers

A number of chemical compounds have been investigated as potential radiosensitizers. As a class, the most widely studied have been the **nitroimidazoles.** These drugs owe their radiation sensitizing properties to their oxygenlike electron affinic nature and, therefore, sensitize only hypoxic cells. A common antimicrobial agent, metronidazole, belongs to this group and has radiosensitizing properties when given in very large doses. Another drug of this class, misonidazole, has been studied thoroughly and been the subject of several phase III trials by the Radiation Therapy Oncology Group.

The study of two new nitroimidazoles, SR2508 primarily in the USA and RO-03-8799 primarily in Great Britain, is being conducted in hopes of achieving clinically significant levels of radiation sensitization along with tolerable levels of toxicity. Neurotoxicity, primarily peripheral in nature, has been the major stumbling block to the integration of these agents into the clinical management of patients receiving radiation.

Many cytotoxic chemotherapeutic agents also sensitize tissues to radiation effects. The mechanisms by which certain chemotherapeutic agents may act as radiosensitizers are diverse. Halogenated pyrimidines such as 5-bromodeoxyuridine (BUDR) and 5-iododeoxyuridine (IUDR) when incorporated into the DNA molecule may make chromosomal DNA inherently more susceptible to chemical bond breaks owing to incident radiation. Other agents may inhibit the repair of sublethal radiation damage. Drugs that have been shown to potentiate the effects of radiation included actinomycin, doxorubicin, bleomycin, cisplatin, hydroxyurea, methotrexate, and fluorouracil.

CLINICAL RADIATION ONCOLOGY

Process of Radiation Oncology

The practice of radiation oncology involves many discrete activities. The steps involved often occur concurrently rather than sequentially.

A. Consultation: The delivery of radiation for therapeutic purposes is a multistep process; it begins with the consultation. The radiation oncologist should independently evaluate the patient, confirm the diagnosis, verify the stage of the tumor, and determine whether additional diagnostic studies are necessary or desirable to evaluate the patient as a candidate for radiation. On the basis of these studies, the radiation oncologist will determine whether the goal of therapy will be cure or palliation. Preferably, a multidisciplinary tumor board will convene to discuss the integration of surgery, chemotherapy, and radiation for optimal effect.

B. Definition and Localization of Treatment Volume: Once radiation has been determined to be appropriate for a given patient, the next step is definition and localization of the treatment volume (Figure 11–4). This step begins with careful clinical evaluation, palpation of the tumor if possible, and critical interpretation of all imaging studies. The culmination occurs in the radiotherapy simulator, where the physician, radiation physicist, and technologist combine their expertise to localize the treatment volume, consider the optimal patient position during treatment, and begin to design the shape, size, and direction of the treatment portals. Careful localization and measurement of the tumor dimensions and shape, and the position of limiting normal anatomy are essential to this step.

C. Treatment Planning: The radiation physicist using all the measured parameters of the tumor and the patient's anatomy constructs several computer simulations of treatment approaches. Such trial plans may include multiple fields, mixed photon and electron beams, dynamic therapy, custom blocks, wedges, tissue compensators, and other beam modification devices. The physician reviews these plans to select the one that combines the best dose distribution to define tumor volume along with optimal protection from overdosage to critical normal structures (Figure 11–5).

D. Verification of Treatment Plan: This step may require another session in the simulator to obtain diagnostic quality verification films. Alternatively, for simple plans, a verification or port film might be taken on the therapy machine (Figure 11–6). Radiation dosimeters may be applied to the patient to verify

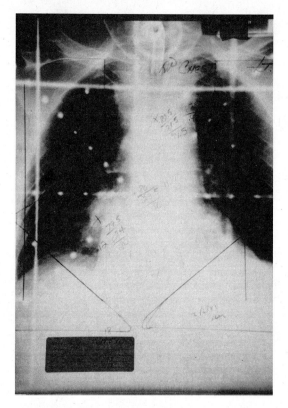

Figure 11–4. Simulator film defining treatment volume for a bronchogenic carcinoma. In addition to the primary tumor, both hili and mediastinum are included in the initial radiation treatment volume.

that the dose predicted by the computer plan is accurate for a particular anatomic location. A phantom such as that shown in Figure 11–7 can be used in a mock treatment to ensure that the desired dose is delivered to the tumor while critical normal structures are protected. Phantoms can be as simple as water tanks or they can be complex synthetic structures designed to mimic human anatomy. In either case, they permit the placement of dosimeters for direct measurements to verify calculated doses in human tissues.

E. Construction of Beam-Modifying Devices: Wedges or custom tissue compensators that make up for differences in body part thickness or density are often fabricated or added at this stage. If custom blocks are required, they are drawn by the physician on the verification films and molded by a trained technician.

F. Treatment: During the treatment phase, it is essential that continuous quality assurance checks be made. All ancillary treatment devices must be properly used. The patient and treatment portals must be

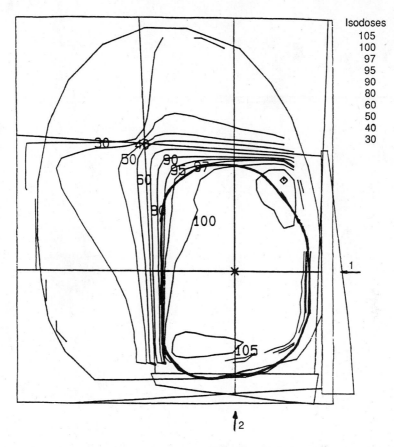

Isodoses
105
100
97
95
90
80
60
50
40
30

Figure 11–5. Plot demonstrating relative radiation dose delivered to a primary brain tumor and the surrounding normal brain parenchyma. Doses are normalized to the 100% dose line labeled "100." Other doses are indicated as percentages of the 100% isodose. The treatment target volume is delineated by the bold line, and the entire plot is a representation of the brain in cross section. The technique demonstrated here is called the wedged pair technique and is simple but useful. When the tumor is located in a quadrant, two perpendicular radiation beams are designed to intersect within the tumor. The beams are attenuated by the wedges in proportion to the thickness of the wedge. In this fashion, the radiation dosage is concentrated within the tumor and an abrupt decrease in the dose beyond the tumor volume spares normal brain tissue.

accurately and reproducibly positioned. Figure 11–8 shows the relation of the simulation film to the template and special blocks constructed to treat a specific patient. For curative treatments, especially when radiation portals are small or difficult to reproduce, weekly verification portal films should be obtained. During the treatment phase, the patient must be continually evaluated for both tumor response and untoward effects of treatment. Convention requires a weekly evaluation. However, the patient must be assured that the radiation oncologist is available at any time to deal with complications of treatment.

G. Posttreatment Evaluation: Initially, the patient is followed at frequent intervals varying from 1 week to 2–3 months, depending on the clinical situation and tumor type and stage. Once the patient is fully recovered from any acute complications, does not show any troublesome chronic effects, and dem-

onstrates durable control of the tumor, the interval of follow-up appointments may be increased. However, even after 5 years of tumor control, it is recommended that the patient continue to be seen once a year. This continued evaluation is important to detect any late complications. It also serves to encourage the clinician, as well as patients who are currently under treatment, that cancer often is a curable disorder.

Equipment Required

A modern radiation oncology center contains a wide variety of therapy units to individualize treatment to a given tumor in a given anatomic site.

A. Simulator: The radiation therapy simulator is a diagnostic x-ray unit having the same geometry as therapy units. Most patients begin radiotherapy treatment by entering the simulator to have their tumor localized and radiation ports designed. With precise

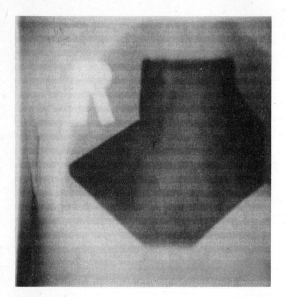

Figure 11–6. This x-ray is a specialized image commonly called a port film, which is generated by exposing an x-ray film cassette to the treatment beam. Since the x-ray energies used for therapy are much higher than the optimal energies used for imaging, such a port film does not show good diagnostic detail. However, since it is taken on the treatment machine during the treatment, it is the best assurance to the radiation oncologist that the desired volume of tissue is receiving a therapeutic dose of radiation. The radiation oncologist will compare such a port film to the diagnostic quality simulator film (Figure 11–4).

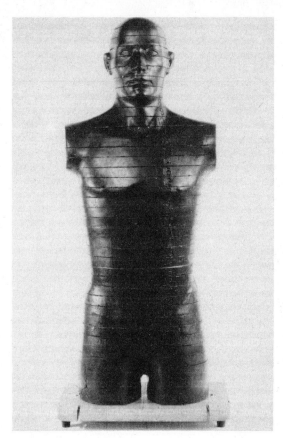

Figure 11–7. This phantom is constructed of thin slabs of tissue-equivalent material stacked to form a three-dimensional facsimile of the human anatomy. Within the slabs composing the phantom, hundreds of small wells are provided into which dosimeters may be placed. Without any exposure to a patient, a radiation therapy plan can be precisely verified by "treating" the phantom. During this mock treatment, dosimeters are placed in the phantom in locations equivalent to the position of the tumor and normal tissues of concern within the patient. The measured doses are compared to those predicted by the plan to verify the accuracy of the treatment plan.

measurements, x-ray imaging verification, and a thorough understanding of anatomy, the radiation oncologist with the support of the radiation physicist and technologist designs a treatment plan that may involve multiple fields with intersecting beams or even dynamic treatment in which the therapy unit rotates around the patient to deliver the appropriate dose to a tumor and at the same time protect vital normal structures.

B. Orthovoltage: Orthovoltage machines typically produce x-rays in the 100- to 250-kVP range. Although for most applications they have been replaced by more modern units, they are still used to treat skin cancers and other superficial disorders.

C. Teletherapy: Teletherapy machines, today essentially consisting only of cobalt units, contain a very high activity radioisotope source in the machine head. In order to treat, a shutterlike device is opened exposing the patient to the gamma rays produced by the isotope. The radiation field can be shaped or collimated to deliver the desired treatment volume. Cobalt units are dependable and relatively inexpensive. They still have application in treating tumors in body parts that are not too thick. Typically, tumors of the brain, tumors of the head and neck, and certain bone metastases are treated with cobalt. Since the photons

produced are in the mid energy range, these units provide some skin sparing and improved depth dose characteristics over orthovoltage.

Cobalt units do not have the same penetrability as higher energy units and are not generally suited for treating deep-seated tumors in thick body parts. Cobalt units also have fixed outputs leading to dose rate deliveries that are not variable and decrease as the source decays. Because of cobalt's half-life of less than 6 years, cobalt sources are typically replaced every 3–5 years.

Because the cobalt source is not a point source but rather a cylinder with a diameter of 1–2 cm, the edge of the cobalt treatment beam is not sharp. This char-

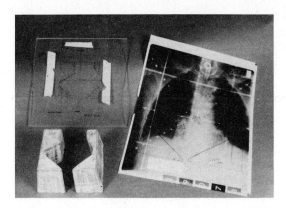

Figure 11–8. At right is the simulator film defining treatment volume (Figure 11–5). In the upper left is a template produced from the simulator film. It is inserted into the blocking tray on the head of the therapy machine. Custom lead alloy blocks are then molded from the simulator film. During treatment they are positioned by placing them on the template. In this way, the radiation field is shaped to deliver radiation to the target volume and protect nearby normal structures.

acteristic is called the beam's penumbra. It is the penumbra that makes it difficult to match two adjacent radiation ports without either a "cold spot" of underdosage or a "hot spot" of overdosage.

D. Linear Accelerator: Linear accelerators are state-of-the-art radiotherapy equipment. They produce x-rays by accelerating electrons and focusing them on a target. These electrons interact with the nuclei of the target material to produce x-rays. By using a wave guide rather than electrical potential differences, accelerators can produce electrons possessing

many million electron volts of energy. These high-energy electrons produce x-rays with a peak energy equal to their own kinetic energy. A wide selection of x-ray energies are commercially available ranging from about 4 to 25 MeV.

For high-energy x-rays produced in this fashion, both depth dose and skin sparing are improved over cobalt and orthovoltage units. Dose rate is also variable and may be adjusted typically from 100 to 1000 cGy per minute.

A final advantage of the x-ray beam produced by the linear accelerator is that the beam edge is very sharp. This is especially useful when matching adjacent fields over a critical organ such as the spinal cord where neither an underdosage nor an overdosage can be tolerated. For this reason, extended field radiotherapy such as total nodal treatment for Hodgkin's disease requiring the matching of adjacent fields should be given by linear accelerator rather than cobalt teletherapy.

A comparison of depth-dose characteristics and skin sparing for orthovoltage, cobalt, and linear accelerator energies was given in Figure 11–1. By removing the target from the stream of electrons, high-energy linear accelerators usually have the capability of producing an electron beam for therapeutic purposes. A typical machine can produce four or five different electron energies. Electrons are useful primarily in treating superficial tumors. As shown in Figure 11–9, electron beams offer little or no skin sparing. The depth-dose curve plateaus just below the surface, and the extent of the plateau is a function of the electron energy. Beyond the plateau, the dose then falls off rapidly as depth increases. When a superficial tumor is situated over an organ with poor radiation tolerance or little remaining tolerance owing to previous treatment, the electron beam energy with the ap-

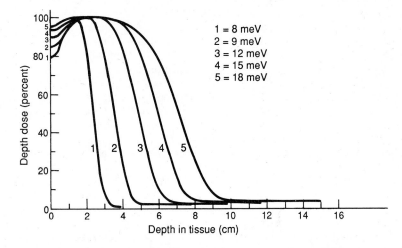

Figure 11–9. Depth-dose plot for electrons. Depending on the depth of the tumor and the tolerance of the tissues lying deep to the tumor, the optimal electron beam energy is selected for a given situation. Compare to the plot shown in Figure 11–1 for differences between electron and photon radiation ports.

propriate depth-dose characteristics can be selected for treatment.

E. Cyclotron: In a very few research facilities, cyclotrons are available to produce particle beams for radiation therapy. Although many particle beams have been produced, including carbon, argon, silicon, and helium ions, only neutron- and proton-beam therapy have had reasonable clinical investigation. A potential advantage for neutron therapy is based on its biologic characteristics of reduced oxygen enhancement ratio and increased relative biologic effectiveness. Proton-beam therapy is attractive because of the sharply focused nature of dose deposition. Neutrons have shown a possible clinical advantage in the treatment of salivary gland and prostate tumors. For protons, the radiation demonstrates a sharp increase in dose as the particle approaches the limit of its range in tissue. This rapid increase of dose deposition is termed the **Bragg peak.** Because of this very concentrated deposition of radiation, protons have their greatest potential in treating a tumor adjacent to a critical organ where the dose must be sharply truncated. Proton therapy appears to have an advantage in treating ocular melanomas and certain tumors involving or adjacent to the spinal cord.

The ultimate role of proton, neutron, and other types of heavy particle beam therapy is not known. It is unlikely that such treatment will in the near future attain wide application owing to its complexity, expense, and marginal advantage over standard radiotherapy in most instances.

Brachytherapy

Brachytherapy, or implant radiation, can be characterized as either intracavitary or interstitial. In either case, a radioactive isotope sealed within a "seed" or a metallic capsule is placed within a body cavity immediately next to the tumor or actually within the tumor itself. The therapeutic advantage of such therapy is based primarily on two factors. First, a high dose of radiation can be delivered to a tumor over a shorter time. Typically, 1000–2000 cGy is delivered in a 24-hour period rather than over 1–2 weeks. Second, the radiation dose can be precisely focused or concentrated within the tumor, with rapid fall-off of radiation dose to surrounding normal structures owing to attenuation and the physical principle of the inverse square law.

Intracavitary brachytherapy can be applied to any accessible body cavity, eg, bronchus, esophagus, uterus, or vagina. The most frequent application has been in the treatment of gynecologic tumors such as cervical and endometrial cancer. Intracavitary brachytherapy is often combined with external radiotherapy and is often utilized as the booster to deliver a higher dose to the volume of gross tumor involvement. By using the intracavitary application to boost such pelvic tumors, a high dose may be given to the tumor while little additional dose is given to critical normal tissues such as the bladder and rectum. Intracavitary radiotherapy has recently received increased application in the treatment of obstructing lesions of the bronchus and esophagus. Such treatment has been particularly advantageous for recurrent tumors that have previously received full-course external radiation. Even though no useful tolerance to further external radiotherapy remains, a palliative course of additional radiation is possible with the precise focusing of the additional dose possible with intracavitary brachytherapy.

Interstitial brachytherapy is the term applied to the insertion of a sealed radioactive isotope directly into the tumor. Interstitial radiotherapy can be accomplished with the insertion of seeds, usually radioactive gold or iodine, as a permanent implant into the tumor volume. Alternatively, a temporary implant can be carried out by first inserting a carrier such as a nylon catheter into the tumor. Once the radiation oncologist is satisfied that the catheters have been optimally located in or near the tumor, these catheters can then be "afterloaded" with the radioactive isotope. This placement of the isotope usually takes place in the patient's room, with radiation exposure to only the individual inserting the isotopes. Exposure to medical personnel is reduced by delaying the loading of the catheters until the patient has been returned to a private, specially shielded hospital room.

Interstitial radiotherapy is commonly used in brain, head and neck, breast, prostate, and bladder tumors. Most frequently the implant is combined with a prior course of external radiation, again with the implant serving as the boost when more than microscopic tumor is present. As with intracavitary brachytherapy, interstitial brachytherapy, because of its closely contained dose, can sometimes be used for tumors recurrent after previous radiotherapy even though little or no tolerance remains for additional external radiotherapy.

Isotopes for permanent implants have either low energy, and therefore limited penetrance in tissue, or short half-lives. One or the other of these characteristics is necessary to make a permanent implant practical from the perspective of safety. The patient must not be a hazard to others once discharged from the hospital.

Radium, once the most frequently used isotope, has fallen out of favor primarily owing to the potential danger of leakage of radon gas from the radium capsule if the integrity of the radium tube is damaged. Table 11–1 describes the common radioisotopes used for brachytherapy.

Radiation Dose Fractionation & Time-Dose Considerations

A. Standard Fractionation: A standard dose fractionation scheme for a curative course of external radiation is one treatment per day, 5 treatments per week, consisting of 180–200 cGy per treatment.

Table 11–1. Common radioactive isotopes used for brachytherapy.

Isotope	Effective Energy	Half-Life	Application	Source Configuration
Radium (^{256}Ra)	0.83 meV	1622 years	Intracavitary gynecologic Interstitial head and neck Breast and others No longer popular because of radiation safety concerns	Needles, tubes
Cesium (^{137}Cs)	0.6 meV	30 years	Intracavitary gynecologic	Tubes, needles
Iodine (^{125}I)	0.035 meV	60 days	Permanent implant Prostate and others Special high-activity source Temporary brain implants Temporary eye plaque for melanoma	Seeds
Gold (^{198}Au)	0.42 meV	2.7 days	Prostate and other Permanent implants	Plaque Seeds
Iridium (^{192}Ir)	0.38 meV	74 days	Temporary implants Breast, brain, prostate, others	Wire, seeds Ribbon
Cobalt (^{60}Co)	1.25 meV	5.3 years	Ocular melanoma High-activity source in remote afterloading system applied to many tumors.	Plaque Tube

Total dose may range from 2500 cGy for subclinical disease in seminomas to 7000 cGy for sarcomas or bulky carcinomas (Table 11–2). Not only tumor histology but also tumor size determines the appropriate dose. For implant radiation therapy (brachytherapy), tumor doses may range as high as 15,000–20,000 cGy; however, the radiation in this case is given slowly and continuously. It takes nearly a year to deliver the dose with a permanent implant with an isotope such as ^{125}I, which has a half-life of about 60 days.

When patients are irradiated for palliative rather than curative intent, the radiation course is usually shortened by increasing the dose per treatment (fraction size) from 180–200 cGy to 300–400 cGy. The intent of such alteration is to complete treatment

Table 11–2. Typical radiation doses for selected tumors.

Tumor	Dose	Remarks
Wilms'	1000–2000 cGy (occasionally up to 3800 cGy)	Used as part of combined modality approach; limited usually to residual disease or patients with unfavorable prognostic signs.
Seminoma	2500–3500 cGy	Primarily applied in stage I or II macroscopic nodal disease or potential microscopic disease below the diaphragm.
Hodgkin's disease	3500–4500 cGy	Used primary modality in most stage I and II and some stage III disease; used for consolidation of some with bulk disease treated with primary chemotherapy.
Non-Hodgkin lymphoma	3000–5000 cGy	Employed as primary therapy in rare stage I; combined with chemotherapy for cure of certain aggressive histologic types; used as palliation for certain indolent histologic types.
Head and neck	5000–7000 cGy	Used primary treatment for certain stage I and II patients. Combined with surgery in most stage III and IV patients. Offered as palliation in advanced inoperable cases.
Breast	5000–6000 cGy	Combined with lumpectomy for tumors ≤ 4 cm. Used postmastectomy for select patients at high risk for local recurrence.
Esophagus	5000–7000 cGy	Often used alone or with chemotherapy as primary treatment; also as adjunct to surgery pre- or postoperatively.
Cell lung	5000–7000 cGy	Employed as adjunct to surgery with positive nodes or margins, as primary treatment for certain stage I, II, and III patients, as palliation in stage IV.
Small-cell lung	5000–6000 cGy (lung) 2400–3000 cGy (brain)	Used as adjunct to chemotherapy in limited disease with chest consolidation and brain prophylaxis; palliative in extensive stage.
Pelvic (cervix, endo-metrium, bladder, prostate, rectum, anus)	5000–7000 cGy	Whole pelvis often treated to 5000 cGy with boost to macroscopic disease. Often used as adjunct to surgery with positive margins or nodes. Often used externally combined with brachytherapy.
Brain	5000–7000 cGy	Generally combined with surgery and often chemotherapy. Lower doses given for lymphomas and higher doses for gliomas.
Sarcoma	6000–7000 cGy	Used as adjunct to surgery pre- or postoperatively. Sometimes combined with chemotherapy.
Brain and bone metastases	3000–5000 cGy	Accelerated course often appropriate in patients with poor performance status and short longevity.

quickly in order to alleviate pain or improve organ or tissue function. It is also desirable to complete treatment rapidly and not exhaust a patient with terminal disease by a protracted course of irradiation. A typical palliative dose for brain or bone metastases is 3000 cGy in 10 treatments over 2 weeks. Such a scheme has a stronger biologic impact on both the tumor and surrounding normal tissues than 3000 cGy given at 200 cGy/d. In terms of tumor effect it may be equivalent to 3600–4000 cGy given at a normal daily dose. It is also likely to cause a higher incidence of late complications if the patient survives more than 1 year. By carefully assessing the patient and understanding the short-term prognosis, the radiation oncologist can select those patients who will best be served by a course of radiation consisting of a higher dose per fraction and a lower number of treatments.

B. Altered Radiation Fractionation Schemes: Since the mid 1970s, a serious reexamination of the optimal dose fractionation scheme for radiation therapy has taken place.

1. Split Course Radiotherapy–Beginning about 20 years ago, a variation of radiation fractionation termed split-course radiotherapy was investigated in several cooperative group trials. Often fraction size was increased over the usual 200 cGy. A planned break from treatment lasting 2–3 weeks was introduced about midway through the treatment course. This interruption of treatment was intended to prevent or minimize acute reactions. It was also believed that during this period tumor shrinkage would result in reoxygenation and increased radiosensitivity. Such a treatment course was tolerated better acutely; however, local tumor control was usually worsened, and this regime has been largely abandoned.

2. Hyperfractionation–In hyperfractionated regimens, approximately the same daily dose is given but the dose is divided into more than one fraction—usually two—per day. A common treatment regimen is 120 cGy twice a day. The treatment course is accomplished in about the same overall time as a standard course, and the total dose is increased by 10–20%. Daily treatments should be separated by at least 4 and preferably 6 hours to allow for the repair of sublethal damage of the so-called late tissues. Late tissues are tissues such as those of the central nervous system that are not actively cycling. These tissues do not generally demonstrate much acute toxicity owing to little or no mitotic activity but may show significant late complications. Since the dose per fraction of radiation is a large determinant of late radiation damage, late complications are reduced by hyperfractionation. Malignant cells do not appear to possess repair mechanisms that are as good as those of normal tissues, and because of this relatively poor repair capacity, tumors may be more successfully irradiated by hyperfractionated regimens. Several studies report

improved tumor control when hyperfractionated radiation is given.

3. Accelerated Fractionation–Accelerated fractionation occurs when nearly the same total dose as in a standard radiation regimen is given over a shortened period of time. Accelerated treatment is usually given by treating the patient more than once per day on at least a few days per week. A common treatment protocol is two treatments of 160 cGy/d with each fraction delivered to the same radiation target volume. Another regimen, termed the concurrent boost, delivers 180–200 cGy per day to a larger radiation field, with a smaller dose of 150 cGy or so given to a reduced boost volume as a second treatment 2 or 3 days per week. As with hyperfractionated courses, when more than one treatment is given per day, treatments should be separated by at least 4 and preferably 6 hours. Because of increased acute toxicities (mucositis and radiation dermatitis), such a treatment regimen may necessitate a break from treatment during the third or fourth week of treatment. This break must be kept as short as possible to ensure the best therapeutic result. Accelerated radiation is most useful in rapidly growing tumors for which, by shortening an overall treatment course by about 1 week, the additional repopulation and growth that would occur during the additional week is avoided.

Radiation Complications

Ionizing radiation is a potent therapeutic modality with attendant potentially serious or lethal complications when improperly utilized. Even when scrupulously administered, therapeutic radiation can cause troublesome or debilitating morbidity. Such serious complications occur in about 5% of patients receiving therapeutic radiation. A few broad principles to apply when considering radiation complications are presented below.

Such a general principle requires that in order to assess an untoward reaction in a given anatomic site as a radiation side effect that part must be receiving or have received radiation in the past. It is frustrating for the radiation oncologist and unproductive for the patient when all untoward symptoms experienced by the patient are attributed to radiation. For example, a patient receiving radiation for a lung cancer will not become nauseated or vomit as a result of radiation exposure, since neither the stomach nor the small bowel is commonly included in a radiation portal for bronchogenic cancer. Such a patient, however, may be nauseated owing to unknown hepatic metastases, and the discovery of these metastases may be delayed if the symptoms are mistakenly attributed to a radiation effect. Although radiation and chemotherapy often cause similar complications, eg, nausea, alopecia, marrow suppression, and mucositis, radiation can only do so when the affected target organ is included in the radiation portals. Chemotherapy is potentially systemic in therapeutic effect and complications, whereas radiation has local or regional therapeutic effects and side effects.

Radiation effects should also be classified as **acute** or **late reactions.** Acute reactions generally have their onset either during the later phases of treatment or just after completion of treatment. Late reactions may occur 6 months to 1 year after completion of therapy or any time thereafter. Acute reactions occur predominantly in tissues with a high level of mitotic activity. These tissues, like tumors, are sensitive to immediate radiation effects in direct proportion to their frequency of mitotic activity. Skin and the mucosa of the gastrointestinal tract from the mouth to the anus are tissues that cycle rapidly. Acute radiation dermatitis, mucositis, pharyngitis, proctitis, and enteritis generally occur during or just after the completion of radiation. They can be severe enough to interrupt the course of treatment. They are treated symptomatically. Typically, they are self-limited and resolve within about 2–4 weeks after completion of radiation.

Late radiation complications are not self-limited and tend to progress with time. The most serious include transverse myelitis of the spinal cord, brain necrosis, and severe radiation cystitis or enteritis. In general, no treatment is available to restore function, and often removal of the damaged part, if possible, is the only option. Some promising experience using hyperbaric oxygen to support debridement or removal of necrotic irradiated mandible and to support bony reconstruction of the mandible has been reported.

Late radiation complications are thought to be due to an indirect effect secondary to vascular compromise as a result of radiation-induced end arteritis and stromal fibrosis. Some experts now believe that at least some late radiation damage is due to a delayed direct effect on parenchymal cells, with a resultant decrease in cellularity and degradation of function.

Because no broadly effective treatment for chronic radiation complications is available, the radiation oncologist must anticipate the possibility of late damage and prevent its occurrence. Prevention is usually accomplished by reduction in radiation dosage. When a resistant tumor, such as a sarcoma requiring at least 7000 cGy, is located next to a tissue such as the spinal cord that the radiation oncologist is unwilling to treat to a dose in excess of 4500 cGy, the obvious result is a dissatisfying underdosage to the tumor. Table 11–3 lists the practical tolerance doses for common limiting organs. These tolerances assume a standard dose fractionation scheme consisting of 180–200 cGy per day, 5 days per week. For each tissue, the tolerance is applicable to either the entire organ or a specific length or cross-sectional area of the organ.

Furthermore, it must be remembered that the tolerance of certain tissues to radiation is lowered when treatment is combined with either surgery or chemotherapy. For example, the heart of a patient who has

Table 11–3. Practical radiation tolerance of common dose-limiting organs.

Organ	Practical Tolerance	Potential Toxicity
Brain (whole)	6000 cGy	Necrosis, infarction, leukoencephalopathy
Spinal cord (10-cm length)	4500 cGy	Transverse myelitis, necrosis, infarction
Heart (entire organ) (25%)	4000 cGy 7000 cGy	Pericarditis, myocardiopathy Pancarditis
Lung (whole)[1]	2000 cGy	Pneumonitis, fibrosis
Small bowel (400 cm² cross section)	4500 cGy	Ulcer, perforation, fistula, necrosis
Stomach (100 cm² cross section)	4500 cGy	Ulcer, perforation, necrosis
Rectum (100 cm² cross section)	6000 cGy	Stricture, ulcer, necrosis
Liver (whole)	2500 cGy	Acute and chronic hepatitis
Kidney (whole)	2000 cGy	Hypertension, chronic renal failure, proteinuria
Bladder (whole)	6000 cGy	Contracture, ulcer, necrosis
Lens of the eye (whole)	500 cGy	Cataract
Retina (whole)	5500 cGy	Infarction, necrosis
Cornea (whole)	5000 cGy	Ulceration, necrosis
Bone marrow[2]	250 cGy (whole) 4000 cGy (segmental)	Pancytopenia Myelofibrosis

[1]Smaller segments of the lung may be treated to higher doses without symptomatic pneumonitis. Significant fibrosis and permanent hypofunction occurs for those portions of the lung treated to doses greater than 2000 cGy, but adequate reserve may be available outside the radiation ports.

[2]If doses to the whole body and therefore to all the marrow exceed 400 cGy, approximately 50% of those so irradiated will die without marrow transplant. For segmental radiation, it is possible that portions of the marrow that exceed 4000 cGy are never repopulated successfully by marrow stem cells owing to myelofibrosis.

received doxorubicin chemotherapy will not tolerate as high a radiation dose as the heart of a patient who has not. In addition, when a patient is receiving preoperative irradiation for a head and neck tumor prior to a neck dissection, most radiation oncologists will limit the dose to 5000 cGy in order to prevent an unacceptable incidence of surgical complications.

Future Directions

Common misconceptions hold that therapeutic radiation has only palliative benefit and that radiation will be made obsolete by improved systemic therapies. In fact, about half of patients who receive radiation today are treated with curative intent. As new chemotherapeutic agents and biologic response modifiers are developed to treat tumors with potentially systemic extension, radiation as a local and regional control modality will assume an even more vital role in the curative treatment of malignancies. A need for consolidative radiation to sites of bulk disease following effective systemic treatment is already established in small-cell lung cancer and certain lymphomas.

Research areas of promise include altered fractionation schemes, particle beam therapy, radiation sensitizers, extended field radiotherapy, intraoperative radiation, and radiolabeled monoclonal antibodies. Monoclonal antibodies tagged with radioactive isotopes will carry radiation selectively to the tumor. This approach has both therapeutic and diagnostic applications. More closely than any other approach it approximates the development of the "magic bullet"

that attacks only the tumor and has little or no toxicity for normal tissues.

In the short run, increased use of radiotherapy often combined with chemotherapy and limited surgery in lieu of radical resection or amputation offers much promise. The intent is not improved cure rates but rather comparable cure rates accompanied by improved quality of life due to the preservation of a functional limb or organ. Such an approach has come to fruition in breast conservation and limb preservation with sarcomas. There are expectations of similarly successful approaches to the management of anal, esophageal, and early rectal cancers.

REFERENCES

Biologic Effects of Ionization Radiation Committee: *The Effects on Populations of Exposure to Low Levels of Ionizing Radiations.* National Academy of Sciences/National Research Council, Washington DC, 1980.

Brady LW: The changing role of radiation oncology in cancer management. *CA* 1983;**33**:2.

Coleman CN et al: Phase I trial of the hypoxic radiosensitizer SR 2508: The results of the five to six week drug schedule. *Int J Radiat Oncol Biol Phys* 1986;**12**:1105.

Cox JD et al: Complications of radiation therapy and factors in their prevention. *World J Surg* 1986;**10**:171.

Hall EJ: *Radiobiology for the Radiologist.* Harper & Row, 1988.

Johns H, Cunningham J (editors): *The Physics of Radiology,* 4th ed. Charles C Thomas, 1983.

Khan FM: *The Physics of Radiation Therapy.* Williams & Wilkins, 1984.

Kinsella TJ et al: Continuous intravenous infusions of bromodeoxyuridine as a clinical radiosensitizer. *J Clin Oncol* 1984;**2**:1144.

Knee R, Fields RS, Peters LJ: Concomitant boost radiotherapy for advanced squamous cell carcinoma of the head and neck. *Radiother Oncol* 1985;**4**:1.

Laramore GE et al: Fast neutron radiotherapy for advanced carcinomas of the prostate: Results of an RTOG randomized clinical trial. *Int J Radiat Oncol Biol Phys* 1985;**11**:1621.

Moss WT, Cox JD (editors): *Radiation Oncology: Rationale, Technique, Results,* 6th ed. Mosby, 1989.

Order SE, Leibel S: Radiolabeled antibodies in the treatment of primary liver cancer. *Appl Radiol* 1984;**15**:67.

Perez CA, Emmami B, Von Gerichten D: Clinical results with irradiation and local hyperthermia in cancer therapy. In: *Proceedings of Fourth International Symposium on Hyperthermic Oncology,* Vol 1, Summary Papers. Overgaard J (editor). 1984.

Perez CA, Brady LW (editors): *Principles and Practice of Radiation Oncology,* 2nd ed. Lippincott, 1991.

Rubin P: Late effects of chemotherapy and radiation therapy: A new hypothesis. *Int J Radiat Oncol Biol Phys* 1984;**10**:1.

Tucker M et al: Bone sarcomas linked to radiotherapy and chemotherapy in children. *N Engl J Med* 1987;**317**:588.

Wang CC, Blitfer PH, Swit H: Twice-a-day radiation therapy for cancer of the head and neck. *Cancer* 1985;**55**:2100.

Medical Oncology

12

Daniel D. Von Hoff, MD

The practicing oncologist is often at the center of the patient management team and as such is looked upon to design and coordinate the management plan. This chapter briefly outlines certain principles under which the medical oncologist should operate in this role.

NEVER TREAT WITHOUT A HISTOLOGIC DIAGNOSIS

The first critical step in evaluating the patient is to determine if the patient has cancer and, if so, of what histologic type. The diagnostic procedure to obtain tissue for histologic diagnosis should be the safest, least invasive procedure possible. However, the material obtained must be adequate to make the diagnosis with absolute certainly. Extreme caution in making the diagnosis of cancer is necessary when the diagnosis is based on only a few cells obtained for cytologic study (sputum, urine, etc) or a few cells obtained by a needle aspiration. When there is any doubt, obtain tissue for examination.

The principle of obtaining a histologic diagnosis is particularly important in the evaluation of a person who has had a cancer in the past and develops a new symptom or sign (eg, a new pulmonary nodule). It is important to document whether this new symptom or sign represents a recurrence of the patient's original tumor, represents a different type of cancer, or perhaps is not cancer at all. This determination can be made only by a biopsy of the suspicious area.

ALWAYS CAREFULLY STAGE THE PATIENT

This principle seems obvious, but in the physician's zest to want to do something for the patient it often is not adhered to. Once the presence of a malignancy has been established, the patient should have all necessary procedures to document where the tumor is. Not only will this help determine the most appropriate treatment, but it may also prevent future complications that could seriously affect the patient's quality of life (eg, an unsuspected lytic lesion in the femur that could go on to fracture and incapacitate an otherwise mobile patient).

In carrying out the staging procedures, keep in mind the natural history of the disease. For example, it is extremely unusual for colorectal cancer to be metastatic to the skeleton, so a bone survey would not be indicated in the initial staging procedure. That is, of course, unless the patient is complaining of bone pain in a certain area, in which case a film of that area should be obtained.

In planning the staging workup, keep in mind the various treatments for the various stages of the disease. For example, in staging a patient with lymphoma, if bone marrow aspiration and biopsy are performed and a tumor is found in the bone marrow, it is not necessary to obtain a lymphangiogram. The treatment for the patient would have to be chemotherapy because of the organ (bone marrow) involvement, and performing a lymphangiogram would not help in the patient's management.

The stage of the patient should be carefully recorded to avoid confusion about how treatment decisions were made. In addition, tumor measurements recorded by the staging procedures provide an important baseline for determining whether the patient is responding to the selected therapy.

USE A COMBINED MODALITY APPROACH

The most obvious individuals involved in the care of the cancer patient are the medical oncologist, the radiation oncologist, and the surgical oncologist. Other members of the combined modality team include the oncology nurse, the psychological support representative, and the social worker. The best way to foster the combined modality approach forum is the use of a special conference (also called a combined modality conference or tumor board in some hospitals) at which all patients and their management are discussed in detail. This approach provides for optimal patient care.

REMEMBER COMPASSION & QUALITY OF LIFE

The issues of quality of life and the impact of the treatment on quality of life are always issues for discussion between the patient and the physician. It has been well documented that physicians tend to overestimate the survival of their patients by a factor of 3 or 4 times the actual survival of the patient. Obviously this optimism plays some role in the selection of treatment for the patient. Remember that an important aspect of whether or not a treatment can help a patient is the condition of the patient at the time of treatment initiation. One measure of the patient's overall condition is the patient's performance status. This simple measure has been clearly documented to correlate with patient survival and chance for a response to treatment. Performance status as measured by the Karnofsky scale, Eastern Cooperative Oncology Group (Zubrod) scale, or Southwest Oncology Group criteria should be assessed and should be a major factor in determining the patient's management.

The issues of quality of life and pain control are rapidly developing areas of research in medical oncology. The major problem has been development of instruments to measure these two parameters. Clinical trials to validate such instruments are ongoing.

MAXIMIZE THE PATIENT'S TREATMENT

If the decision is made to treat, treatment should be given with the maximum intensity possible. The relationship between dose-intensity and response to chemotherapy has been well documented, and therefore administering as much treatment in as short a period as possible is an important concept.

MAKE THE PATIENT COUNT

Only about 3% of patients who are eligible for organized clinical trials are actually placed on those studies. The National Cancer Institute has started new programs to encourage entry of patients onto high-priority clinical trials. However, the most important person in initiating this process is the clinician seeing the patient. It is essential that the patient be counted somewhere and treated in a standardized manner so that more effective treatment can be provided in the future.

REFERENCES

Amer MH, Al Sarraf M, Vaitkevicius VK: Factors that affect response to chemotherapy and survival of patients with advanced head and neck cancer. *Cancer* 1979;**43**:2202.

Coates A et al: On the receiving end. 2. Linear analogue self-assessment (LASA) in evaluation of aspects of the quality of life of cancer patients receiving therapy. *Eur J Cancer Clin Oncol* 1983;**19**:1633.

Finkelstein DM, Ettinger DS, Ruckdeschel JC: Long term survivors in metastatic non-small cell lung cancer: An Eastern Cooperative Oncology Group study. *J Clin Oncol* 1986;**4**:702.

Hryniuk WM: More is better. *J Clin Oncol* 1988;**6**:1365.

Parker CM: Accuracy of predictions of survival in later stages of cancer. *Br Med J* 1972;**2**:29.

Tannock IF et al: A randomized trial of two dose levels of cyclosphosphamide, methotrexate, and fluorouracil chemotherapy for patients with metastatic breast cancer. *J Clin Oncol* 1988;**6**:1377.

Wooley PV, Schein PF: *Methods in Cancer Research*. Academic Press, 1979.

Bone Marrow Transplantation

13

William P. Peters, MD, PhD

Bone marrow transplantation is a medical supportive procedure in which hematopoietic stem cells, usually as bone marrow, are administered to patients to treat a bone marrow production deficiency state. This procedure is used in the treatment of primary marrow deficiency states such as aplastic anemia and paroxysmal nocturnal hemoglobinuria, in the treatment of several inborn errors of metabolism, and as a rescue procedure during the intensive treatment of various malignant conditions, including the acute and chronic leukemias, lymphoma, myeloma, neuroblastoma, and certain solid tumors, The application of bone marrow transplants has become widespread, the technology is generally well established, and for selected patients it represents state-of-the-art therapy.

Rationale

For nonmalignant disorders, bone marrow transplantation is intended to provide a functional bone marrow capable of restoring normal hematopoietic or enzymatic function. For example, in primary immunodeficiency diseases such as severe combined immunodeficiency disease (SCID) or Wiskott-Aldrich syndrome, bone marrow transplantation is capable of restoring normal immunologic function by supplying a replacement for a genetically defective precursor in the immune system. In this setting, the restoration of normal immunologic function can usually be complete. In other nonmalignant settings, such as aplastic anemia, in which immunologic function is not fully deficient, immunosuppression is required for administration of an exogenous graft in order to prevent the development of immunologically mediated adverse consequences. When donor stem cells are transplanted, transfer of immunocompetent lymphocytes and macrophages also occurs. Not only is there danger of rejection of the graft by the host but also of rejection of the host by the graft, ie, graft-versus-host disease (GVHD), which exists in both chronic and acute forms.

Marrow transplantation has found its widest application in the treatment of malignant diseases in which dose escalation of chemotherapy and radiation therapy has enabled improved antitumor results at the price of marrow ablation. The ability of high-dose therapy to eradicate malignant cells has resulted in attempts to utilize allogeneic, syngeneic, or autologous marrow as rescue techniques to permit the successful application of this treatment. In the acute and chronic leukemias, involvement of bone marrow with malignant cells led to the early development of the use of HLA-matched allogeneic marrow (obtained from another individual) or syngeneic marrow (obtained from an identical twin) as the primary rescue technique. More recently, with the development of immunologic and pharmacologic methods of "purging" bone marrow (ie, removing malignant cells from a person's own [autologous] marrow or of T-cell depletion from mismatched allogeneic bone marrow), improved methods of immunosuppression, and an in vivo treatment with anti-T-cell immunotoxins, the extension of this technique to patients not having an identical HLA-matched sibling donor has been possible. Critical to the development of these techniques has been the recognition that effective therapy for various diseases can be achieved by dose escalation. The infused bone marrow, of allogeneic, syngeneic, or autologous source, will restore hematopoietic and immunologic function in the transplanted individual. With allogeneic bone marrow, a therapeutic effect against the malignancy itself (graft-versus-leukemia effect) may occur from the use of transplanted bone marrow. Selected patients with malignant lymphoma (Hodgkin's and non-Hodgkin's) neuroblastoma, breast cancer, ovarian cancer, and small-cell lung cancer (Table 13–1) have also been considered for bone marrow transplant procedures.

Technique

A. Autologous Marrow Grafting: The general criterion for acceptance of a patient for autologous marrow transplantation is a malignancy that is dose-sensitive to the therapy proposed and a marrow free of malignant involvement or an ability to remove the malignant cells from the bone marrow. Animal experiments suggest that use of a cellular infusion for a marrow transplant should include 1×10^8 nucleated cells/kg. Bone marrow generally is aspirated (10–15 mL/kg) from the posterior iliac crest, and the nucleated cell fractions are separated and cryopreserved. Since small numbers of "stem cells" circulate normally, an alternative method is to harvest peripheral

Table 13–1. Diagnoses for which bone marrow transplantation is considered.

Malignant disease
    Acute nonlymphoblastic leukemia
    Acute lymphoblastic leukemia
    Chronic myelogenous leukemia
    Non-Hodgkin's lymphoma
    Hodgkin's disease
    Breast cancer
    Testicular cancer
    Ovarian cancer
    Myeloma
    Neuroblastoma
Nonmalignant disease
    Aplastic anemia
    Paroxysmal nocturnal hemoglobinuria
Genetic disease
    Severe combined immunodeficiency disease (SCID)
    Wiskott-Aldrich syndrome
    Thalassemia major
    Severe sickle-cell disease
    Selected inborn errors of metabolism (eg, Hunter's syndrome)
    Primary lysosomal storage disorders

blood progenitor cells via leukapheresis. This approach obviates the need for marrow harvesting, but it usually requires multiple procedures to obtain sufficient cells to ensure stable and reliable hematopoietic reconstitution. Recently, hematopoietic colony-stimulating factors have been used to prime the bone marrow for collection of peripheral blood progenitor cells. Patients are administered granulocyte colony-stimulating factor (G-CSF) or granulocyte-macrophage colony-stimulating factor (GM-CSF) either during or after recovery from prior chemotherapy. These cells represent primarily mature progenitors but appear to contain increased numbers of earlier hematopoietic progenitors as well. They are cryopreserved as bone marrow.

B. Syngeneic Marrow Transplantation: Syngeneic bone marrow is obtained from the donor who is a genetically identical twin. The usual criteria for establishing this status are HLA, ABO, and minor red cell antigen identity as well as the description of the placenta at the time of birth.

C. Allogeneic Marrow Transplantation: In this setting, the marrow is obtained from a donor of differing genetics. Because of the problems associated with GVHD, most marrow transplants are obtained from HLA-matched siblings. HLA-A, -B, and -Dr are defined serologically, and reactivity of the HLA-D locus is determined by a mixed leukocyte culturing technique. The genetics of the HLA system provide that one-half of a phenotype is inherited from the mother and one-half from the father; hence, within a given family, there are four possible haplotypes (assuming that low-frequency crossovers have not occurred in this region). Therefore, the chance of having an HLA-identical match in the family is approximately one in four if the number of siblings is large enough. Since family size often is lim-

ited and an HLA match cannot be identified, efforts to use alternative donor sources have been undertaken. These include identification of phenotypically identical donors from an international bone marrow transplant registry, and the use of partially matched donors in which patients who possess one haplotype genotypically identical with the parent and another haplotype phenotypically compatible with at least one of the three major loci are considered for transplantation. In these settings, the incidence of GVHD is increased, but the overall treatment results obtained thus far have not been meaningfully different from those of patients receiving an HLA identical matched transplant in some studies.

Methods for reducing the incidence of GVHD by selective removal of T cells using monoclonal antibodies have resulted in an increased incidence of graft rejection, suggesting the importance of the T cell in the engraftment process. In addition, there has been an increased frequency of relapse, again pointing to a potential role for graft-versus-leukemia as a result of allogeneic transplantation therapy. The ability of systemic infusion of anti-CD4 antibodies to suppress the GVHD process has enabled the use of allogeneic marrow transplantation across wider HLA barriers. Further studies are underway.

Marrow & Peripheral Blood Progenitor Cell Collection

Bone marrow is harvested from the posterior iliac crests under general or regional anesthesia using multiple aspirations of bone marrow. The marrow is generally screened to remove bone particles and to create a single-cell suspension. For allogeneic marrow transplantation, the marrow usually is not processed further, except when mismatching requires T-cell depletion of the marrow. For autologous bone marrow transplantation, the marrow is generally centrifuged to obtain a buffy coat preparation, mixed with 10% dimethylsulfoxide (DMSO), and cryopreserved in liquid nitrogen until use. Usually, $1–4 \times 10^8$ nucleated cells/kg are collected in this manner.

Peripheral blood progenitor cells (PBPCs) are collected via leukapheresis. The leukapheresis collections are made either at the time of measured PBPC release during recovery from a course of chemotherapy or after full hematopoietic recovery with release of PBPCs stimulated by administration of hematopoietic colony-stimulating factors, usually either G-CSF or GM-CSF. The number of cells collected is generally much higher than that obtained via bone marrow harvesting and is usually $10–80 \times 10^8$ nucleated cells/kg in most series. Cryopreservation is undertaken as described for bone marrow without further processing except for the addition of cryoprotectant.

Ex vivo treatment of the marrow by physical separations or with drugs, lectins, or antibodies may be undertaken to remove either malignant cells or immunologic subsets of cells.

While all cytotoxic drugs are being administered, the marrow is rapidly thawed to 37 °C and infused intravenously without further treatment. Infused marrow stem cells circulate through the pulmonary circulation and "home" to marrow cavities.

Treatment of Recipient

Successful bone marrow transplantation depends on (**1**) adequate treatment of the underlying neoplasm, if necessary; (**2**) a source of hematopoietic stem cells free of clonogenic malignant cells; (**3**) adequate immunosuppression to prevent rejection of allogeneic marrow; and (**4**) adequate supportive care during hematopoietic recovery.

After satisfactory collection and storage of hematopoietic progenitors, high-dose chemotherapy with or without total body irradiation is used to treat the malignancy or provide the requisite immunosuppression for marrow engraftment. Following intensive chemoradiation therapy, rapid and profound myelosuppression ensues. Hematopoietic reconstitution to a neutrophil count of >500/mm^3 usually requires 15–19 days, with thrombocytopenia persisting generally longer. Supportive care techniques vary from center to center but generally include reverse isolation, transfusional therapy, and empiric and therapeutic antibacterial and antifungal therapy. Radiation of blood products is performed to eliminate the potential for GVHD resulting from transfused blood products. Parenteral nutrition frequently is utilized, since many patients, particularly those treated with total body irradiation or with certain alkylating agents such as thiotepa or melphalan, experience severe mucositis. Recommendations for hospital facilities and for transplant team capabilities have been developed by the American Society of Clinical Oncology and the American Society of Hematology.

Results

A. Acute Leukemia: In early studies of allogeneic bone marrow transplantation in patients with acute nonlymphoblastic leukemia (ANL) or acute lymphoblastic leukemia (ALL) transplanted in resistant relapse, approximately 12% of patients remained in continuous unmaintained remission over 10 years from treatment. Transplantation is now generally performed in patients with ANL in first remission of early relapse or in patients with ALL in second or subsequent complete remission. Extended disease-free survival is seen after an allogeneic bone marrow transplant in approximately 45% of patients with AML in first complete remission with better results seen in young patients (<20 years). Results of allografting in ALL have resulted in extended disease-free survival in 27% of patients.

Autologous bone marrow transplantation has also been used in these diseases. Interpretation of avail-

able studies is complicated by differences in therapeutic regimens, differences in the interval between complete remission and autografting, and inadequate descriptions of the patient populations. Results in advanced resistant disease indicate that although complete responses occurred in more than 50% of patients, relapses were nearly universal. More recent efforts have concentrated on patients in first or second complete remission using purged or nonpurged bone marrow. A recent analysis of 263 patients with acute myelocytic leukemia, autografted in first complete remission between 1982 and 1987, reports leukemia-free survival at 3 years to be 39%, with the time to transplant from achievement of complete remission being important for studies using marrow purging. Results of autologous bone marrow transplantation in patients with acute lymphocytic lymphoblastic leukemia are less satisfactory. In a comparison of autografting to allografting in 91 patients with ALL in first through fourth remission, 20% of autografted and 27% of allografted patients became long-term disease-free survivors.

B. Lymphoma: In patients with relapsed lymphoma, many centers now indicate that the expected results are superior to those achieved with any salvage chemotherapy. In patients with high-grade malignant lymphoma, the therapeutic result of bone marrow transplantation in patients with non-Hodgkin's lymphoma appears to be related to the grade and extent of disease and its resistance to previous chemotherapy. In advanced-stage intermediate- and high-grade lymphoma, 3-year progression-free survival ranges from 20% to 60%, reflecting small study numbers and selection effects. In general, results appear superior in patients with smaller volume disease and those who respond to induction therapy.

C. Chronic Myelogenous Leukemia: Allogeneic bone marrow transplantation for chronic myelogenous leukemia (CML) in chronic phase or early relapse results in long-term disease-free survival in over 50% of treated patients. On the basis of the proposition that normal clones may exist within CML marrow, autologous bone marrow transplantation in patients with chronic myelocytic leukemia was attempted using either CML remission marrow or peripheral blood stem cell collections. Remissions of short duration were achieved, but relapse of chronic-phase leukemia is the rule.

D. Breast Cancer: Most studies in solid tumors have utilized autologous bone marrow transplantation, since marrow contamination is not universal and treatment can be targeted at the disease without the need for immunosuppression. In selected poor-prognosis patients with metastatic breast cancer, high-dose combination alkylating agent therapy results in 15–25% of patients remaining in extended remission. Patients with limited volume disease and less prior chemotherapy respond better. High-dose consolidation with cyclophosphamide, cisplatin, and carmustine with autologous bone marrow and peripheral blood progenitor cell support in the setting of high-risk primary breast cancer involving 10 or more axillary lymph nodes has been studied with an apparent benefit derived from this approach compared with contemporary or historical series. Prospective, randomized, comparative trials are in progress.

E. Other Malignancies: Autologous bone marrow transplantation has been utilized in other chemotherapy sensitive malignancies, eg, ovarian cancer, small-cell lung cancer, testicular cancer, and myeloma, with selected patients able to achieve remissions apparently superior to those with less intensive approaches. Results, however, are limited to small series often in heterogeneous patient populations.

The prognosis for children with neuroblastoma over the age of 1 year is poor, with most relapsing and dying of disease. The use of phenylalanine mustard and total body irradiation in patients with neuroblastoma, with or without marrow purging, demonstrates that 25–40% of children with neuroblastoma can remain continuously disease-free after this treatment. Relapses after 21 months have not been observed.

Complications

Complications resulting from treatment depend on the source of the marrow used, the preparative regimen, the duration of myelosuppression and immunosuppression after the transplant, and the underlying condition of the patient at the start of the transplant. Allogeneic bone marrow transplantation is associated with acute graft-versus-host disease in 20–50% of patients receiving HLA-identical transplants, which is associated with a 2.5-fold increased transplant related mortality. Patients developing acute GVHD are at higher risk for chronic GVHD, which occurs in 25–35% of patients with HLA-identical matched grafts.

Extended myelosuppression that occurs with both autologous and allogeneic bone marrow transplantation is associated with frequent bacterial and fungal infections. The incidence and frequency of these infections has been reduced by the use of the hematopoietic colony-stimulating factors, particularly G-CSF and GM-CSF, and the use of better prophylactic antibiotic regimens. Viral and protozoan infections occur most frequently during the first 6 months after transplant in recipients of both autologous and allogeneic grafts but are more common and more severe in allogeneic bone marrow transplantation. Herpes virus types 1 and 3 and cytomegalovirus are the predominant viral agents. *Pneumocystis carinii* is now less often a source of morbidity owing to effective prophylaxis with trimethoprim-sulfamethoxazole or pentamidine.

Nonhematologic toxicity resulting from the preparative regimens reflects the agents employed and their intensity. In the early period following therapy, hemorrhagic myocarditis, renal insufficiency, severe mucositis, enterocolitis, and toxic hepatitis predominate. Veno-occlusive disease, which presents clinically as right upper quadrant pain, jaundice, hepatomegaly, and ascites may be seen in 15–25% of patients. Pulmonary toxicity resulting from either radiation therapy or drugs frequently occurs 1–4 months posttransplant and is often exquisitely sensitive to corticosteroid therapy.

REFERENCES

American Society of Clinical Oncology and American Society of Hematology Recommended Criteria for the Performance of Bone Marrow Transplantation. *J Clin Oncol* 1990;**8**:563.

Dunphy FR et al: Treatment of estrogen receptor–negative or hormonally refractory breast cancer with double high-dose chemotherapy intensification and bone marrow support. *J Clin Oncol* 1990;**8**:1207.

Franzone P et al: Chemo-radiotherapy and autologous bone marrow transplantation in poor prognosis neuroblastoma. *Radiother Oncol* 1990;**18**:102.

Gale RP, Armitage JO, Dicke KA: Autotransplants: Now and in the future. *Bone Marrow Transplantation* 1991;**7**:153.

Gianni AM et al: Growth factor–supported high-dose sequential (HDS) adjuvant chemotherapy in breast cancer with ≥10 positive nodes. *Proc Am Soc Clin Oncol* 1992;**11**:60.

Gorin NC et al: Autologous bone marrow transplantation for acute myelocytic leukemia in first remission: A European survey of the role of marrow purging. *Blood* 1990;**75**:1606.

Gratwohl A et al: Bone marrow transplantation for leukemia in Europe: Report from the Leukemia Working Party 1987. *Bone Marrow Transplantation* 1987;**2(Suppl 1)**:15.

Peters WP et al: Adjuvant chemotherapy involving high-dose combination cyclophosphamide, cisplatin and carmustine, and autologous bone marrow support for stage II/III breast cancer involving ten or more lymph nodes (CALGB 8782): A preliminary report. *Proc Am Soc Clin Oncol* 1990;**9**:22.

Peters WP et al: High-dose alkylating agents and autologous bone marrow support (ABMS) for Stage II/III Breast Cancer involving 10 or more axillary lymph nodes. *Proc Am Soc Clin Oncol* 1992;**11**:58.

Peters WP et al: High-dose combination alkylating agents with bone marrow support as initial treatment for metastatic breast cancer. *J Clin Oncol* 1988;**6**:1368.

Peters WP et al: Strategies in the treatment of breast cancer with intensive chemotherapy and autologous bone marrow support. Pages 465–474 in: *Autologous Bone Marrow Transplantation: Proceedings of the Fourth International Symposium.* Dicke KA et al (editors). MD Anderson Hospital Press, 1987.

Pinkerton CR et al: High-dose chemo-radiotherapy with bone marrow rescue in stage IV neuroblastoma: EBMT Survey, 1988. Pages 543–548 in: *Autologous Bone Marrow Transplantation: Proceedings of the Fourth International Symposium.* Dicke KA et al (editors). MD Anderson Hospital Press, 1989.

Thomas ED et al: Marrow transplantation for the treatment of chronic myelogenous leukemia. *Ann Intern Med* 1986;**104:**155.

Thomas ED et al: Marrow transplantation for patients with acute lymphoblastic leukemia: A long-term follow-up. *Blood* 1983;**62:**1139.

Section IV.
Drugs in the Treatment of Cancer

Chemotherapy

14

Geoffrey R. Weiss, MD

Chemotherapy broadly includes the use of anticancer pharmaceuticals that possess cytotoxic or cytocidal activity. As a discipline of anticancer therapy, chemotherapy shares a position with surgery and radiation therapy as a primary form of treatment. Over more than 40 years of evolution, chemotherapy has emerged as the major systemic weapon against cancer. In that time, it has moved from a form of treatment relegated to the management of only advanced or disseminated cancers to become additionally an important component of the multidisciplinary care of the early cancer patient. This chapter is intended to provide the fundamental concepts and tools necessary to the aggressive and effective use of chemotherapy in the safest manner possible.

The wartime use of chemical weapons, in particular mustard gases with very high tissue alkylating and cytotoxic activity, was accompanied by the clinical observation that potent systemic effects occurred in the victims suffering skin or respiratory exposure. Bone marrow suppression and lymphoid cytotoxicity were the major consequences of exposure that stimulated the greatest clinical interest. Gilman conducted the first clinical trials of nitrogen mustard for cancer treatment. Farber at the Boston Children's Hospital was among the first clinicians to explore the utility of antifols in childhood leukemia. The effects were prompt and dramatic. Leukemias frequently entered remission for short periods. However, the brevity of remission and the uniformly fatal outcome for the treated patients led to the creation of anticancer drug screening programs devoted to the systematic evaluation of these cytotoxic agents alone and in combination with other anticancer agents. More recently, chemotherapy has proved its value in the palliative and in the curative treatment of childhood leukemias, some adult leukemias, Hodgkin's and non-Hodgkin's lymphomas, testis cancer, and a small proportion of small-cell lung cancers. In the USA, large cooperative organizations of cancer treatment facilities have been sponsored by the National Cancer Institute to conduct major studies of high-priority clinical cancer trials. These organizations are designed to rapidly test new concepts in cancer treatment, to provide definitive answers to important therapeutic questions, and to develop treatment concepts that will have impact upon cancer treatment in general. It is now clear from the work of cooperative groups that chemotherapy is unlikely to stand alone as a treatment for the most common cancers afflicting patients today but will serve as a systemic component of the multidisciplinary management of cancer.

PHARMACOLOGIC PRINCIPLES OF ANTICANCER DRUG USE

Therapeutic Index

Anticancer agents are unique among pharmaceutical products insofar as they are applied with the intent of exploiting subtle differences in cell biology between the malignant cell and the normal cell. Both types of cells exist in a host whose aggregate physiology and metabolism affect the behavior of systemically administered drugs, including anticancer agents. The purpose of chemotherapeutic treatment is to administer the largest dose of drug possible that will be effective in killing the largest number of cancer cells while inducing reversible and tolerable toxicity in the host. For most anticancer agents, there is a very narrow margin between doses of an agent that produce significant toxicity in the host and those that achieve important cancer-killing results. The theoretical width of this margin is termed the **therapeutic index** of a drug and is a reflection of a variety of host, tumor, and drug interactions (Figure 14–1). The margin between the induction of host toxicity and the accomplishment of maximum anticancer effect is not fixed for drug, host, or type of cancer. It is conditioned by route and schedule of drug administration, drug metabolism, intrinsic sensitivity of the tumor to the agent, and health of the patient, among other factors. The clinician's responsibility is to assess as much as possible the contribution of all these factors and to administer treatment in a manner that maximizes tumor killing and minimizes host toxicity.

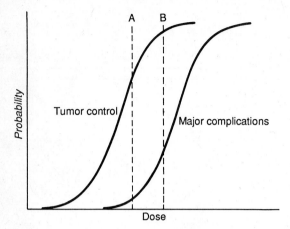

Figure 14–1. Sigmoid curves of tumor control and complications. **A:** Dose for tumor control with minimum complications. **B:** Maximum tumor dose with significant complications. (Reproduced, with permission, from Hellman S: Principles of radiation therapy. Page 263 in: *Cancer: Principles & Practice of Oncology,* 3rd ed. DeVita VT, Hellman S, Rosenberg SA [editors]. Lippincott, 1989.)

Kinetics

It has been well documented experimentally and clinically that anticancer agents do not destroy all cancer cells in the host following each administered dose. Rather, each dose of drug will kill a fixed proportion of the tumor cells in the host. The manner in which an anticancer agent produces tumor cell killing follows "first-order kinetics", ie, tumor killing is dependent upon drug dosage, and a given dosage of drug will kill a constant fraction of the remaining tumor cells. Consequently, complete eradication of tumor will not occur until sufficient drug has been administered to accomplish theoretical destruction of a "fraction" of the last remaining cell (Figure 14–2). In practice, it is extraordinarily difficult to document the fraction of tumor cells killed with each dose of the drug, and it is extremely unlikely that the proportion of destroyed tumor cells remain constant with continued treatment. The theoretical destruction of all tumor cells in the host is a consequence of multiple factors and reflects a complex set of interactions between the host and the tumor. The interaction may include or may be modified by (**1**) acquisition of resistance to the anticancer drug by the tumor, (**2**) acquisition of cumulative toxicity to the drug by the host, (**3**) presence of tumor in anatomic sites that are sanctuaries from drug effect, (**4**) expression of host drug metabolism unfavorable to optimal drug effect, (**5**) suboptimal health of the host, (**6**) alteration of the rate of growth of the tumor, and (**7**) other unknown or undefined factors.

Anticancer Drug Resistance

The inability to achieve complete tumor destruction and cure of cancer in patients afflicted with the commonest tumors appears to be largely a manifestation of preexisting or acquired anticancer drug resis-

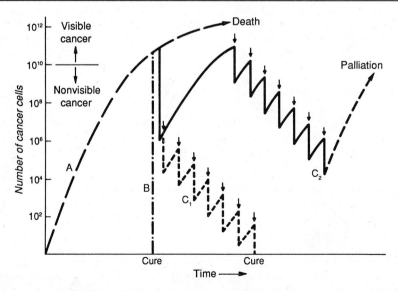

Figure 14–2. Schematic representation of heterogeneity of drug response in human cancer. Curve A shows the growth curve for an untreated cancer. Line B shows the result of successful local treatment prior to metastatic spread. Lines C_1 and C_2 illustrate two ways of adding systemic chemotherapy (vertical arrows) to local treatment. Line C_1 shows the effect of systemic chemotherapy used immediately after local treatment in patients at high risk of recurrence from occult micrometastases (adjuvant treatment). (Reproduced, with permission, from Haskell CM: Introduction. Page 5 in: *Cancer Treatment,* 3rd ed. Haskell CM [editor]. Saunders. 1990.)

tance in the tumor. Tumor cells may effectively utilize existing cellular detoxification mechanisms to avoid the adverse effects of the drugs. In fact, tumor cells may acquire the ability to amplify these detoxification mechanisms above basal levels. Tumor drug resistance may involve single or multiple contributions from the following recognized mechanisms: (1) reduction of drug entry or transport into tumor cells, (2) increased drug efflux from the tumor cell, (3) increased intracellular degradation of the drug, (4) increased production of tumor target proteins of the drug, (5) enhanced repair of drug injury to the tumor cell, (6) inadequate conversion of the drug to the active derivative, and (7) utilization of alternative biochemical pathways not inhibited by the drug.

An understanding of anticancer drug resistance is currently a focus of clinical and experimental cancer research. Insights into the manner by which tumor cells accomplish resistance to anticancer agents may help develop strategies for overcoming these impediments to effective cancer treatment. For example, a protein of MW170 (P-170) has been detected in some tumor cells that have acquired resistance to the drugs doxorubicin and the *Vinca* alkaloids. It has been learned that the P-170 protein is a transport protein responsible for the enhanced efflux of these drugs from the cancer cell. Conceivably, a monoclonal antibody might be raised against this protein, be delivered to the host bearing a tumor expressing P-170, and thereby effectively restore tumor sensitivity to the drugs.

Pharmacokinetics

Although the development of anticancer drug resistance may render an agent impotent in the clinical setting no matter how aggressively or innovatively the agent is delivered, the routine administration of drug therapy for cancer demands a basic knowledge of pharmacology to exploit the full potency of the available agents against drug-sensitive cells. Anticancer agents may be broadly categorized into two groups: (1) cycle-specific agents, ie, drugs that exert their antitumor activity at certain phases of the cycle of the dividing cancer cell and (2) cycle-nonspecific agents, ie, drugs that possess antitumor activity against tumor cells in any state of cellular division or rest. In general, nearly all anticancer agents exhibit some dependence on the fraction of cells in the proliferative state although radiation and alkylating agents have the capacity to kill cancer cells in all phases of the cell cycle. Antimetabolites and some antitumor antibiotics exhibit specific tumor killing only on cells that have entered certain phases of the cell cycle.

Another important concept applicable to both experimental and clinical situations is the observation that the same degree of cytotoxicity and toxicity may occur over a considerable range of drug concentrations (C) and durations of exposure (T), ie, $C \times T =$ Constant. Alterations in drug dosages and in times of administration may be accomplished with equivalent toxicity or with no loss in cytotoxic potency if the $C \times T$ constancy is preserved.

Finally, because most anticancer agents used in clinical practice kill tumor cells consistently with first-order kinetics, slight variations in dosage may have profound effects on the efficiency of cell destruction. Specifically, a linear increase or decrease in drug dosage may produce a log increase or decrease in tumor cell killing, respectively (log-linear relationship). For example, if a given dose of drug kills 9% of the cells in a tumor, a doubling of the drug dosage will kill 99% of the cells. Consequently, drug dosage and scheduling should strive to achieve maximum drug exposure ($C \times T$) on a schedule (dose-rate) consistent with the best host tolerance of toxicity.

Although drug administration might reasonably be scheduled to exploit drug-sensitive cellular events and thereby enhance tumor cell killing, in practice, drug administration schedules have been empirically derived to permit sufficient time for host recovery from toxicity and to comply with patient and physician schedules.

Combination Chemotherapy

It is now well recognized that combinations of anticancer agents may more than additively increase the cytotoxic potency of each of the agents alone. This is particularly clear in the chemotherapeutic treatment of breast cancer, lymphoma, testis cancer, bladder cancer, small-cell lung cancer, and acute leukemia. However, in order to preserve the individual utility and potency of each agent alone, the following principles must be adhered to:

(1) Drugs that are reasonably active against a cancer when used alone should be included in the combination regimen.

(2) Drugs whose toxicities do not overlap should be utilized.

(3) Dose rate for the combination regimen should remain as consistent as possible and the interval between courses of treatment as tight as possible.

(4) Drugs should be used in a manner reproducing their optimal dosage and schedule as single agents.

The above approach ensures exploitation of all the factors contributing to maximal cell kill, best tolerance of toxicity in the host, and least opportunity for development of tumor resistance.

ANTICANCER AGENTS

The commonly used anticancer agents fall into several broad groups whose component drugs share similar mechanisms of action. The common theme among most anticancer agents is a capacity to induce, either directly or indirectly, potentially lethal damage upon tumor cell DNA. These groups are classified as plant alkaloids, antibiotics, antimetabolites, alkylating agents, and enzymes. The specific mechanisms of action, toxicities, and pharmacology of the drugs within each group are discussed generally in the following paragraphs. Each drug is listed specifically in Table 14–1.

Plant Alkaloids

Alkaloids isolated from many plant species have provided potent and useful natural products for a variety of clinical conditions for centuries. The major anticancer alkaloids include the *Vinca* alkaloids (vincristine, vinblastine, vindesine), isolated from *Vinca rosea*, and the epipodophyllotoxins (etoposide, teniposide), isolated from the mandrake plant. The *Vinca* alkaloids bind to tubulin, the protein that forms the spindle along which chromosomes migrate during mitosis, and lead to its dissolution. The epipodophyllotoxins do not appear to bind to tubulin but are more directly toxic to DNA, causing strand breaks. The alkaloids act predominantly during metaphase and are therefore cell cycle–specific agents.

The *Vinca* alkaloids vary in the types of toxicities they produce. Vincristine may induce peripheral and autonomic neuropathies. Vinblastine causes primarily bone marrow toxicity, oral mucositis, and less commonly neuropathy. Vindesine produces myelosupression and neurotoxicity intermediate between that of vincristine and vinblastine. The dose-limiting toxicity for both epipodophyllotoxins is leukopenia. They may also produce mild thrombocytopenia, mild nausea and vomiting, and mild peripheral neuropathy.

The *Vinca* alkaloids are excreted in very small amounts in the urine. All drugs appear to undergo metabolism before excretion, vincristine by the liver with excretion in the feces, vinblastine and vindesine by less well defined methods. The epipodophyllotoxins are more extensively excreted in the urine (up to 45%), and both drugs undergo some hepatic metabolism before excretion although up to one-third of etoposide may be excreted unchanged.

Antibiotics

The anticancer antibiotics are a group of drugs derived from the fungus genus *Streptomyces*. Additional antibiotic drugs have been made synthetically to exploit known chemically active nuclei of these agents. The antibiotics exhibit a wide range of biologic and biochemical properties but appear to share characteristics of DNA intercalation and free-radical formation that individually or together induce DNA damage leading to failure of DNA replication and transcription or RNA translation. Among the most clinically important antibiotics are bleomycin (a mixture of small-molecular-weight peptides), anthraquinones (including the anthracyclines daunomycin and doxorubicin, and mitoxantrone), mitomycin, and dactinomycin (actinomycin D).

The toxicities of these agents vary, are sometimes severe, and are some of the major reasons for limitations to the clinical usefulness of these agents. Except for bleomycin, all of the antibiotics are myelosuppressive (usually maximal 10–20 days after drug administration, delayed 20–35 days for mitomycin). Nausea, vomiting, oral mucositis, alopecia, and tissue necrosis with subcutaneous extravasation are toxicities frequently but variably observed following use of these agents (Table 14–1). A specifically noteworthy toxicity of bleomycin is chronic pneumonitis that may progress to pulmonary fibrosis. It may be particularly severe in elderly individuals, those with chronic lung disease, recipients of lung or mediastinal irradiation, and patients exposed to high oxygen tensions (during surgery with endotracheal anesthesia or during mechanical ventilation). A similar but infrequent pneumonitis may be observed after mitomycin administration. Dactinomycin may also interact with radiation to produce not only a delayed or "recall" pneumonitis but may also produce independently hepatotoxicity, gastrointestinal toxicity, and skin toxicity. As well, skin toxicity is not uncommonly observed with bleomycin administration. It may cause marked peeling of the skin, increased pigmentation, and erythema. The anthraquinones cause both acute and chronic cardiotoxicities. The acute toxicities may manifest as rhythm disturbances, conduction abnormalities, acute heart failure, myocardial infarction, or pericarditis. The chronic cardiomyopathy is cumulative and dose-related; when the dosage of doxorubicin reaches or exceeds 550 mg/m^2, the incidence of cardiotoxicity increases exponentially. Mitomycin causes an acceleration of cardiotoxicity when coadministered with doxorubicin. This antibiotic may also cause a rare nephrotoxicity, at times associated with a microangiopathic hemolytic anemia that can be fatal.

All of the antibiotics may be administered by intravenous injection; bleomycin is the only antibiotic that may be injected intramuscularly or subcutaneously. Bleomycin is excreted largely unchanged in the urine, and dosage should be altered in patients with impaired renal function. None of the other antibiotics undergoes significant renal excretion, and dosage is not routinely adjusted for renal impairment. The anthraquinones are metabolized in the liver, and the native drugs and their matabolites are predominantly excreted in the bile and feces and in smaller quantities in the urine. Consequently, hepatic dysfunction demands dosage reduction or avoidance of anthraquinone administration. The clinical pharmacologies of dactinomycin and mitomycin are insufficiently defined to provide guidelines for dosage adjustment in the setting of liver or renal impairment; for both agents, clearance is rapid and defined by rates of tissue binding or metabolism.

Table 14–1. Common anticancer chemotherapeutic agents.[1]

Note: The drug dosages in this table are ranges used in clinical practice and are not offered as recommended dosages. The administration of these drugs should be under the supervision of physicians experienced in their clinical use.

Agent	Dosage	Category and Action	Common Toxicities	Other Toxicities	Metabolism	Disease
Asparaginase (Elspar)	1000–20,000 IU/m² IV daily for 1–40 days	Enzyme. Depletion of nonessential amino acid L-asparagine; inhibition of protein synthesis.	Nausea, vomiting, fever, chills; inhibition of protein synthesis (albumin, insulin, clotting factors); disorientation, coma, seizures; liver function abnormalities	Hypersensitivity (urticaria, bronchospasm, hypotension), pancreatitis	Unclear; trace excretion in urine	Chilhood acute leukemia
Azacytidine	150–300 mg/m² IV daily for 3–5 days	Antimetabolite. Substrate for RNA synthetase, incorporated into RNA.	Myelosuppression, nausea, vomiting	Liver function abnormalities, fever, rash myalgias	Unclear; rapidly removed from plasma	Adult nonlymphocytic leukemia
Bleomycin (Blenoxane)	5–15 units/m² IV, IM, or SC weekly	Antibiotic. DNA strand breakage.	Pneumonitis, pulmonary fibrosis; skin erythema, peeling, hyperpigmentation	Hypertension, fever, hypersensitivity, hyperbilirubinemia	Renal excretion, drug unchanged	Testicular cancer, malignant pleural effusions, Hodgkin's disease, non–Hodgkin lymphoma
Busulfan (Myleran)	0.05–0.2 mg/kg PO daily continuously	Alkylating agent. Alkylation of DNA.	Myelosuppression	Pulmonary fibrosis, addisonian state (skin pigmentation, weakness)	Renal excretion of metabolite	Chronic myelogenous leukemia, preparative regimens for bone marrow transplantation
Carboplatin (Paraplatin)	200–400 mg/m² IV every 28 days	Alkylating agent. DNA binding.	Myelosuppression, nausea, vomiting		Renal excretion	Advanced ovarian cancer, testicular cancer
Carmustine: See Nitrosoureas						
Chlorambucil (Leukeran)	0.05–0.2 mg/kg PO daily continuously	Alkylating agent. Alkylation of DNA.	Myelosuppression	Acute leukemia	Metabolic transformation	Chronic lymphocytic leukemia, low-grade non–Hodgkin lymphocytic lymphoma
Cisplatin (Platinol)	30–120 mg/m² IV every 3–4 weeks	Alkylating agent. DNA binding.	Renal toxicity, hypomagnesemia, nausea, vomiting, myelosuppression (platelets and leukocytes)	Peripheral neuropathy, hypersensitivity, ototoxicity	Renal excretion of native drug and metabolites	Advanced ovarian cancer, advanced bladder cancer, testicular cancer, small cell lung cancer, advanced non–small-cell lung cancer, head and neck cancer, advanced esophageal carcinoma, advanced gynecologic cancer
Cyclophosphamide (Cytoxan, Lytoxan, Neosar)	500–1500 mg/m² IV every 3–4 weeks; 60–100 mg/m² PO daily for 1–14 days	Alkylating agent. Alkylation of DNA.	Myelosuppression, nausea, vomiting, alopecia, immunosuppression, sterility	Hemorrhagic cystitis, renal tubular water retention, acute leukemia, pulmonary fibrosis, myocardial necrosis	Unclear: metabolism of drug to active agents by the liver	Breast cancer, soft tissue sarcoma, plasma cell myeloma, small cell lung cancer, advanced non–small-cell lung cancer, non–Hodgkin lymphoma, childhood solid tumors

(continued)

Table 14–1. Common anticancer chemotherapeutic agents. (continued)

Note: The drug dosages in this table are ranges used in clinical practice and are not offered as recommended dosages. The administration of these drugs should be under the supervision of physicians experienced in their clinical use.

Agent	Dosage	Category and Action	Common Toxicities	Other Toxicities	Metabolism	Disease
Cytarabine (Cytosar, others)	100 mg/m^2 IV or SC every 12 hours or continuous infusion for 7–21 days; 2–3 g/m^2 IV every 12 hours for 3–4 days	Alkylating agent. Alkylation of DNA.	Myelosuppression, nausea, vomiting, diarrhea, gastrointestinal mucositis, hepatotoxicity	Seizures with intrathecal use	Hepatic metabolism	Acute non-lymphocytic leukemia, meningeal cancers, non–Hodgkin lymphoma
Dacarbazine (DTIC-Dome, others)	150–250 mg/m^2 IV daily for 5 days every 28 days	Alkylating agent. Alkylation of DNA.	Nausea, vomiting, myelosuppression	Flu syndrome, toxic synergy with doxorubicin	Hepatic activation; excretion unclear	Malignant melanoma, Hodgkin's disease, soft tissue sarcoma
Dactinomycin (Cosmegen)	0.5 mg/m^2 IV daily for 5 days	Antibiotic. DNA intercalation, strand breakage.	Myelosuppression, gastrointestinal mucositis, alopecia, skin toxicity	X-ray interaction	Bile and urinary excretion, drug unchanged	Ewing's sarcoma, embryonal rhabdomyosarcoma, Wilms' tumor, gestational trophoblastic tumor, Hodgkin's disease
Daunorubicin (Cerubidine)	30–60 mg/m^2 IV for 1–3 days every 3–4 weeks	Antibiotic.	Myelosuppression, oral mucositis, alopecia, skin damage with extravasation, cardiac toxicity (acute and chronic)	X-ray toxicity synergy	Hepatic metabolism; biliary and renal excretion of metabolites	Acute nonlymphocytic leukemia
Doxorubicin (Adriamycin, many others)	25–90 mg/m^2 IV every 3–4 weeks	Antibiotic. DNA intercalation; DNA strand breakage.	Myelosuppression, oral mucositis, alopecia, skin damage with extravasation, cardiac toxicity (acute and chronic)	X-ray toxicity synergy	Hepatic metabolism; biliary and renal excretion of metabolites	Breast cancer, small-cell lung cancer, advanced non–small-cell lung cancer, Hodgkin's disease, non-Hodgkin lymphoma, soft tissue sarcoma, plasma cell myeloma, gastric cancer, acute nonlymphocytic leukemia, neuroblastoma, advanced ovarian cancer, embryonal rhabdomyosarcoma, thyroid cancer, bladder cancer, hepatocellular carcinoma
Etoposide (VePesid)	50–150 mg/m^2 IV daily for 1–5 days; 200–250 mg/m^2 IV weekly	Plant alkaloid. Action unknown; perhaps inhibition of DNA synthesis.	Leukopenia, thrombocytopenia, nausea, vomiting, mild peripheral neuropathy		Metabolic degradation; 45% excreted in urine as native drug and metabolites	Small-cell lung cancer, testicular cancer

(continued)

Table 14–1 Common anticancer chemotherapeutic agents. (continued)

Note: The drug dosages in this table are ranges used in clinical practice and are not offered as recommended dosages. The administration of these drugs should be under the supervision of physicians experienced in their clinical use.

Agent	Dosage	Category and Action	Common Toxicities	Other Toxicities	Metabolism	Disease
Fluorouracil (many)	7–15 mg/kg IV daily for 5 days or once weekly	Antimetabolite. Inhibition of thymidylate synthetase and synthesis of DNA.	Oral and gastrointestinal mucositis, myelosuppression (mild)	Cerebellar ataxia, myocardial necrosis syndrome, conjunctivitis, tear duct stenosis, phlebitis with protracted infusion, dermatitis	Hepatic metabolism	Breast cancer, gastrointestinal cancer, head and neck cancer, hepatocellular carcinoma
Hexamethylmelamine (Hexastat)	6–12 mg/kg PO daily 14–21 days or continuously	Investigational triazene alkylating agent. May act by alkylation of DNA.	Nausea, vomiting, neurotoxicity, peripheral neuropathy		Metabolism in plasma; <15% excreted in urine	Uterine cervix cancer
Hydroxyurea (Hydrea)	25 mg/kg PO daily continuously	Antimetabolite. Inhibition of nucleotide reductase and DNA synthesis.	Myelosuppression, nausea, vomiting, oral mucositis, skin rash	Convulsions	Hepatic metabolism	Chronic myelogenous leukemia, preparative regimens for bone marrow transplantation
Ifosfamide (Ifex)	0.8–1.2 g/m² IV daily for 5 days; 3–4 g/m² IV every 3 weeks	Alkylating agent; alkylates DNA, produces strand breaks.	Bone marrow suppression, hemorrhagic cystitis (must be coadministered with MESNA), alopecia	Nephrotoxicity, confusion, hepatotoxicity, nausea, vomiting	Activation by liver; catalysis in liver and kidneys	Advanced testicular cancer, soft tissue sarcoma
Interferon-2α (Intron A, Roferon A)	3 million IU given IM or SC daily or 3 times weekly (up to 30 million IU or more for investigational use)	Biologic agent. Direct antitumor activity and immunologic modulation.	Fever, chills, flulike symptoms, myalgias, headache, anorexia, nausea, leukopenia, thrombocytopenia, anemia, SGOT elevation	Diarrhea, vomiting, dizziness, central nervous system abnormalities	Renal clearance and renal tubular degradation	Hairy cell leukemia, renal cell carcinoma, malignant melanoma, Kaposi's sarcoma, refractory Hodgkin's disease and non–Hodgkin lymphoma
Lomustine: See Nitrosoureas						
Mechlorethamine (Mustargen)	6 mg/m² IV on days 1 and 8 every 4 weeks	Alkylating agent. Alkylation of DNA, RNA, protein.	Myelosuppression, nausea, vomiting, skin necrosis with extravasation, alopecia	Dermatitis, sterility	Rapid tissue binding and inactivation; metabolites excreted in urine	Hodgkin's disease
Melphalan (Alkeran)	0.05–0.2 mg/kg PO daily for 5 days	Alkylating agent. Alkylation of DNA.	Myelosuppression, alopecia, nausea, vomiting		Metabolism in plasma; <15% excreted in urine	Advanced ovarian cancer, plasma cell myeloma, breast cancer

(continued)

Table 14-1. Common anticancer chemotherapeutic agents. (continued)

Note: The drug dosages in this table are ranges used in clinical practice and are not offered as recommended dosages. The administration of these drugs should be under the supervision of physicians experienced in their clinical use.

Agent	Dosage	Category and Action	Common Toxicities	Other Toxicities	Metabolism	Disease
Mercaptopurine (Purinethol)	1–2 mg/kg PO daily for 5 days	Antimetabolite. Inhibition of de novo purine synthesis; incorporation into DNA.	Myelosuppression, hepatotoxicity, gastrointestinal mucositis, inhibition of cell-mediated immunity, increased toxicity with allopurinol	Dermatitis, fever, Budd-Chiari syndrome	Metabolism in liver to inactive thiopurine	Adult acute non-lymphocytic leukemia
Methotrexate (many)	20–100 mg/m² IV, IM, PO by a variety of schedules; 3–12 g/m² IV with leucovorin	Antimetabolite. Inhibition of formation of tetrahydrofolate by dihydrofolate reductase.	Myelosuppression, gastrointestinal mucositis, nausea, vomiting, alopecia, dermatitis	Renal tubular necrosis, pulmonary fibrosis, cirrhosis, osteoporosis, transverse myelitis and microcalcific leukoencephalopathy with radiation, fever	Renal excretion, drug unchanged	Osteogenic sarcoma, breast cancer, non-Hodgkin lymphoma, head and neck cancer, meningeal cancers, bladder cancer, adult leukemia, gestational trophoblastic cancer, ovarian cancer
Mitomycin (Mutamycin)	10–20 mg/m² IV every 6–8 weeks	Antibiotic. Alkylation of DNA and inter- and intrastrand cross-linkages.	Myelosuppression (cumulative), nausea, vomiting, cutaneous necrosis, alopecia, oral mucositis, skin rash	Pulmonary fibrosis, renal failure, microangiopathic hemolytic anemia, cardiomyopathy	Metabolism in liver and other tissues; minor renal excretion	Gastrointestinal cancers, non–small-cell lung cancer
Mitotane (Lysodren)	2–10 g PO daily continuously	Adrenal cytotoxic agent. Adrenocortical atrophy; inhibition of mitochondria.	Nausea, vomiting, diarrhea, lethargy, somnolence, skin rash	Leukopenia, hepatic toxicity	Hepatic and renal metabolism; excretion of metabolites in urine	Cancer of the adrenal cortex
Mitoxantrone (Novantrone)	10–14 mg/m² IV every 3–4 weeks	Antibiotic. Action unclear; may cause DNA breaks.	Myelosuppression, skin necrosis with extravasation	Nausea, vomiting, cardiotoxicity, alopecia		Acute nonlymphocytic leukemia, breast cancer, ovarian cancer, non–Hodgkin lymphoma
Nitrosoureas: Carmustine (BiCNU), Lomustine (CeeNu), Semustine (Methyl-CCNU; investigational)	100–200 mg/m² every 4–6 weeks	Alkylating agents. DNA strand breakage and cross-linkages.	Myelosuppression (delayed), alopecia, nausea, vomiting, oral mucositis, pain with intravenous injection (carmustine)	Bone marrow aplasia, acute leukemia, pulmonary fibrosis, renal toxicity (semustine), central nervous system and peripheral nerve toxicities	Spontaneous decompensation to active intermediates in aqueous solution; urinary excretion	Primary brain cancer, non-Hodgkin lymphoma, gastrointestinal cancers, malignant melanoma, metastatic brain cancer, plasma cell myeloma
Plicamycin (Mithracin)	0.025–0.05 mg/kg IV daily for 1–3 days, or IV every other day to toxicity	Antibiotic. Inhibits DNA-directed RNA synthesis.	Nausea, vomiting, thrombocytopenia, prolonged prothrombin time, hemorrhage, renal toxicity, liver toxicity	Fever, myalgias thrombosis	Unknown	Testicular cancer, chronic myelogenous leukemia in blast crisis Malignant hypercalcemia

(*continued*)

Table 14–1. Common anticancer chemotherapeutic agents. (continued)

Note: The drug dosages in this table are ranges used in clinical practice and are not offered as recommended dosages. The administration of these drugs should be under the supervision of physicians experienced in their clinical use.

Agent	Dosage	Category and Action	Common Toxicities	Other Toxicities	Metabolism	Disease
Procarbazine (Matulane)	100–200 mg/m^2 PO daily continuously or for 14 days	Radiomimetic with alkylating ability. Alkylation of DNA.	Myelosuppression (delayed), nausea, vomiting, flulike syndrome, lethargy, oral mucositis, diarrhea	Peripheral neuropathy, dermatitis, radiation sensitizer, MAO inhibition and medication interactions	Liver metabolism and renal excretion of inactive metabolites	Hodgkin's disease, non-Hodgkin lymphoma
Semustine: See Nitrosoureas						
Streptozocin (Zanosar)	0.5–1.5 g/m^2 IV daily for 5 days or weekly for 6 weeks	Nitrosourea; inhibition of DNA synthesis; damage to pancreatic B cell.	Nausea, vomiting, nephrotoxicity (hypophosphatemia, renal tubular defects)	Mild myelosuppression, liver toxicity, alteration of glucose metabolism, burning of vein	Rapid biotransformation after intravenous injection; renal excretion of 15% of total dose	Pancreatic islet cell tumors, pancreatic carcinoma, carcinoid tumors
Taxol	135 mg/m^2 IV 24-hr infusion	Plant alkaloid. Stabilizes tubulin polymerization.	Leukopenia, alopecia, anaphylaxis	Cardiac arrhythmias, peripheral neuropathy oral mucositis	Unknown, probably hepatic metabolism.	Ovarian cancer, breast cancer
Thioguanine	100 mg/m^2 IV daily for 5 days	Antimetabolite. Inhibition of de novo purine synthesis; incorporation into DNA.	Myelosuppression, nausea, vomiting	Hepatotoxicity, inhibition of cell-mediated immunity	Hepatic metabolism; renal excretion	Adult acute non-lymphocytic leukemia
Thiotepa	0.2–0.5 mg/kg IV or IM daily for 5 days or once weekly	Alkylating agent. Alkylation of DNA.	Myelosuppression, nausea, vomiting		Renal excretion, drug unchanged	Breast cancer, malignant effusions, superficial bladder cancer
Vinblastine (Velban) others	1.5–2 mg/m^2 IV daily for 5 days; 4–6 mg/m^2 IV weekly	Plant alkaloid. Binding of tubulin; mitotic arrest.	Leukopenia, constipation, skin necrosis with extravasation, alopecia, peripheral neuropathy (loss of reflexes, nerve palsies, muscle wasting, paresthesias)	Nausea, vomiting	Hepatic metabolism and biliary excretion	Testicular cancer, Kaposi's sarcoma, Hodgkin's disease, non-Hodgkin lymphoma, non–small-cell lung cancer
Vincristine (Oncovin) Vincasar others	0.5–2 mg/m^2 IV weekly	Plant alkaloid. Binding of tubulin; mitotic arrest.	Peripheral neuropathy (see vinblastine), leukopenia, constipation, skin necrosis with extravasation	Alopecia, nausea, vomiting	Hepatic metabolism and biliary excretion	Acute lymphocytic leukemia, acute non-lymphocytic leukemia, plasma cell myeloma, Hodgkin's disease, non-Hodgkin lymphoma, Wilms' tumor
Vindesine	2–3 mg/m^2 IV weekly	Plant alkaloid. Binding of tubulin; mitotic arrest.	Peripheral neuropathy, leukopenia, skin necrosis with extravasation	Thrombocytosis, alopecia, nausea, vomiting	Hepatic metabolism and biliary excretion	Non–small-cell lung cancer

[1]Reproduced, with permission, from Weiss GR: Oncology. Pages 458–465 in: *Internal Medicine: Diagnosis & Therapy,* 2nd ed. Stein JH (editor). Appleton & Lange, 1991.

Alkylating Agents

The alkylating agents make up a large group of drugs with major clinical utility. Alkylating drugs for human administration were among the first chemotherapeutic agents to be studied in the post–World War II era, and in many malignant condition they are the foundation of effective treatment. Although the term alkylation reflects the fact that many of these drugs attach alkyl ligands to the DNA of malignant cells, the emergence of more drugs with alkylatinglike activity has shown that their cytotoxic capacity is accomplished by heterogeneous means. Within the class of drugs known as alkylating agents are included the nitrogen mustards (mechlorethamine and the more stable substituted mustards, cyclophosphamide, ifosfamide, melphalan, and chlorambucil), the nitrosoureas (lomustine, carmustine, semustine, and streptozotocin), cisplatin and its analogs, and busulfan. Although alkylation may occur on many sites in biologic substances (proteins, amino acids, and nucleic acids), the most important action from the anticancer standpoint seems to be that which affects DNA integrity and function. As a group, these agents can form electrophilic moieties that react with nucleic acids on DNA, adding organic groups to DNA, producing DNA strand breaks, or cross-linking DNA strands with other strands, other proteins, or the alkylating agent itself.

Mechlorethamine (nitrogen mustard) is soluble in aqueous solution and must be administered by intravenous injection. It is rapidly reactive with many tissues and may produce severe local skin destruction if extravasated. Nausea, vomiting, myelosuppression, alopecia, and diarrhea are among its toxicities. Cyclophosphamide, a more stable substituted mustard, must undergo in vivo hepatic activation to the very potent phosphoramide mustard. Cyclosphosphamide may be given intravenously or orally. Its toxicities also include myelosuppression, nausea, vomiting, local skin toxicity with extravasation, and alopecia; however, its unique toxicities include hemorrhagic cystitis, pneumonitis or pulmonary fibrosis, cardiac necrosis when administered in very high dosage, immunosuppression, and carcinogenesis. Similarly melphalan may be administered orally or intravenously and shares many toxicities of cyclophosphamide except for cystitis, pneumonitis, and cardiac necrosis. Chlorambucil is administered only by the oral route, causing myelosuppression, and rarely pneumonitis and second malignancies. Ifosfamide is a more recent addition to the collection of substituted mustards, its dominant nonhematologic toxicity a troublesome hemorrhagic cystitis requiring coadministration of sodium 2-mercaptoethanesulfonate (mesna). The nitrosoureas are lipid soluble and are variably soluble in aqueous solution. These agents produce profound and delayed myelosuppression (nadir at 14–28 days after drug administration),

pulmonary fibrosis, renal failure, and rarely carcinogenicity.

Cisplatin is an extremely active and perhaps the most widely and routinely used anticancer agent in modern cancer therapy. Its toxicities are well recognized and include renal azotemia (abrogated by coadministration of large volumes of aqueous saline), severe nausea and vomiting, neurotoxicity, and mild myelosuppression. Finally, busulfan is an orally administered methanesulfonate. Its toxicities are modest (myelosuppression, skin pigmentation) except for the infrequent production of pulmonary fibrosis.

The clinical pharmacology of the alkylating agents is varied and often complex. Each of the mustards is extensively metabolized and is excreted by various and poorly understood means. Hepatic transformation is a major means of transformation of the nitrosoureas; their lipid solubility ensures ready movement of these agents into the central nervous system after systemic administration. Cisplatin is heavily tissue bound and is excreted by glomerular filtration. The drug must be withheld or its dosage severely reduced where there is preexisting renal toxicity.

Antimetabolites

Like the alkylating agents, the antimetabolites are classical anticancer agents whose mechanisms of action are, for selected agents, well known. Indeed, many of these agents have been rationally designed based on known biochemical targets in cancer cells. This group of drugs is large, receiving frequent contributions of new agents with improved biochemical or toxicity profiles. The antifols are led by methotrexate as the best known and most durably active agent of this type. Methotrexate exerts its action by inhibiting dihydrofolate reductase, the enzyme necessary for maintaining cellular levels of reduced folates, substrates for single carbon contribution to the synthesis of certain amino acids, thymidylic acid, and purine bases. Inhibition of these processes is ultimately cytotoxic to the malignant cells (as well as normal cells) by virtue of interference with DNA synthesis. Although the inhibition of dihydrofolate reductase is shared by both malignant and normal cells, qualitative differences in this inhibition can be exploited to advantage by administering huge doses of methotrexate to cancer patients, then administering leucovorin (N^5-formyl-tetrahydrofolic acid), a form of reduced folate more effectively transported in normal cells (which are then "rescued" from the toxicity) than in malignant cells.

Another well-studied group of antimetabolites is the pyrimidine analogs. This group includes cytarabine (ara-C) and vidarabine (ara-A). These agents are the product of the rational synthesis of drugs likely to confer cytotoxic effects preferentially greater upon malignant cells than upon normal cells. Ara-C acts as an inhibitor of DNA polymerase, competing with its analog deoxycytidine triphosphate (dCTP). Ara-C is incorporated into DNA and inhibits chain elongation. Consequently, this agent is a selective cytotoxin in the S-phase of the cell cycle (cell cycle–specific). Ara-A is an analog of adenosine. It is more commonly used as an antiviral agent, and it is less useful as an anticancer agent because it is poorly soluble in aqueous solutions and because it is rapidly metabolized by adenosine deaminase, which is found in high concentration in gastrointestinal epithelium, bone marrow, and certain hematologic tumors (T cell leukemia and acute myelogenous leukemia). Ara-C is commonly used in the treatment of acute myelogenous leukemia and occasionally in the management of chronic myelogenous leukemia and acute lymphoblastic leukemia. Analogs of the pyrimidine bases include 6-thioguanine (6-TG) and 6-mercaptopurine (6-MP), synthetic derivatives of guanine. These agents require conversion to monophosphate nucleotides before they become active as inhibitors of de novo purine biosynthesis. As triphosphates, these agents may be incorporated into DNA. The thiopurines possess poor activity against solid malignancies but have significant utility in the management of childhood leukemias.

6-TG, ara-C, and ara-A must be administered intravenously and tend to be more active and more toxic when administered by prolonged infusion. 6-MP is administered orally, and its dosage must be reduced for patients receiving allopurinol, an agent that inhibits its metabolism to 6-thiuric acid by xanthine oxidase. Both 6-TG and 6-MP undergo extensive metabolic degradation. Similarly, ara-C and ara-A are extensively metabolized. All these agents have elimination half-lives measured in minutes (for 6-MP, up to 45 minutes) to hours (for ara-C, 2 hours; for 6-TG, 90 minutes). Toxicities of these agents include gastrointestinal epithelial injury and bone marrow suppression. All are hepatotoxic to varying degrees. In high dosage, ara-C is neurotoxic, producing ataxia and confusion. Neurotoxicity may be especially prominent in patients receiving this drug intrathecally for meningeal carcinomatosis or leukemic meningitis.

Fluorouracil (5-fluorouracil, 5-FU) is a fluorinated pyrimidine analog that was synthesized to exploit the in vitro observation that malignant cells utilize uracil more efficiently than normal intestinal epithelium of laboratory animals. Fluorouracil may proceed through the pyrimidine synthetic pathways to be converted to FdUMP (5-fluoro-2'-deoxyundine 5'-phosphate), which inhibits thymidylate synthetase and thereby DNA synthesis; as well, it is converted to FUTP (fluorouridine triphosphate), which may be incorporated into RNA. The agent is almost always administered intravenously, although it is also active when administered by other routes (intra-arterial, intraperitoneal, oral). The drug is cell cycle–specific and more active when administered more frequently or by infusion. Fluorouracil is rapidly metabolized by the liver, and therefore its half-life is measured in minutes. Toxicities include frequent oral and gastrointestinal mucositis (oral ulceration and diarrhea), myelosuppression that is milder with continuous infusion, central nervous system toxicity (ataxia and stupor or somnolence), conjunctivitis, rarely myocardial ischemia or infarction, and occasionally nausea and vomiting. Fluorouracil is frequently used in the treatment of gastrointestinal malignancies, head and neck cancer, breast cancer, and less frequently other adult solid tumors.

RATIONALE FOR COMBINATION CHEMOTHERAPY

The modern use of chemotherapy in the treatment of cancer depends on the judicious combination of multiple anticancer agents administered simultaneously or sequentially. Such use is a result of the recognition that many agents are ineffective when used singly. The effectiveness of therapy utilizing drugs in combinations is attested to by the development of curative regiments in leukemias, lymphomas, childhood cancer, and germ cell malignancies. Furthermore, drug combinations have had important impact on the survival of patients afflicted with combination chemotherapy-responsive diseases such as breast, ovary, bladder, and small-cell lung cancer.

The principles underlying combination drug use include the following:

(1) The selected drugs should possess some (if incomplete) anticancer activity against the disease to be treated.

(2) Drugs whose toxicities do not overlap should be combined.

(3) The selected drugs should be administered in their highest effective dosage and on their most active regimen.

(4) The schedule of administration should be at the closest frequency allowed by the toxicities of the combined drugs.

If the principles are adhered to, a major strength of combination chemotherapy may be exploited, ie, avoidance of the emergence of tumor resistance to the combined agents. Limitations of the effectiveness of combination chemotherapy, particularly for most of the common malignancies managed by the cancer specialist, are the dearth of active single agents against most of these diseases, shared toxicities among the most useful agents, and the rapid development of resistance to the agents by the treated malignancies. A theoretical derivative of these principles has been the development of the Goldie-Coldman hypothesis, a mathematical model that estimates the rapidity of onset of drug resistance in tumors as a function of tumor size and the tumor's likelihood of spontaneous mutation to resistance. This hypothesis suggests that the potential for complete eradication of a malignancy may be accomplished by the incorporation of as many effective drugs as are available against a given type of cancer in at least two non–cross-resistant combination regimens.

MANAGEMENT OF DRUG EXTRAVASATION

Many anticancer agents are vesicants and are extremely irritating to soft tissues. Intravenous administration of these drugs is not infrequently accompanied by accidental paravenous extravasation followed by the abrupt or gradual onset of pain, marked skin erythema and swelling, and occasionally tissue necrosis, ulceration, scarring, and infection. When such agents are administered, extraordinary efforts should be exercised to avoid extravasation. These efforts should include the following:

(1) A fresh intravenous line should be established at the time of injection. Intravenous fluid should be started through the line, and good blood return should be ensured before the drug is injected.

(2) The anticancer agent should be injected by piggyback or sideport injection as rapidly as feasible into the running intravenous line.

(3) Intravenous fluid should be continuously infused through the line after drug injection to ensure clearance of the line or needle of residual drug.

(4) Patient complaint of local pain, dislodgment of the intravenous line, skin changes at the injection site, or loss of blood return should stimulate concern about the possibility of extravasation and should lead to discontinuance of the infusion until venous patency is assured.

Should drug extravasation occur, the following maneuvers should be applied to limit tissue injury and to relieve patient discomfort:

(1) The drug infusion should be stopped immediately and the needle removed.

(2) An icepack should be applied to the affected area to induce vasoconstriction and to limit tissue injury.

(3) Local anesthesia may be induced by infiltration of the affected tissues with 2% lidocaine or topical ethyl chloride.

(4) Injection of other pharmaceuticals into the area may be attempted but remains a controversial approach. Such methods are best left to individuals experienced in their use.

(5) If extravasation is greater than very mild and self-limited, surgical consultation is warranted, since resection of damaged tissue and skin grafting may be required.

SPECIAL CONSIDERATIONS

Intracavitary Chemotherapy

Limitations to the effectiveness of the available chemotherapies are related to the toxicities of the drugs to the host and to the resistance (acquired with treatment or present at the outset of treatment) of tumors to these agents. Efforts to overcome these limitations are numerous, but a noteworthy approach that is entering clinical practice involves administration of drugs to certain body cavities or hollow organs which harbor tumor and which may protect the host from exposure to toxic concentrations of the drugs. For example, clinical trials are in progress to explore the value of administering anticancer agents to the bladder, peritoneal cavity, and pleural cavity. Intrathecal chemotherapy has long been successfully utilized for the treatment of hematologic and lymphomatous malignancies involving the meninges. Cytarabine, methotrexate, and thiotepa have separately been employed for administration to the cerebrospinal fluid because of pharmacokinetics favoring high local concentrations for prolonged periods of time, substantial antitumor activity against malignancies with a tropism for the central nervous system, and mild-to-moderate toxicity to the meningeal space.

Intraperitoneal chemotherapy is being scrutinized as a potentially efficacious method for treating advanced ovarian carcinoma, a variety of gastrointestinal malignancies, and peritoneal malignant mesothelioma, among other cancers. The criteria for selection of this form of therapy have been fairly well defined and include the following requirements:

A. The peritoneal tumor should be distributed in small deposits (no deposit >2 cm in greatest diameter).

B. The chemotherapy selected for intraperitoneal use should be of relatively high molecular weight, which favors longer retention in the peritoneal cavity.

C. The systemic clearance of drug that diffuses into the circulation should be high compared with the clearance of the agent from the peritoneal cavity. This relationship favors a reduction in the systemic exposure to drug that is likely to induce toxicity.

D. The intraperitoneal drug should be delivered in high volume (at least 2 L) to ensure adequate distribution of the drug to all areas of the peritoneum.

Although the full potential of intraperitoneal chemotherapy has not been entirely defined, many agents have been evaluated for intraperitoneal use and have been shown to be safe: these include cisplatin, mitomycin, methotrexate, fluorouracil, etoposide, melphalan, interferon, interleukin-2, mitoxantrone, carboplatin, and cytarabine.

Similarly, intrapleural chemotherapy is being evaluated for its role in the control of pleura-based malignancies such as malignant mesothelioma, ovarian cancer, breast cancer, and lymphoma. The behavior of drugs placed in the pleural cavity shares many of the pharmacokinetic features of intraperitoneal therapy. However, this approach remains investigational at present.

Intra-arterial Chemotherapy

Another regional approach to the treatment of cancer exploits the vascular isolation of certain anatomic sites from the rest of the body. For example, the arterial supplies to the brain, head-and-neck region, liver, and extremities provide little perfusion to other organs or anatomic sites. These areas, if bearing tumor, may be cannulated with catheters through which chemotherapeutic agents may be delivered specifically to the tumor-bearing site. Several principles should be observed when utilizing this form of therapy.

A. At equivalent dosages, chemotherapy administration via the arterial supply of the organ bearing the tumor may expose the tumor to drug concentrations several orders of magnitude greater than drug concentrations accompanying systemic administration.

B. If the perfused organ metabolizes the drug, the therapeutic index of the drug may be substantially improved by permitting increased drug dosage and decreased systemic exposure to toxic levels of the drug.

C. New local toxicities may emerge that become dose-limiting (instead of dosage limitation due to systemic toxicities).

Hepatic arterial infusion of chemotherapy has long been used to treat liver metastases. This method exploits the knowledge that hepatic tumors are predominantly perfused by the hepatic artery while the liver parenchyma receives its dominant blood supply from the portal vein. Floxuridine (FUDR) and fluorouracil have long been infused via the hepatic vein for the treatment of liver metastases from gastrointestinal malignancies. These fluorinated pyrimidines are avidly extracted from the hepatic blood supply with little drug remaining in the hepatic vein blood. Dose-limiting toxicity of hepatic arterial FUDR is gastric ulceration and biliary sclerosis, as opposed to diarrhea, nausea, and vomiting for systemically administered FUDR. Recent advances in hepatic arterial catheter and infusion pump technology have permitted the evaluation of the long-term infusion of these agents at maximal dosage without the need for frequent percutaneous catheter placement. It appears that the anticancer effect is improved, but it is not as clear that patient survival has equally improved.

Arterial infusion is employed for treatment of extremity melanoma and sarcomas, squamous malignancies of the head and neck, and metastatic and primary cancers of the brain and liver.

REFERENCES

Chabner B: *Pharmacologic Principles of Cancer Treatment.* Saunders, 1982.

Chabner BA, Myers CE: Clinical pharmacology of cancer chemotherapy in cancer. Pagers 287–328 in: *Principles and Practice of Oncology,* 3rd ed. DeVita VT, Hellman S, Rosenberg SA (editors). Lippincott, 1989.

DeVita VT: Principles of chemotherapy in cancer. Pages 257–286 in: *Principles and Practice of Oncology,* 3rd ed. DeVita VT, Hellman S, Rosenberg SA (editors). Lippincott, 1989.

Dorr RT, Fritz WL: *Cancer Chemotherapy Handbook.* Elsevier/North-Holland, 1980.

15

Hormonal Therapy

Suzanne M. Fields, PharmD, & Jim M. Koeller, MS

Tumor response to hormone manipulation was first reported in the late 1800s when significant regression of breast cancer occurred following oophorectomy. However, it was not until almost 40 years later that estrogen was discovered and the logic behind tumor regression following oophorectomy was delineated. Since that time, the hormonal management of cancer has progressed dramatically owing to the understanding of endogenous steroid synthesis and metabolism, the development of new synthetic hormonal agents, and the discovery of steroid hormone receptors. Hormone-dependent tumor growth is inhibited when endogenous hormone production is stopped by surgical removal of the hormone source (eg, ovary, testis, adrenal). Similarly, the administration of pharmacologic doses of hormones or hormone antagonists will cause tumor regression with certain types of cancers. The most common malignancies treated with hormonal therapy are listed in Table 15–1.

The mechanism of action of most hormonal agents is unknown. However, structural similarity to endogenous steroid hormones is important for their activity. Estrogens, androgens, progestins, and glucocorticoids are all derivatives of steroid hormones and possess the same basic chemical structure: a five-sided ring attached to 3 six-sided rings (Figures 15–1 and 15–2). In the body, these hormones are produced in the adrenal cortex, ovaries, testes, and placenta and circulate in the bloodstream bound to plasma proteins. Target tissues in the body, both normal and tumor, contain receptors in their cytosol that are specific for hormonal agents. The hormone and the receptor bind to form a hormone-receptor complex that is translocated to the nucleus of the cell where it affects DNA synthesis, RNA synthesis, protein synthesis, and cell division (Figure 15–3). **Hormone antag-**

onists, such as the antiestrogens and antiandrogens, have a different mechanism of action in that they exert their effect by interfering with the normal binding process between the hormone and the target cell receptor. This action is known as **competitive binding.**

However, the binding of sex hormones to tumor cell surface receptors is not the only process that promotes and regulates tumor cell growth. Tumor cells also secrete **growth factors** such as transforming growth factor (TGF)-alpha or epidermal growth factor that stimulate their own growth. These factors are known as **autocrine** factors. Tumor cells may also secrete growth factors known as **paracrine** factors that will inhibit the growth of other cells. TGF-beta is an example of a paracrine growth factor. Hormonal agents that are utilized in cancer therapy are thought to produce their antitumor effects through alterations in receptor binding as well as changes in the secretion of autocrine and paracrine growth factors.

The discovery of steroid hormone receptors on tumor cells has led to significant advances in the hormonal management of certain tumors, best demonstrated with breast cancer. The response rate in breast cancer patients treated with endocrine therapy is approximately 30%. However, this response rate increases to 50–60% when only patients having estrogen receptor–positive tumors are evaluated. This response rate increases further to about 85% when women with both estrogen and progesterone receptor–positive tumors are treated with hormonal therapy. Additionally, tumor response appears to be directly related to the number of hormone receptors, since women with higher estrogen receptor values demonstrate higher response rates to hormonal ther-

Table 15–1. Malignancies treated with hormonal therapy.

Breast cancer
Prostate cancer
Renal cell cancer
Endometrial cancer
Leukemia
Lymphoma
Multiple myeloma

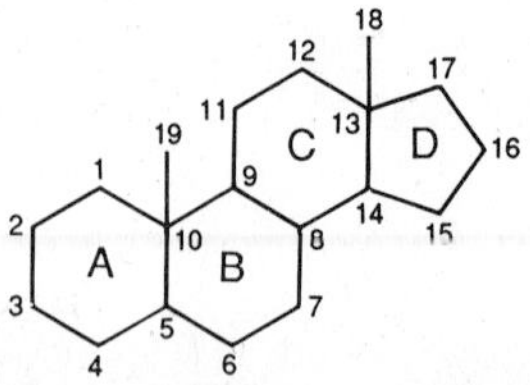

Figure 15–1. Basic hormone ring structure.

Estrogen

Antiestrogen

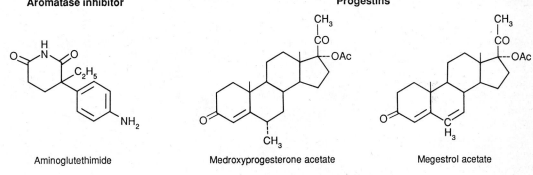

Diethylstilbestrol (DES)

Tamoxifen

Aromatase inhibitor

Progestins

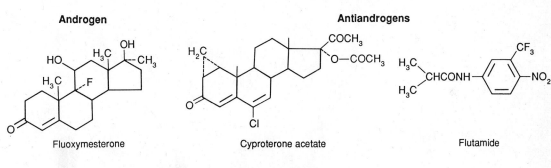

Aminoglutethimide

Medroxyprogesterone acetate

Megestrol acetate

Androgen

Antiandrogens

Fluoxymesterone

Cyproterone acetate

Flutamide

Glucocorticoids

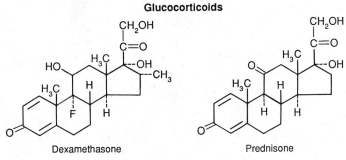

Dexamethasone

Prednisone

Figure 15–2. Chemical structures of hormonal agents.

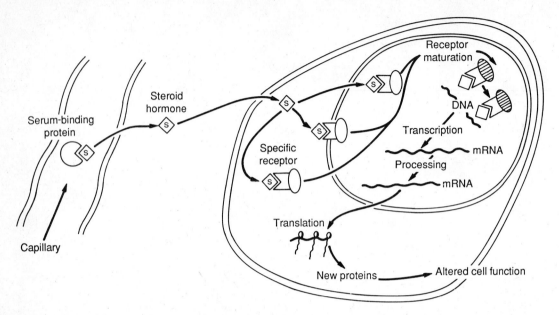

Figure 15–3. Steroid hormone-receptor binding complex. (Reproduced, with permission, from Sutherland DJ: Hormones and cancer. Page 210 in: *The Basic Science of Oncology*. Tannock E, Hill RP [editors]. McGraw-Hill, 1987.)

apy. Only 5–10% of patients with estrogen receptor–negative tumors will respond to hormonal manipulation. Unfortunately, the presence of hormone receptors does not always indicate that a tumor will respond to endocrine therapy. Additionally, tumors may consist of both hormone-dependent and hormone-independent subsets of cells, thus limiting the response of the tumor to hormonal therapy. However, receptor positivity does help guide the oncologist's decision for initial antitumor therapy. Hormone receptors have also been identified for prostate, endometrial, and renal cell carcinoma, but their clinical utility is not yet recognized.

Another good example of hormonal therapy is the management of metastatic prostate cancer. The goal of therapy is to ablate androgen production from all sources, since the growth of prostate cancer cells is dependent on androgens. This goal can be accomplished in several ways, since there are numerous sites in the male reproductive system for hormonal intervention (Figure 15–4). Hormonal manipulation is never curative in this population, but it induces remission in 40–80% of patients and improves well-being and quality of life. The initial response to hormonal therapy usually has a duration of 2–3 years. Upon symptomatic relapse, additional salvage hormonal therapy may be tried, but only 10–20% of patients will experience clinical improvement. Most patients die within 6–9 months of treatment failure.

The various hormonal agents used in cancer treatment, including standard doses and side effects, are discussed briefly below. The recommended treatment

regimens for specific cancers are given in chapters pertaining to those diseases.

ESTROGENS

Diethylstilbestrol (DES), the most frequently utilized synthetic estrogen, is used for the palliative treatment of metastatic prostate and breast cancer. In men with prostate cancer, DES produces symptomatic relief of bone pain as well as decreases in bony metastases and serum acid phosphatase concentrations. The proposed mechanism for this activity is a decrease in serum testosterone concentrations due to inhibition of the release of luteinizing hormone from the pituitary gland. Initial studies conducted by the Veterans Administration Cooperative Urological Research Group comparing 0.2-mg, 1-mg, and 5-mg doses per day showed that a DES dose of 5 mg/d was effective in decreasing serum testosterone concentrations to castrate levels (<50 mg/m), but the risk of cardiovascular mortality (myocardial infarctions, stroke, cerebrovascular accidents, congestive heart failure, and pulmonary embolism) was increased in these patients (25% for 1 mg/d versus 55% for 5 mg/d). This study also showed that lower doses of DES are as effective as higher doses. However, at doses of 1 mg/d, castrate levels of serum testosterone may not be reached by all patients. As a result, an intermediate dose of DES of 3 mg/d is commonly used for the treatment of prostate cancer, but it has not been tested in formal clinical trials.

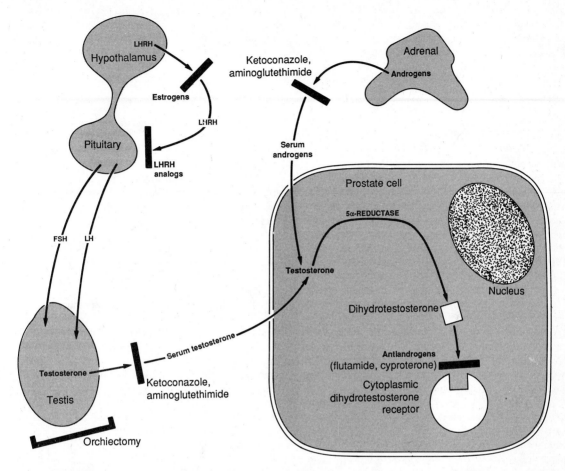

Figure 15–4. Pathways for androgen deprivation in prostate cancer. (Reproduced, with permission, from Garnick MB: Urologic cancer. Page 6 in: *Scientific American Medicine,* Section 12, Subsection IX. Rubenstein E, Federman D [editors]. © Scientific American, 1991.)

DES has also been used as alternative therapy for the treatment of metastatic breast cancer in postmenopausal women. The recommended oral dose of DES in this situation is 5 mg three times daily. However, tamoxifen or progestins have become the preferred agents for hormonal therapy of breast cancer because of their decreased toxicity profile.

Common side effects associated with DES therapy are listed in Table 15–2. In males, estrogen therapy causes impotence, testicular atrophy, and gynecomastia. However, low-dose radiation therapy to the breast prior to therapy can prevent the development of painful gynecomastia. Side effects specific to females receiving DES include endometrial hyperplasia and breakthrough vaginal bleeding.

ANTIESTROGENS

The antiestrogens antagonize the effects of estrogen on tumor cells by binding with estrogen receptors and producing conformational changes and depletion or down-regulation of the receptor. Currently, three antiestrogens are available in the USA: nafoxidine, clomiphene, and tamoxifen. Tamoxifen is by far the most frequently utilized agent. FDA-approved indications for tamoxifen include the treatment of metastatic disease in postmenopausal women with hormone receptor–positive tumors as well as adjuvant

Table 15–2. Side effects associated with diethylstilbesterol (DES).

Nausea and vomiting
Fluid retention
Hot flashes
Anorexia
Thromboembolism
Hepatic dysfunction

therapy for postmenopausal women with either node-positive or node-negative disease. It may also be used in patients with ovarian or endometrial carcinoma, but these indications are not approved by the FDA. Further trials are currently being conducted to determine other patients who may benefit from tamoxifen therapy.

Tamoxifen is effective in the management of metastatic breast cancer in both premenopausal and postmenopausal women. The response rate with tamoxifen therapy is approximately 50–60% in estrogen receptor–positive patients, with a median response duration of 12–18 months. Several trials have also demonstrated the efficacy of tamoxifen as adjuvant therapy for breast cancer. Significant improvements in survival have been reported in postmenopausal estrogen receptor–positive women receiving tamoxifen as adjuvant therapy. However, the recommended duration of adjuvant therapy with tamoxifen remains to be determined. Currently, adjuvant tamoxifen therapy should be continued for at least 2 years. Clinical trials comparing long-term (5 years) and short-term (2 years) adjuvant tamoxifen therapy are being conducted to determine the optimal duration of therapy. Trials are also being conducted to evaluate the use of tamoxifen in premenopausal women as well as the combination of chemotherapy plus tamoxifen as adjuvant therapy.

Tamoxifen is the treatment of choice for breast cancer in older patients because it is extremely well tolerated; less than 3% of patients discontinue therapy owing to side effects, the most common of which are listed in Table 15–3. Patients with bone metastases may experience a disease flare (ie, worsening bone pain and hypercalcemia) during the first few weeks of tamoxifen therapy, but this can usually be managed symptomatically and is self-limiting. Less common side effects include bone marrow suppression (leukopenia and thrombocytopenia), thrombophlebitis, rash, headache, and depression.

The recommended oral dose of tamoxifen is 10 mg twice daily. The drug possesses several active metabolites and undergoes extensive enterohepatic recirculation resulting in an activity half-life of approximately 14 days. Consequently, a once daily dose should be equally effective and easier to take than a twice daily dose. The necessity of the administration of a loading dose has been raised owing to the long half-life of the drug, but the clinical benefit has not been proved. Clinical trials have not shown that increasing the dose of tamoxifen (>20 mg/d) increases the response rate to therapy. Trials are being conducted to determine the optimal duration of therapy with tamoxifen.

PROGESTINS

Medroxyprogesterone acetate and megestrol acetate are two progestins currently used to treat breast, endometrial, prostrate, and renal cell carcinoma. Medroxyprogesterone possesses slightly more androgenic effects than megestrol, but megestrol is slightly more antiestrogenic. The mechanism of action of these agents is unknown, but progesterone receptors located on the surface of tumor cells are thought to play an important role. Direct cytotoxicity to the tumor and changes in hormone levels may also be involved in their antitumor activity. Tumor response to therapy appears to correlate with the presence of progesterone receptors on tumors. The response rate for patients with breast cancer to progestin therapy is approximately the same as the rate obtained with tamoxifen therapy, and as a result progestins are considered first- or second-line therapy for metastatic breast cancer. With endometrial tumors, approximately one-third of patients will experience tumor regression with progestin therapy. Less than 10% of patients with renal cell carcinoma will respond to therapy, and the response in previously treated patients with prostate cancer is minimal. As a result, progestins are used only as a final option in these patients.

Side effects associated with progestin therapy are listed in Table 15–4. Both medroxyprogesterone and megestrol have been associated with increased appetite and an average weight gain of 2 kg (4.5 lb) with or without fluid retention. This finding has prompted researchers to conduct studies using megestrol for cachexia associated with malignancy and the acquired immunodeficiency syndrome (AIDS). The doses employed in these studies are significantly higher than the ones used for hormonal treatment of cancer.

Megestrol, available as 20- and 40-mg tablets, is administered orally 3–4 times a day. Medroxyprogesterone is administered by the intramuscular route as a weekly dose of 400–1000 mg.

Table 15–3. Common side effects associated with tamoxifen.

Toxicity	Incidence
Hot flashes	10–30%
Nausea and vomiting	10–25%
Vaginitis	10%
Edema	5–10%

Table 15–4. Side effects associated with progestins.

Toxicity	Incidence
Weight gain	20–50%
Hot flashes	5–10%
Vaginal bleeding	5–10%
Impotence	10–20%

AROMATASE INHIBITORS

Aminoglutethimide is used in the management of breast and prostate cancer to produce a "medical adrenalectomy" by blocking central and peripheral steroid synthesis. In the adrenal gland, aminoglutethimide blocks the enzymatic conversion of cholesterol to pregnenolone, resulting in decreased production of estrogens, androgens, glucocorticoids, and mineralocorticoids. Additionally, the aromatase inhibitor acts peripherally in the tissues by blocking the conversion of androstenedione and testosterone to estrogens. Figure 15–5 illustrates the steroidogenesis and sites of action of aromatase inhibitors. Following several days of aminoglutethimide therapy, the drug-induced adrenal blockade may be reversed by compensatory negative-feedback increases in ACTH production. The concurrent administration of hydrocortisone, 40 mg/d (10 mg twice a day, 20 mg at bedtime), will prevent this from occurring. Dexamethasone should not be substituted for hydrocortisone in this treatment setting, since aminoglutethimide increases the metabolism of the dexamethasone. Some patients also require mineralocorticoid replacement with fludrocortisone acetate, 100 µg/d.

During the first 6 weeks of aminoglutethimide therapy, approximately 50% of patients will experience some of the side effects listed in Table 15–5. These effects usually are self-limiting and improve within 2–6 weeks from the initiation of therapy. A generalized macular pruritic rash also commonly occurs during the first 2 weeks of therapy. It resolves spontaneously within 5–8 days and is not cause to discontinue treatment.

Aminoglutethimide is generally initiated at a dose of 250 mg orally twice daily along with hydrocortisone, 50 mg orally twice daily. A lower aminoglutethimide dose combined with an increased hydrocortisone dose may help to minimize some of the side effects experienced during the first weeks of treatment. After 2 weeks, the aminoglutethimide dose should be increased to 250 mg 4 times a day and the hydrocortisone dose decreased to 40 mg/d in divided doses (10 mg in the morning, 10 mg at 5 PM, and 20 mg at 10 PM). However, preliminary data suggest that 250 mg twice a day may be as effective as 250 mg 4 times a day. The concomitant administration of dexamethasone should be avoided. Coadministration of warfarin and theophylline should also be avoided owing to decreased pharmacologic effects secondary to hepatic microsomal enzyme induction.

ANDROGENS

Androgens have been utilized as third- to fourth-line treatment of breast cancer but are not first-line agents because other hormonal agents and chemotherapeutic agents have greater activity. Their mechanism of antitumor activity is unknown. Fluoxymesterone is the most frequently prescribed androgen for the treatment of breast cancer. Its main drawback is its virilization effects on women that occur in more than 50% of patients. Table 15–6 lists the side effects associated with androgen therapy. The recommended dose of fluoxymesterone is 10 mg orally twice daily.

ANTIANDROGENS

Flutamide and cyproterone are antiandrogens that have demonstrated activity in the management of prostate cancer. These drugs act by blocking the binding of androgens to androgen receptors located on target tissues (Figure 15–4). Flutamide was approved for the treatment of advanced prostate cancer when used in combination with a luteinizing hormone–releasing hormone (LHRH) analog owing to its comparable efficacy with diethylstilbestrol. The incidence of patients responding to flutamide therapy alone is 50–80%, which is approximately equivalent to the response seen with DES. Cyproterone acetate also produces a response rate of approximately 80% in patients who have not received previous endocrine therapy. This agent, however, possesses orphan drug status in the USA.

Common side effects associated with both flutamide and cyproterone include gynecomastia, hot flashes, decreased libido, decreased spermatogenesis, and testicular atrophy (Table 15–7). Both agents are available for oral administration. The recommended dose of flutamide is 250 mg three times a day, and the dose of cyproterone is 200–300 mg/d.

Megestrol (see above) may also be classified as an antiandrogen owing to its interference with androgen receptor complexes.

GONADOTROPIN-RELEASING HORMONE AGONISTS

Synthetic analogs of the naturally occurring gonadotropin-releasing hormone (GnRH) have been administered to patients to produce medical castration. GnRH is normally produced in pulses by the hypothalamus and stimulates the release of follicle-stimulating hormone (FSH) and luteinizing hormone (LH). Both leuprolide and goserelin are synthetic analogs of GnRH in which the amino acid sequence has been altered either at position 6 or at the N terminus (Figure 15–6). The repeated or sustained administration of either of these agents causes an initial increase in LH and testosterone levels that is followed by an inhibition of the release of both LH and FSH. This inhibition is thought to be due to receptor down-regulation. The antitumor activity of these drugs in hormone-dependent tumors such as prostate and breast cancer is probably due to the decreased levels of es-

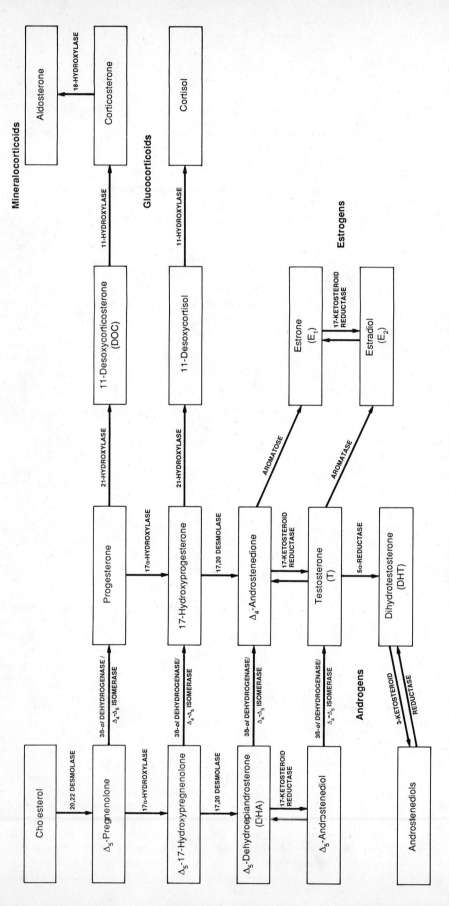

Figure 15–5. Enzymatic steps for normal steroidogenesis.

Table 15–5. Side effects associated with initiation of aminoglutethimide therapy.

Toxicity	Incidence
Lethargy	10–40%
Skin rash	30%
Postural hypotension	10–15%
Ataxia	10%
Nystagmus	5%

Table 15–7. Incidence of side effects associated with leuprolide.

Toxicity	Leuprolide plus Flutamide	Leuprolide plus Placebo
Hot flashes	61%	57%
Loss of libido	36%	31%
Impotence	33%	29%
Diarrhea	12%	4%
Nausea and vomiting	11%	10%
Gynecomastia	9%	11%

trogen, progesterone, and testosterone that occur secondary to receptor down-regulation.

The objective response rates obtained with leuprolide and goserelin in men with advanced-stage prostate cancer are approximately equivalent to the results obtained with orchiectomy or diethylstilbestrol. Furthermore, the combined administration of luteinizing hormone-releasing hormone (LHRH or GnRH) agonist and an antiandrogen (such as flutamide) may cause an increased benefit owing to total androgen blockade. The LHRH agonists are also being studied in premenopausal women with breast cancer.

Common side effects that occur following the administration of both leuprolide and flutamide are listed in Table 15–7. Because of the initial rise in testosterone levels that occurs with both drugs, patients may also experience a "tumor flare" or worsening of symptoms. Dysuria, hematuria, urinary retention, and increased bone pain may all be exacerbated after drug administration. As a result, the LHRH agonists should be used with extreme caution in patients with impending spinal cord compression or urethral obstruction. The concomitant administration of the antiandrogen flutamide may help minimize the tumor flare symptoms that occur with the LHRH agonists. A short-acting and a long-acting formulation of leuprolide are commercially available. The recommended dose for the short-acting agent is 1 mg/d subcutaneously. The long-acting preparation should be administered intramuscularly in a dose of 7.5 mg every 4 weeks. Goserelin is available as a unique copolymer preparation that releases a specific amount of drug daily for 28 days. A dose of 3.6 mg should be administered subcutaneously every 4 weeks with concomitant lidocaine administration because of the pellet of drug that must be injected. Following administration, the polymer drug vehicle degrades into lactic and glycolic acids in the tissues. Both agents may cause minor irritation around the injection site.

Table 15–6. Side effects associated with androgens.

Deepening of the voice
Alopecia
Hirsutism
Facial and truncal acne
Fluid retention
Menstrual irregularities
Cholestatic jaundice

GLUCOCORTICOIDS

Prednisone and dexamethasone are two glucocorticoids commonly employed in pharmacologic doses for the treatment of lymphomas, leukemias, and multiple myeloma owing to their antilymphocytic effects. They may also be used in combination with other antitumor agents for the treatment of some solid tumors. High-dose steroids (eg, dexamethasone) are also used for the management of disease complications such as spinal cord compression and increased intracranial pressure. In addition, prednisone is used in some settings to manage hypercalcemia. The cytotoxic effect of these agents is thought to be due to their affinity for glucocorticoid receptors located in normal lymphocytes and some tumor cell populations.

The side effects associated with glucocorticoids are dependent upon both the dose and the duration of drug administration (Table 15–8). Adrenal insufficiency may occur upon the abrupt withdrawal of glucocorticoids following prolonged administration. However, most of the antitumor regimens using glucocorticoids require supraphysiologic pulse doses of the drug to be administered at prescribed intervals.

Prednisone is available in tablet form in doses from 1 to 50 mg. Dexamethasone is available in various strength tablets (0.25–4 mg) and in an intravenous formulation (4 mg/mL). Doses in excess of the normal equivalent physiologic amount secreted daily by the adrenal gland (prednisone, 5 mg, and dexamethasone, 0.75 mg) are administered according to the pre-

Table 15–8. Side effects associated with glucocorticoids.

Short-term use
  Hypokalemia
  Edema
  Hypertension
  Hyperglycemia
  Euphoria
  Psychosis
Long-term use
  Increased susceptibility to infection
  Cushing's syndrome
  Osteoporosis
  Hirsutism
  Acne
  Striae/ecchymoses
  Muscle weakness
  Cataracts

Gonadotropin-releasing hormone

Pyro Glu-His-Trp-Ser-Tyr-Gly-Leu-Arg-Pro-Gly-NH$_2$
  1   2   3   4   5   6   7   8   9   10

Leuprolide

Pyro Glu-His-Trp-Ser-Tyr-D-Leu-Leu-Arg-Pro-Ethylamide
  1   2   3   4   5   6   7   8   9   10

Goserelin

Pyro Glu-His-Trp-Ser-Tyr-D-Ser (*tert*-butyl)-Leu-Arg-Pro-Azagly
  1   2   3   4   5   6   7   8   9   10

Figure 15–6. Synthetic gonadotropin-releasing hormone analogs.

scribed regimen. When treating a patient with spinal cord compression, an initial loading dose of 10 mg of dexamethasone should be administered followed by a maintenance dose of 4 mg every 6 hours. If steroid therapy is administered for longer than 2–3 weeks, drug discontinuation should be tapered over approximately 1–2 weeks. If the administration period is less than this, the drug can be discontinued abruptly.

REFERENCES

Canellos GP: Hormonal agents and treatment of cancer. *Urology* 1986;**27(Suppl)**:4.

Grayhack JT, Keeler TL, Kozlowski JM: Carcinoma of the prostate: Hormonal therapy. *Cancer* 1987;**60:**589.

Greenberg EJ: The treatment of metastatic breast cancer. *CA* 1991;**41:**242.

Haskell CM: Drugs used in cancer chemotherapy. Chapter 5, pp 44–102, in: *Cancer Treatment.* Haskell CM (editor). Saunders, 1990.

Korman LB: Treatment of prostate cancer. *Clin Pharm* 1989;**8:**412.

Legha SS: Tamoxifen in the treatment of breast cancer. *Ann Intern Med* 1988;**109:**219.

Sutherland DJ: Hormones and cancer. Chapter 13, pp 204–222, in: *The Basic Science of Oncology.* Tannock IF, Hill RP (editors). Pergamon Press, 1987.

Swain SM, Lippman ME: Endocrine therapies of cancer. Chapter 4, pp 59–109, in: *Cancer Chemotherapy Principles and Practice.* Chabner BA, Collins JM (editors). Lippincott Company, 1990.

Biologic Agents

16

Suzanne M. Fields, PharmD, & Jim M. Koeller, MS

Biologic response modifiers (BRMs) are a large group of immune mediators that have the ability to modify the host's biologic response to tumor. These agents are of interest because they provide a new approach to cancer treatment that can be used in conjunction with or supplemented by the more conventional cancer treatments of chemotherapy, irradiation, and surgery.

BRMs have historically been classified as either specific or nonspecific immune modulators. Specific BRMs react with specific tumor antigens. Examples of specific BRMs include monoclonal antibodies, lymphocytes stimulated in vivo, and tumor-derived vaccines. Nonspecific BRMs create an immune response without interacting with a specific antigen. Examples of nonspecific BRMs include the cytokines, bacillus Calmette-Guérin (BCG), and nontumor vaccines.

This chapter reviews the interferons, colony-stimulating factors, interleukins, monoclonal antibodies, tumor necrosis factor, and BCG. Some biologic agents are still in clinical trials and have not been approved for use by the FDA in the USA.

SOME ACRONYMS & ABBREVIATIONS USED IN THIS CHAPTER	
AIDS	Acquired immunodeficiency syndrome
BCG	Bacillus Calmette-Guérin
BRM	Biologic response modifier
CSF	Colony-stimulating factor
EPO	Erythropoietin
G-CSF	Granulocyte CSF
GM-CSF	Granulocyte-macrophage CSF
HAMA	Human antimouse antibody
IL	Interleukin
LAK	Lymphokine-activated killer (cell)
M-CSF	Macrophage CSF
MoAb	Monoclonal antibody
Multi-CSF	Multipotential CSF (IL-3)
NK	Natural killer (cell)
PPD	Purified protein derivative
rTNF	Recombinant TNF
TIL	Tumor-infiltrating lymphocyte
TNF	Tumor necrosis factor

INTERFERON

The interferons are a group of more than 20 proteins and glycoproteins produced in response to viral infections or other interferon inducers (eg, antigens or mitogens). They were discovered in 1957 owing to their antiviral activity. They can be subdivided into three types: alpha, beta, and gamma. Alpha and beta interferon are induced by a variety of cell types and were once referred to as type I interferons owing to their stability in an acid pH environment. Both alpha and beta interferon have similar structures and can competitively bind to a common cell surface receptor, producing similar biologic effects. In contrast, gamma interferon, or type II interferon, is produced by T lymphocytes, is acid labile, and binds to a distinct cell surface receptor. All three types of interferon are now readily producible via recombinant DNA technology and have been used in various clinical trials.

The interferons have a broad range of biologic effects including antiviral, antiproliferative, cytostatic, immunomodulatory, and differentiating. Interferon's antitumor effects are produced directly by cytotoxicity or indirectly through modulation of the immune effector cells. The interferons directly inhibit proliferation of both normal and tumor cells by lengthening all stages of the cell cycle. However, the cells in the G_o (resting phase) of the cell cycle demonstrate the most sensitivity to the antiproliferative effects of interferon.

Another proposed mechanism of action of interferon is interference with oncogene expression. When functioning appropriately, the oncogene regulates cell proliferation, growth, and development. The administration of interferon suppresses oncogene expression, resulting in decreased cell proliferation and differentiation.

A third mechanism by which tumor cells may be affected by interferon is through modulatory effects on the immune system. All cells in the normal host immune system are affected by interferon, including natural killer (NK) cells, killer cells, T cells, B cells, macrophages, and neutrophils. However, all effects are dependent on the timing, dose, route of administration, and duration of exposure to the interferon.

Interferon is administered in various doses and schedules intramuscularly, intravenously, or subcutaneously. The hematologic malignancies are responsive to lower doses of interferon (ie, 2 million units/m² three times weekly or 3 million units daily), whereas solid tumors require much higher doses for a response (ie, 9–20 million units/m²). If a patient experiences severe adverse reactions, the interferon dose should be reduced by 50% or the drug should be discontinued until the adverse effects resolve.

The interferons have been utilized extensively in phase I and II clinical trials for the treatment of hematologic malignancies, lymphomas, acquired immunodeficiency syndrome (AIDS), and certain other malignancies. At present, the only FDA-approved uses for alpha interferon are for the treatment of hairy cell leukemia, Kaposi's sarcoma, condylomata acuminata (genital warts), and chronic hepatis C. Gamma interferon is approved for the treatment of chronic granulomatous disease owing to decreased incidence in serious infections in patients receiving the drugs. However, both alpha and gamma interferon have demonstrated antitumor activity in several other disease states. Phase I studies with beta interferon are too preliminary to determine its antitumor activity.

The use of relatively low doses of alpha interferon (ie, 2–3 million units administered daily or three times weekly) has produced objective response rates of over 70%, with complete response rates of 5% reported in patients with hairy cell leukemia. However, even patients who demonstrate only a partial response to interferon therapy experience a prolongation in survival with fewer complications such as opportunistic infections. Treatment responses usually occur within 4–6 months of initiation of therapy, with improved quality of life, nomalizing peripheral blood counts, and decreased numbers of hairy cells in the bone marrow. However, a transient decrease in the peripheral counts may occur early in the course of therapy, so patients should be monitored closely during this time period.

Response rates of long duration (approximately 18 months) of 25–30% have been seen when alpha interferon is used in treating AIDS-related Kaposi's sarcoma. The dose employed in this patient population is 20–30 million units m² three times per week, although most patients require dosage reduction owing to toxicity of this high dose. Specific subsets of patients are more likely to respond to interferon therapy, such as patients with less severe immune dysfunction, earlier less bulky disease, and fewer disease complications. Patients who do respond to therapy experience fewer opportunistic infections and survive longer. The combination of alpha interferon and zidovudine is being investigated in patients with AIDS-related Kaposi's sarcoma in an attempt to potentiate antitumor and antiviral activity. Antitumor responses of 45–50%, decreased serum HIV p24 antigen levels, and increased CD4+ lymphocyte counts have been reported in the trials to date.

Impressive response rates have also been observed in patients treated with low-dose interferon for chronic myelogenous leukemia, especially patients who are in the early phase of chronic disease. Following a dose of 5 million units/d, approximately 75% of patients will have clearance of malignant cells from their peripheral blood and 5% will experience cytogenetic remission in the bone marrow with the disappearance of the Philadelphia chromosome clone. These response rates are somewhat decreased in patients in the late chronic phase or accelerated/blast phase of the disease. The median survival of patients with chronic myelogenous leukemia following interferon therapy is significantly longer than that obtained with chemotherapy.

Partial response rates have also been obtained with interferon in patients with non-Hodgkin's lymphoma, cutaneous T cell lymphoma, multiple myeloma, malignant glioma, carcinoid tumors, renal cell carcinoma, ovarian cancer, and malignant melanoma. Most doses of interferon utilized for these malignancies are close to the maximum tolerated dose. Various routes of administration, including intraperitoneal and intravesical, as well as various combinations of treatment modalities (ie, immunotherapy plus radiation therapy or chemotherapy), have also been used in clinical trials. Preliminary results utilizing the combination of fluorouracil and alpha interferon in the treatment of advanced colorectal cancer are promising (>60% partial response rate). Controlled trials are being conducted to verify these results and determine the role of interferon in combination with fluorouracil in the treatment of colorectal cancer.

The final clinical situation in which alpha interferon has been shown to have activity is in the treatment of hepatitis. Patients with either hepatitis B or hepatitis C have shown clinical improvement in liver function tests and hepatic histology following treatment with interferon.

The toxicities associated with the interferons appear to increase in frequency and severity with increasing dose and patient age (Table 16–1). The most common side effect is an acute influenzalike syndrome consisting of fever, fatigue, chills, myalgias, headache, and nasal congestion. These symptoms occur in more than 95% of patients with the first course of therapy and are usually controllable with acetaminophen. Repeated dosing leads to the development of tachyphylaxis to these side effects, but the adverse effects may flare on the first day of interferon therapy following a drug holiday. Nighttime adminis-

Table 16–1. Common toxicities associated with interferon therapy.

Acute
  Influenzalike syndrome
  Cardiovascular effects (hypotension, tachycardia, arrhythmias)
  Neurologic toxicities
  Elevated hepatic transaminases
  Nausea and vomiting
Chronic
  Anorexia
  Weight loss
  Malaise
  Fatigue
  Depression, personality changes

tration of interferon may improve tolerance to therapy in some patients. Dose reduction is seldom necessary for the acute side effects experienced with interferon. However, with chronic dosing, patients may experience anorexia, weight loss, malaise, fatigue, and depression, and these symptoms can be severe enough in some patients to warrant dose reduction or discontinuation of drug therapy.

Other side effects that have been reported with interferon therapy include central nervous system, hematologic, cardiovascular and gastrointestinal toxicities, mucocutaneous side effects, and mild proteinuria. The central nervous system toxicities are manifested as dizziness, lethargy, depression, mild confusion, and decreased ability to concentrate, which reverse following discontinuation of the drug. Dose-related decreases in white blood cell, lymphocyte, and granulocyte counts also occur and appear to be more dramatic in patients who have previously received intensive chemotherapy or radiation therapy or in patients who have disease in the bone marrow. Thrombocytopenia and a normochromic normocytic anemia may also occur in a small percentage of patients. All of these hematologic toxicities are reversible with drug discontinuation and have not resulted in increased infection rates in patients.

The development of serum neutralizing antibodies following the administration of human proteins has been demonstrated with insulin, growth hormone, and interferon. The development of these antibodies could interfere with the clinical effectiveness of interferon and limit its usefulness, but this has not been proved. Neutralizing antibody formation and measurement varies markedly among patients and may be affected by numerous factors including route of drug administration (greater for subcutaneous and intramuscular administration than for intravenous administration), duration of treatment and cumulative dose, tumor type (more rapid for patients with renal cell carcinoma and Kaposi's sarcoma), and different assay methodologies. Whether the development of serum neutralizing antibodies influences the clinical effect of interferons is controversial, but reports suggest that some patients who become antibody-positive do experience a concomitant decreased antitumor response. Others have reported continued response even with the development of neutralizing antibodies.

COLONY-STIMULATING FACTORS

The hematopoietic colony-stimulating factors (CSFs) are a group of glycoprotein growth factors that were discovered when scientists attempted to grow normal human bone marrow cells in vitro. These growth factors are essential for the proliferation, differentiation, and maturation of the various stem cells involved in hematopoiesis. Several growth factors working either individually or in combination with other factors are reported to be involved in this complex process (Figure 16–1). The human hematopoietic growth factors that have been identified and cloned via recombinant DNA technology are erythropoietin (EPO), granulocyte-macrophage colony-stimulating factor (GM-CSF), granulocyte colony-stimulating factor (G-CSF), macrophage colony-stimulating factor (M-CSF), multipotential colony-stimulating factor or interleukin-3 (multi-CSF or IL-3), interleukin-1 (IL-1), interleukin-4 (IL-4), interleukin-5 (IL-5), and interleukin-6 (IL-6) (Table 16–2). EPO, GM-CSF, and G-CSF are the only hematopoietic growth factors currently commercially available, but interleukin-2 (IL-2) is awaiting FDA approval. M-CSF, IL-3, and IL-1 have only recently entered clinical trials, so commercial availability will be delayed. The development of CSFs will have a major impact on the practice of hematology and oncology in that previously untreatable diseases may become treatable while the toxicity and morbidity associated with cancer therapy may be decreased.

EPO was the first CSF identified and has primarily been employed for the treatment of anemia associated with end-stage renal disease. EPO is normally produced mainly by the kidneys and induces the proliferation, differentiation, and maturation of red blood cells. Doses ranging from 50 to 500 IU/kg three times weekly following dialysis have decreased transfusion requirements and improved quality of life in patients with dialysis-dependent renal failure. The main side effects are mild hypertension and arteriovenous fistula clotting. The production of erythropoietin antibodies in response to therapy have not been reported. EPO may also prove effective in other types of anemia such as aplastic anemia, myelodysplasia, the anemia of chronic disease (eg, rheumatoid arthritis or cancer), and drug-induced anemias (eg, cisplatin or zidovudine).

IL-1 (see also below) is released by monocytes and other cells and plays an important role in inflammatory reactions. It also is important in the hematopoietic process, since it sensitizes early progenitor cells

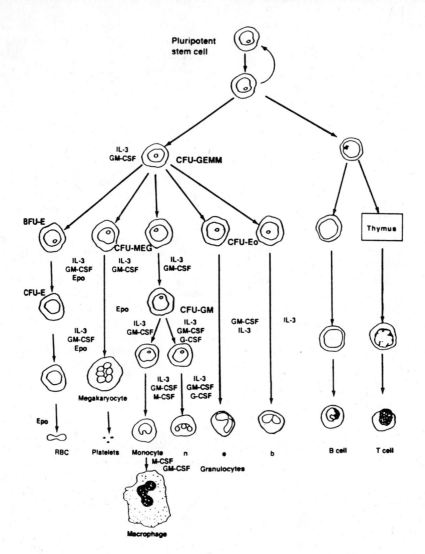

Figure 16–1. Hematopoietic cascade. CFU-GEMM, colony-forming unit, granulocyte-erythrocyte-monocyte-megakaryo-cyte; CFU-Meg, CFU-megakaryocyte; CFU-Eo, CFU-eosinophil; CFU-GM, CFU-granlocyte/monocyte; CFU-E, CFU-ery-throid; BFU-E, burst-forming unit–erythroid; CSF, colony-stimulating factor; n, neutrophil; e, eosinophil; b, basophil; m, monocyte/macrophage; E, erythrocyte; M, megakaryocyte; Epo, erythropoietin; IL-3, interleukin-3. (Reproduced, with permis-sion, from Clark SC, Kamen R: The human hematopoietic colony-stimulating factors. *Science* 1987;**236**:1231.)

to the later effects of more lineage specific colony-stimulating factors such as G-CSF or GM-CSF. Consequently, the combination of IL-1 with G-CSF, M-CSF, or GM-CSF may be useful in patients receiving intensive chemotherapy. IL-1 also has the unique ability to accelerate hematopoietic regeneration in normal cells that have been exposed to either irradiation or chemotherapy, which could prove beneficial in cancer patients by decreasing mucositis and other toxicities. IL-6 is similar to IL-1 in that it also primes the early bone marrow progenitor cells so that they proliferate upon later exposure to G-CSF, GM-CSF, or M-CSF and potentiate cell colony formation.

Other actions of IL-6 are described in the section on interleukins.

IL-3 or multi-CSF is produced by T cells and stimulates the differentiation of early progenitor cells and is much less lineage specific, causing an increase in red blood cells, platelets, monocytes, basophils, eosinophils, and mast cells. Interestingly, the genes that code for IL-3, GM-CSF, and M-CSF are all located on the q arm of chromosome 5. Abnormalities of this region of chromosome 5 are present in some anemias and acute myeloid leukemia. Phase I and II trials have been initiated to determine the dosing and clinical utility of IL-3. It appears that IL-3 will need to be

Table 16–2. Hematopoietic growth factors.

Growth Factor[1]	Target Cell
Erythropoietin (EPO)	Erythrocytes
Granulocyte-macrophage CSF (GM-CSF)	Granulocytes, macrophages
Granulocyte CSF (G-CSF)	Granulocytes
Macrophage CSF (M-CSF)	Macrophages
Multipotential CSF or interleukin-3 (Multi-CSF or IL-3)	Erythrocytes, granulocytes, basophils, eosinophils, megakaryocytes, mast cells
IL-1	Early bone marrow progenitor cells
IL-4	Basophils, mast cells
IL-5	Eosinophils
IL-6	Early bone marrow progenitor cells

[1]CSF = colony-stimulating factor; IL = interleukin.

given in combination with a more committed cell stimulant such as GM-CSF, G-CSF, or M-CSF for marked hematopoietic stimulation to occur. Clinical trials are also being conducted to determine if platelets can be stimulated in patients with severe aplastic anemia who are receiving chemotherapy, because of the very early effects of IL-3 on progenitor cells.

GM-CSF is similar to IL-3 in that it is produced by T cells, is located on the 5q chromosome, and stimulates the production of neutrophils, basophils, eosinophils, monocytes, and early erythroid and megakaryocyte progenitors. As a result, GM-CSF has been used in numerous clinical trial situations including treatment of the leukopenia associated with AIDS, bone marrow failure due to myelodysplasia and aplastic anemia, and the leukopenia associated with cancer chemotherapy and bone marrow transplantation. However, the only FDA-approved indication for GM-CSF is the acceleration of myeloid engraftment in patients undergoing autologous bone marrow transplantation for the treatment of non-Hodgkin's lymphoma, acute lymphoblastic leukemia, and Hodgkin's disease. Various doses have been utilized in these studies via the intravenous or the subcutaneous route. The use of GM-CSF in AIDS patients resulted in an increase in functional neutrophils and monocytes, but the leukocyte count returned to baseline values after drug therapy was discontinued. A possible drawback to the use of GM-CSF in AIDS patients is that it could modulate HIV activity; however, this is controversial. GM-CSF may also improve AIDS patients' tolerance to zidovudine and antibiotics required for the management of infections that are myelosuppressive (eg, trimethoprim-sulfamethoxazole, ganciclovir). Patients with myelodysplastic syndromes have also experienced increased white blood cell counts, hematocrit, and platelet counts during therapy with GM-CSF. However, treatment with GM-CSF may stimulate the proliferation of leukemic cell populations because of its proliferative effects.

Patients having high numbers of blast cells in the bone marrow (>15%) have been shown to progress more frequently to acute leukemia during treatment with GM-CSF.

On the other hand, the stimulation of leukemic cell formation could be beneficial in some cases. If GM-CSF is given along with chemotherapy, the blast cells in the resting phase of the cell cycle can be recruited to the active phase and, as a result, cell kill may be increased. Increased white blood cell counts have also been reported with GM-CSF in aplastic anemia, but the results have not been as impressive as the ones obtained in myelodysplastic syndromes. Positive results in the form of shortened duration of neutropenia and hospitalization have also been reported with the administration of GM-CSF during autologous bone marrow transplantation. Overall, GM-CSF administration is well tolerated at lower doses (≤10 µg/kg) and has mild side effects such as low-grade fever, myalgias, phlebitis or pain at the injection site, bone pain, and nausea. Most of these symptoms are transient and can be managed with acetaminophen and supportive care. At higher doses (>32 µg/kg/d) large vessel thromboses, pleuropericarditis, fluid retention, and adult respiratory distress syndrome have been reported.

G-CSF differs from GM-CSF in that it selectively stimulates neutrophil production. The duration of neutropenia and the incidence of mucositis both were reduced in patients receiving methotrexate, vinblastine, doxorubicin, and cisplatin (M-VAC) for bladder cancer when G-CSF was administered concomitantly. A shortened period of neutropenia was noted in patients receiving combination chemotherapy plus G-CSF for small-cell lung cancer. As a result, G-CSF is approved by the FDA for the neutropenia associated with cancer chemotherapy. G-CSF has also been effective for the treatment of congenital neutropenia, whereas GM-CSF was found to be ineffective. G-CSF has been associated with minimal side effects including bone pain, myalgias, and skin rash. The serious side effects reported with high-dose GM-CSF have not been reported with G-CSF at any dose.

M-CSF stimulates monocytes and macrophages and the release of numerous other cytokines (G-CSF, GM-CSF, IFN, IL-1, and TNF). Animal models and in vitro studies with M-CSF have demonstrated tumoricidal activity against melanoma, antimicrobial activity against bacteria and fungi, and terminal differentiation and destruction of leukemic cell clones. Preliminary phase I trials are being conducted to delineate the therapeutic role of M-CSF.

INTERLEUKINS

The interleukins are a group of proteins secreted primarily by activated lymphocytes and macrophages involved in the immune response that promote cell growth, differentiation, and functional activity. Over the past two decades, 12 different interleukins have been described, and the genetic code for the DNA sequence of the interleukins and some of the interleukin receptors has been determined. This has allowed for the production of interleukins via recombinant DNA technology and has further aided in the determination of individual interleukin activities.

The mechanism of action of the interleukins is characteristic of a true biologic response modifier in that all the antitumor effects occur via complex indirect effects of immune effector cells. These agents do not possess any direct cytotoxic effect on tumors. Both IL-1 and IL-6 are produced by macrophages and stimulate cells involved in both immune and inflammatory reactions. IL-2 through IL-6 and IL-10 are produced by T cells, while IL-7 and IL-11 are produced by bone marrow stromal cells. IL-5 stimulates eosinophil growth and differentiation and induces B cell proliferation with increased immunoglobulin secretion. IL-4 and IL-6 also stimulate B cells, leading to antibody production, while IL-1, -3, -4, -7, and -11 stimulate various hematopoietic precursors. IL-8 stimulates granulocyte activity and induces chemotactic migration of cells. IL-9 causes proliferation of the megakaryoblastic leukemia cell line and may also induce erythroid precursors. IL-10 is known as a cross-regulatory cytokine because it is produced by a subset of activated T lymphocytes and inhibits cytokine production by other T lymphocyte subsets. IL-12, which was originally called cytotoxic lymphocyte maturation factor, stimulates the growth of activated human T cells and NK cells. IL-2, also known as T cell growth factor, stimulates antibody-dependent T lymphocytes, B lymphocyte proliferation, and nonantibody-dependent lymphokine-activated killer (LAK) cells (eg, NK cells, T cells). IL-2 also enhances the differentiation of B lymphocytes and the tumoricidal activity of macrophages, with increased production of tumor necrosis factor (TNF). A final mechanism by which IL-2 exerts its activity is by increasing the production of other lymphokines such as gamma interferon and GM-CSF. Recombinant forms of both IL-2 and -3 have been extensively studied in clinical trials and will probably be the first commercially available interleukins. As a result, the remainder of this section focuses on the clinical uses and toxicity of IL-2. IL-1, -3, -6 are discussed further in the section on hematopoietic colony-stimulating factors.

Numerous dosing schedules and routes of administration of IL-2 have been investigated in an attempt to find the most effective dose having tolerable side effects. Bolus intravenous infusions, continuous infusions, intrathecal injections, intravesical injections, subcutaneous injections, and direct intraperitoneal infusions have all been used. Continuous intravenous infusion, intraperitoneal administration, and subcutaneous injection all produce lower sustained serum levels than intermittent bolus injections and result in more biologic activity owing to greater rebound lymphocytosis following the dose. Unfortunately, the therapeutic effectiveness obtained with high-dose continuous intravenous infusions is accompanied by increased toxicities. The intraperitoneal route has not decreased the systemic toxicities associated with IL-2. The most common dosing regimens range from 10,000–100,000 U/kg intravenously every 8 hours for 5 days to 1–7 million $U/m^2/d$ by continuous infusion. The optimal dose, rate, and schedule of IL-2 administration remains to be determined. The coadministration of LAK cells, cyclophosphamide, interferon, TNF, monoclonal antibodies, and tumor-infiltrating lymphocytes (TILs) is also being investigated in an attempt to improve the activity of IL-2.

IL-2 has primarily been studied in patients with advanced cancers who have failed to respond to standard therapy or in those for whom no standard therapy is available. To date, 20–30% of the patients treated with IL-2 have experienced objective responses (defined as a 50% decrease in tumor size for a duration of at least 1 month). Many of these responses have been durable (>12 months). All of the responding patients had either renal cell carcinoma or malignant melanoma, most of which were resistant to chemotherapy. However, a small subset of patients (5%) have obtained complete remission following IL-2 therapy.

In an attempt to increase the clinical response with IL-2, the surgical branch of the National Cancer Institute conducted a trial comparing high-dose IL-2 alone or in combination with alpha interferon, TNF, LAK cells, or TILs. The combination of IL-2 and LAK cells is referred to as adoptive immunotherapy. This combination has produced responses in additional tumor types including colorectal cancer, lung cancer, and non-Hodgkin's lymphoma. Similar objective response rates (20–35%) were again reported in patients with renal cell carcinoma or malignant melanoma receiving either IL-2 alone or in combination with LAK cells. No improvement was seen with the coadministration of TNF, but additional trials are being conducted with the combination of IL-2 and interferon.

The administration of high-dose recombinant IL-2 is associated with a broad range of toxic side effects in a variety of organ systems that frequently require management in an intensive care setting. Most organ toxicities are probably the result of lymphoid infiltrates in vital organs as well as fluid retention and interstitial edema associated with IL-2–induced capillary leakage. The toxicities of IL-2 appear to be dose and schedule dependent, with the greatest toxicities occurring with the high-dose continuous infusion and bolus administration schedules. Combination therapy with IL-2/LAK has also been associated with numerous serious side effects, but most of these have been attributed to IL-2. Following discontinuation of IL-2 administration, the toxicities quickly resolve, and the average time period between the last IL-2 dose and hospital discharge is 5 days.

Systemic symptoms including chills and fever occur early after the administration of IL-2 and probably are due to the induction of secondary cytokines such as IL-1, IL-6, TNF, and gamma interferon. These side effects can be minimized with concomitant administration of acetaminophen or nonsteroidal anti-inflammatory agents. Patients may also develop diffuse macular erythema that progresses to a desquamating rash with pruritus. The mechanism for the development of this rash is unknown, and patients can generally be managed symptomatically with antipruritics. Nausea, vomiting, diarrhea, and anorexia are common gastrointestinal side effects. The anorexia may be caused by the induction of TNF, a cytokine identical to cachectin (see below).

Cardiovascular side effects also occur acutely following drug administration, producing a clinical picture similar to septic shock. These symptoms include decreased systemic vascular resistance, hypotension, tachycardia, and increased cardiac output. The hypotension may respond to intravenous fluid challenges but usually requires management with pressors such as dopamine and phenylephrine because of the pulmonary edema and fluid overload that occur secondary to IL-2–induced capillary leak syndrome. The loss of albumin and fluid into interstitial tissues also causes an intravascular volume depletion that may be associated with oliguria and prerenal azotemia. The precise mechanism for the capillary leak syndrome is unknown, but direct toxic effects of cytokines on endothelial cell surfaces have been proposed. Cardiac arrhythmias and myocardial infarction have also been associated with IL-2 therapy, so patients with a previous cardiac history should be carefully evaluated before treatment.

Neuropsychiatric changes manifested as hallucinations, disorientation, delusions, personality changes, and behavioral changes have been reported to occur near the end of a treatment course of IL-2. These symptoms warrant discontinuation of the drug and usually resolve within 24–48 hours. Endocrine effects such as increased circulating levels of adrenocorticotropic hormone (ACTH), cortisol, prolactin, and growth hormone have been measured following IL-2 administration. The development of hypothyroidism has occurred in 20% of patients 6–11 weeks following high-dose IL-2/LAK therapy.

IL-2 therapy has several adverse effects on the hematopoietic system. In addition to the immediate lymphopenia followed by lymphocytosis that occurs with therapy, patients may develop a progressive anemia requiring blood transfusions. Moderate thrombocytopenia (platelet count 25,000–50,000) occurs in approximately 30% of patients, while severe thrombocytopenia (platelet count <25,000) may occur in as many as 15% of patients. Eosinophilia is a frequent side effect of IL-2 therapy and is thought to be caused by increased eosinophilopoietin owing to IL-5 or IL-6 induction. Prolonged prothrombin times and partial thromboplastin times are also a common side effect experienced by patients receiving IL-2 therapy. As in the case of the interferons, the production of serum neutralizing antibodies against interleukin have been seen following prolonged administration of the drug.

Preliminary results with this therapy are promising, and IL-2 has been approved for the treatment of advanced or metastatic renal cell carcinoma. Further studies are necessary to determine other indications, doses, and route and schedule of administration. Further characterization of the other interleukins may result in the discovery of additional agents with cytotoxic activity against various cancers.

MONOCLONAL ANTIBODIES

Since the development of monoclonal antibody technology in 1975 by Kohler and Milstein, there has been a surge of research involving the use of monoclonal antibodies (MoAbs) for the diagnosis and treatment of cancer. The intention behind using MoAbs in cancer therapy is to develop an antibody against an antigen that is specific to tumor cells, resulting in immune mediated tumor cell killing. MoAbs may be utilized in various ways for the treatment of malignancies. The MoAb may be administered alone, causing direct or indirect cytotoxicity, or it can be conjugated with radiolabeled isotopes, toxins, or drugs in an attempt to target drug delivery to malignant cells.

Several problems are inherent to the development of tumor-directed antibodies. First, the heterogeneity of tumor cells within a single patient or among patients makes it impossible to develop a single tumor-specific antibody. In efforts to overcome this obstacle, researchers are using combination monoclonal antibodies (or "cocktails") to increase the activity against human tumors. The ideal method for increasing antitumor activity would be to develop individual monoclonal antibodies for patients based on biopsy samples of their own tumor. This is not currently practical on a large scale.

A second problem is the possibility of organ toxicity due to sequestration of antibody conjugates in the lungs, liver, and spleen. Some of these problems may be eliminated by pharmacologic manipulation of the immunoconjugate. Another significant problem is the development of human antimouse antibodies (HAMAs) following administration of murine MoAbs. The development of HAMAs occurs rapidly in most patients who are not immunosuppressed and prohibits the repeated administration of MoAbs owing to neutralization of the therapeutic effects.

Several solutions have been proposed for minimizing the development of HAMAs. The best solution would be the development of human MoAbs, but mass production of human MoAbs for clinical trials has not been accomplished to date. Through genetic engineering, monoclonal antibodies that consist of murine fragments spliced into human immunoglobulins have been produced. These antibodies, known as chimeric antibodies, have proved to be less immunogenic than pure murine MoAbs in preliminary studies, but their clinical utility remains to be determined. The administration of immunosuppressive agents such as cyclophosphamide and cyclosporine prior to MoAb treatment may also delay the development of HAMAs and allow the administration of repeated doses of murine MoAbs. Clinical trials utilizing these techniques are being conducted.

MoAbs (both alone and conjugated to a toxin) have been used in the treatment of numerous cancer types including breast, lung, colon, and ovarian and melanoma, lymphoma, and leukemia. The main side effects consist of fever, chills, flushing, urticaria, nausea, and vomiting. In patients with high levels of HAMAs, life-threatening anaphylactic reactions have been reported. Unfortunately, MoAbs have not turned out to be the "magic bullets" for cancer treatment that researchers had hoped. However, research and development are still in the early stages. With more time, MoAbs may prove to be important tools for the diagnosis and treatment of malignancies.

TUMOR NECROSIS FACTOR

Nearly a century ago scientists first observed tumor necrosis and regression in cancer patients with concomitant bacterial infections. Since that time, there have been numerous attempts to identify the protein responsible for this phenomenon. In 1975, tumor necrosis factor (TNF) was identified. TNF-alpha, also called **cachectin,** is a cytokine that is produced and released primarily by macrophages as part of the general immune response. A protein with similar homology and biologic functions is produced by lymphocytes and is referred to as **lymphotoxin** or TNF-beta. Both compounds are available in large quantities as a result of recombinant DNA technology and are in clinical trials.

In vitro and in vivo studies have demonstrated that TNF produces numerous biologic effects in addition to its cytotoxic/cytostatic effects on tumor cells, including inflammatory reactions, the septic shock syndrome associated with acute infections, and the anorexia and altered metabolism associated with chronic disease. These biologic effects occur secondary to immune cell activation and release of other cell mediators (such as IL-1 and G-CSF) induced by the TNF. The antitumor mechanisms of TNF are not fully elucidated, but direct cytotoxicity on tumor cells owing to free-radical induction, DNA fragmentation,

and breakdown of the nuclear membrane have been proposed.

Phase I and II clinical trials of **recombinant TNF** (rTNF) have utilized various doses, schedules, and routes of administration. Single intravenous doses up to 200 $\mu g/m^2$ and subcutaneous doses up to 250 $\mu g/m^2$ have been given. Continuous intravenous infusions have also been tried with rTNF in an attempt to maximize drug exposure because of the short half-life of the drug. The toxicities reported with either route are similar except that bolus intravenous administration produced more severe systemic toxicities. Severe inflammation at the injection site was the dose-limiting side effect for the subcutaneous route of administration. Fever, chills, and rigors were the most common side effects reported in phase I trials. Other reported side effects include headache, fatigue, hypotension, thrombocytopenia, leukopenia, hepatotoxicity, and altered lipid metabolism. Serum antibodies against rTNF have not been reported in the clinical trials to date.

The tumor responses reported in phase I clinical trials were minimal; phase II trials are under way to determine the specific antitumor activity of rTNF. The data for single agent rTNF are somewhat disappointing, but the combination of other biologic response modifiers or chemotherapeutic agents with rTNF may improve the activity of the drug. Gamma interferon, IL-2, and GM-CSF have demonstrated synergism with rTNF, and there is speculation that cell cycle–specific chemotherapeutic agents may enhance the cytotoxicity of rTNF.

BACILLUS CALMETTE-GUÉRIN

Bacillus Calmette-Guérin (BCG) is an attenuated strain of *Mycobacterium bovis* that was originally developed as a vaccine against tuberculosis. Because of its stimulatory effects on the immune system, BCG has also been used in clinical trials for the treatment of various malignancies including acute leukemia, malignant melanoma, and colon, breast, renal cell, and bladder carcinoma. The only significant responses so far have been seen in the treatment of superficial bladder cancer. Two BCG products are commercially available for the intravesical treatment of bladder carcinoma in situ.

The mechanism of action of BCG is unclear, but nonspecific immune stimulation leading to lymphocyte and macrophage activation has been reported. BCG cytotoxicity may also be due to endogenous production of other biologic response modifiers such as gamma interferon, tumor necrosis factor, and interleukin-2. BCG has demonstrated the most activity following direct intravesical administration for the treatment of superficial bladder cancer. Furthermore, several criteria are required for a tumor response to occur. They include small tumor size, immunocompetence of the host, drug administration in close proximity to the tumor, and administration of adequate numbers of mycobacteria.

The recommended intravesical dose of BCG varies according to the mycobacterium strain being utilized. From 10 million to 100 million BCG bacilli have been administered as a single dose. The dose is commonly diluted in 50–60 mL of normal saline and administered directly into the bladder via a catheter. The solution is retained in the bladder for 1.5–2 hours. Weekly doses of intravesical BCG are currently recommended for a total of six treatments followed by maintenance therapy at 1-, 2-, or 3-month intervals. Patients who do not respond to BCG initially or have an early recurrence may benefit from a second trial of therapy. After two treatment failures, the patient should be treated with an alternative regimen. BCG has also been administered by the subcutaneous, intradermal, intratumoral, intrapleural, and intravenous routes.

The side effects of BCG appear to be dose and route related, with repeated doses resulting in increased toxicity. Most patients experience a local reaction in the form of bladder irritability, frequency, urgency, and dysuria. These symptoms may be increased in patients who have decreased bladder capacity owing to surgery or radiation treatment. These local reactions can often be paralleled by systemic symptoms resembling an influenzalike reaction including fever, chills, malaise, headache, and weakness. All these symptoms occur within 6–12 hours of the dosing of BCG and usually resolve within 48 hours following treatment. Both local and systemic toxicities can be decreased with a reduction in BCG dose. Antipyretics and antihistamines may also help minimize these effects. Because the possibility exists that patients may experience a transient systemic BCG infection following treatment with BCG, prophylactic isoniazid has been given in some clinical trials. Serious disseminated BCG infections have also been reported with this therapy but primarily in patients who are immunosuppressed. Patients may convert from a negative to a positive PPD test following treatment with BCG. Interestingly, this conversion and the development of bladder granulomas occur most frequently in patients who exhibit a tumor response to BCG therapy. A final side effect that has been suggested is the accelerated growth and development of second primary malignancies following therapy with BCG. While animal studies have shown that the timing of the administration of BCG may result in tumor enhancement, data to support this effect in humans are lacking. Further investigation is warranted.

REFERENCES

Interferon

Davis GL et al: Treatment of chronic hepatitis C with recombinant interferon alpha: a multicenter randomized, controlled trial. *N Engl J Med* 1989;**321**:1501.

Krown SE et al: Interferon-α with zidovudine: Safety, tolerance, and clinical and virologic effects in patients with Kaposi sarcoma associated with the acquired immunodeficiency syndrome (AIDS). *Ann Intern Med* 1990;**112**:812.

Nelson BE, Borden EC: Interferons: Biological and clinical effects. *Semin Surg Oncol* 1989;**5**:391.

Quesada JR et al: Clinical toxicity of interferons in cancer patients: A review. *J Clin Oncol* 1986;**4**:234.

Thompson JA, Fefer A: Interferon in the treatment of hairy cell leukemia. *Cancer* 1987;**59**:605.

Colony-Stimulating Factors

Bajorin DF et al: Macrophage colon-stimulating factor: Biological effects and potential applications for cancer therapy. *Semin Hematol* 1991;**23 (Suppl 2)**:42.

Gabrilove JL et al: Effect of granulocyte colony-stimulating factor on neutropenia and associated morbidity due to chemotherapy for transitional-cell carcinoma of the urothelium. *N Engl J Med* 1988;**318**:1414.

Mertelsmann R et al: Hematopoietic growth factors in bone marrow transplantation. *Bone Marrow Transplant* 1990;**6**:73.

Miles SA et al: Combined therapy with recombinant granulocyte colony-stimulating factor and erythropoietin decreases hematologic toxicity from zidovudine. *Blood* 1991;**77**:2109.

Peters WP: The myeloid colony-stimulating factors: Introduction and overview. *Semin Hematol* 1991;**28 (Suppl 2)**:1.

Interleukins

Kintzel PE, Calis KA: Recombinant interleukin-2: A biological response modifier. *Clin Pharm* 1991;**10**:110.

Oster W et al: Interleukin-3: Biologic effects and clinical impact. *Cancer* 1991;**67**:2712.

Rosenberg SA et al: Experience with the use of high-dose interleukin-2 in the treatment of 652 cancer patients. *Ann Surg* 1989;**210**:474.

Siegel JP, Puri RK: Interleukin-2 toxicity. *J Clin Oncol* 1991;**9**:694.

Starnes HF Jr: Biological effects and possible clinical applications of interleukin-1. *Semin Hematol* 1991;**28 (Suppl 2)**:34.

Monoclonal Antibodies

Dillman RO: Monoclonal antibodies for treating cancer. *Ann Intern Med* 1989;**111**:592.

Harris DT, Mastrangelo MJ: Serotherapy of cancer. *Semin Oncol* 1989;**16**:180.

Hertler AA, Frankel AE: Immunotoxins: A clinical review of their use in the treatment of malignancies. *J Clin Oncol* 1989;**7**:1932.

Kosmas C, Kalofonos H, Epenetos AA: Monoclonal antibodies: Future potential in cancer chemotherapy. *Drugs* 1989;**38**:645.

Vaickus L, Foon KA: Clinical applications of monoclonal antibodies in oncology. *Hosp Formul* 1990;**25**:50.

Tumor Necrosis Factor

Beutler B: The tumor necrosis factors: Cachectin and lymphotoxin. *Hosp Pract* (Feb. 15) 1990;**25**:45.

Cerami A: Cachectin/TNF and the immune response. *Adv Oncol* 1990;**6**:5.

Grunfeld C, Palladino MA: Tumor necrosis factor: Immunologic, antitumor, metabolic, and cardiovascular activities. *Adv Intern Med* 1990;**35**:45.

Schiller JH et al: Biological and clinical effects of intravenous tumor necrosis factor-α administered three times weekly. *Cancer Res* 1991;**51**:1651.

Wanebo HJ: Tumor necrosis factors. *Semin Surg Oncol* 1989;**5**:402.

Bacillus Calmette-Guérin

Bohle A et al: Elevations of cytokines interleukin-1, interleukin-2, and tumor necrosis factor in the urine of patients after intravesical bacillus Calmette-Guérin immunotherapy. *J Urol* 1990;**144**:59.

Lamm DL et al: Complications of bacillus Calmette-Guérin immunotherapy: Review of 2602 patients and comparison of chemotherapy complications. European Organization for Research on Treatment of Cancer Genitourinary (EORTC GU) Group Monograph 1989;**6**:335.

Martinez-Pineiro JA et al: Bacillus Calmette-Guérin versus doxorubicin versus thiotepa: A randomized prospective study in 202 patients with superficial bladder cancer. *J Urol* 1990;**143**:502.

Orihuela E et al: Toxicity of intravesical BCG and its management in patients with superficial bladder tumors. *Cancer* 1987;**60**:326.

Sarosdy MF, Lamm DL: Long-term results of intravesical bacillus Calmette-Guérin therapy for superficial bladder cancer. *J Urol* 1989;**142**:719.

Pain Management

Nicolas E. Walsh, MD, & Janna S. Blanchard, MD

Pain is a source of fear and morbidity for the patient with cancer. It is one of the most dreaded complications of the disease, and many cancer patients spend the last weeks, months, or even years of their lives in discomfort and suffering that greatly compromise the quality of their lives. Early recognition, thorough understanding, and aggressive treatment of pain should be a major concern for the physician who cares for these patients.

Clinical experience suggests that a multidisciplinary approach, which may include physical therapy modalities, analgesic drugs, neurosurgical and anesthetic procedures, psychological intervention, and supportive care, is most effective. A primary goal is significant relief of pain so that the patient can attain an acceptable functional status, a reasonable quality of life, and a death relatively free of pain.

Incidence

In the USA in 1991 there were an estimated 1.1 million new cases of cancer and over 500,000 deaths due to cancer. No comprehensive epidemiologic studies on the prevalence and impact of pain associated with cancer are available; however, several major cancer treatment centers have conducted surveys that provide some indication. Approximately 70–95% of terminal cancer patients have frequent or persistent pain before death. Moderate to severe pain occurs in 40–50% of cancer patients with early or intermediate stage cancer and in 60–90% of patients with advanced cancer.

Cancer can be painful at onset, and pain was an early symptom, present when the cancer was first diagnosed, in 40–50% of patients who had cancer of the breast, prostate, colon, rectum, ovary, or cervix and in 60–70% of those with cancer of the lung or pancreas. Pain is eventually experienced by approximately 85% of patients with primary bone tumors, 70% of patients with cancer of the genitourinary tract, 50% of patients with breast cancer, 45% of patients with lung cancer, 20% of patients with lymphoma, and 5% of patients with leukemia. Based on World Health Organization (WHO) data, it is estimated that over 9 million people in the world suffer from cancer pain.

Although it has been suggested that cancer pain can be adequately controlled with current therapies in 90–95% of patients, at least 25% and, in some parts of the world, as many as 80% of these patients are not adequately treated for their pain. Twenty-five percent of cancer patients worldwide die in severe pain without relief.

The medical community has been admonished for generally failing to adequately deal with the often excruciating pain that these patients suffer. Certainly one of the main reasons why cancer patients suffer from pain is undertreatment of pain by health care providers. Some physicians may not use analgesics and adjuvants appropriately owing to an incomplete understanding of their pharmacology. Often there is fear of patient addiction, respiratory depression, or other side effects that may interfere with correct dosing. In addition, beyond the standard modalities for pain control, many physicians are not aware of the variety of treatment options available for cancer patients with pain problems.

Etiology

Pain directly related to the disease accounts for approximately 75% of pain in cancer patients. The pain associated with cancer results from tumor invasion into normal tissues. Infiltration and compression of nerves produce a severe neuropathic pain, while tumor infiltration of blood vessels and lymphatics can result in edema, engorgement, and painful ischemia. If the tumor obstructs a hollow viscus or ductal system, there can be severe pelvic or abdominal pain. Pain also occurs in any area of the body from cancer-related tissue damage secondary to ulceration, necrosis, or infection. Bone pain results when the tumor activates nociceptors locally, stretches and distends well-innervated periosteum, or results in pathologic fractures. Most cancer patients display multiple mechanisms for their pain, and a mixed picture of bone destruction, nerve compression, and tissue damage is not unusual (Table 17–1).

Pain associated with cancer therapy accounts for 20% of the pain reported by cancer patients. Injury to pain-sensitive structures secondary to lumbar puncture, bone marrow harvests, surgical procedures, radiation therapy, and chemotherapy are included in this category (Table 17–1).

Table 17–1. Causes of pain in cancer patients.

Directly related to cancer
  Pressure from tumor growth in tight compartments (organ capsule, periosteum, fascia)
  Venous engorgement (blockage of egress)
  Arterial ischemia (blockage of egress)
  Obstruction of hollow viscus (colic, retrograde tissue destruction)
  Tissue damage (necrosis, infection, ulceration, inflammation) in pain-sensitive structure
  Bone pain (periosteal irritation, fracture)
  Neuritis pain (infiltration, distant effect, extrinsic pain, pressure, postherpetic pain, phantom limb pain, causalgia, postcordotomy pain)
  Mixed
Associated with cancer therapy
  Surgical procedures
  Radiotherapy
  Chemotherapy
Unrelated to cancer per se
  Constipation
  Peptic ulcer
  Pressure sores
  Cystitis
  Musculoskeletal disorders
  Pain syndromes not due to cancer

Pain unrelated to cancer or the therapy accounts for 5% of the pain reported by cancer patients. It may be due to constipation, peptic ulcers, pressure sores, musculoskeletal disorders secondary to disuse, or coincidental pain such as that due to degenerative joint disease, herniated disk, or diabetic neuropathy (Table 17–1).

Anatomy & Physiology of Pain

Pain results from the activation of nociceptors in cutaneous, superficial, or deep tissues. Nociceptors are sensory receptors that are sensitive to a variety of tissue-damaging (noxious) stimuli (eg, mechanical, thermal, or chemical). When activated, nociceptors conduct painful impulses to the spinal cord by two types of afferent nerve fibers: A delta fibers are thinly myelinated, conduct impulses rapidly, and are associated with sharp, initial pain, while C fibers are unmyelinated and conduct dull, boring pain more slowly. Both these fibers enter the spinal cord through the dorsal horn and terminate in various areas of Rexed's lamina. In this area, interposed neurons modulate the nociceptive signals. These pain signals are eventually transmitted via a variety of routes to the brain. The main route for conduction involves the spinothalamic system in the anterolateral portion of the cord. Although detailed mechanisms are yet unclear, there appears to be a descending control system that can modify the painful transmissions. There is also a system of endogenous opiatelike peptides (endorphins and enkephalins distributed throughout the entire body, spinal cord, and other areas of the central nervous system. In these locations, they may modulate and inhibit neural activity and play a role in pain control.

The pain of malignant disease may be classified as **somatic, visceral,** or **deafferentative.** Somatic and visceral pain result from activation of nociceptors. Somatic pain is typically well localized, whereas visceral pain is poorly localized and often referred to cutaneous sites that are remote from the lesion. Somatic pain is described as aching or gnawing and occurs in the cancer patient as a result of bone metastasis, ulceration, or musculoskeletal pain. Visceral pain is often described as deep and sickening with pressure that results from tumor invasion of thoracic or abdominal viscera from either primary or metastatic growth.

Pain due to deafferentation occurs following damage to either the peripheral or the central nervous system caused by invading tumor, surgical trauma, chemotherapy, or irradiation, resulting in neuropathies, plexopathies, or spinal cord compression. The quality of this pain is described as burning, electrical, or constant aching.

A general understanding of the anatomy and physiology of pain will help the physician understand its cause.

Evaluation of Pain

A. Believe That a Pain Problem Exists: Paramount to an effective working relationship with the cancer patient is belief by the physician in the pain complaint. The physician must take the patient's pain problem seriously and assess its severity with professionalism and compassion.

B. Take a Thorough History: The diagnostic evaluation begins with a thorough history of the patient's cancer and any other systemic illnesses. Use the PQRST mnemonic to help guide the patient in describing the pain: P = provocative and palliative factors; Q = quality; R = region; S = severity; and T = temporal relationships of the pain. The influence of the pain on routine daily activities and the sleep-wake cycle should be specifically noted as well as the success or failure of medications or therapies previously prescribed. Several types of pain intensity scale have been used to help quantitate the amount of pain the patient is experiencing. They include visual analog, numeric color, and categoric scales. The patient can be asked to rate the pain on a scale of zero to ten, with zero representing no pain and ten representing the worst possible pain. A baseline value is obtained at the initial evaluation, and at each subsequent office visit the patient can rate the pain and the progress of therapy can be gauged. A complete review of the patient's records, the staging of the patient's disease, and previous diagnostic studies can provide additional information.

C. Perform a Thorough Physical Examination: A physical examination of the painful region as well as a general physical examination with particular attention to the neurologic and musculoskeletal systems is essential for clinical correlation with the patient's complaints. Since cancer usually is not a static disease, it is also important to document all physical abnormalities, particularly neurologic, and follow them closely with frequent reexamination and reassessment.

D. Evaluate Psychological and Social Factors: The cancer patient's emotional state may profoundly influence the perception of pain. Fear, anxiety, changes in body image or functional roles, financial problems, and social isolation may all affect the pain condition. The cancer patient may have ineffective coping skills and severe reactive depression. The patient's support system should be evaluated to assess its role in helping to deal with the stress of cancer and coincident pain. All pertinent psychological and social factors should be identified and considered in the treatment of patients.

Assessment

The physician must determine if the pain is the result of cancer-directed therapy, such as chest wall pain after mastectomy, or if a component of the pain problem can be managed by additional cancer-directed therapy, such as surgery, radiation, or chemotherapy. If there is no therapy option for the cancer, then the pain is approached as a disease itself and treatment is aimed at pain control. When the evaluation is completed, the physician must make an assessment of the cause of the patient's pain and formulate a treatment plan. The approach to pain management in the patient with a curable process may vary completely from the approach used for the same pain problem in a patient with a very limited life span. The physician and patient must decide on realistic goals for pain relief based on the diagnosis and the level of functional activity that the patient wants to maintain or achieve. The patient must be completely informed about all possible risks and benefits of the treatment plan and any options for therapy. The physician should outline an approach to pain management so that the patient will feel confident that, even if complete pain relief is not possible or if the current therapy fails, the physician will sincerely strive to do as much as possible. The physician must be committed to the patient's pain management for as long as is necessary.

Treatment

The therapeutic strategy for the management of cancer pain may rely on the concurrent or sequential use of various treatment modalities adapted to the needs of the individual patient. A wide variety of techniques and modalities are available for cancer pain management. It is advisable to begin with relatively low risk, noninvasive modalities when possible and then progress to higher risk, more invasive technique as appropriate. Oral and parenteral analgesic drugs are the usual first-line treatment and mainstay of cancer pain management. In some situations, how-

ever, it may be appropriate to start with an invasive procedure if it is believed to be the only modality that will provide the patient with maximum pain relief or if the patient is at a crisis stage owing to extreme pain.

A. Pharmacologic Treatment:

1. Three-step management of pain–(See Table 17–2.) WHO recommends a systematic approach to selection of pharmacologic agents for treating patients with cancer pain. The protocol is based on the premise that physicians and health care professionals should know how to use a few simple drugs well. A three-step analgesic ladder is the scheme used for analgesic selection:

a. Step 1–Patients who have mild to moderate pain should initially be treated with a nonopioid analgesic (Table 17–3) such as aspirin or another nonsteroidal anti-inflammatory drug (NSAID) plus an adjuvant analgesic (Table 17–4) if indicated.

b. Step 2–Patients who have moderate to severe pain or who do not achieve adequate relief with step 1 should be started on a weak oral opioids (Table 17–5) such as codeine along with a nonopioid and an adjuvant analgesic if indicated.

c. Step 3–Patients who have very severe pain or who do not achieve adequate relief with the step 2 regimen should be treated with a potent opioid (Table 17–6) such as morphine with or without a nonopioid or with an adjuvant analgesic if indicated.

The nonopioid analgesics act peripherally by interfering with the synthesis of prostaglandins, whereas the opioids act centrally by binding to specific opioid receptors and activating the endogenous pain suppression system in the central nervous system. Because of the this difference, the combination of these

Table 17–2. Clinical classification of pain intensity.

Step	Pain Intensity	Failure to Respond to	Relieved by
1	Mild		NSAID +/– Adjuvant
2	Moderate	Nonnarcotic analgesics	Weak[1] narcotic Codeine Oxycodone Combination with NSAID +/– Adjuvant
3	Severe	Weak narcotic analgesics	Potent[2] narcotic Morphine Hydromorphone Meperidine Methadone +/– NSAID +/– Adjuvant

[1]Although narcotics vary in potency, they are equal in efficacy; ie, increasing the dose of a less potent narcotic can produce the same analgesic effect of the more potent narcotic.
[2]The use of a combination of nonnarcotic and narcotic drugs results in improved pain relief without an increase in the dose of narcotics.

Table 17–3. Nonopioid analgesics for mild to moderate pain (Step 1).[1]

Drug	Plasma Half-life (h)	Peak Effect (h)	Duration of Analgesia (h)	Usual Dose[2] (mg)	Maximum Recommended Dose[3] (mg/d)	Comment
Aspirin	4–16	2	4–12	650 every 4–6 h	6000	Standard of comparison for nonnarcotics.[4]
Acetaminophen	2–4	3	4	650 every 4–6 h	6000	No effect on gastric mucosa, platelet aggregation, or anti-inflammatory response. Increased hepatic toxicity over 4 gld.
Diclofenac (Voltaren)	6–8	2–4	10–12	50–75 every 12 h	150	Decreased gastrointestinal toxicity.
Diflunisal (Dolobid)	8–12	2–3	8–12	500 every 12 h	1500	Decreased gastrointestinal toxicity.
Indomethacin (Indocin, others)	4–5	1–2	4	25–50 every 8 h	200	Greater incidence of gastrointestinal toxicity and central nervous system side effects than for aspirin.
Ibuprofen	2–4	1–2	4–6	400–800 every 6–8 h	3200	
Naproxen (Naprosyn)	12–15	2–4	8–12	250–500 every 12 h	1500	Available in liquid suspension.
Piroxicam (Feldene)	50	3–5	12	20 every 24 h	40	Higher incidence of side effects at dosage of 40 mg for more than 3 weeks.
Salsalate (Disalcid, others)	4–16	2	4–12	1000 every 8 h	6000	Lowest gastrointestinal side effects of the NSAIDs.[5]
Sulindac (Clinoril, other)	14–16	3–4	8–12	150 every 12 h	400	Decreased renal toxicity.

[1]Reproduced, with permission, from Walsh NE: *Rehabilitation of Chronic Pain.* Hanley & Belfus, 1991.
[2]Dosage should be adjusted in the elderly, patients on multiple medications, patients with renal insufficiency or hepatic failure. Doses may be increased at weekly intervals if pain relief is inadequate and dosage is tolerated. Doses and intervals titrated to effect.
[3]Patient should routinely be evaluated for hepatic toxicity. Patients receiving nonsteroidal anti-inflammatory drugs (NSAIDs) should additionally be evaluated for renal toxicity and fecal blood loss due to gastrointestinal irritation. Patients who develop visual complaints during treatment should have ophthalmic evaluation. Gastrointestinal disturbance may be reduced if drug is taken with milk, on a full stomach, or with antacids.
[4]Morphine, 10 mg orally, is approximately equianalgesic to aspirin 650 mg orally.
[5]NSAID = Nonsteroidal anti-inflammatory drug.

Table 17–4. Adjuvant analgesics.[1,2]

Drug Class	Preferred Drugs	Dosing Schedule	Starting Dose (mg)	Comment
Tricyclic antidepressants	Amitriptyline (Elavil, others) Doxepin Imipramine (Tofranil, others) Nortriptyline (Pamelor)	At bedtime (or divide into 2 or 3 doses per day)	10–25 30 20 50	For neuropathic deafferentation pain or pain complicated by insomnia or depression. For the elderly patient, start with 10 mg at bedtime and if daytime somnolence is a problem, give dose earlier in the evening.
Anticonvulsants	Carbamazepine (Tegretol others) Phenytoin (Dilantin) Clonazepam (Klonopin)	Every 6–8 h at bedtime 12 h	200 300 0.5	For neuropathic deafferentation pain with shooting or lancinating quality. May need to follow blood levels.
Neuroleptics	Fluphenazine (Prolixin, others) Haloperidol (Haldol)	8 h 6–12 h	2 2	For refractory deafferentation pain and pain complicated by nausea or delirium.
Antihistamines	Hydroxyzine (Vistaril, others) Diphenhydramine (Benadryl, others)	6–8 h 4–6 h	25–75 25–50	For pain complicated by anxiety, nausea, or insomnia.
Miscellaneous	Dexamethasone (Decadron, others)	Four times a day	4–8	For refractory bone and deafferentation pain.

[1]Reproduced, with permission, from Walsh NE: *Rehabilitation of Chronic Pain.* Hanley & Belfus, 1991.
[2]Drug dosages may need to be modified for the elderly.

Table 17–5. Opioid analgesics for moderate pain (Step 2).[1,2]

| Drug | Equianalgesic Dosage | | | Action Time[5] | | | Usual Initial Dose (mg) | Comment[6] |
	Aspirin[3] PO	Morphine[4] IM	PO	Half-life (h)	Peak Effect (h)	Duration of Analgesia (h)		
Codeine	32	120	200	3	1–2	4–6	32–65 every 3–4 h	Combined with acetamino-phen or NSAIDs
Hydrocodone (Vicodin, many others)	2.5	15	30	3–4	1	3–5	5–10 every 3–4 h	Combined with acetamino-phen or NSAIDs
Meperidine (Demerol, others)	50	90	300	3–4	1–2	2–4	50–100 every 3 h	Short acting, risk of accumula-tion in patients with im-paired renal function
Oxycodone (Per-cocet, others)	2.5	15	30	3–4	1	3–5	5–10 every 3–4 h	Combined with acetamino-phen or NSAIDs
Pentazocine (Talwin, Talacen)	30	60	180	2–5	1–2	4–6	50–100 every 4 h	Not standard for cancer pain
Propoxyphene (Darvocet, others)	100–200	—	300	2–3	1–2	3–6	100–200 every 4 h	Not standard for cancer pain

[1]Reproduced, with permission, from Walsh NE: *Rehabilitation of Chronic Pain.* Hanley & Belfus, 1991.
[2]Drug dosages may need to be modified for the elderly.
[3]Dose providing analgesic equivalent to aspirin, 650 mg orally (PO).
[4]Dose providing analgesic equivalent to single-dose morphine, 10 mg intramuscularly (IM).
[5]Varies with route of administration.
[6]NSAID = Nonsteroidal anti-inflammatory drug.

two types of drugs may produce additive analgesic effects. The adjuvant analgesics are a group of drugs that have various other primary indications and sites of actions but have been shown to be clinically useful for many cancer pain states.

2. Pharmacologic guidelines–
a. The dose of an analgesic should be determined on an individual basis. There is considerable patient-to-patient variation with respect to effective analge-sic dose. Generally, it is better to begin too high rather than too low. Starting suboptimally and titrat-ing upward results in patient anxiety due to a lack of adequate analgesia. The dose of the opioid analgesic should be titrated until the patient has pain relief or

Table 17–6. Opioid analgesics for severe pain.[1,2]

| Drug | Equianalgesic Dosage[3] | | | Action Time[5] | | | Usual[6] Initial Dose (mg) | Comment[7] |
	IM	PO	IV	Half-life (h)	Peak Effect (h)	Duration of Analgesia (h)		
Hydormorphone (Dilaudid, others)	1.5	7.5	1	2–3	1/2–1 1/2	3–4	4–8 every 3–4 h	
Levorphanol (Levo-Dromoran, others)	2	4	1	12–16	1–2	4–6	2–4 every 4–6 h	Increased sedation with re-peated doses.
Methadone (Dolophine, others)	10	20	5	15–57	1–2	6–8	5–10 every 6–8 h	Avoid in patients with signifi-cant respiratory, hepatic, or renal failure.
Morphine	10	30[4]	5	2–4	1/2–1 1/2	4–6	5–10 every 4 h	Standard of comparison for narcotics.
Controlled-release mor-phine		30[4]		2–4	—	8–12	30 mg every 8–12 h	
Oxymorphone (Numorphan)	1	—	0.5	2–3	30–90	4–6		10-mg rectal suppository available.

[1]Reproduced, with permission, from Walsh NE: Rehabilitation of Chronic Pain. Hanley & Belfus, 1991.
[2]Drug dosages may need to be modified for the elderly.
[3]Dose providing analgesic equivalent to single-dose morphine, 10 mg intramuscularly (IM). PO = orally; IV = intravenously.
[4]For chronic dosing only. For single dose, use 60 mg.
[5]Varies with route of administration.
[6]Dosage varies considerably, titrate to control pain.
[7]Most common side effects of opioid drugs include constipation, nausea, and sedation. Less common side effects include urinary retention, bladder spasm, respiratory depression, and intermittent vomiting. Rare side effects include psychotic symptoms, pruritus, orthostatic hypotension, bronchoconstriction, and biliary colic. Dosage should be adjusted in the elderly and patients with impaired ventilation, increased intracranial pressure, liver failure, or bronchial asthma.

intolerable side effects occur. If one drug is ineffective, a stronger one should be prescribed. It is useless to transfer to an alternative drug of similar strength. Avoid drug combinations that increase sedation without improving analgesia.

b. The "as-needed," or prn, schedule does not have a place in the control of chronic pain. The prn schedule results in operant conditioning, craving, a sense of dependence, and anxiety about the drug wearing off. As-needed administration will never relieve cancer pain well enough to erase the patient's memory and fear of the pain. The aim is to titrate the level of analgesic to an optimal dose that prevents the recurrence of pain. The next dose is given before the effect of the previous one has worn off. All medications are given regularly. The time interval for dosing should be consistent with the expected duration of action to maintain steady-state blood levels.

c. Medications are given orally if possible. Oral medications facilitate ambulatory care and independence and do not represent heroic intervention to the patient. Oral administration maintains plasma levels above the concentration necessary for analgesia longer than does parenteral administration. Narcotic elixirs (eg, "Brompton's cocktail") do not decrease toxicities or potentiate pain relief. Injections for pain generally are not required until the last 2–3 days of life if oral medications are given properly. More than four tablets per drug administration is generally unacceptable and stronger forms should be used.

d. The concepts of tolerance, physical dependence, and psychological dependence must be understood when treating cancer patients.

Tolerance means that an increased dose of an opioid is required to achieve the original effect. This usually occurs when the patient's disease process has progressed and the standard dose of analgesic has a shorter duration of action.

Physical dependence is apparent in a patient who has been taking an opioid for more than 2 weeks and the drug is abruptly discontinued. Symptoms can include anxiety, dysphoria, nausea and vomiting, signs of sympathetic nervous system hyperactivity, and seizures depending on the drug involved. If a patient who has been taking narcotics has a nonnarcotic modality instituted for pain control, the narcotic medication must be tapered carefully in order to avoid narcotic withdrawal.

Psychological dependence or addiction is drug-seeking behavior for effects other than pain relief. Anxiety about psychological dependence causes doctors and nurses to use opioids in inadequate doses. Their use should be dictated by the intensity of the patient's pain, and fear of addiction should not be a major concern in cancer patients.

e. Pain is often worse at night and prevents the patient from obtaining adequate sleep, which causes further debilitation. Use of a larger dose of narcotic at bedtime results in more prolonged relief of pain and better sleep. An adjuvant with a sedative effect such as amitriptyline can also be given at bedtime.

f. All clinically useful narcotics produce similar side effects in equianalgesic doses. The most common side effects reported are constipation, nausea and vomiting, and respiratory depression. Almost all patients receiving regular morphine require a laxative, and prophylactic therapy is preferable. About two-thirds need an antiemetic. Clinically important respiratory depression is rare in conjunction with the chronic administration of opioids. Decreased ventilation should be treated with small incremental doses (0.05–0.1 mg) of the antagonist naloxone. If naloxone is carefully titrated to effect (increased respiratory rate) withdrawal and reversal of analgesia can be avoided. Meperidine should not be used chronically because of central nervous system toxicity from its metabolite normeperidine. Pentazocine, a mixed agonist/antagonist, can cause hallucinations before pain relief occurs.

g. Adjuvant drugs can increase the efficacy or reduce the required dose of narcotic analgesics. An antidepressant is indicated for patients who remain depressed despite improved pain control and for those with pain due to deafferentation. An anxiolytic may be used for very anxious patients but should not be used routinely in all cancer patients. Corticosteroids, anticonvulsants, and neuroleptic drugs also have a role to play in selected cases. Barbiturates that do not have analgesic properties should be used infrequently and with caution.

h. Before prescribing pharmacologic agents, the physician must understand the complete prescribing information and possible side effects.

3. Routes of administration–For most situations in cancer pain management, the oral route is preferred for pharmacologic agents. Intravenous routes are indicated when oral intake is not possible. Intravenous agents can be given as a repetitive bolus or continuous infusion. **Patient-controlled analgesia** (PCA) is a newly available technique whereby the patient self-administers up to a preset limit.

The administration of intraspinal opioids has become an efficacious and well-accepted technique. Spinal cord opioid receptors bind the administered narcotics. With intrathecal administration, a very low dose such as 0.5–1 mg of preservative-free morphine can be used, but there is risk of infection or cerebrospinal fluid leak after dural puncture. The epidural route is more often utilized, with starting doses of 5–10 mg of preservative-free morphine. A catheter can be inserted for repeat bolus or continuous infusion administration. It can be placed percutaneously or tunneled under the skin to minimize infection. Delivery systems can be external or implantable infusion pumps. This method of pain control can be effective even in patients who obtain no relief from systemically administered narcotics. It is not uncommon for patients to slowly develop tolerance, and doses must be escalated. Local anesthetics can be substituted or combined with the narcotic to allow the opioid receptors to regain sensitivity.

Cancer patients who have been taking oral or intravenous narcotics may be tolerant to the side effects of urinary retention, pruritus, and respiratory depression, but these potential problems must be considered. The patient who obtains relief from intraspinal narcotics must be tapered carefully from any previous narcotic medications in order to avoid withdrawal problems. Ambulatory infusion pumps are now available for subcutaneous administration of medications by repetitive bolus, continuous infusion, or PCA methods. Narcotics such as morphine and hydromorphone can be administered rectally, which may be an effective route in patients who cannot tolerate oral dosing but do not need repeated injections or are not hospitalized.

Alternative routes of administration may include buccal, transdermal, and intranasal.

B. Noninvasive Measures: Noninvasive measures in the treatment of pain in cancer patients generally have a low risk of complications, are less costly, and produce minimal side effects. They are used singularly for mild pain and in combination with drug therapy for moderate or severe pain.

Psychological intervention and support should be an integral part of each patient's management program. The patient must be reassured that response to these techniques does not mean that the pain is not real or that needed analgesics will be withdrawn or withheld.

1. Cutaneous stimulation–

a. Massage–Massage is often used in conjunction with application of lotion or ointment using a circular stroking motion. Only light pressure is applied over the tumor site.

b. Acupressure–Pressure is applied over traditional acupuncture sites.

c. Vibration–An electric vibrator is used over painful areas of acupressure points but not directly over tumor.

d. Transcutaneous electrical nerve stimulation (TENS)–TENS works best on well-localized moderate pain for limited periods of time. Although the mechanism is not completely understood, TENS is thought to provide stimulation-induced analgesia by inhibiting the nociceptive pathways through a gating mechanism in the spinal cord.

2. Thermal modalities–

a. Heat–Heat is not applied directly over the tumor site or area exposed to radiotherapy but to localized areas of pain.

b. Cold–Ice pack, cold water, or ice massage is applied to the painful area.

3. Activity and function–Cancer patients should maintain functional skills, strength, and mobility. Progressive immobilization is an insidious aspect of this disease that often is iatrogenic. While ra-

diation or chemotherapy may render a patient unable to perform activities for 1 day, the patient should be involved in active physical, occupational, corrective, and recreational therapy programs.

4. Behavioral interventions–

a. Relaxation techniques–Yoga, mediation, biofeedback, and progressive relaxation are techniques that decrease muscle tension. By themselves they will not relieve pain, other than that caused by muscle tension, but when used with other modalities they contribute to decreased pain.

b. Distraction–Increasing attention to activities other than pain is valuable. The activities may be passive or designed to increase daily living or functional skills.

c. Guided imagery–This form of cognitive behavioral modification requires the patient to concentrate on a positive image to help take his or her mind off pain. This technique requires concentration and is usually preceded by a relaxation technique, especially if the patient is tense and anxious.

d. Hypnosis–Deep relaxation and redirection of attention from pain are most useful. Self-hypnosis allows the patient to utilize this technique when required for pain control.

C. Invasive Procedures: More involved modalities or procedures for pain control have to be considered for some cancer patients. Depending on the mechanisms of the pain and its severity, a range of more invasive procedures may be of therapeutic benefit in addition to the usual pharmacologic modalities. The most common is surgical removal of all or part of the tumor in the hope of relieving pain and effecting a cure. Radiation therapy or chemotherapy may relieve pain by shrinking the tumor. In addition, anesthetic and neurosurgical procedures have been used to control cancer pain.

1. Neurolytic blocks–A variety of neurolytic blocks can be performed. They include use of intrathecal phenol or alcohol and trigeminal ganglion, intercostal nerve, or celiac plexus blocks with neurolytic agents. The chemical agent destroys all fibers—sympathetic, sensory, and motor—with which it comes into contact, thus theoretically interrupting pain transmission. The incidence of fair to good results following these blocks is estimated to be 60–70%, but no standardized method of assessing treatment response has been used and no well-controlled studies comparing these techniques to nonsurgical methods for pain control have been performed.

A diagnostic block with local anesthetic is essential before a block is performed with a neurolytic agent. This diagnostic procedure must be carried out with precision for correct needle placement so that therapeutic results can be accurately interpreted. The block will define the dermatomal distribution of the pain and discern the contribution of somatic and autonomic elements. It will also help the patient and family decide if the amount of pain relief and any associated numbness or weakness are acceptable. With neurolytic blocks it may not be possible to control the spread of the chemical agent, and the destructive effects can include loss of bladder, bowel, or motor function and deprive the patient of dignity and quality of life at the end of life.

Neurolytic blocks should be considered only after all other less invasive modalities have been tried. They are indicated for specific pain conditions and should be timed appropriately. Because of the increased life expectancy of patients due to current oncologic therapies, a block may not efficacious for a long enough duration and a fast growing tumor may rapidly extend beyond the limits of the block.

When successful, these blocks can provide impressive pain relief.

2. Neurosurgical procedures–Many types of neurosurgical procedures have been used to control cancer pain. They include neurectomy, rhizotomy, cordotomy, tractotomy, thalamotomy, commissurotomy, and hypophysectomy. The surgical techniques are used to interrupt pain fibers in the brain, spinal cord, or periphery. Reported efficacy ranges from 35% to 100%, but no well-controlled studies have compared these techniques to nonsurgical methods for pain control. Ablative procedures may provide relief for intractable pain, thus improving the quality of life and perhaps reducing the need for pain medications. Such procedures should only be considered after failure of optimal pharmacologic management or less invasive procedures. Any side effects or results must be considered permanent, and for patients having a longer life expectancy, the duration of analgesia may be disappointing.

Before a neurosurgical ablative procedure is done, a diagnostic nerve block with local anesthetic should be performed to determine if the desired effect will be achieved. The patient and family should be comfortable with the side effects of numbness, weakness, or dysfunction if they can result from the procedure. Local anesthetic blocks cannot absolutely predict the long-term benefit of surgical procedures, but they can reliably predict failure if no pain relief is obtained.

3. Treatment for specific pain syndrome–
a. Myofascial pain syndrome–Myofascial pain syndrome is a common cause of somatic pain in cancer patients. It is characterized by exquisitely tender palpable bands in a muscle or its fascia. This painful locus is called a trigger point, and pressure on it results in a characteristic pattern of pain referral.

Cancer patients may develop this syndrome from reflex muscle spasm secondary to their disease. It also occurs in debilitated and sedentary cancer patients who have significant muscle disuse and are susceptible to acute muscle strain or chronic muscle fatigue.

Trigger points can be injected with local anesthetic followed by physical therapy maneuvers with heat application, ultrasound, and gentle stretching and mobilization. Coolant spray and TENS applied over the trigger point can provide additional relief.

b. Sympathetically medicated pain syndromes–Specific pain conditions are associated with dysfunction of the sympathetic nervous system. The three most common syndromes are reflex sympathetic dystrophy, causalgia, and sympathetically aggravated neuralgia. These syndromes can be initiated by nerve damage or irritation due to surgery, radiation, or tumor infiltration.

Sympathetically mediated pain should be suspected when the patient's pain is more severe than anticipated or is resistant to standard therapies or if there is evidence of autonomic instability. The patient complains of intense burning or aching pain with hyperesthesias and periods of warmth and erythema or coolness and cyanosis.

Treatment is more effective if started early. The interruption of sympathetic activity with a local anesthetic block can confirm the diagnosis and is the first-line therapeutic intervention. Blocks that are commonly performed include stellate ganglion, lumbar sympathetic, celiac plexus, and thoracic epidural blocks. Repeated injections may be required for permanent relief depending on the severity of the problem. In some situations, continuous sympathetic block can be provided by placement of a catheter. Surgical or neurolytic sympathectomy may offer relief as may intravenous regional blockade with local anesthetics, corticosteroids, or adrenergic blocking agents. TENS can be a useful adjunct as well as appropriate physical therapy.

c. Neuropathic deafferentation pain syndromes–Tumors can invade or compress nerve roots and the major nerve plexuses, such as the brachial or lumbosacral, or involve peripheral nerves. This action may result in an inflammatory process that can respond to the perineural injection of corticosteroids alone or in combination with local anesthetics.

The cancer process may damage the nervous system in such a way that there is abnormal increased sensitivity and spontaneous activity of the neurons peripherally and centrally. This deafferentation pain can be difficult to treat. The patient may complain of crushing pain or dysesthesias. Adjuvant analgesics such as tricyclic antidepressants, anticonvulsants, and neuroleptics are standard therapy. Systemic intravenous local anesthetics may benefit some patients. Neurolysis procedures that cause additional peripheral denervation are usually of no value and may increase pain.

REFERENCES

Incidence

Bonica JJ, Ventafridda V, Twycross RG: Cancer pain. In: *The Management of Pain*. Bonica JJ (editor). Lea & Febiger, 1990.

Baines M, Kirkham SR: Cancer pain. In: *Textbook of Pain*. Wall PD, Melzack R (editors). Churchill Livingstone, 1989.

Etiology

Abram SE: Pain—Acute and chronic. In: *Clinical Anesthesia*. Barash PG, Cullen BF, Stoelting RK (editors). Lippincott, 1989.

Bonica JJ: A short course on the management of cancer pain. *J Pain Symptom Management* 1987;**2:**S3.

Foley KM: Cancer pain syndromes. *J Pain Symptom Management* 1987;**2:**S13.

Morris J et al: The effect of treatment setting and patient characteristics on pain in terminal cancer patients: A report from the national hospice study. *J Chronic Dis* 1986;**39:**27.

Anatomy & Physiology of Pain

Payne R: Anatomy, physiology and neuropharmacology of cancer pain. *Med Clin North Am* 1987;**71:**153.

Raj PP: Basic functions and organization of the nervous system. In: *Practical Management of Pain*. Raj PP (editor). Year Book, 1990.

Evaluation

Foley KM: Pain syndromes in patients with cancer. *Med Clin North Am* 1987;**71:**169.

Payne R: Cancer pain mechanisms and etiology: In: *Cancer Pain*. Abram SE (editor). Kluwer Academic, 1989.

Zimmerman M, Drings P, Wagner G: Pain in the cancer patient: Pathogenesis, diagnosis, and therapy. Recent Results Cancer Res 1984;**89:**1.

Treatment

Brescia FJ (editor): A short course on the management of cancer pain. *J Pain Symptom Management* 1987;**2:**S2.

Cleeland C: Nonpharmacological management of cancer pain. *J Pain Symptom Management* 1987;**2:**S23.

Cleeland C: Psychological aspects of pain due to cancer. In: *Cancer Pain*. Abram SE (editor). Kluwer Academic, 1989.

Coyle N: A model of continuity of care for cancer patients with chronic pain. *Med Clin North Am* 1987;**71:**153.

Ferrer-Brechner T: Neurolytic blocks for cancer pain. In: *Cancer Pain*. Abram SE (editor). Kluwer Academic, 1989.

Ferrer-Brechner T: Rational management of cancer-related pain. In: *Management of Pain*. Raj PP (editor). Year Book, 1990.

Foley KM: The treatment of cancer pain. *N Engl J Med* 1985;**313:**84.

Jessup BA: Relaxation and biofeedback. In: *Textbook of Pain*. Wall PD, Melzack R (editors). Churchill Livingstone, 1989.

Levy MH: Pain management in advanced cancer. *Semin Oncol* 1985;**12:**394.

Orne MT and Dinges DF: Hypnosis. In: *Textbook of Pain*. Wall PD, Melzack R (editors). Churchill Livingstone, 1989.

Payne R: Oral and parenteral drug therapy for cancer pain. In: *Cancer Pain*. Abram SE (editor). Kluwer Academic, 1989.

Quimby PR: Ablative neurosurgical procedures in pain related to malignancy. In: *Cancer Pain*. Abram SE (editor). Kluwer Academic, 1989.

Racz GB: *Techniques of Neurolysis*. Kluwer Academic, 1989.

Wall PD: The dorsal horn. In: *Textbook of Pain*. Wall PD, Melzack R (editors). Churchill Livingstone, 1984.

Woolf CJ: Segmented afferent fibre-induced analgesia: Transcutaneous electrical nerve stimulation (TENS). In: *Textbook of Pain*. Wall PD, Melzack R (editors). Churchill Livingstone, 1989.

World Health Organization: *Cancer Pain Relief*. WHO (Geneva), 1982.

Section V.
Malignant Diseases & Their Treatment

Breast Cancer

18

Peter M. Ravdin, MD, PhD

Of all the common adenocarcinomas for which individuals are at risk in the USA, breast cancer is the one for which the greatest advances in understanding have been made in terms of early diagnosis, treatment, and molecular characterization. Clinical trials evaluating the treatment of breast cancer have demonstrated two principles of oncology: (1) cancer (in particular breast cancer) often is a systemic disease whose prognosis is governed by initially clinically occult systemic metastatic disease and (2) patients with early disease have a lower systemic tumor burden and a better prognosis with or without systemic therapy. Thus, basic strategies in the treatment of breast cancer are early discovery and initiation of definitive local therapy and, for women at high risk of systemic relapse, an attempt to prevent relapse by means of adjuvant therapy.

Essentials of Diagnosis
- Mass or lump within the breast.
- Skin dimpling of area on the breast.
- Retraction of nipple.
- Discharge from nipple (especially bloody).
- Reddening of skin of the breast.
- Change in breast skin texture ("peau d'orange").
- Enlarged axillary lymph nodes.

Epidemiology
Breast cancer is one of the most common cancers in the USA; more than 160,000 women develop this cancer each year, and 40,000 women die annually of this malignancy. Approximately 1 out of 9 women in the USA will develop breast cancer sometime during their lives. Breast cancer primarily affects women although 1% of cases occur in men. Risk increases with age, rising rapidly up to menopause and continuing to rise thereafter although at a slower rate. The risk is large. Women aged 60 years and older have 3–4% chance of developing breast cancer during each decade of life.

Several factors appear to affect the risk of developing breast cancer. One is cultural and environmental (probably diet). The risk of women in the USA is 5 times higher than for women in most Asian and African countries. When people from low-risk countries immigrate to the USA, they acquire the higher risk within 1–2 generations.

Major statistically significant and independent risk factors for developing breast cancer relate to the family history, history of prior breast disease, and reproductive and menstrual history. There appears to be a genetic risk factor for developing this cancer although its magnitude is debated and it does not correlate with ethnic or racial background. A woman may have 2–10 times the average risk if several first-degree relatives develop breast cancer, particularly if these relatives developed cancer before menopause or in both breasts. A woman's own history of breast disease is associated with increased risk of developing breast cancer if the problem disease leads to breast biopsy, even if the results are benign. Menstrual and reproductive history correlate with risk of developing breast cancer. Women with onset of menses before the age of 12 are at increased risk. Another factor that affects risk is the age at which a woman has her first child. Women who have their first full-term pregnancy before 18 years of age have less than half the risk of women who have their first child at more than 30 years of age or who have no children.

Several factors do not appear to correlate independently with the risk of developing breast cancer. Use of oral contraceptives does not seem to affect risk. Fibrocystic disease of the breast is not a risk factor. Smoking cigarettes does not appear to increase the risk of breast cancer. Although epidemiologically defined risk factors help identify women at high risk, 75% of breast cancers occur in women with no recognized major risk factor.

Pathogenesis
A single pathogenic factor does not appear to be responsible for all breast cancers. Animal models provide some clues about the causes of breast cancer. In general, animal models suggest that the risk of developing breast cancer is the result of a complex interplay of genetic, mutagenic, endocrinologic, and dietary factors. In animal models, genetics is known to play a major role in the risk of developing breast can-

cer. In humans, the genetic alleles that place women at risk for breast cancer have yet to be identified, except in some families with the Li Fraumeni syndrome in which an aberrant form of the tumor suppressor P53 has been identified. In animal models, mutagenic insults such as radiation and chemical mutagens have been shown to cause breast cancers. Exposure to chemical mutagens is probably also important in some women, but no chemical mutagens have yet been identified. Breast cancer risk was shown to correlate with radiation exposure in women exposed to radiation during the bombing of Hiroshima and with thymic irradiation during childhood. In animal models, viruses have been shown to cause breast cancer with direct transmission from mother to offspring. No human mammary cancer virus has been identified at this time. The endocrinologic status of the host is also important in defining risk. The protective change that occurs after pregnancy has not yet been identified.

Histopathology

Most breast cancers arise within the ductal epithelium of the breast. Several histologic abnormalities of the ductal epithelium of the breast suggest the possibility of evolution of many breast cancers through the stages of hyperplasia (proliferative disease without atypia), dysplasia (atypical hyperplasia), noninvasive neoplasia (ductal carcinoma in situ or intraductal carcinoma, DCIS), and finally neoplasia (infiltrating ductal carcinoma, IDC) with high metastatic potential. Each stage is associated with an increased risk of developing an infiltrating ductal carcinoma: two-fold for hyperplasia, four-fold for atypical hyperplasia, and ten-fold for ductal carcinoma in situ. Carcinomas, both intraductal and invasive, demand definitive local treatment, while hyperplasia and dysplastic changes require close follow-up. Ductal carcinoma in situ is distinguished from invasive or infiltrating carcinoma by a lack of penetration through the basement membrane into the breast parenchyma. Ductal carcinoma in situ itself is rarely associated with spread to regional lymph nodes and subsequent systemic relapse.

The most common type of invasive breast cancer is infiltrating ductal carcinoma without further histologic subtyping. Less common invasive subtypes such as mucinous, papillary, tubular, and lobular invasive breast cancers are in general treated in the same way as infiltrating ductal carcinomas but may have a better prognosis.

Histopathologic features relating to tumor differentiation are important in predicting prognosis in breast cancer. However, intra-observer variability among pathologists makes it difficult to use this information in a generalizable manner. An example of the uncertainties in grading histopathologic features is the fact that none of the major national trials of the treatment of breast cancer uses this information to assign patients to prognostic groups. Nonetheless, most studies suggest that histopathologic grade is important, with grade 1 tumors being well differentiated and carrying a better prognosis than grade 3 anaplastic tumors. Nuclear grade has also been defended as being of prognostic significance, with grade 1 nuclei being anaplastic and carrying a graver prognostic significance than grade 3 more normal nuclei. Again, this feature is not routinely used for prediction of prognosis, since it is not easily reproducibly evaluated by different pathologists.

Other features that are reported but not routinely used for staging or the prediction of prognosis are tumor necrosis (unfavorable), local lymphatic invasion (unfavorable), and sinus histiocytosis (unfavorable). These features seem to correlate with and therefore do not add information to the more easily assessable characteristics of tumor size and lymph node involvement.

Clinical Findings

Because of the better outcome when breast tumors are discovered when they are small in size, great efforts have been made to educate women and healthcare professionals about the clinical signs of breast cancer (Table 18–1) and to initiate screening programs (Table 18–2). These efforts have two main foci: **physical examination** and **mammography.** Breast self-examination should be conducted on a monthly basis by women. Most breast lesions are discovered in such a way by women themselves. The other part of the early detection program is breast examination by the physician during routine physical examinations. Signs of breast cancer include a new or enlarging lump or thickening within the breast. Dimpling of an area on the breast or a change in the contour of the breast also require additional evaluation. Changes in texture of the skin or its color are also worrisome. The classic Paget's "peau d'orange" texture of the skin suggests an underlying breast cancer. Reddening of an area of skin is sometimes a sign of inflammatory breast cancer. Another sign is a discharge, particularly a bloody discharge, from the nipple.

The second focus of early detection is the mammogram. According to the guidelines of the American Cancer Society, screening mammography should be offered to all women over the age of 40 irrespective of their risk factors for developing breast cancer. Screening mammography allows detection of many

Table 18–1. Clinical signs of breast cancer.

Mass or lump within the breast
Skin dimpling of area on the breast
Retraction of nipple
Discharge from nipple (particularly bloody)
Reddening of skin of the breast
Change in breast skin texture ("peau d'orange")
Enlarged axillary lymph nodes

Table 18–2. Guidelines of the American Cancer Society (ACS) for screening mammography.

Age	Recommendation
>20 years	Breast self-examination monthly
20–40 years	Physical examination every 3 years
35–40 years	Baseline mammogram
40–50 years	Mammogram every 1–2 years based on risk factors
>40 years	Physical examination every year
>50 years	Mammogram every year

breast cancers before they would otherwise be detectable and results in an approximately one-third reduction in mortality due to breast cancer. Improvements in mammographic techniques have led to minimization of radiation exposure, and this objection to routine use of the test is no longer of great concern.

New breast abnormalities, whether reported by the woman herself, found on physical examination, or detected by mammography, must be thoroughly evaluated. The simplest technique is thin needle aspiration. If clear fluid is obtained and the abnormality does not recur, it is likely that the abnormality is a benign cyst. If the mass is solid and does not resolve within a menstrual cycle, a biopsy should be performed. The first step can be needle aspiration, but if the cytologic specimen does not show cancer, a larger volume (incisional or excisional) biopsy should be done. While mammography is helpful in assessing abnormalities found on physical examination, it must not be used in the place of biopsy to rule out malignancy, since it is frequently falsely negative.

Staging

The most commonly used staging system for breast cancer is shown in Table 18–3. This staging system incorporates both pathologic and clinical information but is most heavily dependent on direct pathologic information. Pathologic information include whether the tumor is intraductal or invasive, tumor size as measured at biopsy, and whether tumor is present in

Table 18–3. Pathologic staging system for breast cancer.

Stage	Primary Tumor	Lymph Nodes	Distant Disease
0	Carcinoma in situ	None	None
1	<2 cm	None	None
2	<5 cm	*or* Ipsilateral axillary nodes positive but not fixed	None
3	>5 cm[1]	*or* Ipsilateral axillary nodes positive and fixed[2]	None
4	Any size if skin involvement or if fixed to chest wall	*or* Supraclavicular involvement	*or* Present

[1]Subclass (b) if fixed to pectoral fascia or muscle or (a) if not.
[2]Fixed to each other or to skin or other structures.

the axillary lymph nodes or more distant sites. Clinical staging information includes whether the tumor is fixed to other structures and whether the axillary lymph nodes are matted or fixed to other structures. The staging of breast cancer has the goal of identifying patient subsets that require similar treatments and have a similar prognosis.

Stage 0 patients with preinvasive cancer have local disease and are usually cured by local measures. Stage 1 breast cancers are invasive without high metastatic potential as indicated by the lack of axillary lymph node involvement. These patients are often cured by local measures alone, although they have a substantial risk of systemic relapse and death. Most stage 2 and stage 3 patients have systemic disease that will become manifest at some time following local treatment. Stage 4 patients either have systemic disease that is manifest or have such signs as inflammatory breast cancer involving the skin of the breast, which leads to early systemic relapse even with meticulous local treatment. The chances of surviving 10 years after diagnosis are >90%, 75%, 50%, 25%, and <5% for stage 0, 1, 2, 3, and 4, respectively.

Axillary lymph node involvement in staging of all but intraductal carcinomas is based on direct histopathologic examination (intraductal carcinomas are excluded because of their very low rate of axillary lymph node involvement). Clinical assessment of lymph node involvement is notoriously inaccurate (frequent false positives and false negatives) and should not be used for staging. Biopsy proof of inflammatory disease or spread of cancer beyond the breast should be available before a patient is assigned the prognosis of stage 4 disease.

Other Prognostic Factors

Breast cancer is unique among adenocarcinoma types in that there are well-established biochemical markers and other tests to help in the assessment of prognosis and the selection of optimal treatment options (Table 18–4). Breast cancer treatment planning in part depends on the chemical analysis of the tumor proteins. Tumor specimens are routinely examined for the presence of hormone receptors for estrogen and progesterone.

Estrogen receptors (ERs) and progesterone receptors (PgRs) are proteins that have the ability to bind their respective hormones and also to DNA. Steroid hormones acting through receptors are thought to control the transcription of defined subsets of genes. Primary breast tumors that express ERs, PgRs, or both are less likely to recur than tumors that do not express these proteins. Steroid hormone receptor levels are also used to predict the probability that a breast tumor will regress during treatment with a hormonal agent. If the tumor tissue has less than 10 femtomoles (fmol) per milligram of the estrogen receptor protein and progesterone receptor protein, it is unlikely (<10%) that hormonal treatments will cause

Table 18–4. Additional prognostic tests.

Conventional biochemical
  Steroid receptor status
    Estrogen receptor
    Progesterone receptor
Conventional histologic
  Nuclear grading
  Pathologic subtype
Flow cytometry
  Ploidy (DNA index)
  S phase (a measure of proliferative index)
Investigational
  Peptide hormone receptors
    Her-2/neu, EGF-R
  Peptide hormones
    PS2
  Proteases
    Cathepsin-D
  Tumor suppressors
    P53
  Proliferation antigens
    Ki-67

the tumor to regress. If the tumor has either more than 10 fmol/mg of ER or PgR protein, there is an approximately 40% chance that the tumor will respond to hormonal manipulation. If the tumor is positive for both ER and PgR, there is a 70–80% chance of response to hormonal therapy. Thus, knowledge of the hormone receptor status can help in the selection of therapy as either hormonal manipulation or chemotherapy in both the immediate postoperative setting for the prevention of recurrence (adjuvant therapy) and in the treatment of advanced disease.

The expression levels of a number of other proteins in tumors have been shown to correlate with risk of recurrence, eg, the peptide hormone receptor Her-2/neu and the epidermal growth factor receptor, the peptide hormone PS2, the protease cathepsin-D, and the proliferation antigen Ki-67.

Additional information can be gained by flow cytometry. With this technique, individual nuclei of cells from the tumor can be analyzed for DNA content. This information can be used to estimate the mitotic rate of the tumor (the number of cells in S phase, or replicating their DNA) and whether the cells have the normal diploid DNA content or are aneuploid. Relapse is more likely when tumors are found at the time of resection to have higher than average S phase fractions or to be aneuploid.

Although the levels of a large number of tumor proteins and other information about tumor properties have been shown to be of prognostic significance, what information should be obtained and the optimal combinations have yet to be defined.

Major Treatment Modalities

The treatment of breast cancer proceeds in two distinct phases. The first phase is removal of the primary tumor, if possible, and the second phase is aimed at eradicating systemic disease. Thus, in patients without signs of overt systemic disease, the goals of treatment are control of local disease and in some cases eradication of micrometastatic systemic disease by chemotherapy or hormonal therapy. The postoperative therapy aimed at preventing recurrence is referred to as adjuvant therapy.

A. Surgery: The mainstay of local treatment is surgery and in some situations radiotherapy. More patients are cured by surgery than by any other treatment modality, and it is imperative that definitive surgical resection be performed if possible. The most commonly performed surgery for definitive local control of disease is the modified radical mastectomy. However, major clinical trials, most notably those of the National Surgical Adjuvant Breast Program (NSABP), have shown that for patients with tumors smaller than 4 cm segmental mastectomy followed by radiation therapy offers similar local control and survival rates. The lesser procedure often is cosmetically more acceptable and should be considered in all women with small primary tumors.

B. Radiation Therapy: The role of radiation therapy in the local control of breast cancer is that of eradicating microscopic residual disease within the breast. Radiation therapy is no longer routinely used following modified radical mastectomy in all stage 1 and stage 2 patients because local recurrence rates are low in this group and overall survival is defined by recurrence at distant sites. Local recurrence rates are high following segmental resections, and this group routinely receives radiation therapy. Other situations in which the risk of early local relapse is high warrant consideration of postoperative radiation therapy, eg, large primary tumors (>5 cm), questions of tumor involvement at the resection margins, and involvement of the pectoral fascia. Optimal timing for administration of radiation to postoperative patients who will also receive adjuvant chemotherapy has not been established, but it is often given following the adjuvant chemotherapy. Radiation therapy plays an important role in the treatment of metastatic breast cancer. It is primary therapy for brain metastases, is often used to control local recurrences, and is used to treat painful or structurally threatening osseous lesions.

C. Chemotherapy: The third major modality in the treatment of breast cancer is chemotherapy (Table 18–5). Chemotherapy is used to eradicate micrometastatic disease and, in women with metastatic disease, to attempt to delay progression of the cancer. Breast cancer responds to a large number of chemotherapeutic agents, and the highest response rates have been noted in clinical trials employing combinations of these agents. A large number of different treatment regimens have been used. The most common are based on the drugs cyclophosphamide, methotrexate, and fluorouracil (CMF) or cyclophosphamide, doxorubicin (Adriamycin), and fluorouracil (CAF).

Table 18–5. Some effective chemotherapeutic agents.

Single agents
  Doxorubicin
  Mitoxantrone
  Cyclophosphamide
  Melphalan
  Thiotepa
  Fluorouracil
  Methotrexate
  Vinblastine
Most commonly used multiagent therapy
  Cyclophosphamide, methotrexate, fluorouracil (CMF)
  Cyclophosphamide, doxorubicin (Adriamycin), Fluorouracil
    (CAF)

Table 18–6. Hormonal therapy options.

Steroid hormone antagonists or agonists
  Tamoxifen (antiestrogen)
  Megestrol acetate (progestin)
  Fluoxymesterone (androgen)
  Diethylstilbestrol (estrogen)
Aromatase inhibitors
  Aminoglutethimide
LHRH analogs
Surgical ablative procedures
  Oophorectomy
  Adrenalectomy
  Hypophysectomy

When CMF- or CAF-based regimens are used for the treatment of metastatic breast cancer, response probability rates (partial remission plus complete remission) range from 30% to 70% depending on details of the therapeutic regimen and the patient's clinical history. In adjuvant treatment regimens, these agents can delay relapse and improve overall survival in some patient subsets. Chemotherapeutic regimens often cause troublesome and occasionally life-threatening but reversible toxicities. These include neutropenia (with the associated risk of sepsis), thrombocytopenia, alopecia, nausea and vomiting, and general fatigue.

Dose intensity may play an important role in the chance of response to chemotherapy in the treatment of metastatic disease and in the improvement of prognosis in patients receiving adjuvant treatment. Very high dose chemotherapeutic regimens, with and without autologous bone marrow rescue, and trials in which colony-stimulating factors (CSFs) are used to attempt to decrease hematologic toxicity will explore whether such regimens further improve treatment outcomes. This question is important because at this time, although adjuvant conventional chemotherapy appears to have some modest curative potential when used against micrometastatic disease, it does not have curative potential when used against systemic recurrence.

D. Hormonal Therapy: The fourth type of treatment for primary breast cancer is hormonal manipulation. This treatment modality should be considered for women who have Er- or PgR-positive primary tumors. The main treatment options for hormonal therapy are shown in Table 18–6. There is no compelling evidence that any of these options has a higher response rate than any other. Therefore, selection is largely defined by the relative amount of risk or toxicity. The most commonly employed hormonal therapy is the steroid analogue tamoxifen, which is a competitive antagonist with estrogen for binding to the estrogen receptor. Tamoxifen (10 mg twice daily) is the primary hormonal therapy because it has the mildest side effects.

Other steroid analogs such as megestrol acetate are widely used. Megestrol acetate, a progestin, is usually used as second-line hormonal therapy because it is slightly more toxic than tamoxifen. Other pharmaceutic agents used include diethylstilbestrol and aromatase inhibitors such as aminoglutethimide, which interferes with steroid production in the adrenal and blocks peripheral tissue aromatization of steroids to estrogen. This compound has the effect of causing a medical adrenalectomy; because of the fall in glucocorticoid levels, patients are concurrently treatment with hydrocortisone. Luteinizing hormone–releasing hormone (LHRH) analogs have been used to cause a failure of gonadotropin production in the pituitary with a secondary fall in steroid production in the ovary. This class of agents has potential in treating premenopausal women. The surgical ablative therapy oophorectomy is an effective hormonal therapy in premenopausal women, and clinical responses to adrenalectomy and hypophysectomy have been noted in postmenopausal women. Surgical ablative surgery has become infrequent with the introduction of a large number of effective pharmacologic agents, but oophorectomy is still performed as second- or first-line endocrine therapy in premenopausal women, and trials are assessing whether it is equivalent to or better or worse than tamoxifen in this patient population.

Treatment Recommendations

A. General Recommendations: The strategy for the treatment of breast cancer has three basic levels: (1) removal and control of the primary cancer at the earliest possible time and assessment of the probability of systemic recurrence, (2) use of adjuvant chemotherapy or hormonal therapy to eradicate any micrometastatic systemic disease with the intention of curing the patient or markedly delaying relapse, and (3) use of treatment modalities to lessen symptoms and delay death when there is systemic recurrence.

B. Recommendations for Healthy Women: Can breast cancer be prevented? In animal studies, the antiestrogen tamoxifen, retinoic acid analogs, and dietary manipulation have been shown to decrease the risk of developing breast cancer. There is indirect evidence in humans that some or all of these strategies may be effective. For example, women taking adjuvant tamoxifen after a first breast cancer had a 39% reduction in the rate of occurrence of contralateral breast cancer. This observation led to the design of a major breast cancer double-blind placebo-controlled prevention trial in the USA in which healthy women with a 0.35% or higher risk of breast cancer will receive tamoxifen or placebo for 5 years. It is not yet known whether the benefits (expected reduction in breast cancer occurrence rate by 40%) will outweigh the risks (increased thrombotic events and increased uterine cancer).

C. Stage 0: For intraductal carcinoma, the main goal is removal of local disease. Conventional therapy has been modified radical mastectomy. Lesser surgeries such as segmentectomy may have a role, but local recurrence rates are high unless local radiation therapy is also given. Patients with small intraductal carcinomas need not undergo axillary dissection, since less than 5% show evidence of axillary lymph node involvement. Adjuvant chemotherapy is not warranted. Adjuvant hormonal therapy with tamoxifen may be of use in preventing local recurrence and second primary breast cancers.

D. Stage 1: Patients found to have primary tumors smaller than 2 cm and no axillary lymph node involvement have an approximately 66% chance of being cured by surgery alone. Use of adjuvant chemotherapy or hormonal therapy in these patients improves average disease-free and overall survival. However, the meta-analysis of all clinical adjuvant trials suggests that adjuvant chemotherapy or hormonal therapy prevents only about 1 in 6 of the deaths that would have occurred by 10 years (Table 18–7). Thus, stage 1 patients who receive therapy do not need it, and of those who are destined to relapse, the majority will experience relapse despite the adjuvant therapy. In stage 1 patients with positive steroid receptors and a low proliferative rate as measured by flow cytometry, the relapse risk may be so low as to not warrant the use of adjuvant therapy, and the 1990 National Institutes of Health (NIH) Consensus Conference suggested that axillary node–negative patients with tumors smaller than 1 cm do not need treatment.

E. Stage 2: Patients who have stage 2 disease have only a 25% chance of cure by surgery alone, and 75% will relapse. Because the majority will develop life-threatening recurrence, adjuvant therapy to attempt to prevent or delay recurrence is indicated in all

these patients. Over the last 20 years, numerous randomized clinical trials have examined a number of adjuvant therapeutic regimens. Overview meta-analysis suggests that appropriate adjuvant therapy can modestly delay recurrence and death. In order to decide which adjuvant therapy is most appropriate for an individual patient, it is important to take into account the menopausal status of the patient and the ER status of the tumor. Most clinicians would agree that in premenopausal patients, the adjuvant therapy is chemotherapy irrespective of hormone receptor status. The role of additional hormonal therapy in that population is being defined. In postmenopausal patients who are ER-positive, the most widely used adjuvant therapy is tamoxifen, but whether additional aggressive chemotherapy further improves outcome is under investigation. The optimal therapy for postmenopausal patients who have ER-negative tumors is not well established. Some studies suggest a benefit from adjuvant chemotherapy in this group, but the benefit seems more modest than in premenopausal patients.

F. Stage 3 or Stage 4 Locally Advanced Disease (Without Overt Metastatic Disease): In patients with locally advanced disease but without overt evidence of metastatic disease, surgical cure should be attempted. Because of the large size of most patients' tumors, breast-conserving therapy is not possible, and in many cases initial resection of the tumor is also not possible. Initial options include modified radical mastectomy if possible and neoadjuvant chemotherapy, in which curative surgery is attempted after the use of chemotherapy to decrease the size of the primary tumor. Postoperative radiotherapy should be considered. Depending on menopausal status and steroid hormone receptor status, all patients should receive adjuvant therapy with the same general considerations for stage 2 disease.

G. Stage 4 Initially Metastatic or Recurrent Cancer: Except for occasional patients with solely local recurrence (which can be cured by local therapy), systemic metastatic breast cancer is not curable by present conventional treatment modalities. Two very different approaches to the treatment of metastatic disease exist. The more conventional is to achieve disease stabilization or regression with the least toxicity for as long as possible. The second approach is to attempt to achieve a durable complete remission of the disease with as high a probability as possible but at the cost of substantial treatment-related toxicity due to the intensive therapy.

Figure 18–1 illustrates a conventional strategy for the treatment of the metastatic disease. The clinician must address the following: (1) Is the tumor likely to be ER- or PgR-positive, was the initial tumor ER- or PgR-positive or unknown, or was the disease-free interval better than 1 year, or did biopsy of the recurrent disease confirm the disease to be hormone receptor positive? (2) Does the disease have immediately life-

Table 18–7. Effect of adjuvant therapy on clinical outcome at 10 years' follow-up (percent relative reduction of risk).

Treatment	Risk of Relapse	Risk of Death
Tamoxifen	25% Reduction	17% Reduction
Polychemotherapy	28% Reduction	16% Reduction

Steroid hormone receptor–positive or indolent disease

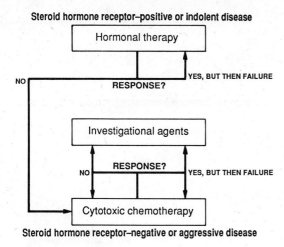

Figure 18–1. Algorithm for general conventional treatment strategy for metastatic disease.

threatening consequences? Because it often takes 8–12 weeks before the most commonly used endocrine therapy, tamoxifen, causes tumor regression, while the effects of chemotherapy are apparent within 4 weeks, chemotherapy is the treatment of choice in situations in which the patient has immediately life-threatening disease such as lymphangitic pulmonary disease or massive hepatic recurrence, even if the tumor is thought to be hormone receptor positive.

In patients having hormone receptor–positive tumors who are thought to have indolent disease with a good probability of hormonal response, the first-line therapy is hormonal therapy. The usually selected therapy is either tamoxifen or oophorectomy in premenopausal women and tamoxifen in postmenopausal women. If there is a response but eventual progression of disease or if there is no response, the second-line therapy is either hormonal therapy or chemotherapy depending on whether or not the disease is immediately life-threatening. In patients who have hormone receptor–negative tumor recurrence or aggressive life-threatening disease, the initial therapy is chemotherapy. If there is a response but eventual progression of disease or if there is no response, the second-line therapy is again chemotherapy.

For some patients, a more aggressive initial approach is preferred. In this approach, intensive chemotherapy is given irrespective of steroid receptor status. The goal is to achieve a long-term complete remission during which no therapy is necessary except hormonal therapy. In some autologous bone marrow trials, a substantial minority (10–20%) of the patients appear to achieve a complete remission of <5 years' duration, a better result than that achieved by conventional therapy, but this result awaits confirmation in randomized clinical trials.

REFERENCES

Bonadonna G, Valagussa P: The contribution of medicine to the primary treatment of breast cancer. *Cancer Res* 1988;**48**:2314.

Early Breast Cancer Trialist's Collaborative Group: Systemic treatment of early breast cancer by hormonal, cytoxic, or immune therapy. *Lancet* 1992;**339**:1,71.

Fisher B: Ten-year results of a randomized clinical trial comparing radical mastectomy and total mastectomy with or without radiation. N Engl J Med 1985;**312**:674.

Fisher B et al: Five-year results of a randomized clinical trial comparing total mastectomy and segmental mastectomy with or without radiation in the treatment of breast cancer. *N Engl J Med* 1985;**312**:665.

Gail MH et al: Projecting individualized probabilities of developing breast cancer for white females who are being examined annually. *JNCI* 1989;**81**:1879.

Harris JR et al: *Breast Diseases.* Lippincott, 1991.

Henderson IC: Adjuvant systemic therapy for early breast cancer. *Curr Probl Cancer* 1987;**44**:128.

Hryniuk W, Levine MN: Analysis of dose intensity for chemotherapy in early (stage II) breast cancer and advanced breast cancer. National Cancer Institute Monograph No. 1, 1986, p. 87.

McGuire WL, Clark GM: Prognostic factors and treatment decisions in axillary node–negative breast cancer. *N Engl J Med* 1992;**326**:1756.

19 Central Nervous System Cancer

Pamela Zyman New, MD

Intracranial neoplasms are classified as **primary tumors** (those arising from structures within the intracranial cavity) and **secondary** or **metastatic tumors.** This chapter discusses primary brain tumors.

Approximately 17,030 new cases of primary central nervous system (CNS) neoplasms are diagnosed annually in the USA, an occurrence rate of 8.2 per 100,000 persons. The incidence steadily increases with age, being 2.3 per 100,000 in childhood, with a peak rate of 20.4 per 100,000 in the 55- to 64-year-old age group, and remains constant at this rate for the next decade (ages 65–74). Over age 75, the incidence declines to 15.4 per 100,000. A review of autopsy records reveals that primary intracranial neoplasms account for 1–2.7% of autopsied deaths, 9–10% of cancers seen at autopsy at all ages, but 50–55% of malignant neoplasms in autopsied deaths between ages 10 and 19.

Certain tumor types are more common to some age groups. For instance, cerebellar astrocytoma and medulloblastoma characteristically occur in childhood, whereas glioblastoma, meningioma, and neuroma increase in frequency with advancing age. Over age 65, more than half of intracranial tumors will be gliomas and one-third meningiomas. Glial tumors as a whole account for more than half of all brain tumors at all ages.

The distribution of primary intracranial tumors with regard to sex reveals little difference except for certain specific tumor types. Females seem more susceptible to meningiomas and pituitary adenomas, whereas males over age 40 show a preponderance of gliomas and neurinomas.

Etiology

No conclusive causes for central nervous system cancer have been isolated. However, there are several predisposing syndromes, including neurofibromatosis (von Recklinghausen's disease) and tuberous sclerosis (Bourneville's disease), in which there is a definite increase in tumors of glial and neuronal cell lines. Extensive research has been performed to link such factors as maldevelopment, chromosomal aberrations, viruses, chemical compounds, and immunologic dysfunction to CNS cancer, but no causal relationships have been established.

Pathogenesis

Parenchymal brain tumors are believed to develop from the neoplastic transformation of differentiated cells at loci of glial and neuronal cell development. These neoplasms are rarely encapsulated but most often are diffusely infiltrative. Dividing cells spread through the normal environment of nondividing or slowly proliferating glial and neuronal cells. For this reason, total resection of an intrinsic brain tumor is usually not feasible. A radical procedure may remove at most 90–99% of a glial tumor.

Metastatic spread is most often limited to the neuraxis (axon) and occurs via the cerebrospinal fluid pathways. Metastases outside the central nervous system are rare and most often occur in the childhood tumors (40% of reported metastases) or following craniotomy or a shunting procedure and involve lungs, bone, liver, or lymph nodes. The pathogenesis of tumors that arise spontaneously involves invasion of vessels by tumor with subsequent dissemination into the systemic circulation and arrest in distant target organs.

Clinical Findings

A. Symptoms and Signs: The most common presenting symptom in the patient with an intracranial mass is headache. Patients may complain of this being worse upon arising and improving as the morning wears on, if there is involvement of the cerebrospinal fluid pathways and resultant obstructive hydrocephalus. In this situation, headache is usually accompanied by nausea and vomiting, particularly upon arising in the morning. Relief may be obtained by resuming a supine position. Headaches may also be more regional in location in some cases. A history of recurring headache in the same location should prompt radiologic evaluation.

A second prominent early feature is seizure, which may be focal or grand mal epileptic or consist of a slight loss of awareness that goes unrecognized by the patient. Seizure is a positive prognostic factor in that it frequently is an early warning of CNS dysfunction and may allow for early diagnosis and treatment.

Other focal neurologic symptoms include weakness, sensory loss, and visual or hearing deficits. Increased intracranial pressure may present as lethargy, drowsiness, or irritability and represent either a significant mass effect or increasing cerebral edema. At this point, urgent management is required, and lethargy carries an unfavorable prognosis.

The neurologic assessment of these patients should encompass level of consciousness; evaluation of speech, memory, mathematic, and verbal skills; and multiple-step commands. Speech tests assess repetition, content, and appropriateness. Cranial nerve findings are also of localizing value. Motor strength is important, since it is graded on a numeric scale and is an easy measurement to follow. Sensory functions may be more complex to grade and localize, but a lesion should be able to be placed along the pathway from the parietal lobe to the spinal cord.

The crucial clues to diagnosis are symptoms of headache, seizures, or focal deficits. A relentless progression differentiates evolving mass lesions from a vascular accident.

Clinical manifestations of tumor depend on its size, location, and growth rate regardless of cell type. Presenting symptoms usually involve progressive dysfunction confined to a single area of the brain. A knowledge of functional neuroanatomy is necessary for diagnosis and follow-up.

A simple approach to anatomic localization in the brain refers to the tentorium as the most important divider in the cranium (Figure 19–1). Lesions above and below produce distinctive syndromes. In laterally located supratentorial tumors, over 50% of patients present with seizures initially, and 80% of those who have had tumors for 2 years develop seizures. The focality of the seizure is of further localizing benefit (eg, in which limb did the seizure begin?). There are six types of focal epilepsy relating to the area of the brain from which they arise:

1. Precentral gyrus–Twitching of one side of the body may eventually spread to all four limbs. The first part to move is a clue to localization. The first part initially affected may be paralyzed for minutes to hours after the seizure (Todd's palsy).

2. Left temporal lobe–Aphasia or speech arrest spread usually involves the face next.

3. Frontal eye fields–Head and eyes turn to the opposite side, consciousness is lost, and activity may spread to limbs.

4. Postcentral gyrus–Sensory epilepsy, numbness, and tingling of limbs occur on one side.

5. Visual cortex–Seizures in occipital lobes cause hallucinations of light or colors, not objects or people, in opposite visual field from the lesion.

6. Temporal lobe epilepsy–

a. Momentary absence, lapse of consciousness.

b. Psychic phenomena, eg, olfactory hallucination, fear, déjà vu experiences.

c. Automatisms, eg, complex, perfectly executed activities.

The nondominant parietal lobe is necessary for orientation in space and appreciation of body image. A tumor here may cause a patient to neglect a limb, especially on the left. Even if the limb is not weak, the patient may fail to use it for bimanual skills. The patient may not be able to recognize common landmarks and get lost or may not be able to draw a clock or copy diagrams.

Lesions of the dominant (most commonly the left) parietal-temporal lobe result in the patient being unable to recognize parts of the patient's own body or to distinguish right from left. Inability to calculate may also be demonstrated.

Anterior fossa masses may damage olfactory bulbs and tracts, causing anosmia, while the sign of hemianopsia speaks for involvement of the optic radiations. A high parietal lesion causes loss of the lower quadrant of the visual field. A lesion involving the lower area of the optic radiations (temporal lobe) produces an upper quadrant anopsia.

Centrally located supratentorial tumors may involve the anterior third ventricle, the sellar region, or the cavernous sinus. When the cavity of the anterior third ventricle is involved, tumors cause only increased pressure by occluding the foramen of Monro. This may be intermittent, causing episodic headaches, hydrocephalus, or drop attacks. Masses above the ventricle involve the corpus callosum, producing profound dementia, drowsiness, and yawning. Patients may seem mentally inaccessible and may have bilateral hemiplegia. Sellar and suprasellar tumors cause compression of the chiasm. The central pressure from below (tumor growing up from the sella) causes bitemporal hemianopia, beginning in the upper quadrants. It is important to test visual acuity in these patients, since blindness may ultimately result as the chiasm is compressed. Endocrine abnormalities may also occur secondary to pituitary and hypothalamic nuclei involvement, causing hypogonadism, hypothyroidism, or adrenocortical deficiency, with diabetes, obesity, or dwarfism. Cavernous sinus syndromes involve the third to sixth cranial nerves. Proptosis may occur as well as fifth cranial nerve dysfunction. This presents as facial pain in the first division (forehead); loss of sensation over trigeminal branches is less common. It is important to check corneal function. Cranial nerve III is more commonly involved than IV or VI; symptoms may begin with what appears as a squint before full ocular palsy is detected. Diplopia is an early sign of extraocular motion imbalance; visual "blurring" may be the first sign.

The earliest signs of an infratentorial tumor are those of increased intracranial pressure. These tumors occur mostly in children; two-thirds of intracranial tumors in patients under age 15 occur in the posterior fossa. The general presenting symptoms are vomiting and headache in occipital region with radiation down the neck. Centrally located tumors involve the cerebellar vermis and fourth ventricle. The masses produce hydrocephalus and increased intracranial pressure. Nystagmus and limb ataxia are seldom seen, but

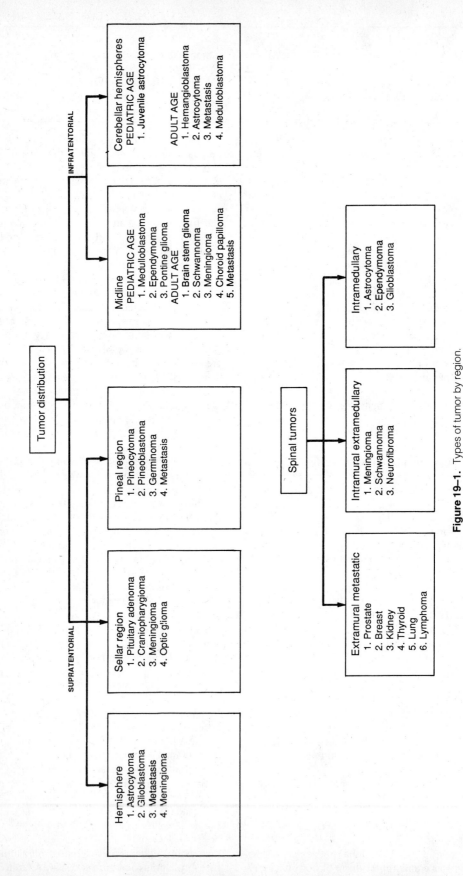

Figure 19–1. Types of tumor by region.

truncal ataxia may be disabling. Vomiting as the only sign reflects involvement of the floor of the fourth ventricle, which can also give nuclear facial palsy and respiratory irregularities. Laterally located (cerebellar hemisphere) masses produce ataxia of limbs as the presenting sign. Nystagmus may also be present. Dysarthria may be due to cerebellar disease or bulbar palsy from a tumor in the medulla. Cranial nerve palsies from masses in this area are most constant in the cerebellopontile angle and include deafness, vertigo, and facial palsy.

Tumors in the jugular foramen region affect cranial nerves IX–XII; dysphagia and dysarthria are presenting signs.

Transtentorial tumors lie laterally along the brain stem and may go above and below the tentorium, indenting occipital lobes and upper cerebellar hemisphere. Patients develop palsies of cranial nerves VII and VIII combined with symptoms of hemianopsia/dysarthria associated with an ataxic syndrome. Centrally located tumors may arise in the pineal gland or tectal plate, then spread more widely to cause hemianopsia or hemiplegia. Hydrocephalus from obstruction of the aqueduct occurs early. Other signs include third nerve dysfunction (sluggish, dilated pupils, mild ptosis, and impaired upward gaze [Parinaud's phenomenon]).

B. Imaging Techniques: The CT scan is about 96–97% sensitive for all histologic groups and locations of brain tumors. MRI is even more sensitive when gadolinium enhancement is used. MRI is also more sensitive than CT in delineating anatomic distortion caused by masses, especially when multiple imaging planes are utilized. Imaging techniques can give accurate estimates of tumor size. However, neuropathologic studies confirm that the limits of microscopic disease cannot always be delineated by the tumor boundaries that appear on the CT scan. There is a great deal of variation in how far outside the contrast-enhancing area tumor cells may actually exist. A combination of imaging and stereotaxic biopsy data is needed to more accurately define tumor size.

Edema of the vasogenic type is the response of normal brain to the presence of a tumor. Neuroimaging techniques have been used to examine edema and the effect of dexamethasone. Positron-emission scanning studies reveal that its effect may be based on reduction in blood-to-tissue transport. Experimental work suggests that dexamethasone may cause a large decrease in size of the extracellular space or a decrease in pore size of tumor capillaries.

Following identification of an intracranial mass on CT scan or MRI, the next step is to determine if it is intra- or extra-axial. Placing the lesion in the correct compartment markedly reduces the diagnostic possibilities. MRI combined with multiple imaging planes and paramagnetic contrast agents provides better detail than the CT scan.

Pathology

Most brain tumors display an abnormal microvasculature with hyperplasia and endothelial proliferation. In normal brain, capillaries have a continuous lining of endothelial cells joined by tight junctions, lacking gaps and fenestrae, but containing a few pinocytotic vesicles. The effect of this lining is to restrict the passage of proteins and large molecules from the circulation into brain parenchyma. In contrast, malignant brain tumors display vascular hyperplasia, large sinusoids, hyperplastic capillaries, and adjacent areas of necrosis. The vascular endothelium may contain fenestrations, gaps, and junctional abnormalities, resembling systemic vasculature. However, this is not the case throughout the neoplasm, and large portions of the microvasculature may be normal or deviate only slightly. The outer layers of vessel walls are composed of pericytes and tumor cells surrounded by a basement membrane, having large perivascular spaces. All these features account for the regional variability in vascular permeability. Studies using the protein tracer horseradish peroxidase have verified this, revealing a permeability range in the vasculature of the average tumor to be from 50% to 100%. In the central bulk of these tumors, there is also decreased blood flow, whereas at the edge of the tumor flow rates approach normal. These differences, together with the changes in the blood-brain barrier described above, provide important background for treatment.

The presence of various primary and secondary tumors in the intracranial cavity seems to elicit an immunologic response. Mononuclear lymphocytic infiltrates similar to those encountered in allergic encephalitis are observed by usual histologic techniques in 30–60% of well and poorly differentiated gliomas as well as sarcomas, metastases, germ cell tumors, and meningiomas. Mononuclear cell infiltrates also occur in the perivascular regions in or adjacent to Virchow-Robin spaces, within the tumor tissue itself, and in surrounding brain parenchyma. These infiltrates include macrophages, T lymphocytes of the suppressor/cytotoxic type or mixed suppressor/cytotoxic type with helper cell phenotypes. The presence of B lymphocytes is very rare. The suppressor/cytotoxic cell activity may actually be a reflection of immune suppression rather than cytotoxic effect. Lymphocytes at various tumor sites have been shown to have either an inhibitory or an enhancing effect on tumor progression. Their functional activity seems to depend on the stage of tumor growth.

The question of the value of mononuclear cell infiltrates in glioma is not resolved. Some investigators correlate increased survival and decreased metastatic potential in systemic tumors with such infiltrates. T cells alone are not sufficient defense against tumor cells but may help to destroy circulating tumor cells and prevent their proliferation to metastases. Other researchers have shown that in some malignant glioma cell lines an interaction between lymph cells and tumor cells results in a "cell coat" production, which may account for the suppressor effect and malignant behavior. This "coat" can allow escape from immune attack by impairing the generation of reactive lymphocytes. It consists of hyaluronidase- sensitive sulfated glycosaminoglycans, which tend to decrease with increasing anaplasia, suggesting a progressive cellular degeneration. No data substantiate a link between lymphocytic invasion and survival. Fortunately, glioblastoma has a lower incidence and intensity than well-differentiated or anaplastic gliomas and brain metastases. Preoperative corticosteroids seem to decrease the intensity but not the frequency of the infiltrate. There is also a documented decrease in lymphocytic invasion following irradiation and chemotherapy.

Differential Diagnosis

The differential diagnosis of any intracranial neoplasm is that of other space-occupying lesions including subdural hematoma, brain abscess, and other inflammatory masses such as tuberculoma. Degenerative neurologic diseases such as dementia of the Alzheimer type, multiple sclerosis, and other demyelinating diseases may need to be considered. Connective tissue disorders such as systemic lupus erythematosus with CNS involvement may mimic the presence of a mass lesion. Likewise, vasculitis involving the CNS may produce similar findings. Lastly, arteriovenous malformations of the brain may present as mass lesions both clinically and radiographically. MRI is helpful in evaluating and ruling out all of these entities.

Nomenclature

In an effort to obtain a uniform nomenclature for international use in classifying brain tumors, the World Health Organization (WHO) composed a histologic classification of tumors of the central nervous system (Table 19–1). Several criticisms have been made of this classification, and revisions have been proposed. It is included here because of the frequency with which it is referred to in the literature and as an aid to understanding the derivation of these tumors. All tumors are routinely assigned to a cell of origin. The actual tumor type is usually identified by cytoplasmic features, eg, the "fried egg" cells of oligodendrogliomas, "pseudorosettes" (a perivascular orientation of cells) in ependymomas, and neuroblastic rosettes in medulloblastomas. The glioblastoma is identified by the presence of necrosis and orientation of cells referred to as pseudopalisading. The WHO revised classification of pediatric brain tumors incorporates the newer classification concept of primitive neuroectodermal tumors (PNET) (Table 19–2).

Sequelae of CNS Radiation

The treatment of primary brain tumors is not without adverse effects especially within the pediatric population.

Three types of CNS radiation injury occur, named according to the time interval from treatment to occurrence.

A. Acute: Acute changes occur within 24 hours and are rare. Symptoms include nausea and vomiting, headache, and lethargy. Herniation may occur if significant edema is present. This syndrome is infrequent with the use of conventional fractionation and also with dexamethasone therapy. Treatment involves reduction of intracranial pressure.

B. Subacute: Subacute radiation encephalopathy occurs within 2–4 months. Symptoms include fatigue, anorexia, somnolence, low-grade fever, and in 40% exacerbation of focal neurologic signs, such as ataxia and cranial nerve findings. This picture is important to recognize because it can resemble recurrent tumor. Symptoms may persist for 1–2 months, after which time the patient either recovers or dies. Autopsy reveals demyelination.

C. Delayed: Delayed radiation necrosis appears after 6–24 months following cranial radiation for brain tumor, CNS prophylaxis, or a course of therapy that includes the brain within its portals. Tolerance for the adult brain is estimated to be about 5000–5500 cGy with fractions of 150–180 cGy. Radiation necrosis is thought to occur in almost 5% of patients who receive 5000–6000 cGy. Fraction size is the dominant factor influencing postradiation necrosis at levels up to 6000–6300 cGy; fractions greater than 220–250 cGy have been implicated in cases of necrosis at levels below 6000 cGy.

Again, findings may resemble tumor recurrence. Symptoms include headache, mental status changes, loss of bladder function, focal deficits, and at times seizure activity. The diagnosis depends on brain biopsy, since CT scan and MRI may reveal a hypodense lesion with necrosis, compatible with tumor. Patients may have a prolonged course or progress rapidly to severe disability and death. Treatment options include surgical resection of necrotic foci and dexamethasone; results are minimally beneficial.

Brief mention should be made of the neuropsychiatric changes that have been described in long-term survivors of childhood brain tumors. IQ levels in this population are 10–20 points below those of the normal population. Memory and attention span are decreased, especially for children who were under age 4–8 at the time of diagnosis. The decline seems to begin at 2–5 years following treatment. These factors need to be considered when designing therapy for this age group. Studies involving children who have undergone both radiation and chemotherapy are still to be done.

Table 19–1. WHO histologic classification of tumors of the central nervous system.

	Grade
I. Tumors of neuroepithelial tissue	
A. Astrocytic tumors	
1. Astrocytoma	II
(a) Fibrillary	
(b) Protoplasmic	
(c) Gemistocytic	
2. Pilocytic astrocytoma	I
3. Subependymal giant cell astrocytoma (ventricular tumor of tuberous sclerosis)	I
4. Astroblastoma	II–IV?
5. Anaplastic (malignant) astrocytoma	III
B. Oligodendroglial tumors	
1. Oligodendroglioma	II
2. Mixed oligo-astrocytoma	II
3. Anaplastic (malignant) oligodendroglima	III
C. Ependymal and choroid plexus tumors	
1. Ependymoma	I
Variants:	
(a) Myxopapillary ependymoma	I. II
(b) Papillary ependymoma	I
(c) Subependymoma	I
2. Anaplastic (malignant) ependymoma	III. IV
3. Choroid plexus papilloma	I
4. Anaplastic (malignant) choroid plexus papilloma	III. IV
D. Pineal cell tumors	
1. Pineocytoma (pinealocytoma)	I–III
2. Pineoblastoma (pinealoblastoma)	IV
E. Neuronal tumors	
1. Gangliocytoma	I
2. Ganglioglioma	I. II
3. Ganglioneuroblastoma	III
4. Anaplastic (malignant) gangliocytoma and ganglioglioma	III. IV
5. Neuroblastoma	IV
F. Poorly differentiated and embryonal tumors	
1. Glioblastoma	
Variants:	
(a) Glioblastoma with sarcomatous component (mixed glioblastoma and sarcoma)	IV
(b) Giant cell glioblastoma	
2. Medulloblastoma	
Variants:	
(a) Desmoplastic	
(b) Medullomyoblastoma	IV
3. Medulloepithelioma	
4. Primitive polar spongioblastoma	
5. Gliomatosis cerebri	?
II. Tumors of nerve sheath cells	
A. Neurilemoma (schwannoma, neurinoma)	I
B. Anaplastic (malignant) neurilemoma (schwannoma, neurinoma)	II
C. Neurofibroma	I
D. Anaplastic (malignant) neurofibroma (neurofibrosarcoma, neurogenic sarcoma)	III. IV
III. Tumors of meningeal and related tissues	
A. Meningioma	
1. Meningiotheliomatous (endotheliomatous, syncytial, arachnotheliomatous)	
2. Fibrous (fibroblastic)	
3. Transitional (mixed)	I
4. Psammomatous	
5. Angiomatous	
6. Hemangioblastic	
7. Hemangiopericytic	II
8. Papillary	II. III
9. Anaplastic (malignant) meningioma	II. III
B. Meningeal sarcomas	
1. Fibrosarcoma	III. IV
2. Polymorphic cell sarcoma	III. IV
3. Primary meningeal sarcomatosis	IV
C. Xanthomatous tumors	
1. Fibroxanthoma	?
2. Xanthosarcoma (malignant fibroxanthoma)	?
D. Primary melanotic tumors	
1. Melanoma	IV
2. Meningeal melanomatosis	IV
E. Others	

(continued)

Table 19–1. WHO histologic classification of tumors of the central nervous system. (continued)

	Grade
IV. Primary malignant lymphomas	III. IV
V. Tumors of blood vessel origin	
A. Hemangioblastoma (capillary hemangioblastoma)	I
B. Monstrocellular sarcoma	IV
VI. Germ cell tumors	
A. Germinoma	II. III
B. Embryonal carcinoma	IV
C. Choriocarcinoma	IV
D. Teratoma	I
VII. Other malformative tumors and tumorlike lesions	
A. Craniopharyngioma	I
B. Rathke's cleft cyst	
C. Epidermoid cyst	
D. Dermoid cyst	
E. Colloid cyst of the third ventricle	
F. Enterogenous cyst	I?
G. Other cysts	
H. Lipoma	
I. Choristoma (pituicytoma, granular cell "myoblastoma")	
J. Hypothalamic neuronal hamartoma	
K. Nasal glial heterotopia (nasal glioma)	
VIII. Vascular malformations	
A. Capillary telangiectasia	
B. Cavernous angioma	
C. Arteriovenous malformation	
D. Venous malformation	I
E. Sturge-Weber disease (cerebrofacial or cerebrotrigeminal angiomatosis)	
IX. Tumors of the anterior pituitary	
A. Pituitary adenomas	
1. Acidophil	I
2. Basophil (mucoid cell)	I
3. Mixed acidophil-basophil	I
4. Chromophobe	I
B. Pituitary adenocarcinoma	III
X. Local extensions from regional tumors	
A. Glomus jugulare tumor (chemodectoma, paraganglioma)	?
B. Chordoma	See similar
D. Chondrosarcoma	tumors
E. Olfactory neuroblastoma (esthesioneuroblastoma)	elsewhere
F. Adenoid cystic carcinoma (cylindroma)	in the
G. Others	body
XI. Metastatic tumors	
XII. Unclassified tumors	

GLIOMA

The most common tumors in all age groups, gliomas account for 45–55% of all brain tumors in children and adults. This category is further subdivided into astrocytoma, accounting for 20–30%, glioblastoma, 40–50%, oligodendroglioma, 15%, and ependymal tumors, 5%.

Essentials of Diagnosis

- Progressive neurologic deficit.
- Generalized or focal seizures.
- Organic mental changes.
- Mass lesions on CT scan or MRI.

1. ASTROCYTOMA

This tumor (often referred to as low-grade astrocytoma) is composed of astrocytes containing var-

ious numbers of intracytoplasmic intermediate filaments. Glial fibrillary acidophilic protein (GFAP) is the major protein component of these glial intermediate filaments, and it is a useful marker for astrocytic differentiation when determining the cell of origin in tumors with complex histologic features. It can also be found in the other glia-derived tumors mentioned above and, if found, provides definite evidence that a malignancy is primary rather than metastatic. There are various subgroups of astrocytoma, identified on the basis of their cellular appearance and the patterns they form. These include fibrillary, protoplasmic, pilocytic, gemistocytic, and xanthomatous.

Grading

The grading of astrocytomas is based on nuclear characteristics. It relies on cell density, chromatin density and coarseness, mitotic activity, and nucleolar prominence. Several numerical grading systems have come into use, adding to the confusion of clini-

Table 19–2. WHO revised classification of brain tumors in children.

I. Tumors of neuroepithelial tissue
  A. Glial tumors
    1. Astrocytic tumors
      (a) Astrocytoma (fibrillary, protoplasmic, gemistocytic, pilocytic, and xanthomatous)
      (b) Anaplastic astrocytoma
      (c) Subependymal giant cell tumors (tuberous sclerosis)
      (d) Gigantocellular glioma
    2. Oligodendroglial tumors
      (a) Oligodendroglioma
      (b) Anaplastic oligodendroglioma
    3. Ependymal tumors
      (a) Ependymoma
      (b) Anaplastic ependymoma
      (c) Myxopapillary ependymoma
    4. Choroid plexus tumors
      (a) Choroid plexus papilloma
      (b) Anaplastic choroid plexus tumor (carcinoma)
    5. Mixed gliomas
      (a) Oligoastrocytoma
        1. Anaplastic oligoastrocytoma
      (b) Astroependymoma
        1. Anaplastic ependymoastrocytoma
      (c) Oligoastroependymoma
        1. Anaplastic oligoastroependymoma
      (d) Oligoependymoma
        1. Anaplastic oligoependymoma
      (e) Subependymoma-subependymal glomerate astrocytoma
      (f) Gliofibroma
    6. Glioblastomatous tumors
      (a) Glioblastoma multiforme
      (b) Giant cell glioblastoma
      (c) Gliosarcoma
    7. Gliomatosis cerebri
  B. Neuronal tumors
    1. Gangliocytoma
    2. Anaplastic gangliocytoma
    3. Ganglioglioma
    4. Anaplastic ganglioglioma
  C. "Primitive" neuroepithelial tumors
    1. "Primitive" neuroectodermal tumor, not otherwise specified (NOS)
    2. "Primitive" neuroectodermal tumor, with
      (a) Astrocytes
      (b) Oligodendrocytes
      (c) Ependymal cells
      (d) Neuronal cells
      (e) Other (melanocytic, mesenchymal)
      (f) Mixed cellular elements
    3. Medulloepithelioma
      (a) Medulloepithelioma, NOS
      (b) Medulloepithelioma with
        (1) Astrocytes
        (2) Oligodendrocytes
        (3) Ependymal cells
        (4) Neuronal cells
        (5) Other (melanocytic, mesenchymal)
        (6) Mixed cellular elements
  D. Pineal cell tumors
    1. "Primitive" neuroectodermal tumor (see C) (pineoblastoma)
    2. Pineocytoma
II. Tumors of meningeal and related tissues
  A. Meningiomas
    1. Meningioma, NOS
    2. "Papillary" meningioma
    3. Anaplastic meningioma
  B. Meningeal sarcomatous tumors
    1. Meningeal sarcoma, NOS
    2. Rhabdomyosarcoma or leiomyosarcoma
    3. Mesenchymal chondrosarcoma
    4. Fibrosarcoma
    5. Others

(continued)

Table 19–2. WHO revised classification of brain tumors in children. (continued)

   C. Primary melanocytic tumors
     1. Malignant melanoma
     2. Melanomatosis
     3. Melanocytic tumors, miscellaneous
III. Tumors of nerve sheath cells
   A. Neurilemoma (schwannoma, neurinoma)
   B. Anaplastic neurilemoma (schwannoma, neurinoma)
   C. Neurofibroma
   D. Anaplastic neurofibroma (neurofibrosarcoma, neurogenic sarcoma)
IV. Primary malignant lymphomas
   Classify according to local current standards
V. Tumors of blood vessel origin
   A. Hemangioblastoma
   B. Hemangiopericytoma
   C. Neoplastic angioendotheliosis-angiosarcoma
VI. Germ cell tumors
   A. Germinoma
   B. Embryonal carcinoma
   C. Choriocarcinoma
   D. Endodermal sinus tumor
   E. Teratomatous tumors
     1. Immature teratoma
     2. Mature teratoma
     3. Teratocarcinoma
   F. Mixed
VII. Malformative tumors
   A. Craniopharyngioma
   B. Rathke's cleft cyst
   C. Epidermal cyst
   D. Dermoid cyst
   E. Colloid cyst of third ventricle
   F. Enterogenous or bronchial cyst
   G. Cyst, NOS
   H. Lipoma
   I. Granular cell tumor (choristoma)
   J. Hamartoma
     1. Neuronal
     2. Glial
     3. Neuronoglial
     4. Meningioangioneurinomatosis
VIII. Tumors of neuroendocrine origin
   A. Tumors of anterior pituitary
     1. Adenoma
     2. Pituitary carcinoma
   B. Paraganglioma
IX. Local extensions from regional tumors
   Type to be specified according to primary diagnosis
X. Metastatic tumors
XI. Unclassified tumors

cal trial and study results when investigators do not name the system being used or when histologic features are not adequately described. The two most commonly used grading systems for astrocytoma are shown in Table 19–3. The purpose of these grading systems is to aid the clinician in delivering treatment and to provide a prognosis. They are ultimately based on the histologic type and degree of differentiation. The grading of an isolated biopsy specimen can be misleading, since poorly differentiated areas commonly coexist with well-differentiated areas in these tumors. Because of the close association between histology and length of survival, if a specimen is taken from a more benign area, adequate treatment measures may not be undertaken and an inaccurate prog-

nosis assigned. Other techniques and variables must be considered in the overall diagnosis and treatment of the individual patient.

Pathology

Major topographic sites of these tumors are (1) cerebral hemispheres. Diffuse and ill-defined, solid or cystic tumors of the fibrillary or mixed cell type are most often found. They may invade the leptomeninges and occasionally undergo dedifferentiation (into an anaplastic astrocytoma or glioblastoma). The average doubling time for most of these tumors is 36 days. Recurrences usually reveal more malignant histologic characteristics. Only 40% will be histologically unchanged at the time of recurrence, and these

Table 19–3. Major histologic grade coding systems for gliomas.

Four-tiered grading system (Kernohan Classification, 1949)
Grade I Benign: Isomorphic, differentiated tissue picture of low cellularity, no pleomorphism, no hyperchromatic nuclei, no or rare mitotic activity. Gliosis versus glioma.
Grade II Semibenign: Moderate cellularity, slight pleomorphism, mild nuclear hyperchromasia, occasional mitotic activity, no or only mild vascular proliferation, no necrosis.
Grade III Semimalignant: Moderate to marked hypercelluarity and pleomorphism but cellular origin of many neoplastic cells still recognizable (positive GFAP), hyperchromatic nuclei, high mitotic activity, vascular proliferation and rare necrosis.
Grade IV Malignant: Extreme hypercellularity, marked cellular and nuclear pleomorphism, hyperchromatic nuclei, abundant mitotic activity, necrosis with or without pseudopalisading, marked vascular proliferation. Glioblastoma.
Three-tiered grading system (Ringertz Classification, 1950)
Grade I Isomorphic, benign: Differentiated tissue picture of low to moderate cellularity, no or only slight pleomorphism, no mitoses, vascular proliferation or necrosis.
Grade II Intermediate: Less well differentiated tissue pattern, moderate hypercellularity, moderate pleomorphism, moderate number of mitoses, vascular proliferation, no or only few necroses.
Grade III Anaplastic: Dedifferentiated picture, marked hypercellularity, extreme cellular and nuclear pleomorphism, abundant pathologic mitoses, true necrosis, and massive capillary endothelial proliferation.
Histologic criteria of astrocytomas (used by the Brain Tumor Study Group; most commonly used current classification)
I. Astrocytoma Moderate to high cellularity, slight pleomorphism, no hyperchromatic nuclei, no vascular proliferation, no necrosis.
II. Anaplastic astrocytoma Moderate hypercellularity, moderate pleomorphism, hyperchromatic nuclei, vascular proliferation, no necrosis.
III. Glioblastoma multiform Marked hypercellularity, pleomorphism, hyperchromatic nuclei, necrosis with or without pseudopalisading (*required*), vascular proliferation (*not required*). In this classification, the key criterion used to distinguish glioblastoma from anaplastic astrocytoma is *necrosis.*

are of the moderately differentiated type. **(2)** Brain stem. This site is involved more often in children and adolescents than in adults. Astrocytomas constitute 8–12% of brain tumors in this group, and they tend to grow in a diffuse and invasive manner, with enlargement of the brain stem and at times invasion of the fourth ventricle or cerebellum.

Pilocystic astrocytomas consist of elongated cells with unipolar or bipolar processes that form parallel bundles adjacent to loosely structured microcystic areas. They may display Rosenthal's fibers and eosinophilic droplets containing glial filaments that are GFAP negative or only partially positive. This type of astrocytomas is most common in children and seems to localize in midline structures, eg, cerebellum, hypothalamus, optic nerves, chiasm, and brain stem. It is most noted for calcification and large cyst formation, especially in those located in the cerebellum. This specific cerebellar astrocytoma constitutes roughly 12% of brain tumors in children and is the second most common cerebellar tumor affecting the midline and the hemispheres. Likewise, the "juvenile" pilocytic astrocytoma represents 10% of all gliomas of the cerebral hemispheres, including all ages.

The fibrillary or diffuse astrocytoma accounts for greater than 90% of all astrocytomas. It occurs most frequently in the cerebral hemispheres in adults and occasionally in the brain stem or pons in children. In contrast to the pilocytic type, it tends to undergo malignant degeneration. The anaplastic astrocytoma displays various degrees of pleomorphism, increased cellularity, mitotic figures, and possibly vascular proliferation but is without necrosis.

Treatment
See below, under Glioblastoma.

Prognosis
The prognosis for astrocytomas in the cerebral hemispheres is related to morphologic grade and histologic features. Low-grade tumors carry a 5-year survival rate of 30–50% with an average survival rate after surgery of 48 months. There have been long-term survivors exceeding 10 years. Brain stem astrocytomas have a somewhat worse prognosis with a 5–year survival rate of 25–30% despite improvements in radiation therapy and chemotherapy.

Malignant transformation of pilocytic astrocytoma is rare. If it is totally removed, patients are usually recurrence free. Survival rates at 15 years approach 70% and at 25 years, 38%. Prognostic features have been identified in biopsy specimens. Microcysts, leptomeningeal deposits, Rosenthal's fibers, and oligodendroglial foci (present in about 70%) carry an excellent prognosis, with a 10-year survival rate of 94%. Meanwhile, perivascular pseudorosettes, high cell density, necrosis, mitoses, and calcifications (present in 20–30%) are linked to a poor prognosis. Only 29% of this group is estimated to survive 10 years.

The prognosis for anaplastic astrocytoma reflects survival rates approximately half those of lower grade astrocytomas but 50–100% longer than those of glioblastoma irrespective of treatment. A rapid anaplastic transformation can occur spontaneously in supratentorial gliomas of young people. A small number are at risk for an adverse response to chemotherapy and develop focal progression and overgrowth of anaplastic cells. Two studies have shown this increase in anaplasia following radiation therapy and chemotherapy in 3–4.7%.

2. GLIOBLASTOMA

This is the most malignant of the glial tumors, making up 15–20% of all intracranial neoplasms but only 7% of those in childhood. It most often presents in the cerebral hemispheres of adults aged 45–55 and occurs rarely in the posterior fossa.

Pathogenesis

As many as 25–30% may have arisen from preexisting astrocytomas. Others are thought to arise from a primitive stem cell called the "glioblast." Cytokinetic studies show that one-third of the cells in these tumors are in active proliferation, with a cell cycle time of 2–3 days. There is a potential doubling time of 3–8 days. However, a cell loss of 85% maintains the doubling time at 40–55 days. The rate of growth seems to correlate better with the ratio of proliferating cells to total cell number than the actual cell cycle time. This finding, plus the marked heterogeneity with various degrees of drug sensitivity and development of therapeutic resistance, are important prognostic variables.

Pathology

Grossly glioblastomas are large and infiltrative; on microscopic examination, they are remarkable for high cellularity and mitotic rate, necrosis, pseudopalisading, and hypervascularity, with dense coils of hyperplastic vessels. Giant cells may also be present.

Autopsy data reveal that 10–15% of these tumors are invasive to the leptomeninges and ventricular system. Aggressive therapy may be producing an increased survival in this group, and invasion, multifocality, and cerebrospinal fluid spread may actually be more common than was once presumed. Metastases of glioblastoma outside the central nervous system are rare but have been reported to involve lymph nodes, bone marrow, lung, and liver.

There are two variants of glioblastoma. One is the monstrocellular type, which consists predominantly of multinucleated giant cells. It occasionally has a less aggressive behavior. The other variant is the gliosarcoma, which reflects a neoplastic transformation of mesenchymal elements and a vascular endothelial proliferation, thought to represent the final stages in the transformation of capillary hyperplasia. It accounts for 8% of glioblastomas.

Treatment

A. Surgery: Most gliomas are infiltrative and not fully resectable. Rapid reduction of volume (cyto-reduction) is nevertheless of prime importance as first-line treatment, since it provides immediate decompression and relief of symptoms, a tissue diagnosis, and a chance for radiation therapy or chemotherapy to take effect. Areas of tumor with little vascular supply may otherwise be resistant to both these modalities. Gross total or subtotal resection is usually the goal. Patients who undergo biopsy alone generally have a worse course. Surgery also remains the primary treatment for benign tumors, such as meningiomas, cystic cerebellar astrocytomas, and other slow-growing lesions.

A number of technologic developments have allowed for more aggressive resection with less resultant morbidity and mortality, reflecting the remarkable advances in neurosurgery over the last 10 years. These include the use of such devices as the operative microscope, improved CT scan and MRI, and stereotaxic procedures that not only allow approach to otherwise unapproachable areas for biopsy but also allow for better identification of tumor margins and even procedures such as cyst drainage and implantation of radioactive seeds. The use of laser equipment has also proved beneficial.

CT- or MRI-guided stereotaxic procedures begin with placement of the patient's head in a stereotaxic holder while imaging is being performed. Reference rods are attached to the device and also appear on the CT images. Three-dimensional coordinates are obtained for any target point. By means of a computer system in the operating room, reference points can be digitalized and the surgeon can digitalize and the surgeon can digitalize target points. Either the target points themselves or the three-dimensional tumor volume outline can be displayed and rotated in space for any surgical approach. This system can be used for brachytherapy or laser surgery.

The Cavitron ultrasonic surgical aspirator is a device that produces mechanical fragmentation and aspiration without applying traction or heating of the surrounding normal brain. Laser systems operate by vaporizing tissue and can be used as cutting instruments. The CO_2 laser beam is absorbed at the surface, where it is converted into heat. The Nd:YAG laser produces more diffuse scattering, allowing homogeneous coagulation of a larger volume of tissue. This may result in a more edematous boundary but more successfully coagulates vessels than the CO_2 laser.

B. Radiation Therapy: Radiation has been the mainstay of treatment for most types of malignant brain tumors. In glioma it tends to delay progression and recurrence. Early reports by the Brain Tumor Study Group showed an increase in median survival from 14 weeks after surgery to 36 with postoperative radiation. Concurrently 1-year survival increased from 3% with surgery alone to 24%. Clinical improvement occurs in one-fourth to one-half of these patients. Despite this initial response, 100% of glioblastomas and 80% of anaplastic astrocytomas will recur in 2–5 years and result in death.

Indications for radiation therapy are controversial for the low-grade astrocytomas. Data are difficult to interpret owing to variable time courses and a lack of controlled clinical trials. The natural history of this population depends on age at the time of diagnosis, site of presentation, and histologic type. Studies performed in the 1970s showed a greater than twofold increase in 5-year survival rate in patients with incompletely resected grade I or II gliomas and a course of radiotherapy. Positive results have also been reported in biopsy-proved diencephalic lesions as well as in cystic hemispheric astrocytomas. A clear dose-response curve unfortunately does not exist for the low-grade astrocytomas. Major series report doses of 4000–5000 cGy to local fields. Statistical analyses suggest improved survival with these amounts. Recommendations for radiation therapy are based on neurological status and site of origin.

Radiation cell kill is based on the oxygen tension of radiated tissue. With conventional photon radiation, hypoxic cells are only one-third to one-half as sensitive as normally oxygenated tissue. Mechanisms to overcome hypoxic radioresistance of malignant gliomas initially included treatment under hyperbaric oxygen conditions to raise the oxygen tension in poorly vascularized necrotic tumors; however, after 2 years there were still no survivors.

Neutrons interact with matter more densely than do photons and result in high linear energy transfer (LET). They are less dependent on oxygen for cell lethality. Trials show an impressive cell kill, but survival is identical to that of photon-irradiated controls. Autopsies revealed death secondary to cerebral gliosis and demyelination in 90%. Studies are under way to maximize the therapeutic ratio and utilize this apparent neutron efficacy in keeping with CNS tolerance.

Other attempts to add to radiation cell kill utilize so-called radiation sensitizers that affect radiation injury. Cisplatin is one such agent. Actual dosages and timing with respect to radiation are still being evaluated. Altered fractionation schedules are intended to improve the therapeutic ratio by taking advantage of dose-limiting late normal tissue reactions on fraction size. Hyperfractionated radiation involves the use of 2–3 smaller radiation fractions per day, allowing a higher total dose but keeping within the tolerance of normal brain tissue. No obvious advantages have yet been documented.

Routine treatment for most high-grade gliomas remains 4500–6000 cGy delivered in fractions of 180–200 cGy/d, five times a week. This schedule reflects the best tumor kill, with less CNS toxicity.

Recurrence following radiation is at the site of the primary tumor in over 90% of cases.

Brachytherapy is another method to maximize therapeutic ratio and involves implantation of stereotactically placed ^{125}I or iridium, providing localization of high-dose radiation. This technique is particularly of benefit in lesions of limited size (±5 cm), providing good dosimetric distribution with considerable safety. Phase II studies show a high degree of efficacy; the time postimplant to progression exceeds in some cases the interval between primary treatment and recurrence. There is a high likelihood of intralesional necrosis. Patients may need to undergo surgery for removal of this necrotic focus, which in itself can mimic a recurrent mass. Trials are under way to examine the use of both brachytherapy and external beam irradiation to treat malignant glioma.

C. Chemotherapy: Most brain tumors are incurable. Chemotherapy is mainly palliative. In choosing a protocol or specific agent, consider the individual patient and the benefits and risks. The efficacy of various types of protocols should be reviewed as well as the particulars of the one chosen and its toxicities. Most chemotherapy must be given at the highest dose achievable. This dose may be limited by bone marrow suppression, CNS toxicity, or other organ toxicity. Large single or multicenter trials are of importance, since data gathering provides for comparison of multiple treatment arms, allowing sounder conclusions to be drawn regarding the effectiveness of individual therapies. Administration of chemotherapeutic agents requires knowledge of their use, side effects, and toxicities. Familiarity with agents to control pain, vomiting, and infection also is required.

Corticosteroids are one of the earliest and most commonly used agents to treat brain tumors. The original work was accomplished by Galicich and French in the early 1960s. Dexamethasone was used because of its low index of salt/water retention. It is still used for similar reasons as well as for its ability to be absorbed well orally and its long half-life of 50 hours. Its ability to decrease edema makes it an important adjunct to radiation therapy and chemotherapeutic regimens as well. Complications of corticosteroids include gastritis and ulcer disease (advocating a need for antacid therapy), impaired wound healing (important following surgery), myopathy, impaired immunity, and the unmasking or worsening of impaired glucose tolerance (Table 19–4).

Dexamethasone also has an effect on the CT scan of a tumor by decreasing edema and enhancing appearance. For this reason, it is important to correlate changes in dose when comparing tumor size on the scan of a patient enrolled in a chemotherapy protocol.

The vasogenic edema that accompanies brain tumors seems to be related to injury of cerebral vessel walls, causing the escape of water and plasma constituents into the parenchyma. This is different from cytotoxic edema, which is seen when a noxious factor affects structural elements of the brain, producing intracellular swelling. The vascular permeability in the latter case is undisturbed.

Table 19–4. Adverse effects of corticosteroids.

Adrenal supression (Cushing's syndrome)	
Myopathy	Skin fragility
Pathologic fractures	Gastritis/ulcer
Diabetes mellitus	Weight gain
Cataracts	Psychosis
Salt retention	Slowed wound healing
Arthralgias	Infections

Solute transport across capillaries relies on two mechanisms: (1) Substances dissolve in and diffuse through luminal membranes or the cytoplasm of endothelial cells. Blood-to-brain transfer depends on a substance's membrane or lipid solubility and its molecular size. (2) Facilitated or carrier mediated transfer is independent of lipid solubility and molecular size. Normal brain capillaries are impermeable to sodium and chloride ions, preventing the rapid passage of water into the brain. Brain tumors cause an increase in the hydraulic conductivity of the endothelium owing to fenestrations and discontinuities in endothelial walls that allow for bulk flow of fluid from the vascular compartment to the tumor. Experiments suggest that corticosteroids may decrease the extracellular space of a tumor and adjacent brain by decreasing water flow and the influx rate of albumin across capillaries.

The nitrosureas are the best studied chemotherapeutic agents in brain tumor trials and the standard against which other therapy trials are compared. They are ideal CNS drugs because of their high lipid solubility, low ionization at a physiologic pH, and low plasma protein affinity. Carmustine is superior in the treatment of high-grade astrocytomas. Attempts have been made at improving drug delivery to the tumor by intra-arterial injection (carotid and vertebral) and by osmotic manipulation of the blood-brain barrier. The advantage of the former method is the attempt to increase the concentration of drug within the tumor while decreasing the total dose given and theoretically decreasing systemic toxicity, especially to the marrow. Lipid- and nonlipid-soluble drugs can be used with this adjustment. Therapy can be given by infusion pump after placement of a catheter. Carmustine and cisplatin are the best studied in this manner. Response rates are promising with both agents, and phase III trials are under way.

Difficulties with delivering these agents in this manner include the (1) fact that patients must be admitted, (2) association of both carmustine and cisplatin with focal neurologic deficits, both transient and permanent, including ipsilateral blindness and leukoencephalopathy (especially with carmustine), and (3) lack of well-defined infusion rates, dosing intervals, and maximum cumulative doses. Even when catheter placement is above the ophthalamic artery, there is still an increased incidence of focal toxicity and an unacceptable incidence of leukoencephalopathy.

Blood-brain barrier manipulation with mannitol has likewise been attempted. Brain tumors may have areas where the blood-brain barrier is intact but mainly seem to have areas with endothelial fenestrations as do systemic vessels. Mannitol administration disrupts the blood-brain barrier in the neoplasm as well as in normal brain, allowing increased drug delivery throughout and the risk of toxicity to normal brain.

D. Immunotherapy: Because of the impaired immune mechanisms discovered in brain tumor patients as well as the local immune responses frequently seen at the time of biopsy or autopsy, much consideration has been given to manipulation of the immune system as a mode of therapy. As mentioned earlier, malignant gliomas are infiltrative, well beyond the limits defined by CT scan enhancement, making complete resection nearly impossible. What would be a more logical method of eradicating even microscopic disease than to channel the body's own immune defenses against these "foreign" tumor cells?

The defects in immunity that have been described include impaired delayed hypersensitivity, impaired recognition of autologous tumor antigens in culture, and decreased ability to undergo blastogenic transformation when exposed to common mitogens. After several attempts at bolstering patients' immune mechanisms with injections of bacillus Calmette-Guérin (BCG) and even intratumoral injections of autologous lymphocytes with meager results, trials of monoclonal antibodies were begun. Because their specificity would allow for selective tumor cell lysis, it was hoped that normal brain tissue would not undergo toxic changes. However, there is great difficulty in developing monoclonal antibodies with pure glioma specificity, since these tumors are composed of heterogenous cell types and antigens and may demonstrate some cross-reactivity with normal glial cells. Attempts are still being made to link these antibodies to various chemotherapeutic agents or to cell toxins.

Later developments include the biologic response modifiers, or lymphokines. This category includes the interferons, interleukin, and B cell growth factor (Chapter 16).

Course & Prognosis

High-grade astrocytomas form the bulk of primary brain tumors. A better outcome has been noted in patients who develop this disease at a younger age, have a higher performance status, and have a tumor of a lower histologic grade. On the other hand, necrosis seems to consistently forewarn of a poorer prognosis, eg, glioblastoma patients consistently do more poorly than those with anaplastic astrocytoma, with survival rates of 36% and 60%, respectively.

The standard treatment remains surgery plus external beam radiation therapy totalling 6000 cGy. The Brain Tumor Study Group reported an increased survival rate at 18 months with the addition of carmustine from 4% to 19%. This agent still has the highest response rate. Other single agents and multiple-agent combinations have been studied, including doxorubicin, bleomycin, etoposide, fluorouracil, dacarbazine, methotrexate, lomustine, procarbazine, thiotepa, and vincristine. Of these drugs, the most useful as single agents are procarbazine, dacarbazine, and lomustine, the three of which are cell cycle–nonspecific.

The Brain Tumor Study Group was first to show that radiation produced statistically prolonged survival (Table 19–5). Reoperation for these tumors is controversial, though at times it may provide a definite benefit. The median time to recurrence after the first operation is 5–6 months, following which survival generally is limited. With reoperation the median survival is in the range of 14–26 weeks. Most neurosurgeons agree that patients with a rating of 60 or less on the Karnovsky scale (Table 19–6) should not be reoperated.

The management of low-grade astrocytomas has also undergone scrutiny. An early retrospective study spanning 1942 to 1967 revealed that patients with grade I tumors (Kernohan classification) that were resected and treated with irradiation had a 5-year survival rate of 58%, compared with a 25% rate for those not irradiated. Of patients with grade II tumors, 25% survived 5 years with radiotherapy as opposed to 0% without. It must be borne in mind that the radiation techniques of this period were different from those delivered currently. Whether irradiation may induce the tumor to a more malignant transformation with time or whether such malignant transformation is the natural history of these tumors is an unanswered question. Some centers invoke observation alone in this group of patients. A Southwest Oncology Group study is being analyzed in which Kernohan grade I and II astrocytomas were treated with either radiation or radiation plus lomustine; this was the first study to investigate chemotherapy in this group of tumors. The general recommendation, however, remains 5000 cGy for incompletely resected and low-grade astrocytomas. Further large-scale studies need to be undertaken comparing the natural history of these tumors and the effects of treatment.

The prognosis for all glioblastomas is poor; survival time is 4–6 months without treatment and 12–18 months with surgery, irradiation, and chemotherapy. A 30–50% 1-year survival rate has been estimated, and 10–20% at 2 years.

3. OLIGODENDROGLIOMA

Essentials of Diagnosis
- Slow-growing benign tumor of the cerebral hemispheres.
- Calcification on CT scan.
- Infiltration of the cortex.

This is a tumor of adulthood, with prominent sites in the cerebral hemispheres, especially the frontal lobe, and a tendency to infiltrate the cortex.

Pathology
The well-differentiated type consists of round cells with small nuclei and clear cytoplasm, creating the so-called fried-egg appearance. Mitotic activity is minimal, and calcification occurs in 90%. About 3% of all oligodendrogliomas are an anaplastic variant. They are densely cellular, contain pleomorphic nuclei, and have frequent mitotic figures. Vascular proliferation and occasional giant cells are seen. Some may present with necrotic foci and merge with the glioblastoma. A less aggressive course is typified by the presence of microcysts and low cellularity. These tumors do not dedifferentiate to the degree that astrocytic tumors do.

Clinical Findings
These tumors typically calcify. The calcified portions appear hyperintense on a noncontrasted CT scan. The density comparable to bone density on CT scan. MRI is not useful for delineating or detecting calcified lesions and therefore may not be as useful as CT scans performed with and without enhancement.

Treatment
The behavior of oligodendroglioma is difficult to predict on the basis of histologic appearance. Most tumors remain indolent. Following surgery, standard external beam radiation therapy is recommended. Chemotherapy for the more anaplastic variant prolongs time to recurrence and survival. The most beneficial regimen reported thus far is the combination of procarbazine, lomustine, and vincristine. Recurrences of the more benign variant following surgery and radiation are also responsive to this regimen.

Prognosis
The average survival for patients with oligodendrogliomas having a low cell density and isomorphic cell population is 8 years; the 5-year survival rate is 70%. Survivals over 25 years have been noted. Intermediate forms average 4–5 years with a 40% 5-year

Table 19–5. Survival in glioblastoma (Brain Tumor Study Group).

Surgery + supportive care	17	weeks
Surgery + radiation	37.5	weeks
Surgery + carmustine	25	weeks
Surgery + radiation + carmustine	40.5	weeks

Table 19–6. Karnofsky performance scale.

Able to carry on normal activity; no special care is needed.	100	Normal; no complaints; no evidence of disease.
	90	Able to carry on normal activity; minor signs or symptoms of disease.
	80	Normal activity with effort; some signs or symptoms of disease.
Unable to work; able to live at home and care for most personal needs; a varying amount of assistance is needed.	70	Cares for self; unable to carry on normal activity or to do active work.
	60	Requires occasional assistance but is able to care for most needs.
	50	Requires considerable assistance and frequent medical care.
Unable to care for self; requires equivalent of institutional or hospital care; disease may be progressing rapidly.	40	Disabled; requires special care and assistance.
	30	Severely disabled; hospitalization is indicated although death is not imminent.
	20	Very sick; hospitalization necessary; active supportive treatment is necessary.
	10	Moribund; fatal processes progressing rapidly.
	0	Dead.

survival rate. The anaplastic variant has an average survival of 17 months. Half these tumors recur; 75% show the same histologic features on recurrence. Remote extracranial metastases have been described. Many have astrocytic characteristics, including a positive GFAP.

No large studies have been performed comparing radiation with surgery in this group. Reports of 5-year survival rates of 82% with surgery alone are not uncommon, with 45% remaining recurrence free. In one study, the addition of radiotherapy (5300–7000 cGy) produced a 100% survival rate, with 79% free of recurrence.

4. EPENDYMAL TUMORS

Essentials of Diagnosis
- Childhood tumor.
- Fourth ventricular mass on CT scan or MRI (lateral or third ventricle also may be involved).

More commonly seen in childhood, ependymomas arise from the ependymal lining of the following structures (in order of occurrence): floor of the fourth ventricle, the lateral or third ventricles, the cerebellopontile angle, the central canal of the spinal cord, and the filum terminale. They are usually well defined, encapsulated, solid, or cystic.

Pathology
Histologically, ependymomas display high cellularity, a regular pattern of ependymal cells, and often rosettes and pseudorosettes. Perivascular pseudorosette formation is the most common feature. GFAP is often expressed. Several groups of these tumors have been classified by microscopic features: (1) the classic solid, cellular type; (2) papillary type, consisting of papillae and tubules, mimicking the choroid plexus papilloma; (3) myxopapillary type, occurring

exclusively in the region of the cauda equina; and (4) anaplastic ependymomas, which account for 5–10% of all ependymomas. The characteristic features include a high nuclear:cytoplasmic ratio, increased cellularity, multiple nucleoli, increased mitotic figures, necrosis, and vascular proliferation. These occur more commonly in the supratentorial space. Dissemination along cerebrospinal fluid pathways occurs in 20–60%.

"Mixed" glioma tumors, consisting of two or three types of glial cells, occur most often in young people. Any component of the glial cell combination can predominate. Examples include oligoastrocytoma, ependymoastrocytoma, oligoastroependymoma, and oligoependymoma.

Treatment
The ependymoma presents the additional problem of cerebrospinal fluid pathway seeding, the potential for which varies with location. Supratentorial tumors tend to spread in only 8%, whereas those of the posterior fossa seed the leptomeninges in 20%. Histologic grade is an important variable, with 23% of high-grade tumors metastasizing versus only 8% of low-grade tumors. Because of these statistics, a form of therapy has been advocated using whole-brain radiotherapy for low-grade supratentorial tumors, whole-brain radiotherapy to the C5 level for low-grade posterior fossa tumors, and entire craniospinal axis radiation for high-grade ependymomas or low-grade types with definite cerebrospinal fluid spread. A 69% 10-year survival rate has been achieved.

The role of postradiation chemotherapy awaits validation. For recurrence, the use of chemotherapy is experimental—carmustine, vincristine, cisplatin, etoposide, and ifosfamide have produced palliation. Chemotherapy adjuvant to radiation therapy has been active in children.

Prognosis
Overall, the 5-year survival rate in children with

intracranial tumor is 30%. Combination chemotherapy has improved survival to a 20% 10-year rate for the higher grade tumors and 70% for the lower grades. Adults have an even better outcome.

5. TUMORS OF THE CHOROID PLEXUS

Essentials of Diagnosis
- Childhood occurrence.
- Lateral or fourth ventricular mass.

Choroid plexus papillomas occur mostly in children, in the region of the lateral and fourth ventricles. Grossly they appear as a cauliflowerlike mass, with cuboidal cells in a single layer on a basement membrane, which covers a delicate vascular connective tissue core. They do not contain glial fibers as a rule.

Pathology
The expression of carbonic anhydrase is a choroid plexus–specific marker. S-100 protein immunoreactivity is prominent in well-differentiated types. Other markers include cytokeratin, GFAP, and carcinoembryonic antigen (CEA). Aggregates of glycogen granules are often found.

There is a tendency for these tumors to seed the cerebrospinal fluid pathways. Outcome following resection is generally good, although hydrocephalus may develop. There is also an anaplastic variant of choroid plexus carcinoma, which exhibits cellular pleomorphism and mitoses and may even invade the brain parenchyma. It can arise in any ventricle, in adults or children, either de novo or by anaplastic transformation in a benign adenoma.

Treatment
Treatment is generally surgical with the addition of irradiation for the anaplastic variant or for recurrent disease.

PINEAL TUMORS

Essentials of Diagnosis
- Midline enhancing lesion on CT scan or MRI in region of third ventricle.
- Obstructive hydrocephalus—symptoms of raised intracranial pressure.
- Papilledema.
- Perinaud's syndrome.

This rare neoplasm averages 1–2% of all intracranial neoplasms and has a higher incidence in Japan. There are two major types: (1) teratomatous or germ cell tumors, the most common to occur in this area, and (2) tumors of the gland itself— pineocytoma and pineoblastoma.

Pathology
The **pineocytoma** is circumscribed and noninvasive. It can occur at any age and has the appearance of normal pineal gland. Polar processes may radiate toward blood vessels, forming true rosettes. Some may actually show astrocytic or neuronal differentiation. The **pineoblastoma** on the other hand is a highly cellular tumor, is more frequent in infants, and resembles medulloblastoma. It is regarded as a primitive neuroectodermal tumor, and like other neoplasms in that classification, it is poorly differentiated, may infiltrate the cerebrospinal fluid, and often has already disseminated by the time of diagnosis.

Treatment
Treatment consists of surgical excision and possibly radiation therapy as in the case of pineoblastoma. (See also below, under Germ Cell Tumors).

NEURONAL TUMORS

Essentials of Diagnosis
- Slow-growing lesion of cerebral hemispheres.
- Children, young adults affected.

Four types of tumor fall within this category, all containing mature-appearing ganglion cells. (1) Gangliocytomas are composed of ganglion cells with two or more nuclei. They may have abundant neurofilament protein (NFP), and the glial component may be GFAP positive, ie, there are both neuronal and glial features. They occur most commonly in the cerebral hemispheres in childhood, are slow growing, and carry a good prognosis. (2) The dysplastic gangliocytoma of the cerebellum, or Lhermitte-Duclos disease, is a hamartomatous lesion that is more like a malformation than a true neoplasm. It may, however, present as a mass in late childhood. Microscopically there is diffuse scattering of large abnormal neurons thought to be derived from the granular cell layer. (3) The anaplastic gangliocytoma consists of ganglion cells with anaplastic features. (4) Gangliogliomas contain ganglion cells and neoplastic glia (usually astrocytes). They predominantly affect children and young adults, with a preference for the bottom of the third ventricle, hypothalamus, and temporal lobe. They are often cystic and are also slow growing with a good prognosis.

The anaplastic ganglioglioma displays anaplasia of the glial component and may be mistaken for a glioblastoma.

EMBRYONAL TUMORS

Essentials of Diagnosis
- Childhood occurrence.
- Cerebellar mass on CT scan or MRI.
- Gait and limb ataxia.

This class of tumor most commonly occurs in children. They arise in the cerebrum, cerebellum, pineal, or elsewhere in the CNS. Histologic characteristics are undifferentiated cells with some areas of differentiation along glial, neuronal, ependymal, mesenchymal, or pineal lines. More than one mature of immature cell line may be represented. The newer classification for this group of tumors is primitive neuroectodermal tumor (PNET), of which the medulloblastoma is the most common representative. The most primitive type occur in the midline cerebellum, but they may arise anywhere, including the pineal gland. They tend to spread widely by cerebrospinal fluid pathways and may even metastasize outside the CNS, eg, to bone. The cells in this tumor are poorly differentiated neuroepithelial cells with chromatin-rich nuclei and a small rim of cytoplasm. Mitoses are frequent, and necrosis may be present. GFAP and NFP stains are negative.

There is also a more differentiated form of PNET, one of which is the glial type, containing neoplastic glial cells, or ependymoblastomas. The latter is highly cellular, contains poorly differentiated neuroepithelial cells, has frequent mitoses, and may be GFAP positive or negative. Differentiation is restricted to glial precursors with features of ependymal cells. Vascular proliferation, pleomorphism, and multinucleated cells are at a minimum. The median age for this variant is 2, leptomeningeal spread is frequent, and the prognosis is poor. Another PNET with differentiation is the neuroblastoma, consisting of poorly differentiated neuroepithelial cells and mature ganglion cells. This childhood tumor is indistinguishable from peripheral neuroblastomas.

The **medulloblastoma** accounts for 3–5% of all intracranial neoplasms and 20–25% of brain tumors in childhood. The peak age of incidence is 5 years, and 80% occur before age 15. Sites of occurrence are the midline structures, ie, cerebellar vermis and fourth ventricle, in children. There is a predilection for the cerebellar hemispheres in adults.

Pathology

Medulloblastoma is a heterogeneous neoplasm with a variety of histologic features, including small round cells with hyperchromatic nuclei and little cytoplasm. Mitoses are frequent. Homer-Wright rosettes and pseudorosettes are variably present. The tumor is usually well demarcated and is derived from cells of the medullary vellum or multipotential external granular cells (the areas involved in the development of the cerebellum in fetal life). These cells have the capacity to differentiate along glial or neuronal lines. GFAP-positive cells are usually found in young adults with a cerebellar hemisphere tumor, the so-called desmoplastic variant. This is a mixed mesenchymal-ectodermal tumor and has a better prognosis after resection than the more common medulloblastoma. The histologic features also correlate with a better prognosis, revealing fibrillar areas, less cellular density, and glial differentiation.

Medulloblastoma is known for its tendency to seed the subarachnoid space with dissemination to the spinal cord and remaining central nervous system. Several series have documented extraneural metastases in as high as 30%; approximately one-third of these are metastatic to bone. Most of the remaining metastases occur to the peritoneum as the result of the need for shunt placement and subsequent seeding of this space.

Treatment

The 5- to 10-year disease-free interval in this group is 50–60% with surgery and radiation. Because of the propensity to seed the subarachnoid space (mentioned earlier in this chapter), radiation must be directed to the entire craniospinal axis. This point is key to improved disease control. Medulloblastoma has a much higher recurrence rate if the field is limited to the posterior fossa or spine and posterior fossa. Tumor control and survival correlate directly with the dose to the posterior fossa. At more than 5000 cGy there is improved local tumor control, which parallels survival. Amounts of total radiation for the full cranium and spine are less well established; 3000–4000 cGy is used in the studies quoting a 50% survival rate.

Several chemotherapy regimens have shown promising results both for recurrent disease and in the adjuvant setting.

Extent of surgery has great impact on length of survival in this group of patients. Survival rates as high as 60–80% at 5 years have been reported with "total" resections. The question of importance is what constitutes total resection. Is it the observation of the neurosurgeon at the time of surgery or a CT scan that shows no residual disease? Both are necessary. Any enhancement on the CT scan in the surgical bed within the first 48 hours postoperatively is considered tumor. Enhancement occurring during the next few days may be either tumor or postoperative changes. A different problem exists for tumors involving the brain stem, since the CT scan does not delineate this area well.

Is "total" resection ever achievable in this disease? Probably not, when one considers microscopic extension. However, patients who have only a biopsy or a small amount of tumor removed consistently do not survive even after radiation therapy. The attempt at gross total resection, therefore, remains the key to treatment. Other predictors of outcome include the extent of dissemination at the time of diagnosis. As a rule, 20–30% will have dissemination to other CNS sites, and disease-free survival is markedly worse in this group. Myelography plus cerebrospinal fluid cytologic specimen are complementary in making this diagnosis. Up to 50% of patients with leptomeningeal spread will be missed on cerebrospinal fluid examination alone. The optimal timing for lumbar puncture and myelography is unclear. Ten to 14 days seems acceptable. If the cerebrospinal fluid is examined sooner than this after surgery, it may be positive owing to cells that have been shed from surgical resection, and small blood clots may resemble filling defects on myelography.

The desmoplastic variant has a better outcome, as do those tumors that have differentiated along a particular cell line, ie, showing foci of glial, ependymal, or neuronal differentiation. A longer survival is predicted in these tumors than in the undifferentiated type.

Radiation is applied to the entire neuraxis. The usual amounts range from 3000 to 4000 cGy, with a boost of 5500 cGy to the tumor bed. Some older trials incorporated the use of vincristine and lomustine, which seemed to add some benefit to surgery plus radiation. Current studies are investigating MOPP (mechlorethamine, vincristine [Oncovin], procarbazine, and prednisone) and combination lomustine, vincristine, and cisplatin.

Survivors are at risk for cognitive deficits. Pediatric patients should receive neuropsychiatric followup. Radiotherapy takes its toll in this regard, but other factors cannot go unrecognized. These include preoperative and postoperative level of consciousness and any intervening CNS infections. Hormonal deficiencies may occur because of damage to the hypothalamus. Thyroid function should be checked yearly.

Prognosis

With recent therapy, including surgery, irradiation (to include the craniospinal axis), and chemotherapy, a 50–70% 5-year survival rate has been attained and a 10-year survival approaching 30–40%.

TUMORS OF THE NERVE SHEATH

Essentials of Diagnosis

- Occur wherever Schwann cells are present (cranial nerves, spinal roots, peripheral nerves).
- Occur multiply in neurofibromatosis.
- Eighth cranial nerve most common site.

Though usually involving the peripheral nervous system, these tumors are also considered here because of their frequent association with cranial nerves and location within the cranial vault.

1. SCHWANNOMAS

Otherwise known as neurinomas or neurilemoma, this neoplasm originates from Schwann cells and accounts for 6–8% of all intracranial growths. It is a tumor of adulthood. The major locations are the cerebellopontile angle (the acoustic neuroma), followed in frequency by the trigeminal, ninth cranial, and tenth cranial nerves. Schwannomas are firm, encapsulated, and sometimes cystic. Characteristically they displace and compress adjacent brain and are never invasive.

Pathology

The unique histologic pattern of this tumor is one of dense cellular areas arranged in whorls or palisades, the so-called Antoni A pattern. These alternate with a more loosely structured area having a honeycomb appearance with lipid and foam cells, the Antoni B pattern. Nerve fibers themselves are stretched over the capsule but not within the tumor. The S-100 protein is a common marker.

2. NEUROFIBROMAS

Neurofibromas are grossly indistinguishable from neurinomas. They also consist of Schwann cells amid loosely arranged fibroblasts. Antoni A and B patterns are rare, but the S-100 protein is still a marker. They can occur as solitary or multiple lesions of nerve roots. Neurofibromas are usually associated with von Recklinghausen's disease. There are three subtypes: type 1 is encapsulated and plexiform, type 2 is diffuse without a capsule, and type 3 is composed of perineuriumlike cells. Malignant counterparts occur, in particular a recognized complication of von Recklinghausen's disease.

Treatment

Surgical removal is the only treatment. The prognosis is good.

MENINGIOMA

Essentials of Diagnosis

- Benign, slow-growing.
- Symptoms caused by compression rather than invasion.
- Most common in middle-aged women.
- Attached to dura.

Predominantly a tumor of adulthood, meningiomas constitute 13–18% of all intracranial neoplasms. Less than 2% occur in children. The majority occur along the cerebral convexity and the falx (50%) and the remainder at the sphenoid ridge (20%), olfactory groove (10%), suprasellar region (10%), and posterior fossa (10%). Characteristically these are smooth, lobulated masses that attach to the dura with a broad base. They may be intraventricular or located at the epidural space. Most do not invade the brain. Bone, however, can be involved or exhibit an osteoblastic response.

Pathology

There are a number of histologic patterns of little prognostic significance. The common major subtypes are meningotheliomatous (syncytial), fibroblastic (fibrous), transitional, psammomatous, angiomatous, hemangioblastic, hemangiopericytic, papillary, anaplastic, and malignant.

The most frequently occurring subtype is the meningotheliomatous (60%). It consists of sheets of polygonal cells with indistinct borders and oval nuclei containing delicate chromatin and a small nucleolus. The fibrous subtype (6%) has spindle-shaped cells that resemble fibroblasts in interwoven fascicles with a dense collagen network. Arachnoid whorling structures are present in both types.

The transitional subtype (20%) contains transitional and fibrous elements. The bulk of the type referred to as psammomatous consists of psammoma bodies with or without calcification. These occur most often in elderly women in the spinal region. The angiomatous meningioma (8%) has three variants: a highly vascularized but otherwise typical syncytial/transitional type; a hemangioblastic type, equivalent to the hemangioblastoma of the cerebellum but arising in the supratentorial space; and a hemangiopericytic type.

Papillary meningiomas are distinctive because of the orientation of cells to blood vessels, producing radiating perivascular structures similar to the ependymoma. Mitoses, recurrences, and distant metastases are frequent (30%). The anaplastic type (12%) is noted for increased cellularity and mitotic activity. Cells may be elongated and have a sarcomatous appearance. Other malignant features include necrosis, which may be prominent, and invasion of the parenchyma. Recurrences usually do not reflect a change in histologic characteristics.

Treatment

For this common benign tumor, treatment has mainly been surgical. Tumors usually are well circumscribed and easily resected, unless growth involves the venous sinuses and bone or the location is the sphenoid ridge or parasellar region, limiting resectability. Postoperative radiation seems to increase the progression-free survival of these patients as well as limit local recurrence. Objective tumor reduction, however, has not been demonstrated.

Prognosis

The recurrence rate for all types of meningioma is 5–21% after total resection. The figures double after only partial removal. There is no difference in regard to histologic subtype except for the anaplastic and hemangiopericytic variants, which recur with increased frequency at shorter intervals. Nuclear pleo-

morphism, necrosis, and increased vascularity are of no prognostic value in the meningioma. Hypercellularity, mitotic activity, and cortical invasion are the characteristics that denote malignant behavior.

PRIMARY LYMPHOMA OF THE BRAIN

Essentials of Diagnosis

- Occurs spontaneously in fifth to sixth decades of life.
- AIDS patients at high risk.
- Mass of deep cerebral structures.

This rather uncommon tumor (0.5–1.5% of all intracranial tumors) is being reported with greater frequency mainly because of its occurrence in AIDS patients but also in those without known risk factors. The older literature may refer to this tumor as reticulum cell sarcoma, microglioma, or immunoblastic sarcoma. Contributing 1–2% of all malignant lymphomas, the tumor has histologic features identical to those of non-Hodgkin's lymphoma. The peak age of incidence is in the sixth to seventh decades. High-risk groups traditionally include transplant recipients and those with immunodeficiency, whether acquired or intrinsic. The majority are supratentorial; only 25% are infratentorial. Preferred sites are the cerebral hemispheres, basal ganglia, posterior fossa, and corpus callosum (butterfly tumor). At the time of presentation, 20–30% may be multifocal. There may be diffuse infiltration of the brain with spread to meninges and ventricles.

As in non-Hodgkin's lymphoma, most of these tumors are of B cell origin and either diffuse large cell or diffuse mixed cell types. T cell lymphomas of the brain are classically rare, but recently more are being reported, without evidence of systemic T cell lymphoma or AIDS. They tend to begin perivascularly and spread out centripetally. The infiltrates are dense with cells including perivascular histiocytes, microglia, plasma cells, and groups of lymphocytes of the cell type determining the pathologic classification. Unlike the case for malignant glioma, endothelial proliferation is not a feature. There is, however, an intense vascular proliferation with perivascular infiltration. The histologic hallmark is multiplication of the basement membranes of blood vessels involved by the lymphoma. This is best demonstrated by silver reticulum stains.

Etiology

The occurrence of primary lymphoma of the brain is more common in certain clinical settings, including the collagen vascular diseases such as Sjögren's syndrome, systemic lupus erythematosus, and rheumatoid arthritis; in chronic immunosuppression such as in cardiac, thymic, and renal transplants, congenital immunodeficiency syndromes, and AIDS. It is the most common noninfectious space-occupying lesion of the brain in AIDS and the fourth leading cause of death in these patients. As many as 5% will develop this tumor during the course of their illness; it will be discovered in 11% at autopsy. Most patients who are HIV negative are clinically and immunologically normal prior to the abrupt onset of their disease. Since most are over age 50, this finding may reflect decreased immunosurveillance in the older age groups. Other proposed causes include viral induction and chromosome abnormalities. There is not much information to incriminate a hereditary influence at this time.

Clinical Findings

A. Symptoms and Signs: Typical presentation is that of a middle-aged man with nonfocal neurologic symptoms. The peak age of occurrence is 40–60 years, with a 2:1 male-to-female ratio. The symptom duration from onset to diagnosis is about 3 months. Half the patients have nonfocal, nonspecific symptoms, such as headache, nausea and vomiting, and elevated intracranial pressure, and the remaining half show focal signs and symptoms. Mental status changes have been reported in as many as one-third.

Several uncommon syndromes are associated with primary CNS lymphoma, the presence of which may suggest the diagnosis. One of these is uveitis, which may precede the cerebral symptoms by months to years. Eleven percent of patients have uveitis in some series. Other associated syndromes include a subacute encephalitis and a multiple sclerosis–like illness with corticosteroid-induced remissions. Cerebrospinal fluid is abnormal in a nonspecific way. Elevated protein is present in 80% and increased cell count in 40%. About 10% of patients who had cerebrospinal fluid studies had a positive cytologic specimen.

B. Imaging Techniques: There are no typical characteristics on the CT scan, but several features are suggestive. A homogeneously enhancing lesion in the corpus callosum or in the central grey matter is highly suspicious. Less than 10% are hypodense, but isodense lesions are not uncommon. Five to 10% may show a ringlike enhancement or cystic areas. Almost 75% are in contact with the ependymal surface or meningeal surface, suggestive of a meningioma. The distribution favors a peripheral location with 50–60% in the hemispheric grey matter and adjacent white matter. About 25% involve the deep midline, including basal ganglia, septum pellucidum, and corpus callosum. Angiography reveals an avascular mass in almost 60%, whereas 30–40% have a "tumor blush" in the capillary to venous phase, much like meningioma.

Treatment

Aggressive surgery is of little value for this group of patients. Its only role is in biopsy for tissue diagno-

sis. A CT-guided biopsy can give a pathologic diagnosis and histologic subtype as well as specimen for histochemical studies. Radiation therapy improves survival, but the extent and fields are still debated. Chemotherapy prior to radiotherapy is currently advocated with a combination of methotrexate and high-dose cytarabine. This approach yields a median survival of 42 months as compared to a 15- to 18-month median survival with radiation alone. Corticosteroid administration should be withheld until a tissue diagnosis is made, since corticosteroids appear to cause lysis of tumor cells and may render biopsy specimens nondiagnostic as a result.

Prognosis

Survival is estimated at 47% at 1 year and 16% at 2 years with radiation alone. Chemotherapy improves these results (see above). Recurrence after therapy is also high, at 78% by 15 months; it is usually at the original site even if the patient has had a complete response.

TUMORS OF BLOOD VESSEL ORIGIN

Essential of Diagnosis

- Cerebellar mass most common presentation.

Hemangioblastomas and other tumors of endothelial cell origin account for 2% of intracranial tumors. Most occur in the cerebellum, but they may also involve the brain stem, cerebrum, and spinal cord. Though they are most often found in adults, cases have been reported at all ages and may represent Lindau's disease, or von Hippel-Lindau disease. These tumors exist in solid or cystic form and are composed of small blood vessels, separated by stromal cells, which have a clear foamy cytoplasm.

GERM CELL TUMORS

Essentials of Diagnosis

- Enhancing mass on CT scan involving midline regions.
- Children, young adults affected.
- Leptomeningeal metastases common.

Germ cell tumors make up 1–2% of all brain neoplasms, and the highest frequency of occurrence is in Japan. The most common site is the pineal gland; other midline regions that can be involved are the hypothalamus and suprasellar area. This is a tumor of children and young adults. Like medulloblastoma, it has a tendency to seed along cerebrospinal fluid pathways.

Several subtypes fall in this general category:

(1) Germinoma. Germinomas represent 50–75% of CNS germ cell tumors. They occur more commonly in males. They contain large vesicular cells and generally incite an inflammatory reaction of T lymphocytes.

(2) Embryonal cell tumors. The tumor markers AFP and hCG may be present.

(3) Choriocarcinoma. This is a rare, highly malignant tumor that is more primitive than the germinoma. Elements are identical to those of the syncytiotrophoblast and cytotrophoblast; they are strongly positive for AFP and hCG. Metastasis outside the CNS is not uncommon.

(4) Teratomas. These rare childhood lesions involve the pineal area, sellar area, third ventricle, and lateral ventricle.

Treatment

Radiation therapy plays the largest role in treatment. Germinomas are so sensitive to radiation that one method of diagnosis is to initiate therapy totaling 3000 cGy to such a pineal mass. If a response is seen within 2 weeks on CT scan, a reasonable diagnosis of germinoma is made. If there is no response, one may either proceed to biopsy or continue radiation to 5000 cGy. If cerebrospinal fluid spread is documented, complete neuraxis radiation is necessary. Most centers still require a tissue biopsy before initiation of radiotherapy. A rationale for the above-described method of diagnosis and treatment is the fact that these tumors have a remarkably high propensity to spread to the leptomeninges when biopsied or resected. There has been little experience with chemotherapy in these tumors.

Prognosis

Prognosis is related to histologic characteristics. The 10-year survival for patients with pure germinoma who have received radiotherapy is 60–80%. The nongerminoma germ cell tumors are not radiosensitive and are rarely curable with radiation alone. The 5-year survival rate in these is close to zero. Chemotherapy protocols utilizing cisplatin and etoposide combinations are under investigation.

CRANIOPHARYNGIOMA

Essentials of Diagnosis
- Suprasellar mass of childhood.
- Raised intracranial pressure.
- Growth retardation.
- Visual field defects.
- Can invade hemispheres and hypothalamus.

Craniopharyngiomas represent 3% of intracranial

tumors and 6–10% of childhood brain tumors. This tumor, which involves the suprasellar and intrasellar regions, may also extend into the hypothalamus or third ventricle. It is usually cystic but may be partially solid. The cysts are lined by stratified squamous epithelium and often contain colloid, a proteinaceous fluid consisting of carboxymucin. Calcifications are not uncommon, and recurrences average around 50% even with near-total removal.

Treatment

Management is controversial. Total resection has been said to be curative; however, there is a wide variation in the portion of patients whose tumor can be macroscopically resected (10–69%). Recurrences happen in this group. Tumor progression is seen in 70–90% of those treated with incomplete resection, with a median time to progression of 2–3 years. Multiple reports exist, however, of long-term survival in patients who have received high-dose radiation alone. Ultimate survival approaches 90–100% in children and adults. Diabetes insipidus, which occurs in 25–100% following complete surgical resection, and endocrine dysfunction of the pituitary-hypothalamic axis (40–80% of surgically treated patients) are minimal in those who have undergone radiation. Of children who have surgery, 25% complain of decreased vision. This symptom is only anecdotal with radiotherapy. Overall memory and intellectual function seem to be equal or better in the population treated by conservative surgery and radiation.

DERMOID/EPIDERMOID CYSTS

Essential of Diagnosis
- Cerebellar-pontine angle or midline cyst on CT scan or MRI.

These cysts make up 1% of all intracranial tumors. Occurring with equal frequency at any age, they tend to occupy the suprasellar region and cerebellopontile angle. They are lined by a keratin-producing squamous epithelium and are often called pearly tumors or cholesteatoma. Dermoid cysts are essentially the same but may contain skin appendages. They arise more frequently in the midline and in this location may contain hair or teeth. Both types can undergo malignant transformation and meningeal seeding.

Treatment

Surgery is the mainstay of treatment with radiation reserved for those less differentiated and more malignant in appearance.

REFERENCES

Sequelae of Radiation Therapy

Rottenberg DA: Complications of radiation therapy. In: *Neurologic Complications of Cancer Treatment*. Rottenberg DA (editor). Butterworth-Heinemann, 1991.

Gliomas

Kornblith P, Walker M: Chemotherapy for malignant gliomas. *J Neurosurg* 1988;**68**:1.

Leibel S, Sheline G: Radiation therapy of neoplasms of the brain. *J Neurosurg* 1987;**66**:1.

Nazzaro J, Newelt E: The role of surgery in the management of supratentorial intermediate and high-grade astrocytomas in adults. *J Neurosurg* 1990;**73**:331.

Sheline GE: The role of radiation therapy in the treatment of low-grade gliomas. *Clin Neurosurg* 1986; **33**:563.

Walker A, Robins M, Weinfeld F: Epidemiology of brain tumors: The national survey of intracranial neoplasms. *Neurology* 1985;**35**:219.

Walker M et al: Randomized comparisons of radiotherapy and nitrosoureas for the treatment of malignant gliomas after surgery. *N Engl J Med* 1980;**303**:1323.

Oligodendroglioma

Cairncross G, Macdonald D: Successful chemotherapy for recurrent malignant oligodendroglioma. *Ann Neurol* 1988;**23**:360.

Mork S et al: Oligodendroglioma: Incidence and biological behavior in a defined population. *J Neurosurg* 1985;**63**:881.

Reedy DP, Bay JW, Hahn JF: Role of radiation therapy in the treatment of cerebral oligodendroglioma: An analysis of 57 cases and a literature review. *Neurosurgery* 1983;**13**:499.

Ependymomas

Goldwein J et al: Recurrent intracranial ependymomas in children: Survival, patterns of failure, and prognostic factors. *Cancer* 1990;**66**:557.

Kun L, Kovnar E, Sanford R: Ependymomas in children. *Pediatr Neurosci* 1988;**14**:57.

Choroid Plexus Tumors

Cohen ME, Duffner PK: *Brain Tumors in Children: Principles of Diagnosis and Treatment*. Raven, 1984.

MvGirr SJ et al: Choroid plexus papillomas: Long-term follow-up results in a surgically treated series. *J Neurosurg* 1988;**69**:843.

Pineal Tumors

Bruce DA, Allen JC: Tumor staging for pineal region tumors of childhood. *Cancer* 1985;**56**:1792.

Packer RJ, Siegel KR, Sutton LN: Leptomeningeal dissemination of primary central nervous system tumors of childhood. *Ann Neurol* 1985;**18**:217.

Packer RJ et al: Pineal region tumors of childhood. *Pediatrics* 1984;**74**:97.

Neuronal Tumors

Jellinger K (editor): *Therapy of Malignant Brain Tumors*. Springer-Verlag, 1987.

Embryonal Tumors

Friedman HS, Oakes WJ: The chemotherapy of posterior fossa tumors in childhood. *J Neurooncol* 1987;**5**:217.

Hershatter BW, Halperin EC, Cox EB: Medulloblastoma: The Duke Medical Center experience. *Int J Radiat Oncol Biol Phys* 1986;**12**:1771.

Packer RJ, Siegel PA, Sutton LN: Efficacy of adjuvant chemotherapy for patients with poor risk medulloblastoma: A preliminary report. *Ann Neurol* 1988; **24**:503.

Nerve Sheath Tumors

Baptiste M et al: Neurofibromatosis and other disorders among children with CNS tumors and their families. *Neurology* 1989;**39**:487.

Meningioma

Barbaro NM, Gutin PH, Wilsom CW: Radiation therapy in the treatment of partially resected meningiomas. *Neurosurgery* 1987;**20**:525.

Jaaskelainen J, Haltia M, Servo A: Atypical and anaplastic meningiomas: Radiology, surgery, radiotherapy, and outcome. *Surg Neurol* 1986;**25**:233.

Rohringer M, Sutherland GR, Louw DF: Incidence and clinicopathological features of meningioma. *J Neurosurg* 1989;**71**:665.

Primary Lymphoma of the Brain

DeAngelis LM: Primary central nervous system lymphoma: A new challenge. *Neurology* 1991;**41**:619.

DeAngelis LM et al: Primary CNS lymphoma: Combined treatment with chemotherapy and radiotherapy. *Neurology* 1990;**40**:80.

Erby NL et al: Increasing incidence of primary brain lymphoma in the US. *Cancer* 1988;**62**:2461.

Hochberg F, Miller D: Primary central nervous system lymphoma. *J Neurosurg* 1988;**68**:835.

Tumors of Blood Vessel Origin

Shimura T, Hirano A, Llena JF: Ultrastructure of cerebellar hemangioblastoma. *Acta Neuropathol* 1985; **67**:6.

Germ Cell Tumors

Allen J: Management of primary intracranial germ cell tumors of childhood. *Pediatr Neurosci* 1987;**13**:152.

Edwards M et al: Pineal region tumors in children. *J Neurosurg* 1988;**68**:689.

Jennings M, Gelman R, Hochberg F: Intracranial germ-cell tumors: Natural history and pathogenesis. *J Neurosurg* 1985;**63**:155.

Craniopharyngioma

Adamson TE et al: Correlation of clinical and pathological features in surgically treated craniopharyngiomas. *J Neurosurg* 1990;**73**:12.

Fischer EG et al: Craniopharyngiomas in children: Long-term effects of conservative surgical procedures combined with radiation therapy. *J Neurosurg* 1990; **73**:534.

Dermoid/Epidermoid Cysts

Jellinger K: Special neurooncology. In: *Therapy of Malignant Brain Tumors*. Jellinger K (editor). Springer-Verlag, 1987.

20

Gastrointestinal Cancer

Thomas D. Brown, MD

On the basis of incidence and mortality, malignancies of the gastrointestinal tract represent one of the most important cancer groups in the USA. Gastrointestinal cancers account for approximately 25% of all new cancer cases and for a similar proportion of all cancer deaths. The major sites include esophagus, stomach, pancreas, liver, biliary tree, small bowel, colon, and rectum. The projected incidence and mortality of these tumor types are shown in Table 20–1.

As a group these tumors are characterized by their refractoriness to therapy once distant metastases occur. Given that most gastrointestinal cancers cannot be cured, supportive care for patients with metastatic disease is a major concern. In approaching the management of gastrointestinal malignancies, it is useful to have clearly defined objectives, specifically whether a given intervention is curative or palliative. The established goals of therapy can then be weighed against the anticipated risk and discomfort to the patient from a particular intervention.

Once a histologic diagnosis is established, a patient's cancer should be clinically staged to assess appropriate treatment options. Routine staging should include a history and physical examination, routine laboratory studies (complete blood count, serum chemistries with liver function studies, and tumor markers if appropriate) and a chest radiograph. Computerized tomographic (CT) scans, in particular of the abdomen, often are helpful both in defining disease extent and in subsequent follow-up of disease. Magnetic resonance imaging (MRI) is undergoing evaluation to determine its role in staging and follow-up of gastrointestinal malignancies. It is often used to complement the evaluation of equivocal findings on CT scan.

The information obtained from these staging procedures can be assembled into an organized staging system by using the American Joint Committee for Cancer Staging criteria. This system employs tumor size (T), status of regional lymph nodes (N), and status of distant metastasis (M) to stage tumors for a particular site. This system is adaptable to both clinical and pathologic staging, though for determining prognosis, it is best applied to pathologic staging. As an example, Table 20–2 provides the AJCC staging criteria for colorectal cancer.

ESOPHAGEAL CANCER

Essentials of Diagnosis
- Dysphagia and odynophagia.
- Weight loss.
- Abnormal upper gastrointestinal series.
- Abnormal upper endoscopy.

General Considerations
The major risk factors for esophageal cancer are smoking and alcohol ingestion. Diseases associated with esophageal cancer include Barrett's esophagus, achalasia, lye stricture, esophageal diverticulae, Plummer-Vinson syndrome, and tylosis. In 1991, 10,900 new cases were diagnosed with 9800 deaths; this disease is over twice as common in men than in women. In the USA, it is the second leading cause of cancer death in black males. Although in most series squamous cell carcinoma is the predominant histologic feature, adenocarcinoma is increasing in frequency in the USA. Distal esophageal presentations are also increasing in frequency. This disease is most common in the Middle East and Far East, where presentation at an early stage is not infrequent. In the USA, most patients have advanced-stage disease at presentation, and therefore only a minority are candidates for therapy with curative intent.

Clinical Findings
A. Symptoms and Signs: Dysphagia, odynophagia, and weight loss are common. Evidence of metastasis is not uncommon, including visceral or skeletal pain, dyspnea, cough, cervical or supraclavicular adenopathy, hepatomegaly, and pleural or peritoneal effusions. Less commonly, nerve involvement can present as hoarseness from recurrent laryngeal nerve involvement, diaphragmatic paralysis due to phrenic nerve involvement, and Horner's syndrome due to sympathetic nerve plexus involvement. Uncommon manifestations of locally advanced disease include hemoptysis and aspiration pneumonia, which can be due to a bronchopleural fistula.

B. Laboratory Findings: An upper gastrointestinal series will reveal esophageal stricture, ulcer, or mass effect. Upper endoscopy with biopsy will document malignancy, usually squamous cell carcinoma

Table 20–1. Incidence and mortality of gastrointestinal malignancies in 1991.

Tumor Type	New Cases	Cancer Deaths
Esophagus	10,900	9,800
Stomach	23,800	13,400
Pancreas	28,200	25,200
Liver/biliary tree	15,000	12,100
Small bowel	2,900	925
Colon	112,000	53,000
Rectum	45,500	7,500

or adenocarcinoma. For gastroesophageal lesions, the endoscope can assist in determining site of origin (esophagus or stomach). Intraluminal ultrasound can be of value in defining the depth of the primary lesion.

Anemia and liver function test abnormalities are common. Plain chest radiograph can demonstrate central adenopathy or esophageal double density. Appropriate radiographic imaging of liver, bone, and lungs can demonstrate evidence of metastases.

Differential Diagnosis

Cancer of the esophagus must be distinguished from benign esophageal tumors, such as leiomyomas, and from benign esophagitis. Distinction must also be made from benign esophageal strictures, including esophageal rings, achalasia associated with stricture, and esophageal webs. All these conditions can be distinguished by upper endoscopy with biopsy. It is often difficult to discern the organ of origin for gastroesophageal adenocarcinomas, and it is unclear whether this distinction is important from a treatment standpoint.

Complications

Esophageal obstruction is a relatively common complication of esophageal cancer, with perforation being less common.

Treatment

Surgery has been the traditional approach to this disease in an attempt at cure. Only about 20% of patients are candidates for an attempt at curative resection; of those undergoing surgery, only 20–30% achieve long-term disease-free survival or cure. Surgical mortality should be less than 5%.

Several uncontrolled trials suggest a benefit from preoperative combined modality therapy. This therapy generally consists of external beam radiation therapy and concomitant chemotherapy with fluorouracil and cisplatin. Trials using surgery and perioperative combined modality therapy generally give results similar to surgery alone. In fact, results with chemotherapy and irradiation, without surgery, are comparable to surgery-based approaches when evaluating long-term disease-free survival.

Advanced disease that is not amenable to curative efforts can be treated with cisplatin and fluorouracil. The majority of patients respond, but responses usually are less than 1 year in duration.

Prognosis

Overall the prognosis for esophageal cancer is poor, with 5-year survival rates of 5–10%. The median survival for all patients with esophageal cancer is less than 1 year.

Table 20–2. American Joint Committee for Cancer Staging criteria for colorectal cancer.

Primary tumor (T)

TX	Primary tumor cannot be assessed
T0	No evidence of tumor in resected specimen
Tis	Carcinoma in situ
T1	Invades submucosa
T2	Invades into muscularis propria
T3	Invades through muscularis propria, into the subserosa, or into nonperitonealized pericolic or perirectal tissues
T4	Perforates visceral peritoneum, or invades other organs or structures

Regional lymph nodes (N)

NX	Nodes cannot be assessed
N0	No node metastases
N1	1–3 positive nodes
N2	≥ 4 positive nodes
N3	Any positive node along a named vascular trunk

Distant metastases (M)

MX	Presence of distant metastases cannot be assessed
M0	No distant metastases
M1	Distant metastases present

	American Joint Committee Stage	Duke's stage
Stage 0	(Tis, N0, M0)	
Stage I	(T1 or T2, N0, M0)	A
Stage II	(T3 or T4, N0, M0)	B
Stage III	(any T, N1, M0; any T, N2, N3, M0)	C
Stage IV	(any T, any N, M1)	D

GASTRIC CANCER

Essentials of Diagnosis
- Abdominal pain.
- Early satiety.
- Nausea and vomiting.
- Weight loss.
- Abnormal upper gastrointestinal series.
- Abnormal upper endoscopy.

General Considerations

Ingestion of smoked or salted foods and of aflatoxins is believed to be the major risk factor for gastric cancer. Pernicious anemia and prior surgery for benign ulcer disease have a controversial association with increased risk of gastric cancer. In 1991, 23,800 new cases were diagnosed with 13,400 deaths; this disease is more common in men than in women by a ratio of approximately 1.5:1. Adenocarcinoma is the most common cell type, accounting for over 90% of cases; other types include lymphomas and leiomyosarcomas. Proximal gastric presentations are becoming increasingly more common. Pockets of high incidence exist in Japan, Scandinavia, Costa Rica, and Chile. In the USA, most patients have advanced-stage disease at presentation, and therefore a minority are candidates for therapy with curative intent. This is in contradistinction to Japan, where early-stage gastric cancers are more commonly encountered, in part owing to aggressive screening approaches.

Clinical Findings

A. Symptoms and Signs: Abdominal pain, early satiety, nausea and vomiting, and weight loss are common. Evidence of metastasis is not uncommon, including visceral or skeletal pain; dyspnea; cervical, supraclavicular, or axillary adenopathy; hepatomegaly; and ascites.

B. Laboratory Findings: An upper gastrointestinal series will often reveal an ulcer crater, mass effect, or loss of or absent gastric motility with delayed gastric emptying. Upper endoscopy with biopsy will document malignancy, with adenocarcinoma being the most common type.

Anemia and liver function test abnormalities are common. Appropriate radiographic imaging of liver, bone, and lungs can demonstrate evidence of metastases.

Differential Diagnosis

Adenocarcinoma of the stomach must be distinguished from other malignancies of the stomach, including gastric lymphomas (see below, under less common malignancies), and leiomyosarcomas. Benign gastric ulcers represent the most difficult distinction, with malignant ulcers often showing transient clinical response to medical ulcer therapies. All these conditions can be distinguished by upper endoscopy with biopsy, though in the case of persistent ulcerating lesions, follow-up endoscopic biopsy may be required despite an initially negative biopsy.

Complications

Gastric obstruction is the most common complication of gastric cancer, with perforation being relatively uncommon.

Treatment

Surgery has been the traditional approach to this disease in an attempt at cure. Approximately 30% of patients are candidates for an attempt at curative resection; of those undergoing surgery, approximately 50% achieve long-term disease-free survival or cure. There is international controversy regarding the extent of surgical resection, with Japanese surgeons favoring a more radical procedure characterized by extensive lymph node dissection; Western surgeons, particularly in the USA, have not yet endorsed this more extensive procedure. A European study is under way, comparing conventional with more radical gastric resection.

At least nine controlled adjuvant trials have been reported evaluating the role of postoperative chemotherapy with fluorouracil chemotherapy, alone or in combination with other agents. All these trials have failed to show a significant survival advantage for postoperative chemotherapy. Therefore, adjuvant chemotherapy cannot be recommended for gastric cancer unless it is part of an ongoing clinical trial. A current intergroup trial is evaluating the role of postoperative fluorouracil plus leucovorin and irradiation.

Advanced disease that is not amenable to curative efforts can be treated with chemotherapy, with response rates of 20–30% and with responses generally of less than 1 year in duration. Single-agent fluorouracil is as active as any other single agent, with a response rate of less than 20%. Multiple-agent chemotherapy such as FAM (fluorouracil, doxorubicin, mitomycin), EAP (etoposide, doxorubicin, cisplatin), or FAMTX (fluorouracil, doxorubicin, high-dose methotrexate with leucovorin rescue) has been advocated; EAP and FAMTX appear to have response rates of at least 30% and occasionally result in complete responses. Both EAP and FAMTX have been associated with substantial toxicities, with the risk of life-threatening toxicity. To date no multiple-agent regimen has shown benefits in survival that would warrant its routine use.

Prognosis

Approximately 15% of patients with gastric cancer will survive for 5 years. The median survival for all patients with gastric cancer is less than 1 year.

PANCREATIC CANCER

Essentials of Diagnosis

- Abdominal pain.
- Nausea and vomiting.
- Anorexia.
- Weight loss.
- Biliary obstruction.
- Pancreatic mass on CT scan.
- Abnormal endoscopic retrograde cholangiopancreatography.

General Considerations

The major risk factor for pancreatic cancer is cigarette smoking; other possible risk factors include alcohol or coffee ingestion and exposure to petroleum products. Chronic pancreatitis and diabetes have been associated with pancreatic cancer. In 1991, 28,200 new cases were diagnosed with 25,200 deaths; this disease is equally common in men as in women. Adenocarcinoma is the most common histologic type. In the USA, most patients have advanced-stage disease at presentation, and therefore only a minority are candidates for therapy with curative intent. Most pancreatic cancers present in the head of the pancreas, and these are most likely to present with symptoms and signs of biliary obstruction.

Clinical Findings

A. Symptoms and Signs: Abdominal pain, nausea and vomiting, anorexia, weight loss, and jaundice due to biliary obstruction are common. Malabsorption due to pancreatic insufficiency can be manifested by diarrhea. Palpation of a pancreatic mass or of associated distention of the gallbladder is sometimes possible. Evidence of metastasis is not uncommon, including visceral or skeletal pain, ascites, or hepatomegaly.

B. Laboratory Findings: Abdominal ultrasound or CT scan of the abdomen often reveals a pancreatic mass; these studies can also demonstrate biliary duct dilatation in association with a pancreatic head mass. In the setting of pancreatic head masses, an upper gastrointestinal series can reveal compression of the duodenal C loop with evidence of delayed gastric emptying. Endoscopic retrograde cholangiopancreatography (ERCP) with aspirate for cytologic study can document malignancy as can a percutaneous needle aspirate directed by ultrasound or CT scan. Laparoscopy or laparotomy is often useful in obtaining pathologic material from the primary mass or from regional sites of metastases such as regional lymph nodes or peritoneal metastases.

Anemia and liver function test abnormalities are common. Liver function abnormalities usually include elevation of serum alkaline phosphatase and total bilirubin, in association with pancreatic head masses and biliary obstruction. Appropriate radio-graphic imaging of liver, bone, and lungs can demonstrate evidence of metastases.

CA-19-9 is a mucinous glycoprotein with a half-life of less than 1 day that is associated with a variety of malignancies (pancreatic, hepatobiliary, gastric, colorectal), but for pancreatic cancer it has a sensitivity of approximately 80% and a specificity of approximately 90%. It therefore is a reasonable marker for diagnosis and postresection follow-up of pancreatic cancer and in the future might help in screening high-risk groups.

Differential Diagnosis

Cancer of the pancreas must be distinguished from chronic pancreatitis. This distinction is especially difficult, since pancreatic cancer is often associated with a marked fibrotic or desmoplastic reaction, and multiple biopsies can be falsely negative. Unusual pancreatic cancer cell types include sarcoma, lymphoma, plasmacytoma, squamous cell carcinoma, and small-cell carcinoma. Cystadenocarcinomas are variants of the uncommon acinar (as opposed to ductal) carcinomas of the pancreas and carry a better prognosis than the common ductal adenocarcinomas of the pancreas.

Complications

Biliary or gastric outlet obstructions represent the most common complications, with biliary obstruction often complicated by sepsis. Pancreatic insufficiency with abdominal distention and diarrhea is not uncommon.

Treatment

Few patients with pancreatic cancer are candidates for an attempt at curative resection. Of the less than 20% of patients who undergo an attempt at resection, most patients have a lesion within the head of the pancreas amenable to performance of a Whipple procedure (ie, a pancreatic head resection with gastrojejunostomy and choledochoduodenostomy). Approximately 25% of patients undergoing radical resection of their malignancy will be alive at 5 years.

One trial reported by the Gastrointestinal Tumor Study Group suggested an improvement in survival with postoperative therapy using fluorouracil and irradiation. The data, however, are very limited.

Chemotherapy has no proved role in the treatment of advanced disease, with response rates for single agents such as fluorouracil or doxorubicin less than 20%. Multiple-agent chemotherapy regimens appear to have no greater response rate. Patients with newly diagnosed advanced pancreatic cancer are encouraged to participate in existing phase II protocols if they wish to pursue anticancer therapy.

Palliative measures include celiac nerve plexus blocks, performed by alcohol injection, to control refractory pain. ERCP or percutaneous approaches can be used to place biliary stents to relieve obstruction. The latter is generally recommended for symptomatic biliary obstruction, eg, associated with biliary sepsis. In selected patients, palliative surgical bypass (eg, gastrojejunostomy, choledochoduodenostomy, or both) can be considered, but the potential benefits to symptomatic patients must be weighed against postoperative morbidity and generally short survivals for most patients.

Prognosis

Overall the prognosis for pancreatic cancer remains poor, with 5-year survival rates of less than 5%. The median survival for all patients is approximately 6 months.

HEPATOCELLULAR CANCER

Essentials of Diagnosis

- Abdominal pain.
- Nausea and vomiting.
- Anorexia.
- Weight loss.
- Jaundice.
- Ascites.
- Hepatic mass on CT scan.
- Enlarging liver in patient known to have cirrhosis.

General Considerations

Worldwide, hepatocellular carcinomas represent a major public health problem, but in the USA, these tumors are relatively rare. The major risk factor for hepatocellular cancer is cirrhosis due to alcohol ingestion or viral hepatitis infection. In the USA, alcoholic cirrhosis is the major risk factor, while in the Far East, hepatitis B and C infections predominate as the major risk factors. Aflatoxin exposure, hemachromatosis, and parasitic infections of the liver have also been associated with hepatocellular carcinoma. In the USA, the incidence of hepatocellular carcinoma is approximately 2 cases per 100,000 population, with a male to female preponderance of approximately 3:1, and with approximately 4000 deaths annually. In the Far East and Africa, incidence rates are more than 50 times greater than in the USA. Hepatocellular cancer is the common histologic type for primary liver cancers. Most patients have advanced-stage disease at presentation, and therefore only a minority are candidates for therapy with curative intent.

Clinical Findings

A. Symptoms and Signs: Abdominal pain, nausea and vomiting, anorexia, malaise, jaundice, ascites, fever, and weight loss are common. Metastatic disease can present as malignant ascites, skeletal pain, dyspnea with pulmonary involvement, and neurologic abnormalities due to brain metastases.

B. Laboratory Findings: Abdominal ultrasound or CT scan of the abdomen reveals a solitary mass or multiple masses. Percutaneous needle aspirate directed by ultrasound or CT scan can be used for a pathologic diagnosis. Laparoscopy or laparotomy can be useful in obtaining pathologic material from the liver or from regional sites of metastases such as regional lymph nodes or peritoneal metastases. Arteriography can be helpful diagnostically by showing a classic capillary blush; it is also helpful in planning surgical strategies by defining the vascular support of the tumor and better delineating its extent.

Anemia and liver function test abnormalities are common. Elevation of serum alpha-fetoprotein occurs in a minority of patients with hepatocellular carcinoma in the USA. Appropriate radiographic imaging of abdomen, bone, lungs, and brain can demonstrate evidence of metastases. Tumor invasion into the inferior vena cava or association with benign inferior vena cava thrombosis is not unusual.

Differential Diagnosis

Hepatocellular carcinoma must be distinguished from adenocarcinoma metastatic to the liver. Clinical evidence of cirrhosis can be confused with the clinical presentation of hepatocellular carcinoma. Benign conditions such as adenomas, hepatic cysts, fatty infiltration of the liver, and parasitic liver disease should also be differentiated initially.

Complications

Hepatic dysfunction, marked ascites, and inferior vena cava thrombosis are among the most common manifestations of hepatocellular carcinomas.

Treatment

Few patients with hepatocellular cancer are candidates for an attempt at curative resection. Approximately 10% of patients undergo an attempt at resection, with less than half having long-term survival. Aggressive surgical options include radical resection or allogeneic liver transplantation.

Pilot experiences have included preoperative use of locoregional therapies such as hepatic arterial chemoembolization. Embolization has been performed with a variety of contrast materials (eg, Ivalon, Lipiodol), and chemotherapeutic agents (eg, fluorouracil or its cogeners, doxorubicin, cisplatin, mitomycin). The role of this therapy as an adjuvant to surgical approaches remains to be defined.

Chemotherapy has no proved role in the treatment of advanced disease, with response rates for single agents such as fluorouracil or doxorubicin less than 20%. Multiple-agent chemotherapy regimens appear to have no greater response rate. In nonresectable disease, chemoembolization has also been used, with response rates from 30% to 50% but with most of these responses being of less than 1 year in duration.

Investigational efforts include radiolabeled immunoglobulin, such as ^{131}I or yttrium-labeled antiferritin.

Prognosis

The prognosis for hepatocellular cancer is poor, with 5-year survival rates of less than 5%. The median survival for all patients with hepatocellular cancer is less than 6 months.

BILIARY CANCER

Essentials of Diagnosis

- Abdominal pain.
- Nausea and vomiting.
- Anorexia.
- Weight loss.
- Jaundice.
- Acholic stools.
- Hepatomegaly or right upper abdominal mass.

General Considerations

Approximately 8000 patients are diagnosed each year in the USA with biliary cancer, and almost as many die each year of this disease. Gallbladder carcinoma is more common in women, while cholangiocarcinoma is more common in men. Risk factors for biliary cancer include cholelithiasis, inflammatory bowel disease, and familial polyposis; in the Far East, liver fluke infestation has been associated with biliary carcinoma.

Clinical Findings

A. Symptoms and Signs: Patients can present with abdominal pain, nausea and vomiting, anorexia, jaundice, palpable gallbladder or hepatomegaly, weight loss, and fever. Metastatic disease can be manifested by ascites and skeletal or visceral pain.

B. Laboratory Findings: Elevation of serum bilirubin and liver function studies, particularly alkaline phosphatase, are frequently manifestations of biliary obstruction.

Ultrasound or CT scan of the abdomen can document biliary dilatation, but tumor mass is not always seen, especially with cholangiocarcinomas. Percutaneous needle biopsy or ERCP can be used to obtain a tissue diagnosis.

Differential Diagnosis

Biliary carcinoma needs be distinguished from pancreatic cancer, other metastatic carcinomas, and benign biliary disease. Malignancies that can metastasize to the biliary tree include gastrointestinal tract malignancies, lymphomas, breast cancer, lung cancer, and melanoma.

Complications

Biliary obstruction and sepsis are the most common complications of biliary cancer.

Treatment

For the rare instances in which curative resection is possible, aggressive surgery is pursued. More often local extension into surrounding structures, such as the liver, stomach, small bowel, or lymph nodes makes resection impossible.

Locally advanced but unresectable malignancy can be palliated with external beam irradiation, with or without concomitant fluorouracil. The response rate with this regimen is 30–40%, with response duration generally less than 1 year. Owing to the partial radiosensitivity of these tumors, novel radiotherapy approaches are being pursued; these include hyperfractionated irradiation, intraoperative irradiation, brachytherapy with intraoperative seed placement, and brachytherapy with biliary catheter placement.

In advanced disease, fluorouracil is as active as any other single chemotherapeutic agent, with expected transient responses around 20%. Multiple-agent chemotherapy has not been shown to be more effective than single-agent chemotherapy. Palliation is often achieved by biliary stent placement with ERCP or with a percutaneous approach.

Prognosis

Since most patients with biliary cancer cannot undergo an attempt at curative resection, most succumb to their disease, with a median survival of less than 1 year.

SMALL BOWEL CANCER

Essentials of Diagnosis

- Abdominal pain.
- Nausea and vomiting.
- Weight loss.
- Jaundice.
- Abdominal mass.
- Anemia.
- Small bowel obstruction.
- Guaiac-positive stools.

General Considerations

Small bowel malignancies are uncommon; in the USA, 2900 cases were diagnosed in 1991 with 925 deaths occurring in that year. The most common histologic type is adenocarcinoma, but lymphomas, sarcomas, and carcinoid tumors are also frequent. Risk factors include Crohn's disease (adenocarcinoma), familial polyposis (adenocarcinoma), celiac sprue (lymphoma), and neurofibromatosis (adenocarcinoma). Location within the small bowel often leads to relative early diagnosis owing to obstruction.

Clinical Findings

A. Symptoms and Signs: Nausea and vomiting, abdominal pain, weight loss, abdominal mass, anemia, and jaundice are common. Manifestations of malabsorption can also be seen with small bowel tumors, including diarrhea and steatorrhea.

B. Laboratory Findings: Anemia and abnormalities in serum liver function studies are common.

Differential Diagnosis

Small bowel malignancies must be distinguished from benign tumors of the small bowel (eg, leiomyomas, hamartomas, adenomas) and from inflammatory bowel disease.

Complications

Bowel obstruction and perforation are the two most important complications of small bowel malignancies. Both are more common with lesions in the jejunum or ileum.

Treatment

Surgery is the cornerstone of treatment. For adenocarcinomas of the small bowel, there is no established role for chemotherapy as an adjuvant or in the advanced-disease setting; this is in part due to the rarity of these tumors. Anecdotally, fluorouracil is presumed to have some activity against adenocarcinomas of the small bowel. Carcinoids and lymphomas are addressed below.

Prognosis

Approximately 60% of patients are cured, presumably because of their relatively early presentation.

COLON CANCER

Essentials of Diagnosis

- Abdominal pain.
- Change in bowel habits.
- Weight loss.
- Hematochezia, melena, guaiac-positive stools.
- Anemia.
- Air contrast barium enema showing stricture or mass effect.

General Considerations

Risk factors for colorectal cancer are thought to include diets high in fat and meat and low in fiber; these associations underlie the current American Cancer Society guidelines for dietary measures to reduce cancer risk (Table 20–3). Associated diseases include familial polyposis, familial cancer syndromes, and inflammatory bowel disease. The familial cancer syndromes include the Lynch syndromes with autosomal dominant inheritance of colorectal cancer; these occur without (Lynch I) or with (Lynch II) other associated malignancies such as endometrial or ovarian cancers. The Lynch syndromes are believed to account for approximately 5% of colorectal cancers and are associated with a normal incidence of polyps.

Polyps are assumed to precede colorectal carcinoma in most cases. Polyps are generally classified as hyperplastic polyps or adenomas. Hyperplastic pol-

Table 20–3. American Cancer Society dietary guidelines for reducing gastrointestinal cancer risk.

Avoid obesity.
Reduce total fat intake to less than 30% of caloric intake.
Consume a variety of vegetables and fruits (eg, dark green and deep yellow vegetables, cruciferous vegetables, citrus fruits).
Consume high-fiber foods (whole-grain cereals, vegetables, fruits).
Limit consumption of alcoholic beverages.
Limit consumption of salt-cured, smoked, and nitrate-cured foods.

yps are rarely associated with malignancy, whereas adenomas are more frequently associated with colorectal cancers. Adenomas have three subtypes: tubular (adenomatous polyps), tubulovillar (intermediate polyps), and villous (villous adenomas). Villous adenomas are most frequently associated with cancer. Although 75% of all polyps are located beyond the splenic flexure, adenomas represent a larger proportion of polyps found within the proximal colon. Polyp size correlates with malignant potential more so than histologic subtype of polyp does, with up to 60% of adenomas greater than 2 cm in diameter being associated with malignancy. For this reason, polypectomy is generally recommended for all hyperplastic polyps of greater than 0.5–1 cm and for adenomas of any size.

Screening for gastrointestinal tumors is of great importance, since curative therapies are applicable only to localized disease. At present, routine screening is recommended for colorectal carcinomas, though the effectiveness of such screening is debated. Several ongoing randomized and controlled clinical trials pertaining to screening for colorectal cancer will clarify this issue. Screening for colorectal cancers in the population at large includes detection of polyps with malignant potential as well as detection of early-stage carcinomas. Screening procedures include the rectal examination, fecal blood testing, radiologic studies (double-contrast barium enema), and endoscopy (rigid or flexible sigmoidoscopy and colonoscopy).

Guaiac-based tests are the most widely used for detecting occult blood in the stool and are based on the pseudoperoxidase activity of hemoglobin. The most widely used guaiac-based test is Hemoccult II, but others are commercially available. In an effort to optimize use of stool guaiac tests, guidelines have been given (Table 20–4). Furthermore, a positive test result should lead to complete study of the colon, consisting of at least proctosigmoidoscopy and colonoscopy. Since the double-contrast barium enema and colonoscopy are complementary studies, the most sensitive evaluation of occult stool blood includes both procedures. A decision of the evaluation to be performed should be based on the patient's other risk factors for colon cancer and the underlying

Table 20–4. Guidelines for use of Hemoccult II cards.

Ingestion of red meat and high peroxidase foods should be avoided for 3 days before and after testing.

Vitamin C, oral iron supplements, and nonsteroidal anti-inflammatory drugs should be avoided.

Two samples should be obtained from three consecutive bowel movements.

The stool should be tested within 6 days of obtaining samples.

Samples should not be rehydrated.

A single positive smear should be interpreted as a positive test result.

Table 20–5. American Cancer Society screening recommendations for colorectal cancer in the general population.

Procedure	Screening Intervention
Digital rectal examination	Yearly, beginning at age 40
Test for occult blood in stool	Yearly, beginning at age 50
Sigmoidoscopy	Every 3–5 years, beginning at age 50

risks for procedures such as colonoscopy. Colonoscopy procedures are associated with a risk of bleeding up to 2.5%, a risk of perforation up to 1.0%, and a mortality risk up to 0.02%. In general, the higher risk patients within these ranges are those undergoing polypectomy. In one set of studies, the positive predictive value of a positive stool guaiac test (percentage of patients with guaiac-positive tests who actually have adenomas or carcinomas) was 30% for adenomas and 10% for carcinomas.

The American Cancer Society has made recommendations regarding screening of the population at large for gastrointestinal cancer (Table 20–5). High-risk groups have been identified, with more aggressive screening recommended for individuals within these groups (Table 20–6). Various techniques are under study to better detect gastrointestinal malignancies, including use of exfoliative cytology, imaging techniques using monoclonal antibodies, and measurement of oncogene expression.

In 1991, 112,000 new cases of colon and 45,500 new cases of rectal cancer were diagnosed with 53,000 and 7500 deaths, respectively; colon cancer is slightly more common in women and rectal cancer is slightly more common in men. By far, the most common histologic type for colon and rectal cancers is adenocarcinoma. With early detection both colon and rectal cancers are potentially curable in a majority of patients. The distinction between colon and rectal cancers is based on treatment considerations; in general, rectal cancers have been defined as having any extension below the peritoneal reflection, or within 12 cm of the anal verge.

Clinical Findings

A. Symptoms and Signs: Abdominal pain, change in bowel habits, melena, hematochezia, and weight loss may occur. Metastatic disease can present as hepatomegaly, malignant ascites, or dyspnea with pulmonary involvement.

B. Laboratory Findings: Air contrast barium enema or colonoscopy is most helpful in localizing the malignancy. These two studies are complementary, with colonoscopy offering the opportunity for biopsy.

Anemia, guaiac-positive stools, and serum liver function test abnormalities are common.

Elevation of serum CEA (carcinoembryonic antigen) occurs in a majority of patients with colorectal cancer; CEA is a glycoprotein with a half-life of approximately 1 week. Serum CEA determination is not a diagnostic test; its value derives from its potential as a tumor marker. Serum CEA has been used to detect early recurrence of colorectal cancer. Several studies have suggested that second surgeries for recurrent disease can result in long-term survival when such surgery is performed based on minimal CEA elevations in patients with no other clinical evidence of recurrence. The value of CEA-directed laparotomies remains controversial, with proponents emphasizing the need to follow CEA levels as often as every month and to respond to CEA elevations before they rise above 10 ng/mL.

Appropriate radiographic imaging of abdomen, lungs, and bone can demonstrate evidence of metastases.

Differential Diagnosis

Colorectal carcinoma must be distinguished from inflammatory bowel disease and other causes of lower gastrointestinal bleeding such as diverticulitis and hemorrhoids. In general, benign explanations for

Table 20–6. Screening guidelines for colorectal cancer in high-risk groups.

Risk Factor	Screening Intervention
History of colon cancer/adenomas	Colonoscopy every year until clear, and then every 2–3 years
History of first-degree relative with colon cancer	Beginning at age 20, as for the population at large
History of breast/genital tract cancer in females	Once cancer diagnosed, as for the population at large
Familial polyposis/Gardner's syndrome	Sigmoidoscopy yearly, beginning at age 12
Familial cancer syndrome	Beginning at age 20, as for the population at large, with colonoscopy every 3–5 years
Ulcerative colitis	Colonoscopy every 2 years in those with colitis for more than 7 years, with sigmoidoscopy during alternate years

lower gastrointestinal bleeding should be diagnoses of exclusion.

Complications

Lower bowel obstruction is the most important complication of colorectal carcinoma.

Treatment

The primary treatment for colorectal carcinoma involves an attempt at curative resection. For carcinomas of the colon, a partial colectomy with primary anastomosis is usually performed. For rectal carcinomas, an abdominal-peritoneal resection has been the classic procedure, but advances in stapling devices have enabled low rectal resections with the possibility of primary anastomosis. Colorectal neoplasms represent the one type of gastrointestinal tumors for which adjuvant therapies have been effective in improving surgical results.

In the past decade, the most important advances in systemic chemotherapy for colorectal cancers and other gastrointestinal malignancies have involved modifications in the use of the antimetabolite fluorouracil. Single-agent fluorouracil has generally shown response rates of up to 10–20% in gastrointestinal cancer. Toxicities are schedule dependent; infrequent bolus schedules are associated with increased myelosuppression, while prolonged bolus or infusion schedules are associated with increased mucocutaneous toxicity. Despite the voluminous literature concerning various schedules, no particular schedule of single-agent fluorouracil is recognized as most effective. However, in a randomized controlled trial, when combined with folinic acid (leucovorin) for the treatment of metastatic colon cancer, the response rate of fluorouracil improved to approximately 40% with a significant improvement in survival. Leucovorin is thought to increase inhibition of thymidylate synthase by providing the folate cofactor necessary for binding of the fluorouracil metabolite, F-dUMP (fluorodeoxyuridine monophosphate), to thymidylate synthase. The optimal doses and schedules of leucovorin and fluorouracil in combination remain to be determined. Regimens that utilize low doses of leucovorin appear as active as regimens employing high doses of leucovorin and are less toxic and less expensive.

Other modifications of fluorouracil administration include protracted intravenous fluorouracil given over 4 weeks, and fluorouracil combined with alpha interferon or with PALA (N-phosphonacetyl)-L-aspartic acid), an inhibitor of de novo pyrimidine synthesis; all these modifications appear to result in approximately 40% response rates. Major studies are under way comparing these various modifications.

In stage III (lymph nodes positive for malignancy) adenocarcinoma of the colon, two major cooperative group studies have demonstrated an improvement in survival with adjuvant fluorouracil in combination with the anthelmintic agent levamisole. The mechanism of action of this combination therapy is unknown. This regimen is begun within 4–6 weeks of surgery and is given over 1 year. At 5 years of follow-up, deaths from colorectal cancer were reduced by approximately 30%. This has resulted in 5-year survival rates for stage III patients in the range of 60–70%. Benefits have not been demonstrated for this treatment in patients with stage II disease (ie, tumor extending through the tunica muscularis propria). These data resulted in a National Cancer Institute recommendation of clinical trial participation or administration of fluorouracil and levamisole over a 1-year period for patients with stage III colon cancer.

In stages II and III (tumor extending through the tunica muscularis propria, or with nodes positive for malignancy) rectal cancers, several major randomized and controlled studies have shown the benefit of adjuvant combined modality therapy consisting of fluorouracil with or without semustine and external beam radiotherapy given within 4–6 weeks following resection. These studies demonstrated an approximately 30% reduction in death at 5 years for patients receiving combined modality therapy. These data resulted in a National Cancer Institute recommendation of participation in ongoing clinical trials or postoperative treatment with fluorouracil and irradiation (fluorouracil is to be given over 6 months with irradiation given over 5–6 weeks of this time).

Prognosis

Approximately 50% of patients with colon cancer and 80% of patients with rectal cancer are cured. With recent advances in adjuvant therapy these figures may improve.

LESS COMMON MALIGNANCIES

Gastrointestinal Lymphomas

Primary gastrointestinal lymphomas account for up to 10% of all lymphomas, with the gastrointestinal tract being the most common site of extranodal lymphomas. In the adult population in the USA, up to half of gastrointestinal lymphomas originate in the stomach and approximately one-third in the small bowel. Chronic gastritis and achlorhydria have been observed in association with gastric lymphomas, though a causal relationship is not clear. Patients with sprue (celiac disease) have an increased risk of gastrointestinal lymphomas, generally of the small bowel. Inflammatory bowel disease (Crohn's disease and ulcerative colitis) has been associated with an increased risk of small and large bowel lymphomas; this risk is less than that of adenocarcinoma of the colon in ulcerative colitis. AIDS-associated gastrointestinal lymphoma is addressed below. Histologically, virtually all gastrointestinal lymphomas are of the non-Hodgkin's type with intermediate- and high-grade lymphomas (eg, diffuse large-cell lymphoma) predominating. Pathologic diagnosis of gastric or large bowel lymphomas is often made by endoscopic biopsy, whereas small bowel lymphomas are usually not diagnosed until laparotomy.

Treatment of gastrointestinal lymphomas is in evolution. Surgery is currently the cornerstone of therapy, especially for locally advanced intermediate- and high-grade lymphomas; resection of the primary appears to reduce the risk of perforation and hemorrhage during subsequent radiation therapy or chemotherapy. Local radiation therapy appears to reduce local recurrence, especially for locally advanced gastric lymphomas. Extensive regional node involvement or metastatic disease merit chemotherapy. For intermediate- and high-grade lymphomas, standard combination regimens such as CHOP (cyclophosphamide, doxorubicin, vincristine, prednisone) are used, whereas for low-grade lymphomas, a single alkylating agent (eg, cyclophosphamide) or an attenuated combination chemotherapy regimen (eg, CVP [cyclophosphamide, vincristine, prednisone]) is used. In general, prognosis correlates best with histologic features and stage; disease confined to the gastrointestinal tract has the best prognosis. Gastric lymphomas are more likely to present with limited stage disease, as opposed to small and large bowel lymphomas. Patients with gastrointestinal lymphomas do not respond as well to chemotherapy as do patients with nodal lymphomas, and less than one-third of patients are cured.

Carcinoid & Islet Cell Tumors

Carcinoid tumors are of neural crest origin and are grouped together with tumors of APUD (amine precursor uptake and decarboxylation) cell origin. Although these tumors can be found throughout the body, over 90% originate in the gastrointestinal tract, specifically the small bowel, appendix, and rectum. Carcinoid tumors are associated with production or induction of a variety of vasoactive peptides, including serotonin and bradykinin. Initial evaluation includes 24-hour urine collection for 5-hydroxyindoleacetic acid (5HIAA), a serotonin metabolite. These tumors are frequently associated with the carcinoid syndrome, which consists of one or all of the following: flushing, diarrhea, bronchospasm, and cardiovascular abnormalities. The latter can include dysrhythmias and endocardial and subendocardial fibrosis with associated valvular dysfunction and cardiomyopathy. Less common conditions associated with carcinoid tumors include pellagra, syndrome of inappropriate antidiuretic hormone (vasopressin) secretion (SIADH), and hyperadrenalism due to ACTH secretion.

Islet cell tumors are also derived from APUD cells and include insulinomas, gastrinomas, glucagonomas, somatostatinomas, and VIPomas (vasoactive intestinal peptide tumors). Islet cell tumors can be part of the multiple endocrine neoplasia (MEN) I syndrome along with pituitary and parathyroid gland tumors. Most of these primary lesions are found in the pancreas, but they can also occur in the stomach, duodenum, and regional lymph nodes; liver metastases are relatively common. As with carcinoid tumors, each of the islet cell malignancies is characterized by its secreted hormones and attendant syndromes. Insulinomas are characterized by hypoglycemia with inappropriately high insulin levels. Glucagonomas are characterized by elevated glucagon levels with insulin-refractory diabetes and a dermatitis known as necrotizing migratory erythema. Somatostatinomas are characterized by elevated somatostatin levels and benign biliary disease, diabetes, and diarrhea. Gastrinomas are characterized by refractory ulcer disease in the setting of hypergastrinemia and elevated basal acid output. VIPomas are characterized by elevation in vasoactive intestinal peptide with refractory diarrhea, hypokalemia, hypochlorhydria, and metabolic acidosis. Radioimmunoassay techniques are used to measure each of the secreted hormones. Since many tumors are smaller than 1–2 cm, the techniques of computerized tomography, arteriography, and ultrasonography are not always helpful in identifying areas of involvement.

Carcinoid and islet cell tumors often grow slowly, and they are relatively refractory to chemotherapy. Approach to management should focus on controlling tumor-associated symptoms and signs while avoiding chemotherapy. This can be achieved through the use of antihistamine/antiserotonin agents (eg, cyproheptadine), conventional antidiarrheal agents, and most recently somatostatin analogs. Systemic therapy with chemotherapy (eg, fluorouracil plus streptozocin) or alpha interferon has demonstrated response rates generally less than 30% and usually of less than 6 months' duration. Recent reports on the use of chemoembolization of hepatic tumors emphasize good palliative results for carcinoid and islet cell tumors metastatic to the liver.

Carcinoma of the Anus

Squamous cell carcinoma of the anus is a rare malignancy that responds well to various modalities of treatment. Initially management was based on surgical resection, with the addition of radiotherapy or chemotherapy, or both, for locally advanced disease. It now appears that combined modality therapy consisting of chemotherapy and concomitant radiation therapy can achieve complete responses in up to 50% of patients with locally advanced disease. Whether such therapy can cure all stages of disease remains to be determined, though early-stage lesions are now being treated with chemotherapy and irradiation alone, while surgery is being reserved for salvage.

Cancers Associated with AIDS

The acquired immunodeficiency syndrome (AIDS)

is associated with several malignancies that either arise from or frequently metastasize to the gastrointestinal tract; these malignancies include Kaposi's sarcoma, lymphomas, and squamous cell carcinomas of the rectum and anus. To the extent that the underlying immunologic deficit will allow, these tumors are managed as they would be in patients without major immune dysfunction. However, the key is to weigh the limited benefits of aggressive anticancer therapy against the possibility of further exacerbating the immunologic deficit. Gastrointestinal involvement with Kaposi's sarcoma and non-Hodgkin's lymphoma are discussed below. Treatment of squamous cell carcinomas of the rectum and anus should follow the guidelines given above, tempered by the status of the patient's underlying immune dysfunction.

Kaposi's sarcoma occurs in approximately one-third of AIDS cases, with half of these demonstrating gastrointestinal involvement. Generally, all of the gastrointestinal tract is at risk of involvement, and the oral cavity frequently is involved. Involvement of the gastrointestinal tract with Kaposi's sarcoma usually is not associated with significant symptoms, but it is associated with increased mortality. When symptoms or signs do occur, they can include diarrhea, protein-losing enteropathy, and intestinal obstruction; bleeding from gastrointestinal lesions is rare. When viewed by endoscopy, lesions usually appear as raised red nodules measuring up to several centimeters in diameter and may demonstrate central ulceration. Diagnosis is best made by endoscopy, although because of the submucosal nature of lesions in Kaposi's sarcoma, a positive biopsy is sometimes difficult to obtain. Treatment options include radiation therapy and chemotherapy. Palliative radiation therapy is often effective, offering pain control and resolution of lesions in half or more of patients. Multiple chemotherapeutic agents (eg, etoposide, bleomycin, vinblastine, vincristine, doxorubicin), as well as alpha interferon, have been reported with response rates ranging from 20% to 80%; the definition of response varies between trials, and most of these responses average just several months in duration. As with all AIDS-associated malignancies, the quality of response must be weighed against the risk of exacerbating the patient's underlying immunosuppression in addition to considering the impact of the usual toxicities of chemotherapy.

Non-Hodgkin's lymphomas occur in up to 10% of AIDS patients. These lymphomas are commonly high grade, including Burkitt's lymphoma, and tend to occur at extranodal sites. In some series, up to 40% of patients with AIDS-associated lymphoma will have gastrointestinal involvement, usually unifocal. The clinical presentation of these patients can often be quite striking, with fever, cachexia, abnormal mental status, or myelosuppression along with a rapidly growing tumor mass. Attempts to treat patients with conventional chemotherapeutic regimens have resulted in complete response rates in the 50% range but with a majority of patients relapsing within months. It is clear that the outcome of patients receiving chemotherapy is dependent on their pretreatment morbidity and performance status. Patients who are HIV positive but have not yet suffered from an infectious complication and have a mild lymphoma presentation are the most likely to benefit from chemotherapy. Conversely, patients who have a long-term history of AIDS-related complications and who have a severe lymphoma presentation are more likely to suffer from attempts at therapy.

SUPPORTIVE CARE

Given the limited success of anticancer treatments in curing gastrointestinal cancers, supportive care takes on special significance with these tumor types. Nutrition is often impaired both by the systemic effects of cancer and often by structural or functional abnormalities of the gastrointestinal tract due to direct involvement with tumor. When nutritional supplementation is deemed appropriate, enteral feeding should be considered if adequate function of the gastrointestinal tract is not at issue. This form of alimentation can be achieved by placement of nasogastric feeding tubes or of gastrostomy or jejunostomy tubes. The latter percutaneous feeding tubes can be placed via laparotomy or laparoscopy or through endoscopic placement. For patients with malignant strictures of the esophagus, dilation appears to be an effective and safe way of maintaining patency of the esophagus. Dilating instruments vary from metal or rubber dilators to balloons. Most patients appear to benefit in terms of resuming some oral intake, and the risk of perforation appears to be small. In patients refractory to mechanical dilation, or those with esophago-pulmonary fistulas, consideration can be given to placement of a prosthetic esophageal tube. One series reported good palliation in a majority of patients, yet with an approximately 10% incidence of procedure-related perforation and a 5% incidence of procedure-related mortality. Additionally, migration or obstruction of the prosthetic tubes is a frequent problem. In patients with obstructing tumors in the upper gastrointestinal tract, laser photocoagulation has been used to regain functional patency. Though this technique shows promise, experience to date is insufficient to know its safety and efficacy as a palliative tool; local complications such as perforation or fistula formation have been reported with this technique. Parenteral hyperalimentation should be utilized only when there are well-defined nutritional objectives. This would apply, for example, to preoperative parenteral hyper-alimentation for the cancer patient with weight loss. In this setting, parenteral nutrition has been found to reduce postoperative morbidity and mortality.

Many patients with gastrointestinal cancer have had surgery resulting in enterostomy placement. Though newer surgical techniques have improved the effectiveness of ostomy surgery, these procedures result in a number of supportive care issues. Before surgery, patients can benefit from counseling by an enterostomy nurse or technician. Complete educational programs have been established for enterostomy patients, emphasizing patient involvement and the goal of independence. Approximately half the patients with descending or sigmoid colostomies will have regular bowel movements not requiring collection appliances. Additional patients will have regular evacuations with regular irrigation. Key elements of ostomy care include keeping the periostomy skin site clear and properly fitting any collection appliance. Periosteal pruritus or burning is likely an indication of leakage around the appliance. Common complications at ostomy sites include maceration, contact dermatitis, and *Candida* infections. Maceration should be managed with nonadherent bandages and topical corticosteroids. Contact dermatitis should be managed by elimination of irritating appliance materials and use of topical corticosteroids. *Candida* infections can be treated with topical antifungal therapy. Patients should be encouraged to maintain contact with an enterostomy specialist and should be made aware of the local Ostomy Association chapter.

In addition to therapy-associated emesis, gastrointestinal tract involvement with tumor can often be the cause of emesis. It is also important to consider emesis as a sign of bowel obstruction. Ileus and bowel obstruction are frequent problems associated with gastrointestinal malignancies, and the aggressiveness of intervention should depend on the prognosis of the underlying disease. Intervention might be restricted to medical efforts (eg, gut rest, nasogastric suction, avoidance of narcotics) or might include surgical decompression (bypass surgery). In patients with gastrointestinal cancer, care should be taken in treating abdominal pain, since aggressive analgesia may result in increased gut dysfunction. Consideration should be given to the use of nonnarcotic analgesics, nerve blocks, or even decompressing surgery if appropriate.

Biliary obstruction is often a result of gastrointestinal cancer due to either a primary tumor or metastatic disease. Approximately 90% of primary tumors causing biliary obstruction arise from the pancreas, with remaining cases arising from the bile ducts or duodenum. Metastatic tumors causing biliary obstruction commonly derive from gastric and colon primaries and are less frequently due to melanoma, breast cancer, lymphoma, and lung cancers. Decompression of the biliary tree can be accomplished surgically, with percutaneous biliary drainage, or with endoscopic placement of a biliary stent. The location of the obstructing mass and the prognosis of the underlying disease dictate the optimal approach. A pancreatic malignancy obstructing the distal end of the common bile duct is best suited to surgical bypass. Conversely, a metastic lesion obstructing the proximal bile duct is best suited to a percutaneous biliary drainage procedure. Metastatic lesions that are responsive to radiotherapy or chemotherapy, such as lymphomas or breast carcinomas, can be treated with these modalities, sometimes obviating the need for biliary drainage. The risks of percutaneous biliary drainage procedures should be emphasized. Estimated rates of catheter-associated cholangitis range up to 50%, with up to a 30% incidence of catheter-associated complications (obstruction or dislodgment) and a 30-day mortality up to 50%. The objectives of biliary decompression procedures must be carefully weighed against the expected morbidity and mortality. Furthermore, it is unclear whether prophylactic decompression of asymptomatic patients is of value or whether in fact it increases the risk of long-term complications due to biliary obstruction.

REFERENCES

Knight K, Fielding J, Battista R: Occult blood screening for colorectal cancer. *JAMA* 1989;**261**:587.

Martin E, Minton J, Carey L: CEA-directed second-look surgery in the asymptomatic patient after primary resection of colorectal cancer. *Ann Surg* 1985;**202**:310.

Moertel C et al: Levamisole and fluorouracil for adjuvant therapy of resected colon carcinoma. *N Engl J Med* 1990;**322**:352.

Krook J et al: Effective surgical adjuvant therapy for high-risk rectal carcinoma. *N Engl J Med* 1991;**324**:709.

Poon M et al: Biochemical modulation of fluorouracil: Evidence of significant improvement of survival and quality of life in patients with advanced colorectal carcinoma. *J Clin Oncol* 1989;**7**:1407.

Weingard D et al: Primary gastric lymphoma: A 30 year review. *Cancer* 1982;**49**:1258.

Moertel C: An odyssey in the land of small tumors. *J Clin Oncol* 1987;**5**:1503.

Shank B: Treatment of anal canal carcinoma. *Cancer* 1985;**55**:2156.

Bartlett J, Laughon B, Quinn T: Gastrointestinal complications of AIDS. Pages 227–244 in: *AIDS—Etiology, Diagnosis, Treatment, and Prevention*, 2nd ed. DeVita V, Hellman S, Rosenberg S (editors). Lippincott, 1988.

Lokich J et al: Biliary tract obstruction secondary to cancer: Management guidelines and selected literature review. *J Clin Oncol* 1987;**5**:969.

Genitourinary Cancer

Michael F. Sarosdy, MD

Cancers of the genitourinary tract account for approximately 18% of new adult malignancies and 10% of adult cancer deaths in the USA. Despite remarkable advances in the treatment of germ cell tumors of the testis and superficial bladder cancer, significant morbidity and mortality still result from the remaining cancers.

RENAL CELL CARCINOMA

Essentials of Diagnosis
- Hematuria, gross or microscopic, usually present.
- Symptoms of metastatic disease as likely to be present as local symptoms.
- "Classic triad" of mass, flank pain, and hematuria present in 10% of cases.
- Often discovered serendipitously on abdominal imaging studies such as gallbladder ultrasonography.

General Considerations
While renal cell carcinoma is said to be relatively rare because it accounts for only 3% of adult malignancies, there are approximately 27,000 new cases and 11,000 deaths due to kidney cancer annually in the USA. It occurs mainly in the fifth to seventh decades, with a male-to-female ratio just under 2:1. It occurs more frequently among those with von Hippel–Lindau disease and polycystic kidney disease and among those living in urban rather than rural areas. The incidence is similar among blacks and whites. The incidence of renal cell carcinoma in the USA is higher than in Japan but lower than in Iceland and Scandinavia.

The administration of diethylstilbestrol can produce renal cell carcinoma in Syrian hamsters, but such a relationship does not appear to exist in humans. Tobacco use has been implicated etiologically in humans, but no other environmental carcinogens have been firmly identified.

Pathologically, adenocarcinoma accounts for 85–90% of all renal parenchymal tumors and is what is referred to as renal cell carcinoma. Other names for this tumor type include clear cell carcinoma, Grawitz's tumor, and hypernephroma. Tumors vary

in size from a few centimeters to as large as 4–5 kg. Most are unilateral, but they may be bilateral, with either synchronous or asynchronous presentation of the latter. Renal cell carcinoma spreads by direct extension as well as by lymphatic and hematogenous routes. A unique feature of renal cell carcinoma is its ability to grow into the lumen of both the renal vein and vena cava, even as far as the diaphragm or into the right atrium. Such growth does not imply a worse prognosis but rather dictates a more complex approach to successful surgical removal of both the tumor thrombus and the involved kidney.

Other solid tumors of the kidney include angiomyolipomas, hemangiopericytomas, sarcomas, lymphoblastomas, oncocytomas, and metastatic tumors. Since most tumors other than angiomyolipomas cannot be distinguished preoperatively, all are approached as if they were renal cell carcinomas.

Clinical Findings
A. Symptoms and Signs: Symptoms range from none to severe symptoms of metastatic disease. Hematuria is the most common single symptom, occurring in roughly two-thirds, either grossly or microscopically. The symptoms of flank pain or a palpable mass are also common. Hematuria, flank pain, and a palpable mass constitute the "classic triad," but this is seen in no more than 10% of patients today.

Fever may be seen in 15%, and anemia unrelated to hematuria may occur in 30%. Paraneoplastic syndromes are not uncommon in renal cell carcinoma and may include polycythemia, hypercalcemia, and a syndrome of reversible hepatic dysfunction that occurs without hepatic metastasis (Stauffer's syndrome) in 20–40% of patients.

Systemic symptoms such as weight loss and fever are not uncommon, nor are symptoms of metastatic disease such as dyspnea due to pulmonary spread. Occasional patients may present with symptoms of renal vein obstruction (sudden onset of a varicocele) or vena cava obstruction (bilateral swelling of the lower extremities). Bone pain may also be a presenting symptom, as may central nervous system findings such as seizure due to brain metastasis.

B. Laboratory Findings: A complete blood count will demonstrate anemia or polycythemia, while a serum chemistry profile will assess renal function and the presence of any hepatic dysfunction or hypercalcemia.

C. Imaging Studies: A urogram or intravenous pyelogram (IVP) will usually demonstrate a mass, but this may not always be apparent in the case of smaller tumors. Sonography will help determine whether a mass is solid or cystic but is often bypassed in favor of a CT scan when a solid mass is highly suspected or obvious. A CT scan will usually distinguish a cystic from a solid mass as well as provide additional information regarding the presence of retroperitoneal lymphadenopathy or liver metastases. While angiography may be confirmatory of a hypervascular neoplastic mass, only 75% of renal cell carcinomas are hypervascular. Angiography is not used often today in the evaluation of solid-appearing renal masses. Ultrasonography of the renal vein and vena cava is usually performed to exclude tumor thrombus. If this cannot be satisfactorily excluded by sonography, cavography may be performed, although magnetic resonance imaging (MRI) may prove to be a better method of assessing the lumen of the vena cava. A liver-spleen scan is rarely positive if an enhanced abdominal CT scan is negative, and bone scans are usually reserved for patients who have an elevated alkaline phosphatase level.

D. Additional Studies: While all patients with hematuria should generally undergo cystoscopy, the value of cystoscopy is debatable when an obvious renal cell cancer has been found. Retrograde pyelography is rarely necessary to aid in the diagnosis of such tumors. In the past, cyst puncture with cytologic and chemical evaluation of aspirated fluid was often performed on equivocal cysts. With the higher resolution of real-time ultrasonography, such studies are rarely necessary today. Finally, percutaneous needle biopsy or needle aspiration cytology is rarely indicated, since most solid renal tumors are malignant, and although reported only rarely in the literature, seeding of the needle tract with tumor cells is an unwarranted risk.

Routes of Dissemination

Renal cell carcinoma spreads by the major routes—lymphatic, hematogenous, and direct spread—as well as by tumor thrombus growth into the renal vein and vena cava. While the last by itself in the absence of other metastatic disease does not seem to worsen prognosis, such growth must be considered preoperatively. Lymphatic spread, even apparently localized to retroperitoneal and perihilar nodes, carries a much worse prognosis. Approximately 25% of patients will have involved lymph nodes. An additional 25% will present with metastatic disease in distant sites, most commonly lung or bone but also the adrenal gland, the contralateral kidney, liver, or brain. Direct spread is not uncommon, with 25% of patients having involvement of the peri-

nephric fat within Gerota's fascia. Direct extension into adjacent organs does occur, but uncommonly. For example, while the colonic mesentery is often involved in large tumors, it is rare that resection of colon is necessary, and liver, pancreas, and adjacent muscle are less often involved.

Staging

A. The Robson system is commonly used in the USA.

Stage A: Tumor confined to the kidney.
Stage B: Tumor through the capsule into the perinephric fat but still contained within Gerota's fascia.
Stage C: Tumor involving the regional lymph nodes, renal vein, or vena cava.
Stage D: Presence of distant metastasis or invasion of contiguous organs.

B. The TNM classification is

T0: No evidence of primary tumor.
T1: Small tumor not enlarging the kidney.
T2: Large kidney with distortion of renal architecture.
T3: Perinephric or peripelvic fat or hilar vessel involvement.
T4: Involvement of adjacent organs or abdominal wall.
N0: No nodes involved.
N1: Single ipsilateral node involved.
N2: Bilateral nodes involved.
N3: Fixed regional nodes.
N4: Juxtaregional nodes involved.
M0: No distant metastases.
M1: Distant metastases.

Treatment

A. Clinically Localized Disease: The treatment of choice for localized disease (pathologic stages A, B, and many C's) is radical nephrectomy. This implies removal of the kidney with Gerota's fascia intact and with early control of the renal artery and vein. This may be accomplished through a variety of incisions, including an anterior subcostal approach, a lateral transperitoneal approach through the bed of the 11th rib, or a thoracoabdominal approach for very large or upper pole tumors. If enlarged periaortic lymph nodes are discovered, they are resected, although such resection now appears to have only prognostic value and no therapeutic value. For this reason, most urologic oncologists have abandoned attempts at regular, orderly lymphadenectomy.

B. Tumors with Vena Cava Extension or Tumor Thrombus: It has been reasonably well documented that tumor thrombus in the caval lumen does not worsen the prognosis for renal cell carcinoma. The worsened prognosis associated with tumor thrombus in the past was mainly secondary to the presence of associated malignant lymphadenopathy. Therefore, surgical resection of such tumors should be pursued aggressively.

C. Metastatic Disease Including Distant Disease or Radiographically Bulky Periaortic Lymphadenopathy: No effective therapies are yet available for metastatic renal cell carcinoma, particularly chemotherapies. Although early work with several immunotherapies appeared promising, additional trials have confirmed only a low level of response. These therapies appear more effective than cytotoxic chemotherapies, with an occasional complete response. Given this state of affairs, the performance of a radical nephrectomy in the face of obvious metastatic disease should be undertaken only under certain circumstances. These include the presence of significant symptoms such as pain, hypercalcemia (if secondary to parathyroidlike hormone secretion rather than osseous metastasis), and anemia or the availability of a therapeutic protocol evaluating the treatment of metastatic disease or the delay of progression in patients with resected high-stage disease. While the argument of "spontaneous regression" of metastases may be raised to justify nephrectomy in such patients, such regression occurs in less than 1% of adequately documented cases. Such an argument should not be used to justify a nephrectomy in an otherwise asymptomatic patient with clinically detected metastatic disease.

D. Tumors in Solitary Kidneys, or Bilaterally Simultaneous Tumors: Renal parenchyma–preserving procedures are gaining in popularity in such cases as these. However, these procedures have not been performed with long enough follow-up to recommend such surgery in patients with a single tumor in one of two otherwise normal kidneys. Such procedures as partial nephrectomy or "lumpectomy" with wide excision of surrounding tissue are justified in solitary kidneys and in the event of multiple tumors in both kidneys. Such surgery is usually feasible in situ, although "bench surgery" with nephrectomy, immediate flushing and cooling of the kidney, followed by rapid excision of the tumor and autotransplantation is a viable alternative when necessary.

Prognosis

Patients with pathologic stage A tumors enjoy a 65% 5-year survival. For those with stage B, survival is still 55–65%. Survival in stage C must be classified by the tissue involved, since nodal spread is much worse than vein or vena cava involvement. Patients with venous or caval involvement only may expect a survival equal to the stage of the primary tumor, ie, A or B. However, if nodes are positive, 2-year survival is only 10–20%, and 5-year survival is near zero. Patients who present with stage D disease generally may expect survival in terms of months rather than years.

CARCINOMA OF THE BLADDER

Essentials of Diagnosis

- Hematuria, either gross or microscopic.
- Cystoscopy and urography required for diagnosis.

General Considerations

Bladder cancers are the second most common urologic malignancy after prostate cancer and account for about 2% of all malignant disease. An estimated 52,000 new cases and 9,500 deaths from bladder cancer occur annually in the USA. The majority (85%) of these tumors are superficial and curable by local excision at the time of initial presentation. However, up to 60% of such patients will experience tumor recurrence. Recurrences are sometimes associated with more aggressive (invasive) tumors. The remaining 15% of patients present initially with either invasive or distant metastatic disease.

Etiology & Risk Factors

The connection between bladder cancer and exogenous carcinogens was made in 1895 by Rehn who noted the disease in workers who manufactured aniline dye. Four compounds have been identified, all having a common aromatic amine structure: β-naphthylamine, 4-aminobiphenyl, 4-nitrophenyl, and benzidine. Workers at risk include those in chemical and dye manufacturing, pigment and patent production, rubber and cable making, textile dyeing, the gas industry, and others who work around high levels of these four compounds.

Cigarette smoking has been linked to bladder cancer in 50% of males and up to 30% of females, probably because naphthylamine and tryptophan are found in the urine of smokers in markedly increased amounts. There does not appear to be an increased risk in pipe and cigar smokers.

Artificial sweeteners have been implicated, but the evidence is controversial. Clinical information is not yet available for cyclamate, and there does not appear to be a clinical risk with saccharine use. Rodent studies that have been positive used dosages 500–700 times those used in humans.

Coffee drinking also has been implicated but no association proved. That may be because a strong link does not exist, or because there is widespread general use of caffeine, or because of its concomitant use with tobacco and sweeteners.

Schistosomiasis is known to be associated with squamous cell carcinoma of the bladder in 15–20% of infected patients.

Chronic irritation and infection have been implicated as risk factors based on the experience with chronic indwelling catheters in patients with neurogenic bladders. Eighty percent will develop squamous cell metaplasia, and a few will progress to squamous cell cancer.

Phenacetin use for long periods of time (up to 10 years) is associated with transitional cell cancer.

Finally, cyclophosphamide has been said to have carcinogenic potential. One report cites a 3% incidence and nine-fold increased risk for patients who have received this drug (usually for arthritis, systemic lupus erythematosus, or other cancers). The association remains to be proved, however.

Clinical Findings

A. Symptoms and Signs: Gross, painless hematuria is the presenting symptom in 80% of patients. It may be intermittent and is usually present throughout the urinary stream (total as opposed to initial or terminal). Irritative or obstructive voiding symptoms may be present in a third of patients. Patients with carcinoma in situ may have no symptoms other than severe dysuria, frequency, and urgency. Bladder carcinoma should be suspected in a patient with recurrent irritative symptoms but persistently negative urine cultures. Patients may present with symptoms of metastatic disease, uremia secondary to advanced local disease obstructing one or both kidneys, or urinary retention due to bladder outlet obstruction.

Cystoscopic inspection of the bladder with transurethral biopsy or resection is the mainstay of diagnosis. This should be preceded by a urogram to rule out upper tract lesions, such as renal cell carcinoma or ureteral or pelvic tumors. If ureteral visualization is not adequate on urography, a retrograde pyelogram should be performed at the time of cystoscopy. If a tumor seen at the time of cystoscopy appears to be low grade and superficial, complete excision is performed, with separate biopsy of the base to look for invasion into muscle. If the tumor appears to be solid or invasive, complete resection is not attempted, and only biopsies adequate for staging are obtained. In either case, "random" (actually systematic and directed) biopsies are also taken from normal-appearing uninvolved areas in order to rule out multicentricity or associated dysplasia or carcinoma in situ. It is also important to perform a bimanual examination under anesthesia, particularly in the patient who has an invasive-appearing tumor. This will help define the extent of spread, in addition to the CT scan.

B. Laboratory Findings: Most values are normal in the majority of patients, since most have superficial tumors. The most common finding is anemia due to blood loss. Azotemia may be present if one or both ureters are obstructed or the patient is in retention. Liver enzymes and alkaline phosphatase levels will be elevated in the uncommon patient with liver or bone metastases.

C. Imaging Studies: Urographic findings on IVP may range from normal to a variable-sized bladder-filling defect to nonvisualization of one kidney due to tumor obstruction at the ureterovesical junction. Patients presenting with the latter finding will have a muscle-invasive tumor in 25% of cases.

D. Additional Studies: Urinary cytology is occasionally helpful in the diagnosis but is more commonly used to follow patients for recurrence. Flow cytometric analysis and quantitative flow image analysis are potentially more accurate and objective methods of surveillance, but large clinical studies confirming these techniques are only now under way.

Pathologic Findings

Transitional cell cancer represents about 95% of bladder cancers, with about 5% squamous and 1% adenocarcinoma. Even so, transitional cell cancer of the bladder does not represent a single entity but rather a spectrum of disease, each with different clinical significance to the physician and patient.

Atypia or dysplasia may be a precursor to frank malignant disease, but conclusive evidence is still lacking. Patients with superficial papillary tumors that have atypia near the tumor base may have a higher rate of eventually developing invasive tumors than do patients with tumors having normal mucosa next to the base.

Carcinoma in situ is a flat, intraepithelial carcinoma, not a premalignant lesions. It has a high rate of spread to lymph nodes, though this usually takes several years to occur. The bladder may look entirely normal or it may have a velvety, erythematous appearance.

Superficial tumors are usually low grade and have a papillary appearance, with a small stalk that may be only 1–3 mm across. A small percentage of these may invade into the muscle, so attention to the base of the stalk is important in accurately staging the patient. These tumors may occur alone, or several may be present in different areas.

Invasive tumors are usually high grade. Most often, they appear to be solid or sessile, and they usually have a broad base in contact with the bladder wall.

Staging & Grading

After tumor resection and the pathologic diagnosis have been made, staging is accomplished according to Marshall's modification of the Jewett-Strong system (TMN system in parentheses).

Stage O: Mucosal involvement only, including both papillary (Ta) and carcinoma in situ (Tis).

Stage A: Penetration into the lamina propria (T1).

Stage B1: Focal invasion into the muscle (T2).

Stage B2: Deep muscle invasion, but not beyond (T3a).

Stage C: Involvement of perivesical fat (T3b).

Stage D1: Direct invasion into other pelvic structures, or nodal spread below the bifurcation of the aorta (T4).

Stage D2: Spread to distant organs or to nodes above the bifurcation of the aorta.

A three-grade system of scoring the degree of anaplasia has generally been adopted:

Grade I: Tumors have the least degree of anaplasia compatible with diagnosis of malignancy.

Grade II: Tumors have a degree of anaplasia between grades I and II.

Grade III: Tumors have the most severe degree of anaplasia.

The grade of the tumor has proved useful in predicting future tumor behavior and is used in conjunction with the stage to help dictate reasonable courses of therapy for individual patients with superficial tumors (stages O and A).

Treatment

Treatment following diagnosis is based on the pathologic stage.

A. Superficial Tumors (Stages 0 and A): Most tumors are superficial and amenable to transurethral resection. While 60–70% of patients will have recurrences, 30% may never have another tumor. No test can yet discriminate who will certainly fall into the latter group. All patients therefore should undergo routine cystoscopy to look for recurrence. In the absence of recurrence, cystoscopy is performed every 3 months for 2 years, then every 6 months for 2 years, then annually. No noninvasive test accurately detects tumor recurrence in all instances. Urine cytologic specimens are helpful, but they are negative in most grade I tumors and may be positive in only 60–80% of grade III tumors. Flow cytometry may have some value, but it is not yet routinely used or widely available. The ABO (H) blood group or cell surface antigens have been shown to be present on noninvasive tumors, and their absence may correlate with eventual recurrence of a tumor that is invasive. At this time, however, the absence of those antigens on a tumor that is otherwise noninvasive does not warrant cystectomy.

For patients who suffer recurrences of superficial tumors, intravesical instillation of various agents may significantly decrease the rate of recurrence. Thiotepa, doxorubicin, and mitomycin are all effective to some degree, but many patients do not respond to these agents, and many who respond initially eventually escape their effect. Bacillus Calmette-Guérin (BCG) causes a significant decrease in the rate of tumor recurrence and often is used after failure of one or more other intravesical agents.

B. Carcinoma in Situ: While carcinoma in situ is not muscle invasive, its pathophysiologic characteristics dictate that it be treated more aggressively than superficial tumors. Although superficial, it is by definition a grade III lesion. Carcinoma in situ may metastasize to lymph nodes without going through another stage. When in multiple areas or associated with papillary tumors, even superficial, cystectomy historically was required in 80% of patients. The treatment of choice today is intravesical BCG. Several centers that have had experience with this agent report complete response rates of 65–90%, including patients followed up to 6 years. Light sensitization with hematoporphyrin derivative followed by ruby-argon laser therapy is an investigational treatment.

C. Invasive Disease (Stages B1, B2, and C): The treatment of choice, if no metastatic disease is found on clinical staging, is radical cystectomy. Attempts at partial cystectomy are usually avoided, since it is not possible to define accurately the intralymphatic spread of tumor within the bladder muscle. For the same reason, repeated transurethral resections to provide local control will not dependably eradicate tumor. Even with negative staging studies and no nodal spread detected by pelvic lymphadenectomy, up to 50% of patients will develop distant metastases within 2 years following cystectomy. Preoperative pelvic radiation was employed in the past but does not appear to have added to survival.

D. Metastatic Disease (Stages D1 and D2): Several anticancer drugs—cisplatin, fluorouracil, methotrexate, cyclophosphamide, doxorubicin, and vinblastine—have some single-agent activity against bladder cancer, but the clinical impact of these agents has been limited. Combinations of these agents generally add little increase in clinical efficacy. The combination of methotrexate, vinblastine, doxorubicin (Adriamycin), and cisplatin (M-VAC) appears to be among the most active. Complete response rates appear to be around 30%, including patients who have undergone pathologic staging with resection of tissue after chemotherapy. Current investigation of M-VAC includes study of its ability to treat bulky disease as well as increase the survival of stage B patients treated with cystectomy.

Other Therapies

Radiotherapy has played a varying role in the treatment of bladder cancer. Interstitial therapy (whereby radioactive seeds are implanted directly into tumor through open cystotomy) has been used in Europe for both invasive and bulky superficial tumors with limited success. External beam therapy went through a period of "definitive" use, but morbidity was not insignificant and true cure or palliation was limited. Despite the absence of controlled studies showing any rationale, external beam therapy was also used as a means of preoperative "downstaging" prior to cystectomy in both "short courses" (2000 cGy in 1 week) and "long courses" (4500 cGy in 4–5 weeks). The most promising role of radiotherapy involves its use in conjunction with fluorouracil in investigative trials of this combination's ability to obtain a response and preserve the bladder.

Nd:YAG lasers represent a new method of treating bladder cancer using photocoagulation rather than electrocautery resection. Potential advantages include treatment without spinal or general anesthesia and no need for catheter drainage postoperatively.

Prognosis

Survival is directly related to stage of bladder cancer at the time of diagnosis. Patients with superficial tumors have an 80–90% 5-year survival. For patients with muscle-invasive tumors, 5-year survival averages 50% over many studies, despite the absence of lymph node metastases. Stage C patients may expect a 20–40% survival, while those with stage D1 have a 0–32% survival.

Rare Bladder Tumors

A. Adenocarcinoma: Less than 1% of bladder cancers are adenocarcinomas. These commonly occur at the trigone or in the dome, with the latter most often representing carcinoma from a urachal remnant. The latter also occur most often in young adults. Patients who fail to have complete surgical excision have an extremely poor outcome, since there is no effective chemotherapy for this disease.

B. Squamous Cell Carcinoma: Approximately 5% of bladder cancers are of this variety. They are associated with chronic inflammation but can occur without it. There is a high association with schistosomiasis where the disease is endemic (eg, Egypt). Again, complete surgical removal is necessary, since effective chemotherapy does not exist for this cancer.

C. Sarcomas: Sarcomas are extremely rare in adults. Leiomyosarcoma is the most common. Rhabdomyosarcoma is a relatively common tumor in children, with rhabdomyosarcoma of the bladder and prostate accounting for about 15% of these tumors in children. Pelvic exenteration and urinary diversion used to be the treatment of choice. However, chemotherapy with vinblastine, doxorubicin, and cyclophosphamide combined with radiotherapy has allowed enough tumor shrinkage and improved survival such that "bladder-sparing" partial cystectomies are now the preferred treatment when deemed surgically feasible.

CANCER OF THE RENAL PELVIS & URETER

Essentials of Diagnosis

- Gross or microscopic hematuria.
- Radiolucent filling defect on urogram or retrograde pyelogram.

General Considerations

Tumors of the ureter are relatively uncommon but not rare, accounting for about 1% of urologic tumors. They occur most often in the distal ureter but can be seen anywhere in the collecting system, from the renal calyces to the ureterovesical junction. Ninety-five percent are transitional, and 5% are squamous, with a rare adenocarcinoma. Sixty to 80% are papillary, and most are grade II or III. They spread by lymphatics and by direct growth into adjacent structures.

Clinical Findings

Presenting symptoms are similar to those associated with bladder cancer. However, hematuria is very common, occurring in up to 90%, and may be intermittent or profuse. Flank pain due to ureteral obstruction may occur in 20–40%.

The critical distinction in patients who present with hematuria and a radiolucent filling defect on the urogram or retrograde pyelogram is whether that defect represents a tumor, blood clot, or lucent stone, such as uric acid. The CT scan is most helpful in making this determination. Ureteral collection of urine for cytologic examination is helpful only when positive, and brush biopsy may be helpful in 50% of cancers. Direct-vision ureterorenoscopy is available and also allows biopsy of any lesion seen.

Staging

The same staging studies should be obtained as in bladder cancer. Tumors of the pelvis and ureter are staged as follows:

Stage O: Confined to the mucosa.
Stage A: Invasion into but not through the lamina propria.
Stage B: Invasion into the muscle but not beyond.
Stage C: Invasion into the adjacent kidney or peripelvic or periureteral fat.
Stage D: Extension into adjacent organs, distant metastases, or lymph node involvement.

Treatment

Treatment has classically been nephroureterectomy with removal of the entire ureter and a "cuff" of bladder. The rationale has been that tumor spillage occurs easily with these tumors, and opening the ureter to perform a partial ureterectomy or local tumor excision led to a high rate of local recurrence. Tumors also recur frequently if a distal stump of ureter is left after nephroureterectomy for an upper tract tumor. This is still the treatment of choice, although there is a trend toward "renal-sparing" procedures when preoperative staging studies (ureterorenoscopy and biopsy) unequivocally demonstrate the tumor to be unifocal and grade I. In a patient with extensive ureteral tumor in a solitary kidney, ureterectomy with autotransplantation of the kidney into the true pelvis is a viable option.

Prognosis

Patients with low-stage disease enjoy a nearly normal life expectancy. Those with disease beyond the ureter locally have only a 40–50% 5-year survival, while those with metastatic disease have a 5-year survival approaching zero.

TESTICULAR CANCER

Essentials of Diagnosis

- Painless, firm mass or enlargement of a testicle.
- Trimodal frequency by age groups—infants, males aged 20–40 (highest frequency), and males over age 60.
- Serum tumor markers—alpha-fetoprotein (AFP) and beta subunit of human chorionic gonadotrophin (hCG)—normal or elevated.
- Symptoms of metastatic disease.

General Considerations

Testicular malignancies are relatively rare, with an annual incidence of 3.7 per 100,000 persons. This translates to an expected 6,500 cases and 350 deaths annually. While the mortality rate has been reversed from what it was 15 years ago, efforts continue at decreasing the morbidity of curative therapy.

Ninety-four percent of testicular cancers are germ cell tumors. Germ cell tumors are classified as seminomas (35%) or nonseminomas (embryonal, 20%; teratocarcinoma, 38%; teratoma, 5%; and choriocarcinoma, 2%). Non–germ cell tumors include Sertoli cell and Leydig cell tumors and are rare as well as usually benign. While testis cancer may occur at all ages, there is a trimodal frequency distribution curve, with peak frequencies in the infant, young adult (aged 20–40), and older adult (over age 60). Certain types have a predilection for specific age groups. Infants tend to acquire teratomas and embryonal carcinomas but not seminomas or choriocarcinomas. Embryonal carcinoma and teratocarcinoma occur primarily between age 25 and 35, choriocarcinoma between age 20 and 30, and seminoma between age 35 and 60. Seminoma is the most common germ cell tumor overall. The most common testicular neoplasm in men over age 60 is lymphoma.

Blacks have an incidence of testis cancer about one-third that of whites, a difference that is found worldwide. The incidence of malignancy is higher in cryptorchidism and does not subside completely following orchiopexy. The risk of tumor development is also higher with greater degrees of cryptorchidism, ie, the rate for malignancy is higher in abdominal cryptorchidism, which has a higher rate than inguinal cryptorchidism. While the true increase in risk is not clear, it is probably on the order of 10 times the risk in a male with normally descended testes.

Several generalizations may be made about testicular malignancies. Spontaneous regression of these tumors is rare, and all germinal tumors in adults should be considered malignant, even those labeled "benign" or "mature" teratoma. The tunica albuginea testis presents a natural barrier to direct spread of the tumor, and local involvement of the epididymis or cord occurs in only 10–15%. On the other hand, lymphatic spread is common to all germinal tumors, and choriocarcinoma spreads by vascular routes as well. The primary route of lymphatic spread is to the interaortocaval and periaortic nodes, with subsequent cephalad extension to the cisterna chyli, thoracic duct, and supraclavicular nodes. Retrograde spread is often seen to the lower lumbar, iliac, and pelvic nodes when massive retroperitoneal disease is present. Scrotal surgery to make the diagnosis is a grave error, and it can result in nodal spread to inguinal lymph nodes also. Most but not all blood-borne metastases occur in conjunction with lymphatic spread. Testis cancers tend to be fast growing, with a doubling time estimated to be 10–30 days; 95% of patients dying from testis cancer do so within 2 years. The rapid doubling time is probably responsible for the fact that 40–50% of patients have metastatic disease at the time of presentation and diagnosis.

Clinical Findings

A. Symptoms and Signs: The most common presentation is that of a painless hard mass or "swelling" noted by the patient. Some patients report a dull ache or sensation of fullness, and occasional patients have acute pain related to hemorrhage into the tumor. About 10% of patients will present with symptoms of metastatic disease, such as cough or dyspnea, abdominal fullness, nausea and vomiting, weight loss, bone pain, central or peripheral nervous system symptoms, and unilateral leg edema. About 5% have gynecomastia or other signs of estrogen excess. A delay in diagnosis is still common, with responsibility for that delay shared by both patients and physicians. A complete physical examination should be performed when testicular cancer is suspected. A testicular tumor is usually firm, relatively nontender, and contained within the tunica of the testis. It may be quite small or very large, but size does not correlate with the presence or absence of metastases.

B. Laboratory Findings: In the absence of significant metastatic disease, serum chemistries and blood count are usually normal. One specific and two relatively nonspecific tumor markers exist, however, and aid in diagnosis as well as in monitoring response to therapy in testis cancer patients.

1. Alpha-Fetoprotein (AFP)–AFP is elevated in about 70% of patients with nonseminoma but is not produced by seminomatous tumors. Elevation of AFP in a patient with a tumor reported histologically as a seminoma should prompt reexamination of the specimen by the pathologist for the nonseminomatous elements that must be present.

2. Beta subunit of human chorionic gonadotropin (β-hCG)–β-hCG is elevated in approximately 65% of nonseminomatous tumors but in only about 10% of seminomas. This marker, unlike AFP, is also specific for testicular cancer.

3. Lactic dehydrogenase (LDH)–LDH, particularly the isoenzyme fraction LDH-1, is elevated in about 60% of patients. Like AFP, it is nonspecific, but it does provide an additional marker with which to follow the patient whose tumor produces it.

Patients undergoing orchiectomy or exploration for possible testis cancer should have a clot drawn before surgery. Should testicular carcinoma be found, this clot allows for serum assays to be performed for these three tumor markers to establish the patient's baseline. A repeat of the assays several weeks later (in those with initially elevated levels) should confirm the progressive return of those values toward normal according to the half-life of each marker (hCG = 24 hours, AFP = 5.5 days). A persistent elevation or slower than expected decay indicates residual metastatic disease, even if all radiographic studies are normal.

C. Imaging Studies: Abdominal CT scan with contrast is the study of choice to stage patients after the diagnosis is made. A CT scan of the chest should be obtained at the same time to rule out thoracic disease that might be present, even in the absence of retroperitoneal lymphadenopathy. Although lymphangiography provides specific visualization of the retroperitoneal lymph nodes, its value over the CT scan is minimal and it is more difficult to obtain. Intravenous urography adds little to the staging of these patients.

D. Ultrasonography: In cases of ambiguous physical findings, ultrasonography may prove useful in the diagnosis of a testicular primary. This imaging technique is useful also to confirm the diagnosis of extragonadal germ cell tumor, a rare tumor that resembles a metastatic germ cell tumor but does not arise from a testicular primary.

Differential Diagnosis

The differential diagnosis includes epididymitis, hydrocele, hernia, hematoma, and spermatocele. If a 2-week course of appropriate antibiotics does not markedly improve the course of presumptive epididymitis, surgical exploration is indicated.

Staging

The most frequently used staging system for testis cancer is that proposed by the Memorial Sloan-Kettering Cancer Center:

Stage A: Tumor confined to testis.
Stage B1: Minimal nodal spread, microscopic only, and with fewer than six nodes involved, none greater than 2 cm.
Stage B2: Grossly positive nodal disease, or more than six nodes positive in retroperitoneum.
Stage B3: Massive retroperitoneal disease, including palpable abdominal mass.
Stage C: Metastases above the diaphragm, or involvement of solid visceral organs, brain, or bone.

Treatment

The diagnosis is confirmed and therapy initiated by an appropriately performed orchiectomy via an inguinal incision. Following diagnosis and clinical staging, treatment varies according to whether the tumor is a seminoma or a nonseminomatous germ cell tumor. Several classification systems have been devised to assign risk to patients as good or poor and to classify the level of disease as minimal, moderate, or advanced. Such systems vary in their accuracy but are generally helpful in selecting initial therapy in some patients.

A. Seminoma: Because of the radiosensitivity of seminoma, clinical stage A patients normally receive 2500–3500 cGy to the aortocaval and ipsilateral inguinopelvic areas. Five-year survival with this therapy is 90–95%.

Without pathologic staging, stage B1 patients are not recognizable clinically, so they are treated as clinical stage A patients. Clinical stage B2 and B3 patients in the past were treated with radiotherapy to the abdomen, with additional treatment to the mediastinum and supraclavicular area. However, survival tacts are better if such patients are treated with the same platinum-based chemotherapeutic agent as is used for nonseminomatous tumors before rather than after major doses of bone marrow–suppressing radiotherapy. The same holds true for stage C patients.

B. Nonseminomatous Germ Cell Tumors: Considerable controversy revolves around the treatment of clinical stage A (pathologic stage A, B1, and many B2's) patients, partly because of the success achieved in treating patients with more advanced disease. In the past, pathologic staging was accomplished by retroperitoneal lymph node dissection. Since only 20–30% of patients had positive nodes, the surgery was negative in the majority, and roughly 8% of the latter patients eventually showed recurrence in the chest. Retrograde ejaculation occurred in most patients owing to interruption of the sympathetic nerves, though improved modified node dissections and nerve-sparing dissections now preserve ejaculation in the majority of node-negative patients. Recurrences were not seen in the retroperitoneum, and those with chest recurrences were detected early. The cure rate for all clinical stage A patients, regardless of pathologic stage, was 100%.

The concept of observation or surveillance for clinical stage A patients was introduced with the hypothesis that 70–80% of patients could be spared a needless lymphadenectomy, while 100% survival would be maintained owing to the efficacy of chemotherapy. To date, no study has achieved that aim, and survival rates have slipped to 95–96%. Reasons include the higher degree of difficulty in detecting retroperitoneal recurrence (or progression) than pulmonary disease, as well as the fast growth of such tumors. Thus, it is necessary to perform an abdominal CT scan every 2 months during the first 2 years of surveillance in all patients, in addition to bimonthly serum marker measurement and chest x-ray. Several factors place a patient at increased risk of retroperitoneal recurrence. These include the presence of embryonal carcinoma in the primary tumor, testicular capsular penetration by the primary tumor, and vascular invasion of the cord. At present, patients having tumors with such histologic features should probably be excluded from surveillance and instead undergo staging retroperitoneal lymphadenectomy. Additional patients who should undergo this procedure are those judged to be poorly compliant for the rigorous follow-up required by surveillance therapy. For the remaining patients, strict adherence to close radiographic follow-up is mandatory. Several centers no longer recommend surveillance therapy for the above-mentioned reasons.

Clinical stage B2, B3, and C patients have retroperitoneal or supradiaphragmatic disease and should receive chemotherapy initially after orchiectomy is performed. If all radiographic studies and markers normalize, they may be followed closely without additional surgery. However, if residual disease is present after adequate chemotherapy as reflected by normalization of markers, resection of that residual tissue should be performed, whether in the lungs, mediastinum, or retroperitoneum. Such residual tissue should be resected because roughly one-third of patients will have scar, one-third teratoma, and one-third active cancer.

C. Chemotherapy: While chemotherapy for testis cancer remains platinum-based, improvement through reduced toxicity continues to occur. The combination of cisplatin, vinblastine, and bleomycin has been replaced by cisplatin, etoposide, and bleomycin, and it now appears that three cycles are as efficacious as four in good-risk patients. Furthermore, early data indicate that four courses of cisplatin and etoposide may be just as efficacious as the three-drug regimen in patients who do not have advanced disease, sparing patients the potentially fatal pulmonary toxicity of bleomycin.

Extragonadar Germ Cell Tumors

These are rate tumors, but their origin distinct from metastases from testicular primaries is clear. They may arise in the mediastinum, retroperitoneum, sacrococcygeal region, and pineal gland. They are thought to arise from either displaced primitive germ cells or the persistence of pluripotential cells in sequestered primitive rests. Both men and women may be affected, and patients tend to present with metastatic disease.

Pediatric Testis Cancers

Testis tumors in children constitute 1–2% of solid childhood tumors. The peak incidence is around age 2. In contrast to the situation for adults, germ cell tumors account for only about 75% of pediatric testis tumors; the rest are a combination of relatively uncommon tumors. Yolk sac tumors account for 75% of these germ cell tumors. This tumor is very similar to embryonal carcinoma and has been termed embryonal, infantile embryonal, endodermal sinus, and Telium's tumor and orchidoblastoma. Yolk sac tumors differ from adult embryonal tumors in that only 15–20% will metastasize. Thus, if there is no evidence on radiographic studies of disease in the chest or retroperitoneum and markers fall to normal after orchiectomy, the current recommendation is for close surveillance for the development of distant disease rather than staging retroperitoneal lymphadenectomy. When chemotherapy is necessary, vincristine, doxorubicin (Adriamycin), and cyclophosphamide (VAC) is the combination employed.

CARCINOMA OF THE PROSTATE

Essentials of Diagnosis

- A palpable, hard nodule or an area of induration in the prostate on rectal examination.
- Pathologic diagnosis confirmed by needle biopsy of the prostate.
- Bony metastatic disease often present at the time of diagnosis.
- Serum acid phosphatase not usually elevated except in advanced disease.

General Considerations

Carcinoma of the prostate is now the most common cancer in men and the number two cause of male cancer deaths in the USA. More than 125,000 new cases of adenocarcinoma of the prostate are diagnosed annually, with about 35,000 deaths. It is seen occasionally in males under age 50, with an increasing frequency in older age groups: up to 35% of men over age 80 have histologic evidence of prostate cancer on postmortem examination. The clinical incidence is much lower, however, at approximately 10% of all men over age 65. A 10% incidence of prostate cancer is found on pathologic examination of tissue resected from palpably benign glands during surgery for bladder outlet obstruction presumed to be secondary to benign prostatic hypertrophy. This rate may be as high as 35% in men over age 80 undergoing transurethral resection of the prostate.

Most (95%) carcinoma of the prostate is adenocarcinoma. It occurs primarily in the peripheral zone of the prostate, as opposed to the central, periurethral zone that gives rise to benign prostatic hypertrophy. While the specific cause is not known, several factors have been implicated. These include genetic, hormonal, and environmental factors as well as infectious agents. While evidence for each of these factors is variable, it is most likely that some interaction of several of them is responsible for the development of prostatic cancer.

Clinical Findings

A. Symptoms and Signs: Up to 50% of men with prostate cancer have no symptoms of the disease. Stage A patients may have bladder outlet obstructive symptoms, but a clinically benign gland by examination allows transurethral prostatectomy to be performed. Up to 40% of patients with stage B or higher disease may be totally asymptomatic. When patients do have symptoms, they are commonly those of bladder outlet obstruction, uremia secondary to ureteral obstruction, or bone pain due to metastatic disease. The most common sign of the disease is the finding of a hard, painless mass in the prostate on digital rectal examination.

B. Laboratory Findings:

1. Prostate specific antigen (PSA) is a serum protease produced only by prostatic epithelial cells. It is thus specific for prostate production but not for prostate cancer. Its use is revolutionizing both the diagnosis and treatment approaches to prostate cancer. However, PSA may be normal in early stages, and 80% of patients with mild elevations (4–10 ng/mL, Hybritech assay) will show only benign hyperplasia on biopsy.

2. In the absence of higher stage disease, serum laboratory findings are usually normal. Patients with advanced local disease may have elevated blood urea nitrogen (BUN) and creatinine if they are azotemic. Those with bony metastases may have elevated alkaline or acid phosphatase levels. Acid phosphatase may also be elevated in some stage C patients with advanced local disease, but most often it is normal.

C. Imaging Studies: X-ray studies are normal in patients with pathologic stage A and B disease, as well as for many with stage C and D1 disease. Plain radiographs of the abdomen are normal in all but those with advanced osteoblastic metastases, and intravenous pyelograms are normal unless ureteral obstruction has occurred. Abdominal and pelvic CT scans may reveal periprostatic, pelvic, or periaortic adenopathy, but many patients with low-volume lymphadenopathy will have normal or equivocal CT scans. MRI may provide a higher degree of accuracy in the clinical assessment of these nodes. Isotopic bone scans (technetium) are more sensitive than plain radiographs in detecting osseous metastasis. They should be performed in all patients undergoing staging, since many patients with bone metastases will be free of bone pain.

D. Additional Studies: Needle biopsy of suspicious areas is performed to obtain histologic confirmation. Pedal lymphangiography is helpful primarily in defining positive lymph nodes in the aortic area and less helpful in the diagnosis of pelvic spread. For this reason, lymphangiography is rarely performed in the staging of patients with prostatic cancer. Fine-needle aspiration with cytologic study is helpful in occasional patients who have visible but not obvious pelvic lymphadenopathy. Such studies, performed under CT scan guidance, will confirm whether a patient has stage D1 disease, and pelvic lymphadenectomy can be avoided in those in whom the aspiration is positive.

Transrectal ultrasound of the prostate is helpful in directing the biopsy of suspicious lesions. Carcinomas generally appear hypoechoic compared to the rest of the prostate, and biopsies under ultrasound guidance can be performed as an outpatient procedure. The routine "screening" of all men over age 50 by ultrasound examination is advocated by some, but the value of ultrasound as sole screening test remains to be proved.

Routes of Dissemination

A. Local Invasion: Extension beyond the capsule of the prostate is common with prostate cancer. Involved tissues may include the seminal vessicles, the bladder, and the external sphincter portion of the urethra distal to the prostate. Actual invasion into the rectal wall is rare because of the barrier called Denonvilliers' fascia.

B. Lymphatic Spread: The initial area of lymphatic spread of prostate cancer is to the nodes around the obturator nerve and internal iliac (hypogastric) artery. Further spread into the common iliac, external iliac, and periaortic nodes then occurs. Lymphatic spread to the supraclavicular nodes is not uncommon in patients with widespread disease.

C. Hematogenous Spread: The most common blood-borne spread is to the bones. Most frequently involved are the central axial bones, including the lumbar vertebrae and pelvis. Long bones, ribs, and skull are also involved in late-stage disease. Bony lesions are usually osteoblastic and occur in 85% of those dying from prostate cancer. Visceral hematogenous spread may occur to the lung, liver, and adrenal gland but is rare in the absence of bone metastases.

Staging

The staging system used most commonly in the USA is the Whitmore-Jewett system.

Stage A: Nonpalpable tumor found incidentally after transurethral prostatectomy for benign prostatic hypertrophy.

Stage A-1: Less than 5% of the resected tissue, and must be low grade or well differentiated.

Stage A-2: More than 5% of the resected tissue, or histologic grade other than well differentiated, or both.

Stage B: A palpable carcinoma on digital examination, confined to the prostate.

Stage B-1: Less than 1.5 cm in diameter and confined to one lobe.

Stage B-2: Greater than 1.5 cm in diameter, or involves both lobes.

Stage C: Local extension through the capsule into periprostatic tissues.

Stage D: Demonstrable distant metastasis.

Stage D-1: Pelvic lymph node involvement only.

Stage D-2: All other distant disease, including periaortic nodes, visceral spread, and osseous metastasis.

Differential Diagnosis

Firm nodules and areas of induration in the prostate may be caused by carcinoma, nodular benign, prostatic hypertrophy, and prostatic calculi or phleboliths. Biopsy is required to distinguish carcinoma from the benign lesions. The presence of prostatic calculi on a plain abdominal film should not preclude performance of a biopsy, since the two entities of stones and cancer can occur together.

Treatment

A. Localized Disease: The decision to treat localized disease should be based on several factors in addition to the histologic diagnosis of cancer. In general, prostate cancer is relatively slow growing, a biologic variability that accounts for its relatively high incidence and increased incidence with advancing age. For this reason, only one-third of men who develop it have clinical evidence of the disease prior to death due to some other unrelated cause. Therefore, age at the time of diagnosis must be considered when determining whether or not to treat a patient with localized disease. In general, a patient should have a 10-year life expectancy if local treatment is to be offered. Thus, most urologic oncologists would not treat a man with localized disease unless he was age 75 or younger. Similarly, treatment of a 68-year-old

man with multiple, severe medical problems may not be warranted. The decision to offer therapy is further tempered by the histologic pattern of the tumor: poorly differentiated cancers appear to progress more rapidly than well-differentiated cancers. The decision to offer therapy is more readily arrived at for those patients with the more poorly differentiated cancers.

Patients with stage A-1 disease generally are thought to have a normal life expectancy without treatment of that cancer. This no-treatment policy is usually predicated on repeat transurethral resection to ensure that additional residual cancer is not present. If additional cancer is found, definitive treatment usually is offered. There is a growing willingness to treat stage A-1 cancers in younger men, ie, aged 55–60.

Patients with clinical stage A-2, B-1, and B-2 disease are generally considered candidates for local therapy within the guidelines above. Whether the intended therapy is surgical or radiotherapeutic, all patients should be staged pathologically by pelvic lymph node dissection, since 20–60% will have positive lymph nodes despite negative radiographic staging studies. This is particularly true in patients with poorly differentiated cancers.

The best treatment for localized prostate cancer continues to be debated. Radiotherapy was popular for many years, but recent data indicate that short-term (5-year) survival rates are not adequate to evaluate results of therapy and that positive biopsies after radiotherapy may well predict eventual disease progression. In addition, "nerve-sparing" radical prostatectomy is now possible, with preservation of potency in about two-thirds of males. For these reasons, radical prostatectomy has gained in popularity in recent years and probably is considered the procedure of choice by urologists. For patients declining radical surgery, radiotherapy is still a reasonable alternative. External beam radiotherapy alone may be utilized, or this may be combined with interstitial radiotherapy using radioactive gold [198]Au. Interstitial therapy alone may be given using radioactive iodine ^{125}I or iridium [192]Ir.

B. Clinical Stage C: Patients with stage C disease are generally not considered surgical candidates owing to the greater risk of complications and the high recurrence rate, both locally in the pelvis and distantly. Treatment of choice is external beam therapy, but this should be used only in those who are shown to be node negative by pelvic lymphadenectomy. There is no evidence that irradiation has survival value in patients with positive lymph nodes.

C. Distant Disease: Patients with stage D disease do not appear to benefit from treatment of the primary tumor, either by surgery or radiotherapy. Significant palliative therapy can be offered by hormonal manipulation (Chapter 15). This may be accomplished by orchiectomy to remove the end organ responsible for most testosterone production or by the administration of exogenous estrogen to block production of testosterone. Castrate levels of testosterone may be predictably achieved by the administration of diethylstilbestrol, 3 mg/d. Estrogen therapy must be used cautiously, since it may cause cardiovascular complications including congestive heart failure, thrombophlebitis, and myocardial infarction, even in patients with no history of cardiovascular disease (10%). For this reason, medical castration now is more often accomplished by the use of luteinizing hormone–releasing hormone (LHRH) analogs, which accomplish a castrate level of testosterone owing to feedback inhibition of the hypothalmic-pituitary axis. They have the advantage of avoiding the cardiovascular side effects seen with estrogen therapy. "Total androgen ablation" using a combination of LHRH analog and flutamide (a nonsteroidal antiandrogen) provides increased benefit over LHRH analog alone. However, the role of flutamide in conjunction with orchiectomy remains to be determined.

The optimal timing of hormonal therapy in asymptomatic patients remains unclear and a matter of physician preference. Many physicians withhold therapy until symptoms develop, so that significant remission will be possible (often 12–24 months) when symptoms do develop. Others feel that early therapy may delay the progression to symptomatic disease, though there is little to offer such patients once they do progress.

Patients failing hormonal therapy may be treated with aminoglutethimide or ketoconazole (both inhibit adrenal testosterone production), with variable response. Radiotherapy to painful bony lesions may provide significant pain control. Occasional patients may require transurethral resection of the prostate to relieve bladder outlet obstruction. Chemotherapy has generally been of little value in prostate cancer, whether as single-agent or combination therapy.

Prognosis

A cure rate of 50–75% can be expected with radical surgery in pathologic stage B-1 patients. This rate decreases in both B-2 and A-2 patients. Since only 10–15% of patients with prostate cancer are stage B-1 at diagnosis, only a small fraction are potentially curable. The greatest improvement in this situation can only be realized by annual screening by digital rectal examination in all men over age 50.

URETHRAL CANCER

Carcinoma of the urethra is rare in both men and woman, with a female-to-male ratio of 3:1. In both sexes, squamous cell carcinomas are the most common, followed by transitional cell carcinomas. Likewise, chronic inflammation has been implicated in etiology, since many patients have chronic infections or a history of urethral strictures.

Signs and symptoms in both sexes are those most commonly associated with infection, namely, bleeding, dysuria, urinary obstruction, or a palpable mass. Lesions in women are often mistaken for urethral caruncle, an inflammatory mass requiring incision and drainage. Delay in diagnosis is common in urethral cancer.

Diagnosis is made by transurethral biopsy. In females, distal cancers may be amenable to wide local excision, though cystourethrectomy may provide safer surgical margins. Proximal lesions or deeply invasive distal lesions are probably best treated by preoperative radiotherapy and anterior exenteration, with urinary diversion, though the value of radiotherapy may be more apparent than real.

In males, urethral cancers occur more commonly in the bulbomembranous or proximal urethra. These often present at higher stages, with invasion of surrounding tissues. Preoperative radiotherapy with widely radical surgery including cystoprostatourethrectomy is required. Distal urethral lesions are more likely to be superficial and may be amenable to treatment by urethrectomy alone or possibly by partial penectomy.

Inguinal lymphadenectomy is not routinely performed but is reserved for those patients who present with palpable adenopathy. If cystourethrectomy is necessary, pelvic lymphadenectomy should be performed at the same time.

Although urethral cancers traditionally have not been responsive to chemotherapy, early data suggest that patients with transitional cell cancer of the urethra might have some response to the combination of methotrexate, vinblastine, doxorubicin, and cisplatin. Whether patients should receive this therapy preoperatively instead of radiotherapy or in lieu of surgery remains to be determined.

The prognosis is good for distal, superficial cancers, approximating 60–75% survival. It is much worse for proximal or extensive lesions, approaching 20% survival in several series.

PENILE CANCER

General Considerations

The incidence of penile cancer is about 1:100,000 males per year in the USA. It occurs primarily in men in the fifth and sixth decades. Its association with noncircumcision is clear. The disease is nonexistent in the Jewish population but may approach an incidence of 20% in some African tribes that do not practice circumcision and also suffer from poor hygiene. Since only 2% of male cancer deaths in the USA are due to penile cancer, much debate has arisen over the value of routine neonatal circumcision, with opponents citing low incidence as poor grounds for routine circumcision. Whether the incidence of penile carcinoma will rise as circumcision is performed less frequently remains to be seen.

Several potentially premalignant lesions have been identified. These include condyloma acuminatum, with a small portion of patients eventually developing carcinoma despite successful therapy of their warts. Buschke-Löwenstein's tumor is actually a giant condyloma that invades and destroys adjacent tissue, despite a benign histologic appearance. Leukoplakia is an additional benign lesion that presents as a white cutaneous plaque. It may be present adjacent to a carcinoma or may antedate the development of a carcinoma. Finally, erythroplasia of Queyrat, or Bowen's disease, is carcinoma in situ of the penile foreskin. While not an invasive lesion, it is probably best treated by aggressive circumcision, although topical medications such as fluorouracil cream may successfully eradicate erythroplasia in occasional patients.

Invasive carcinomas most often originate on the glans or prepuce and only rarely originate on the penile shaft. Ulcerative lesions are common, but exophytic lesions may occur and are difficult to distinguish from Buschke-Löwenstein's tumor except by biopsy. These are almost all squamous cell carcinomas. Delay in diagnosis is common, with many patients presenting with extremely large tumors because of justifiable fear of the diagnosis and treatment. Since primary lymphatic drainage is to the superficial inguinal nodes, these are often enlarged at the time of presentation (25–50%) owing to metastasis (50%) or inflammation due to skin ulceration (50%).

Clinical Findings

Penile cancer begins as a painless nodule with an appearance similar to that of condyloma acumination, ulceration, or blisters. At least half of patients have phimosis. About half of patients will have palpable inguinal lymph nodes at presentation. Since the disease spreads very slowly, laboratory tests should be essentially normal.

The diagnosis is confirmed by a wide excisional biopsy if the lesion is not too large or by an incisional biopsy if it is too large to justify partial penectomy prior to having a histologic diagnosis. Inguinal and pelvic lymph nodes should be assessed by pedal lymphangiography or CT scan. Some favor "sentinel node biopsy," whereas others favor treatment of the primary penile lesion followed by 6 weeks of antibiotic therapy with clinical follow-up of the adenopathy (see below).

Treatment

Most lesions can be successfully treated with local excision including a 2-cm margin. This may require partial penectomy, but compromise to save penile corporeal tissue should be avoided. More proximal tumors or those that are so large that a functional stump will not be left should be treated with total penectomy and perineal urethrostomy.

The treatment of adenopathy is controversial. Debate over the best treatment of clinically palpable inguinal lymph nodes exists for two reasons. The morbidity associated with routine inguinal lymph node dissection is great, with complications including significant skin flap necrosis in up to 50% of patients. On the other hand, this carcinoma is not curable except by surgery, and delay in resection of small amounts of nodal tissue may doom the patient to further progression of disease. A sentinel node biopsy is much more limited than a groin dissection, but the ability of every surgeon to correctly identify and resect the sentinel node (the very first in the chain of lymph drainage) is doubtful. Thus, in an attempt to spare patients morbidity, a nonsurgical conservative approach is usually adopted, whether it is antibiotic therapy with close clinical follow-up or sentinel node biopsy. Conversely, patients with grossly positive nodes that contain cancer probably do not benefit from total groin dissection, since the deep pelvic nodes are usually involved, and survival at this stage of disease is rare.

Prognosis

For patients with superficial lesions, 5-year survival approaches 80%. For those with distant disease or inguinal and pelvic metastasis, it approaches zero. Death is usually due to inanition or hemorrhage and infection due to erosion into local tissues of the groin from pelvic and inguinal foci of the disease.

REFERENCES

Renal Cell Carcinoma

Carini M et al: Conservative surgical treatment of renal cell carcinoma: Clinical experience and reappraisal of indications. *J Urol* 1988;**140:**725.

Novick AC et al: Conservative surgery for renal cell carcinoma: A single-center experience with 100 patients. *J Urol* 1989;**141:**835.

Robson CJ: Radical nephrectomy for renal cell carcinoma. *J Urol* 1963;**89:**37.

Rosenberg SA et al: A progress report on the treatment of 157 patients with advanced cancer using lymphokine-activated killer cells and interleukin-2 or high-dose interleukin-2 alone. *N Engl J Med* 1987;**316:**889.

Trump DL et al: High-dose lymphoblastoid interferon in advanced renal cell carcinoma: An Eastern Cooperative Oncology Group Study. *Cancer Treat Rep* 1987;**71**:165.

Ziegelbaum M et al: Conservative surgery for transitional cell carcinoma of the renal pelvis. *J Urol* 1987;**138**:1146.

Bladder Carcinoma

Brosman SA: The use of bacillus Calmette-Guérin in the therapy of bladder carcinoma in situ. *J Urol* 1985;**134**:36.

Droller MJ: Bladder carcinoma: An overview. Pages 214–220 in: *Current Genitourinary Cancer Surgery.* Crawford EE, Das S (editors). Lea & Febiger, 1990.

Lamm DL, Sosnowski JT: Immunotherapy of bladder carcinoma. Pages 477–492 in: *Current Genitourinary Cancer Surgery.* Crawford EE, Das S (editors). Lea & Febiger, 1990.

Rowland RG et al: Indiana continent urinary reservoir. *J Urol* 1987;**137**:1136.

Skinner DG, Lieskovsky G, Boyd S: Continent urinary diversion. *J Urol* 1989;**141**:1323.

Sternberg CN et al: M-VAC for advanced transitional cell carcinoma of the urothelium. *J Urol* 1988;**139**:461.

Cancer of the Renal Pelvis & Ureter

Babaian RJ, Johnson, DE: Primary carcinoma of the ureter. *J Urol* 1980;**123**:357.

Reitelman C et al: Prognostic variables in patients with transitional cell carcinoma of the renal pelvis and proximal ureter. *J Urol* 1987;**138**:1144.

Zincke H, Neves RJ: Feasibility of conservative surgery for transitional cell cancer of the upper urinary tract. *Urol Clin North Am* 1984;**11**:717.

Testicular Cancer

Birch R et al: Prognostic factors for favorable outcome in disseminated germ cell tumors. *J Clin Oncol* 1986;**4**:400.

Bosl GJ et al: A randomized trial of etoposide plus cisplatin versus vinblastine plus bleomycin plus cisplatin plus cyclophosphamide plus dactinomycin in patients with good prognosis germ cell tumors. *J Clin Oncol* 1988;**8**:1231.

Einhorn LH et al: A comparison of four courses of cisplatin, VP-16 and bleomycin (PVP-16B) in favorable prognosis disseminated germ cell tumors: A southeastern study group (SECSG) protocol. *Proc Am Soc Clin Oncol* 1988;**7**:120.

Jewett MAS et al: Retroperitoneal lymphadenectomy for testis tumor with nerve sparing for ejaculation. *J Urol* 1988;**139**:1220.

Pizzocaro G et al: Difficulties of a surveillance study omitting retroperitoneal lymphadenectomy in clinical stage I nonseminomatous germ cell tumors of the testis. *J Urol* 1987;**138**:1393.

Sarosdy MF: Testicular cancer: An overview. Pages 306–318 in: *Current Genitourinary Cancer Surgery.* Crawford ED, Das S (editors). Lea & Febiger, 1990.

Williams SD et al: Early stage testis cancer: The testicular cancer intergroup study. In: *Adjuvant Therapy of Cancer V.* Salmon SE (editor). Grune & Stratton, 1987.

Carcinoma of the Prostate

Boileau MA et al: Interstitial gold and external beam irradiation for prostate cancer. *J Urol* 1988;**139**:985.

Byar DP: The Veterans Administration Cooperative Urological Research Group's studies of cancer of the prostate. *Cancer* 1973;**32**:1126.

Catalona WJ et al: Measurement of prostatic specific antigen in serum as a screening test for prostate cancer. *N Engl J Med* 1991;**324**:1156.

Cooner WH et al: Prostate cancer detection in a clinical urological practice by ultrasonography, digital rectal examination and prostate specific antigen. *J Urol* 1990;**143**:1146.

Stamey TA et al: Prostate-specific antigen as a serum marker for adenocarcinoma of the prostate. *N Engl J Med* 1987;**317**:909.

Walsh PC, Lepor H, Eggleston JC: Radical prostatectomy with preservation of sexual function: Anatomical and pathological considerations. *Prostate* 1983;**4**:47.

Urethral Cancer

Hopkins SC et al: Carcinoma of the female urethra: Reassessment of modes of therapy. *J Urol* 1983;**129**:958.

Penile Cancer

Cabanas RM: An approach for the treatment of penile carcinoma. *Cancer* 1977;**39**:456.

Mohs PE et al: Microscopically controlled surgery in the treatment of carcinoma of the penis. *J Urol* 1985;**133**:961.

22

Gynecologic Cancer

John J. Kavanagh, MD, Andrzej P. Kudelka, MD, & Creighton L. Edwards, MD

OVARIAN CANCER

Essentials of Diagnosis

- Abdominal fullness, bloating, pain or mass, early satiety, pelvic pressure.
- Elevated serum CA-125 for epithelial tumors and β-hCG or AFP for germ cell tumors.

MALIGNANT EPITHELIAL TUMORS

Epidemiology & Etiology

Ovarian cancer accounts for 4% of malignancies in women and 27% of female reproductive cancers. The mortality rate of over 60% makes it the most lethal of female reproductive neoplasms. One of 70 newborn girls will develop ovarian cancer, with the highest risk occurring at 65–84 years of age. A history of nulliparity and of breast or endometrial cancer doubles the risk.

No clear cause for ovarian cancer has been demonstrated. Transvaginal transport of carcinogens as talc has been considered. Dietary excesses of fat have also been proposed. The process of uninterrupted ovulation has been offered as an explanation for the increased risk in the nulliparous. No preventive measures for the disease are known, and routine pelvic examination and Papanicolaou smear do not reveal early-stage malignancy.

Pathogenesis

After penetration of the ovarian capsule, malignant extension occurs by diffuse intraperitoneal implantation and the development of ascites. There is also local organ invasion of the uterine (fallopian) tube, uterus, bladder, lower colon, and omentum. At presentation, extension to pelvic lymph nodes is common. As the disease progresses, aortic, mediastinal, inguinal, and supraclavicular node involvement occurs. Transdiaphragmatic extension to the pleura may explain the frequency of patients presenting with malignant pleural effusions. Hematogenous metastases

are unusual at presentation. However, with advancing disease and relapse, liver metastases are more frequent. Cutaneous metastases occur late as subcutaneous nodules or erythematous small plaques. Brain and pulmonary metastases are more frequent with increased survival and may occur in the absence of other sites of clinical relapse. Leptomeningeal disease is a clinical curiosity, and symptomatic bone disease is exceedingly rare.

The usual cause of death is a terminal event related to inanition created by persistent ascites and refractory recurrent bowel obstruction. If intra-abdominal disease is modest, then death is due to uncontrolled pulmonary or brain metastases.

Pathology & Grading

Epithelial ovarian tumors are considered adenocarcinomas. **Serous** carcinomas represent about 50% of tumors. **Mucinous** types represent 10–15% and may produce the pseudomyxoma peritonei syndrome. **Endometrioid** tumors resemble endometrial adenocarcinoma, and simultaneous occurrence of both is present in 30% of cases. Concurrent endometriosis is present in 10% of cases. **Clear-cell** carcinomas occur in 5% of cases and are also associated with endometriosis and endometrial cancer. Hypercalcemia may also be seen. **Small-cell** carcinoma is rare, occurs in young women, may cause hypercalcemia, and has a poor prognosis. Malignant **Brenner** tumors are also rare and consist of transitional or squamous epithelium in benign stroma.

Histologic grading is important for prognosis and therapy. Although there is no uniform method, two systems are in common practice. The "pattern" system considers the general microscopic appearance of the lesion. Lesions range from grade I (well differentiated) to grade II (moderately differentiated to grade III (poorly differentiated) depending on a predominantly papillary pattern to a solid pattern, respectively. Broder's grading system ranges from grades I to IV depending on the cytologic and nuclear characteristics, with grade IV being an undifferentiated lesion. Pathologists usually use a combination of both systems. **Borderline** tumors are a distinct entity with complex papillations having a slightly atypical epithelial covering and, most importantly, no stromal invasion. These lesions are usually confined to the ovary, warrant conservative therapy, and are rarely fatal even if disseminated.

Clinical Findings

A. Symptoms and Signs: Symptoms are insidious and indicate advanced disease. The two most common complaints are abdominal distention requiring wardrobe modifications and vague chronic abdominal discomfort. Weight gain with ascites may occur. Menstrual abnormalities and weight loss are *not* the usual presenting complaints. Constipation may indicate extrinsic compression of the lower bowel from tumor. Nausea, vomiting, and borborygmi suggest small bowel obstruction.

Most women appear well nourished and in minimal distress. Palpable supraclavicular lymphadenopathy is found in a small percentage of cases. Pleural effusion may be present. The abdominal examination frequently demonstrates ascites or multiple deep indurated areas suggestive of omental tumor. Abdominal distention with mild tenderness and hyperperistaltic bowel sounds suggests small bowel obstruction. The pelvic examination usually has normal-appearing external genitalia, vaginal mucosa, and cervix. The bimanual and essential rectovaginal examinations reveal an adnexal mass of varying size and consistency. Palpable adnexa in the postmenopausal woman, ovarian adherence to the uterus, and cul-de-sac masses point to malignancy. Part of the examination should include a cervical Papanicolaou smear. If malignancy is strongly suspected, endometrial sampling should be done.

B. Laboratory Findings: There are no predictable abnormalities. A marked deviation should cause consideration of the presence of another disease process or an unusual manifestation of the malignancy, ie, severe anemia secondary to a bleeding gastrointestinal metastasis or renal failure secondary to malignant obstructive uropathy. Hypoxemia may be present in those patients with pleural effusion. An elevated ovarian cancer antigen assay (CA-125) will predict cancer in over 80% of postmenopausal women with a palpable adnexal mass. If it is elevated preoperatively, plans should be made for an appropriate oncologic procedure. The CA-125 is a monoclonal antibody assay that is directed against a large glycoprotein antigen found on the surface of an ovarian cancer cell line. The half-life of the antigen is approximately 5 days. It is not useful as a population screen. The vast majority of epithelial malignancies produce the antigen heterogeneously within the neoplastic cell populations. Serous carcinoma has the highest positivity. The CA-125 may revert to normal after tumor reductive surgery. A persistent or sequentially increasing titer preludes clinical relapse, progression, or persistence of disease. The CA-125 is elevated in several other cancers, particularly of gynecologic origin. Inflammatory processes of the female genital tract also will cause increased measurements.

C. Imaging Studies: These studies should be viewed as diagnostic or as preoperative preparation. The chest x-ray may reveal pleural effusion, which should be tapped for pathologic confirmation. Mammograms may show a second primary. Metastatic breast cancer to the abdomen also is within the differential diagnosis and will cause an elevated CA-125. A barium enema will evaluate the degree of narrowing or the presence of a primary colon cancer. An abdominal ultrasound or CT scan should be done to evaluate the pancreas as a primary neoplastic source and determine the presence of hepatic metastases. A pelvic ultrasound showing a mass with solid components >5 cm in diameter often means malignancy. CT scans and magnetic resonance imaging (MRI) do not have a clearly defined role in the surveillance of patients with ovarian cancer.

D. Other Studies: A cervical cytologic smear and endometrial aspiration should be done. If there are symptoms of early satiety, weight loss, or upper abdominal pain, upper gastrointestinal endoscopy should be considered to rule out gastric carcinoma. Diagnostic paracentesis with a small-gauge needle may confirm the presence of a malignancy and point to a source.

Differential Diagnosis

The differential diagnosis will depend on the menopausal status, age, and presence of extraovarian findings. The young woman with an adnexal mass and no other findings may have a functionally cystic ovary, endometriosis, a benign ovarian tumor as a dermoid, ectopic pregnancy, tubo-ovarian cyst, or cancer including a germ cell tumor. The postmenopausal woman with ascites and a large solid adnexal mass has epithelial ovarian cancer until proved otherwise. The practical differential diagnosis includes malignant sex cord stromal tumors; ovarian metastases from a stomach, colon, pancreas, breast, lung, or melanoma primary; and rare ovarian malignancies such as mixed mesodermal sarcomas, pure sarcomas, and lymphomas. Occasionally, large benign tumors such as serous cystadenomas and fibroma–theca cell tumors are found.

Treatment

The patient with suspected ovarian cancer should undergo laparotomy for three purposes. The first is to accurately diagnose and stage the cancer. The second is to perform maximal debulking of tumor, which has prognostic import. The third is to relieve bowel obstruction caused by tumor even if colostomy and extensive resection are required. A bowel preparation is customary preoperatively. Thoracentesis with chest tube drainage or pleurodesis may be necessary for patients with significant pleural effusions prior to surgery. Central venous access and antibiotic prophylaxis are desirable. The essential steps of the initial laparotomy are set forth in Table 22–1.

Optimal debulking of tumor to <2 cm residual tumor is possible in over 25% of patients with stage III disease. Operative mortality is approximately 2% with acceptable blood loss. Major postoperative morbidity is not uncommon, consisting of congestive heart failure, pulmonary embolus, wound dehiscence, and ileus. Although residual disease clearly prognosticates survival, it is still not clear whether surgery is informational or therapeutic. Nevertheless, successful bulk reduction offers excellent short-term palliation for the patient with symptomatic intra-abdominal disease and allows better patient tolerance to chemotherapy.

In younger patients wishing to retain fertility, a unilateral oophorectomy with complete staging including contralateral ovarian biopsy may be acceptable. However, this applies only if the tumor is confined to one ovary, particularly if it is a borderline or grade I tumor. The development of in vitro fertilization with exogenous hormonal support may make uterus preservation a stronger consideration in this particular group of patients.

After surgery is completed, the patient should be characterized as to histologic grade, stage, and residual disease, ie, <2 cm, <1 cm, <0.5 cm, or none. The term **residual** means the maximum diameter of the largest remaining tumor mass even if multiple in number. The definition of plaquelike lesions varies. The staging criteria are those of the International Federation of Gynecology and Obstetrics (FIGO) (Table 22–2).

Postoperative Therapy

A. Early-Stage Disease: For patients with stage I, grade I (well-differentiated) cancer, no further therapy is necessary. Follow-up consisting of periodic pelvic examinations and CA-125 determinations is

Table 22–1. Essential steps of a staging laparotomy.

1. Midline vertical incision.
2. Evacuation and cytologic analysis of ascites.
3. If ascites absent, cytologic washing of pelvis and paracolonic gutters.
4. Inspection and palpation of the subdiaphragmatic areas, intraperitoneal contents, and retroperitoneal areas including pancreas.
5. Frozen section of ovarian mass (unilateral or bilateral).
6. If carcinoma on frozen section, hysterectomy and bilateral salpingo-oophorectomy.
7. Omentectomy with optimal bulk reduction of remaining tumor masses.
8. Relief of intestinal obstruction by resection or colostomy.
9. If disease limited to ovaries, multiple biopsies including the paracolonic gutters, cul-de-sac, lateral pelvic walls, vesicouterine reflection, subdiaphragmatic sites, and intra-abdominal areas.
10. Ipsilateral and para-aortic lymph node sampling if conservative therapy planned.

Table 22–2. FIGO staging system for ovarian cancer.[1]

Stage	Clinical Findings
I	Tumor limited to the ovaries.
IA	Tumor limited to one ovary; no tumor on ovarian surface, capsule intact; no malignant cells in ascites or peritoneal washings.
IB	Tumor limited to both ovaries; no tumor on the ovarian surface, capsule intact; no malignant cells in ascites or peritoneal washings.
IC	Tumor either stage IA or stage IB but with tumor on the surface of one or both ovaries, or with capsule ruptured, or with malignant cells in ascites or peritoneal washings.
II	Tumor involving one or both ovaries with pelvic extension.
IIA	Extension or metastasis to the uterus or tubes.
IIB	Extension to other pelvic tissues.
IIC	Tumor either stage IIA or IIB with malignant cells in ascites or peritoneal washings.
III	Tumor involving one or both ovaries with microscopically confirmed peritoneal implants outside the pelvis (including the liver capsule) or retroperitoneal or inguinal lymph node metastasis.
IIIA	Tumor grossly limited to the true pelvis with negative nodes but with microscopic abdominal peritoneal metastasis.
IIIB	Macroscopic abdominal peritoneal metastasis 2 cm or less in diameter; lymph nodes negative.
IIIC	Macroscopic abdominal peritoneal metastasis greater than 2 cm in diameter or retroperitoneal or inguinal lymph node metastasis.
IV	Tumor with distant metastasis (excludes peritoneal metastasis). Pleural effusion with positive cytology. Parenchymal liver metastasis.

[1]Modified and reproduced, with permission, form Bearhs OH et al (editors): *Manual for Staging of Cancer,* 4th ed. Lippincott, 1992.

adequate. Patients with less well differentiated cancer present a dilemma. For patients with grade II (moderately differentiated) cancer, conservative therapy is reasonable under the following conditions: (1) lesion confined to ovary; (2) unilaterality; (3) capsule microscopically intact with no tumor excrescences; (4) no operative spillage; (5) no ascites; (6) negative abdominal pelvic washings. Five-year survival should be greater than 90%. Patients who violate these parameters or have grade III (undifferentiated) tumors warrant further therapy.

Therapy may consist of melphalan or 15 mCi of intraperitoneal ^{32}P in early-stage disease. A randomized trial by the Gynecologic Oncology Group comparing these therapies in patients with stage I (Aii, Bii, C), II (A, B, C), or grade III, stage I (Ai or Bi) showed an equal 80% 5-year survival. Relapse usually occurred within 2 years. The ^{32}P is preferred because of the brevity of treatment and absence of leukemogenic risk. Whole-abdomen radiotherapy using 2250 cGy in 22 fractions as an open-field technique, a pelvic boost of 2250 cGy in 10 fractions, and posterior kidney shielding has also been recommended for these patients. The Princess Margaret Hospital of Toronto, Canada, reported a 69% (77:111) 5-year survival in an analogous patient population treated by radiation. More aggressive cytoxic therapy for this category of patients is under investigation.

B. Advanced Disease: Cisplatin-based chemotherapy should be given to patients with stage IV or stage III macroscopic residual cancer. Chemotherapy should be started within 4 weeks of surgery. If ascites is reaccumulating or an overwhelming tumor burden is hindering recovery, therapy may be given 7–10 days after surgery. In the bedridden patient with open wounds or prolonged infections, neutropenia should be avoided. An initial moderate dose of cisplatin, 75 mg/m^2, or carboplatin may be used to gain tumor control and not delay therapy. A standard chemotherapy program is as follows:

Drugs: Cyclophosphamide 500 mg–1g/m^2 intravenously Cisplatin, 75–100 mg/m^2 intravenously
Cycle: Every 21–28 days
Duration: 6–8 cycles

Current available data from randomized trials do not support the use of doxorubicin or hexamethylmelamine in the combination. In addition, dose escalations of cisplatin above 100 mg/m^2 produce significant auditory, visual, and neuropathic toxicity and have not shown long-term benefit as induction therapy. Six to eight cycles of therapy are adequate, with cumulative toxicity necessitating dosage reduction and delays beyond this number. During therapy the major problems are prolonged nausea, anemia, fatigue, peripheral neuropathy, and hearing loss. Combination antiemetics are essential to effectively control vomiting.

Carboplatin is a cisplatin analog with markedly fewer gastrointestinal, neurologic, or ototoxic and nephropathic side effects. However, it causes more myelosuppression, particularly thrombocytopenia, in heavily treated or irradiated patients. It should be used in patients with underlying conditions or side effects (including renal failure) that preclude cisplatin therapy. Fragile elderly or emotionally labile patients may tolerate carboplatin relatively better. Randomized trials comparing carboplatin and cyclophosphamide to cisplatin and carboplatin as primary therapy show equal efficacy. Recommended doses are carboplatin, 300–360 mg/m^2, and cyclophosphamide, 300–500 mg/m^2, on a monthly basis for 6–8 courses. If necessary, lower doses of cyclophosphamide should be used so that the carboplatin dose is not compromised.

For patients with stage III microscopic residual after surgery, the above chemotherapy is also used. Abdominal and pelvic radiotherapy is an alternative, and 10-year survival rates of 42% (27:42) have been reported. This observation is under study in randomized trials.

Intraperitoneal chemotherapy has been utilized for many years with several drugs. Recent efforts have concentrated on cisplatin and etoposide (VP-16). As part of initial therapy it remains unproved. It is not effective in tumor nodules >0.5 cm or for patients with progressive disease while on cisplatin. It may have a role in the palliation of recurrent ascites. Cisplatin-treated patients with partial response have been converted to complete response in about 30% of cases.

Cisplatin-sensitive tumors that relapse after more than a 1-year chemotherapy-free interval will often respond when retreated with systemic cisplatin or carboplatin. The latter will generally be better tolerated if myelosuppression is not a problem.

If the patient's renal function is compromised, the patient may be treated with single-agent carboplatin. The dose is determined using the Calvert formula:

$$TD = AUC (GFR + 25)$$

where TD indicates the total dose of carboplatin infused (not the dose per meter squared of body surface area). AUC refers to the *area under the curve* of serum carboplatin versus time. An AUC of 4–5 is used for previously treated patients and an AUC of 7 for previously untreated patients. GFR indicates the glomerular filtration rate.

C. Restaging Laparotomy: After completing the prescribed therapy, about half of patients will have no clinical evidence of disease, but the status of the cancer is uncertain. Abdominal CT scans will find biopsy-confirmed disease in about 20% of patients. Laparoscopy will be positive in 30–50% of cases with a false-negative rate of 35%. Frequently a restaging or "second-look" laparotomy is done and includes multiple biopsies, particularly of prior disease-bearing sites and peritoneal washings. Approximately 50% of patients will have persistent macroscopic disease, 25% microscopic disease, and 25% negative findings. Patients with macroscopic residual have a median survival of 18–24 months. Microscopic persistence may be associated with prolonged survival, particularly with grade I tumors or biopsies showing glandular inclusions; however, grade III lesions have continuous relapse and few 5-year survivors. Unfortunately, 30–50% of patients with pathologically negative findings relapse, particularly those with grade III cancer.

Selecting meaningful therapy for patients with persistent disease is difficult. Macroscopic disease is particularly resistant, and investigational agents or observation is recommended. Continuing chemotherapy or changing to nonplatinating agents has not proved benefit. Patients with microscopic and negative laparotomies may benefit from intraperitoneal cisplatin, intraperitoneal ^{32}P, or abdominal or pelvic radiotherapy. All these modalities are under study. At present, the restaging laparotomy should be considered investigational surgery of limited prognostic value and capable of stratifying patients for experimental studies.

Patients with recurrent disease resistant to cisplatin or carboplatin reinduction have few options. Chemotherapeutic treatment with alternative agents is not usually successful. Biologic response modifiers have not proved effective. Hormonal therapies with progestational compounds, tamoxifen, or gonadotropin agonists are associated with a low (but definite) response rate and have a palliative role. Estrogen and progesterone receptors are present to some degree in most tumors but do not correlate well with grade or hormonal response. Aggressive surgical procedures in the absence of effective chemotherapy and in the presence of ascites or extensive tumor are associated with significant in-hospital mortality and short survival. Investigational programs (eg, taxol, taxotere, a third-generation platinum compound, a camptothecin derivative) or supportive care are often the only choices.

RARE OVARIAN NEOPLASMS

Germ Cell Tumors

Arising from primordial ovarian germ cells, these tumors most commonly occur in the first two decades of life. No cause has been identified. The malignancy spreads similarly to epithelial ovarian cancer, with visceral metastases occurring late. Patients usually complain of increasing pelvic discomfort, urinary difficulties, and rectal pressure. A pelvic-abdominal mass is found on examination. The ultrasound demonstrates a partially or completely solid adnexal mass. Surgery should remove the primary tumor. Staging should be complete, including pelvic and para-aortic lymph node sampling if conservative therapy is planned. Fertility should be preserved. Dysgerminoma has a significant incidence of bilaterality, and contralateral ovarian biopsy is indicated. The aggressiveness of tumor bulk reduction surgery should be tempered by the exquisite chemotherapy sensitivity of the tumor and the necessity to initiate chemotherapy as soon as possible postoperatively.

Dysgerminomas are analogous to testicular seminomas and are the most common germ cell tumor. Phenotypic females with dysgenetic gonads develop the malignancy in a higher percentage of cases. Accompanying gonadoblastoma or dysgenetic gonadal tissue should be removed. Observation is acceptable for completely staged patients with neoplasms confined to an ovary of less than 10 cm in size and negative pelvic and para-aortic lymph node sampling. Radiation therapy is used only in the management of dysgerminoma. Whole-abdomen doses of 2000–2500 cGy are reserved for those with a high-risk factor or minimum residual disease. Chemotherapy with a platinum-based regimen is acceptable for patients de-

siring fertility, for bulky residual disease, and for extra-abdominal involvement.

Immature teratomas are the second most common germ cell tumor. Histologic grading of the degree of immaturity is critical in determining therapy. This largely depends on the quantity and nature of neutral tissue found within the tumor. Patients with grade 2 or 3 lesions warrant chemotherapy. Stage I, grade I or disseminated mature deposits (grade 0) do not warrant further therapy. **Endodermal sinus (yolk sac) tumors, embryonal carcinoma, nongestational ovarian choriocarcinoma,** and **mixed germ cell tumor** require postoperative chemotherapy (Table 22–3). Restaging laparotomy is not usually done. Prognosis is excellent, with cure rates of 90% for stage I lesions. Stage III disease has a 50–70% disease-free survival. The tumor markers α-fetoprotein (AFP) and the beta subunit of human chorionic gonadotropin (β-hCG) are useful in following the disease and determining remission status (Table 22–4). Most relapses occur within the first year. Salvage therapy is problematic if the patient has received a cisplatin-based regimen.

Rete Cord Stromal Tumors

These neoplasms arise from the rete (sex) cords and mesenchyme. Granulosa cell tumors secrete estrogen and are associated with endometrial cancer or hyperplasia. Presentation and pathogenesis are similar to those of other ovarian malignancies. However, these tumors have a greater tendency toward hemorrhage and late recurrence. Surgery involving unilateral oophorectomy is usually curative in lesions confined to the ovary. Adjuvant radiation or chemotherapy is not recommended. Responses in advanced disease have been reported with cisplatin, doxorubicin, and cyclophosphamide or vinblastine, bleomycin, and cisplatin. Five-year survival is 70–80%. Sertoli–Leydig cell tumors are usually benign, unilateral, and androgen producing and present with clinical virilization. Unilateral salpingo-oophorectomy is adequate therapy. Poorly differentiated tumors have a worse prognosis. Information is limited about the efficacy of irradiation or chemotherapy. Management of problem cases parallels that for granulosa cell or germ cell tumors.

Table 22–3. Chemotherapy program for ovarian germ cell tumors.

Etoposide, 100 mg/m^2 intravenously on days 1–3, 4, or 5[1]
Cisplatin, 100 mg/m^2 intravenously on day 1
±Bleomycin, 15 mg continuous intravenous infusion on days 1–3, or 15 mg/m^2 every 7 days for 5 weeks and on day 1 of course 4
Cycles: Repeated every 28 days
Total cycles: 4–6

[1]Depending on myelosuppression.

Table 22–4. Tumor markers in ovarian germ cell tumors.

Tumor Type	AFP	β-hCG
Dysgerminoma	–	±
Endodermal sinus tumor	+	–
Immature teratoma	±	–
Choriocarcinoma	–	+
Mixed	±	±

Table 22–5. Staging of uterine tube carcinoma.[1]

Stage	Clinical Findings
I	Tumor limited to tubes.
IA	Tumor limited to one tube; no malignant cells in ascites or peritoneal washings.
IB	Tumor limited to both tubes; no malignant cells in ascites or peritoneal washings.
IC	Tumor either stage IA or stage IB with malignant cells in ascites or peritoneal washings.
II	Tumor involving one or both tubes with pelvic extension.
IIA	Extension or metastasis to the ovaries *or*
IIB	Extension to other pelvic tissues.
IIC	Tumor either stage IIA or IIB with malignant cells in ascites or peritoneal washings.
III	Tumor involving one or both tubes with microscopically confirmed peritoneal implants outside the pelvis (including the liver capsule) or retroperitoneal or inguinal lymph node metastasis.
IIIA	Tumor grossly limited to the true pelvis with negative nodes but with microscopic abdominal peritoneal metastasis.
IIIB	Macroscopic abdominal peritoneal metastasis 2 cm or less in diameter; lymph nodes negative.
IIIC	Macroscopic abdominal peritoneal metastasis greater than 2 cm in diameter or retroperitoneal or inguinal lymph node metastasis.
IV	Tumor with distant metastasis (excludes peritoneal metastasis). Pleural effusion with positive cytology. Parenchymal liver metastasis.

[1]Although there is no official FIGO staging for tubal cancer, the FIGO ovarian staging system (Table 22–2) in current use is customarily adopted to apply to uterine tube carcinoma. If there is contiguous macroscopic parenchymal carcinoma involvement of the uterus or ovaries, the cancer may be classified as uterine or ovarian, respectively.

Metastatic Tumors

Uterine tube and endometrial carcinomas involve the ovaries in at least 5% of cases. Metastases from a patient with advanced breast cancer occur in approximately 25% of cases, usually bilaterally and often in an occult manner. Krukenberg's tumors are metastatic mucin-filled signet ring cells usually originating from the stomach. Other sites, particularly gastrointestinal, pancreatic, and bladder, may cause this condition. Carcinoids may be primary or metastatic to the ovary. Bilateral tumors are usually metastatic and have a poor prognosis. Unilateral confined carcinoids with no other primary site identified have a good prognosis. Lymphomas, particularly of Burkitt's type, may involve the ovary.

UTERINE TUBE CANCER

Essentials of Diagnosis

- Abdominal fullness, bloating, pain or mass, early satiety, pelvic pressure.
- Elevated serum CA-125 or CEA.
- No parenchymal involvement of ovaries or uterine corpus.

Tumors involving the uterine (fallopian) tube usually are direct extensions of ovarian or endometrial carcinomas or are metastatic from sites such as the breast or gastrointestinal tract. Primary tumors are rare, have no clear cause, and usually occur in the sixth and seventh decades. They are usually serous, with an occasional sarcoma. Vaginal discharge is the most common complaint. A pelvic mass is usually found on examination. A positive cervical cytologic specimen in the presence of a normal cervix and negative endometrial sampling should raise suspicion. Natural history and management are similar to those of ovarian cancer. The CA-125 measurement may be elevated, but there are no other specific laboratory abnormalities. Ultrasound findings can suggest hydrosalpinx. The differential diagnosis is that of a postmenopausal adnexal mass, with malignancy of primary concern. Staging (Table 22–5) is adapted from the ovarian schema (Table 22–2). Primary therapy consists of surgical removal and tumor reduction, and staging during the laparotomy, analogous to the treatment of ovarian cancer. Therapy thereafter is controversial. Whole abdominal radiation has been employed for selected patients. Patients with gross residual disease should be treated with a cisplatin-based regimen. Responses have been reported with cisplatin, doxorubicin, and cyclophosphamide. Stage I patients have a 60% 5-year survival. Stage II disease recurs in 50% of patients. Higher stages have a 15–20% 5-year disease-free survival.

UTERINE CANCER

Essentials of Diagnosis

Peri- or postmenopausal abnormal vaginal bleeding.
Endometrial cells on Papanicolaou smear.
Pelvic examination often normal.

ENDOMETRIAL ADENOCARCINOMA

Epidemiology & Etiology

Endometrial adenocarcinoma is the most common gynecologic cancer in the USA. However, it is a relatively low cause of mortality, with approximately 75% survival. The prevalence is 7.3:1000 for white women. The disease usually occurs in the seventh decade, particularly in obese women of low parity. Estrogen use has been associated with endometrial carcinoma, while oral contraceptives may offer a protective effect.

Screening for endometrial cancer requires outpatient sampling of endometrial tissue. Approximately 5–20% of the time, adequate tissue cannot be obtained and pathologic interpretation of samples is difficult. Less than 50% of women have a positive Papanicolaou smear. Any abnormal endometrial cells on the smear warrant further evaluation. Screening is recommended for patients with premenopausal anovulatory cycles, late menopause, or postmenopausal obesity or exogenous estrogen use.

Pathogenesis

Cancer arises from the lining of the endometrium. The precursor may be a hyperplastic state that progresses to invasive carcinoma. Direct extension develops into the cervix and through the uterine serosa. As invasion of the myometrium occurs, regional lymph nodes including the paravaginal and para-aortic become involved. Hematogenous metastases develop concurrently. The usual sites of metastatic disease are lung, bone, liver, and eventually brain. The finding of malignant cells in the peritoneal cavity presumably by tubal transport is well documented and is included in staging.

Pathology

Most tumors are pure **adenocarcinomas.** These are graded according to degree of differentiation or resemblance to normal endometrial glands. Grade 1, or well-differentiated, tumors have clearly defined glands. Grade 2 are moderate with glands interspersed among solid tumor sheets. Grade 3 poorly differentiated tumors have solid sheets of cells without recognizable glands. They have a poorer prognosis. **Adenoacanthoma** indicates the presence of benign squamous epithelium within adenocarcinoma. This is not unusual and has no prognostic importance. **Adenosquamous** carcinoma has malignant squamous and glandular components. The latter are often poorly differentiated and carry a poor prognosis. **Papillary serous** carcinomas are associated with advanced disease and poorer prognosis. **Clear-cell** carcinomas represent less than 5% of cases, may have psammoma bodies with early vascular invasion, and have a poor prognosis.

Clinical Findings

A. Symptoms and Signs: Postmenopausal bleeding is the presenting complaint in 90% of women. Premenopausal or anovulatory women may have intermenstrual or heavy bleeding.

The general history and physical examination are usually normal. Obesity is absent in one-third of patients. The pelvic examination is often normal although the uterus may seem bulky. Occasionally the patient will present with an obstructive pyometra. Careful inspection of the genitalia and a rectovaginal examination are important to rule out other disease entities or detect metastatic disease.

B. Laboratory Findings: There are no specific laboratory abnormalities. The CA-125 or CEA (carcinoembryonic antigen) tumor marker is often elevated in advanced cases.

C. X-Ray and other Studies: There are no routine radiologic tests for staging the malignancy. A chest x-ray is usually obtained to rule out pulmonary metastases or pleural effusion. Further evaluations depend on the stage of disease, clinical findings, and planned therapy. Cystoscopy, flexible sigmoidoscopy, and barium enema are used when disease is suspected to involve the bladder or rectum. Suspicion of more advanced disease may require a bone scan and CT scan.

Diagnosis and management require a histologically positive endometrial biopsy. If there is any doubt about the malignant origin or nature of the tissue, fractional curettage under anesthesia is performed. A woman with postmenopausal bleeding and inadequate outpatient biopsy also requires this procedure. This test should clarify whether or not there is an endometrial or endocervical primary.

Differential Diagnosis

The differential diagnosis is that of postmenopausal bleeding. Most women with this complaint will have atrophic vaginitis or endometritis, concurrent estrogen use, cervical or endometrial polyps, or endometrial hyperplasia. Rarer causes include urethral caruncle, trauma, or neoplasms of the urethra, bladder, or rectum.

Staging

Therapy and prognosis are dependent on the stage of tumor (Table 22–6). The staging is clinical and is based on pelvic examination; endocervical and endometrial curettage; endoscopic examination of the bladder, uterus, and rectum; and chest and bone radiographs. Although other studies, including a laparotomy, may show more advanced disease, the original stage designation will remain unchanged. Surgery will reveal that 5–20% of stage I patients have more advanced disease.

Treatment

A. Surgery: Stage I disease confined to the

Table 22–6. FIGO staging for uterine corpus cancer.[1]

Stage	Grade	Clinical Findings
Ia	123	Tumor limited to endometrium
Ib	123	Invasion to ≤ 1/2 myometrium
Ic	123	Invasion > 1/2 myometrium
IIa[2]	123	Endocervical glandular involvement only
IIb	123	Cervical stromal invasion
IIIa	123	Tumor invades serosa and/or adnexae and/or positive peritoneal cytology
IIIb	123	Vaginal metastases
IIIc	123	Metastases to pelvic and/or para-aortic lymph nodes
IVa	123	Tumor invades bladder and/or bowel mucosa
IVb	123	Distant metastases including intra-abdominal and/or inguinal lymph nodes

[1]Adopted at FIGO meeting, Rio de Janeiro, 1988.
[2]Unofficial designation (Society of Gynecologic Oncologists, 1974): Stage II occult—cervical involvement noted by microscopic examination alone. For practical purposes, patients with stage I and stage II occult may be managed alike.

uterus requires a laparotomy with total abdominal hysterectomy and bilateral salpingo-oophorectomy (TAH/BSO). Careful inspection of abdominal contents and peritoneal cytologic specimens are performed. If significant myometrial invasion or a grade III lesion is found, lymph node sampling, including the para-aortics, may be carried out. Gross stage II disease may require radical hysterectomy or preoperative radiotherapy. Stage III and IV patients are difficult to manage. Therapy is aimed at maximizing pelvic control of the primary cancer and palliating the effects of distant metastases.

B. Radiotherapy: Delivery of radiotherapy pre- or postoperatively is controversial. The rate of vaginal and pelvic recurrence may be reduced in high-risk patients, ie, grade III cancer, cervical involvement, or significant myometrial invasion. However, prolongation of survival has not been demonstrated. Radiotherapy options include a preoperative intracavitary system with possible external pelvic radiotherapy of 45–50 cGy. Extended field radiation to include pathologically involved para-aortic nodes has been recommended. Whole abdominal radiotherapy is an option for patients who have adnexal metastases, microscopic abdominal spread, or positive peritoneal cytologic specimens. The last may also be treated by intraperitoneal ^{32}P.

C. Hormonal Therapy: Progestational agents are the mainstay of therapy. There is no clear dose-response relationship although the following schedules are common: medroxyprogesterone acetate, 400 mg intramuscularly every 7 days; medroxyprogesterone, 150 mg orally every day; or megestrol acetate, 160 mg orally every day. Side effects usually are fatigue, weight gain, headache, and occasionally thrombophlebitis. Overall the response rate is 10%. However, usually only grade I cancers are sensitive to this therapy. Most grade I tumors contain estrogen and pro-

gesterone receptors. The value of adjuvant hormonal therapy is unproved. Occasional responses to tamoxifen are seen.

D. Chemotherapy: This is usually reserved for advanced or metastatic disease. Adjuvant therapy has no proved benefit. The primary drugs considered active are cisplatin (50–75 mg/m^2), doxorubicin (40–50 mg/m^2), cyclophosphamide (500 mg/m^2), and carboplatin (200–360 mg/m^2). Single-agent cyclophosphamide has a marginal role in the therapy. Combination therapy is commonly used but has not demonstrated an advantage over single-agent therapy. Response rates range from 20% to 60% and last from 4 to 6 months. The toxicity of the compounds interferes with their utility in the elderly. Carboplatin may be the least toxic alternative.

E. Supportive Care: Metastatic uterine cancer causes proportionately more skeletal and brain metastases requiring radiotherapy. Refractory ascites may require repeated paracentesis.

Prognosis

The prognosis depends on stage, histologic grade and type, presence of myometrial invasion, and presence of lymph node metastases. Higher tumor grade and deep myometrial invasion (outer third) are associated with extrauterine spread in about 40% of cases. The 5-year survival by stage is as follows: I, 75%; II, 58%; III, 30%, and IV, 11%.

UTERINE SARCOMAS

Uterine sarcomas are rare heterogeneous tumors that present in a variety of ways. Leiomyosarcomas are smooth muscle tumors. Prognosis depends on extrauterine spread and number of mitoses per microscopic high-power field (HPF). Tumors with mitotic counts of >10 per 10 HPF are considered malignant. Malignant mixed mesodermal tumors are aggressive lesions with adenocarcinomatous and sarcomatous components. Survival is approximately 50–60% for lesions confined to the uterus. Endometrial stromal sarcomas are of low or high grade depending on mitotic count. Low-grade endometrial stromal sarcoma and endolymphatic stromal myosis have an excellent prognosis. Larger lesions or those penetrating the uterine serosa have a tendency to recur locally. Surgical removal of the primary is the mainstay of therapy. Pelvic radiotherapy reduces pelvic recurrence but does not prolong survival. Adjuvant chemotherapy is of unproved benefit. Chemotherapy for metastatic disease is palliative. Active drugs include doxorubicin for leiomyosarcoma and cisplatin and ifosfamide for mixed mesodermal sarcoma.

CERVICAL CANCER

Essentials of Diagnosis

- Early cancer asymptomatic.
- Postcoital vaginal bleeding, malodorous vaginal discharge, pelvic or sciatic pain, leg swelling in advanced cancer.

Epidemiology & Etiology

Advanced cervical cancer is less common than ovarian or endometrial malignancies. The peak-age incidence is bimodal with peaks at 35–39 and 60–64 years of age. The overall incidence of invasive cancer has been decreasing. Cigarette smoking, early sexual intercourse, high number of sexual partners, and early parity have been associated with the disease. Viruses play a significant role in its development. Human papillomavirus (types 16, 18, and 31) is most commonly implicated. Evidence supporting viral causation includes epidemiologic association, viral antigens in the neoplasia, and genetic integration of viral material into the dysplastic or neoplastic cell. The essential screen for cervical cancer is the Papanicolaou smear. The frequency of examination is somewhat controversial. The American College of Obstetricians and Gynecologists recommends an annual pelvic examination and smear for 3 consecutive years. If normal, the interval may be lengthened. The American Cancer Society allows "low-risk" women to have smears every 3 years. However, the high-risk individual needs an annual examination (high risk is defined as having sexual intercourse before age 20 or a history of more than two sexual partners). False-negative smears occur in 20–30% of cases of squamous cell carcinoma. A common cause of false negativity is improper sampling technique and handling of the specimen.

Pathogenesis

The development of invasive cervical carcinoma is considered to be an orderly process of metaplasia and dysplasia of the epithelium that eventually results in invasion of the basement membrane. The malignancy there may become exophytic or infiltrate and expand the endocervical canal. As volume increases, the parametrial tissues are invaded. Eventually there is further extension and adherence to the pelvic wall resulting in severe discomfort and sciatic type pain. Anterior growth produces a vesicovaginal fistula and obstructive uropathy. Posterior extension causes a rectovaginal fistula. Concomitant with direct extension is lymphatic space involvement resulting in sequential involvement of pelvic, para-aortic, mediastinal, and supraclavicular lymph nodes. Hematogenous dissemination to lungs, liver, and bone are late events. Brain involvement is unusual.

Pathology

Over 90% are **squamous cell** carcinomas that may be subclassified as small- or large-cell nonkeratinizing or keratinizing. This subclassification and tumor grading do not have a clear prognostic role. **Adenocarcinomas** represent about 10% of tumors. *Adenoma malignium* (minimal-deviation adenocarcinoma) is an invasive, potentially metastatic tumor with a benign or dysplastic glandular component. **Adenocarcinomas** occur with squamous components. A benign squamous component is termed *adenocanthoma*. Adenosquamous carcinomas with a malignant squamous component are not rare, particularly in pregnant women. These may have a signet ring component or be undifferentiated and termed glassy cell carcinoma. Mixed adenosquamous carcinomas have a poorer prognosis. **Small-cell** (non–squamous cell) carcinomas are undifferentiated tumors and usually occur in younger women. These uncommon causes have a poorer prognosis and may be accompanied by hypercalcemia or inappropriate secretion of antidiuretic hormone (ADH). **Verrucous** carcinoma is a slowly growing, locally destructive lesion. Choriocarcinoma, malignant melanoma, and sarcomas originate from the cervix and have a poor prognosis. Lymphomas of the cervix are often of a large-cell variety and if confined in the organ have a good prognosis. Metastatic disease in the cervix usually represents direct extension from a neighboring pelvic site but may represent metastatic disease particularly from the stomach, breast, or lung.

Treatment depends on the degree of invasion by the tumor. Microinvasive carcinoma is neoplastic invasion of the stroma ≤3 mm from the basement membrane in the absence of lymphatic or vascular involvement. It rarely involves regional lymph nodes.

Clinical Findings

A. Symptoms and Signs: Most women are asymptomatic and diagnosed by an abnormal Papanicolaou smear. The most common symptom of advanced disease is vaginal bleeding, particularly postcoital. Advanced disease may be accompanied by malodorous vaginal discharge, pelvic sciatic pain, leg swelling, and weight loss. Complaints indicating anemia, renal failure (obstructive uropathy), or pelvic fistulae may be present.

In early disease, the general physical examination with careful attention to the supraclavicular and groin nodes usually is unremarkable. The pelvic examination may be normal owing to a hidden endocervical lesion or occult carcinoma found only on colposcopy. The gross cervical lesion may be a small raised reddish area. However, with increasing size, the cancer may be ulcerative, exophytic and filling the vagina with friable tissue, or infiltrative and causing a hard, expanded cervix. The pelvic examination should include thorough palpation of parametrial tissues to define extracervical extension of the tumor. Careful palpation of vaginal mucosa for rubbery, submucosal infiltration or "skip" metastases is important. Examination under anesthesia may be required. Other signs depend on site of local extension and end organ damage.

B. Laboratory Findings: Routine laboratory tests are usually normal. With advanced disease, there is anemia secondary to blood loss and renal failure due to obstruction. Hypercalcemia indicates skeletal metastases or a small-cell component. The CA-125 and CEA levels may be elevated with adenocarcinoma.

C. X-Ray Studies: Radiologic evaluation is indicated in patients with >3 mm stromal invasion. A chest x-ray may indicate metastatic disease, usually parenchymal nodules. The barium enema and intravenous pyelogram aid in staging. CT scan, MRI, ultrasound, and radionucleotide scan are not routinely recommended. However, these studies may aid in treatment planning for patients with advanced disease.

D. Other Tests: Cystoscopy and proctoscopy should be done to rule out local invasion, particularly with large primaries. Lymphangiography has been advocated to define the presence of malignant disease in the iliac and para-aortic lymph nodes. False-positive rates of 20–40% and false-negative rates of 10–20% are reported. These error rates are analogous to those of CT scan. Abnormal findings should be confirmed by needle aspiration biopsy. Information obtained from these radiographic studies, including MRI, may not be used to stage the patient.

Diagnosing the presence and extent of invasion is essential to therapeutic planning. With a positive Papanicolaou smear and no gross lesion, colposcopically directed biopsies are performed. Abnormalities include looped, branching, or reticular blood vessels; irregular surface contours; and yellow-orange epithelial color. If colposcopy is unsatisfactory or clinical suspicion is high, a diagnostic cone biopsy of the cervix is necessary.

Differential Diagnosis

In the presence of a definitively malignant Papanicolaou smear, the differential is limited to ruling out another source of the abnormal cells. This usually will be a neoplasm of the ovary, uterine tube, uterus, vagina, bladder, or urethra. A gross cervical lesion may represent a benign polyp, ulceration due to chemical or physical trauma, leukoplakia, leiomyoma, or squamous papilloma. Benign fibromas and hemangiomas also occur. Endometriosis, adenomyosis, and mesonephric duct adenoma may confuse the picture. Atypical adenomatous hyperplasia associated with oral contraceptive use resembles clinically

and histologically adenocarcinoma of the cervix. Metastatic tumors are discussed above.

Staging

The staging is clinical (Table 22–7). However, information obtained from the chest x-ray, barium enema, intravenous pyelogram, routine bone radiographs, proctoscopy, and cystoscopy may be used for staging purposes. The MRI, CT scan, ultrasound, lymphangiogram, or nuclear medicine scan may *not* be used for this purpose. Dubious cases are assigned to the earlier stage. The stage once assigned is permanent.

"Barrel" cervix is a clinical description applied to a cervix replaced by tumor in an expansile manner. Commonly a diameter of 6 cm is required for this designation. These lesions have a higher central relapse rate and may warrant more intensive radiotherapy or adjunctive extrafascial hysterectomy. Management is controversial.

Treatment

A. Surgery: The treatment is dependent on stage and bulk of the primary lesion, age of the patient, and concurrent medical problems. The treatment of early invasive disease is primarily surgery (Table 22–8). For lesions that are Stage IB, the options are surgery or radiotherapy. The surgery consists of a hysterectomy of varying degrees of radicality with selective use of lymphadenectomy. The para-aortic lymph nodes should be palpated, and biopsies made of suspicious nodes. The complications of radical hysterectomy include ureterovaginal and vesicovaginal fistulae in less than 3% of cases. Postoperative bladder dysfunction is common but may be a serious persistent problem in about 3% of cases. Lymphocyst formation may occur and rarely causes obstructive uropathy.

B. Radiotherapy: Radiotherapy plays an essential role in the treatment of cervical cancer. It is useful in all stages but is primarily used in stage IB or higher stages of disease not amenable to radical hysterectomy. Primary treatment usually combines 4000–5000 cGy over 4–5 weeks and brachytherapy. Brachytherapy employs an intracavitary device to load a radioactive source into the uterus, cervix, and upper vagina. The intrauterine cylindrical device is known as a tandem. Spherical objects placed in the upper vagina are known as ovoids or colpostats. The radioactive source usually is cesium. These objects are "afterloaded," ie, after satisfactory tandem positioning the radioactive source is placed with minimal exposure to nonpatients. "Remote afterloading" is placement of the source by a machine. Therapy may be expressed in milligrams per hour ie, the total amount of the source and time (hours) in situ. Therapy may also be expressed as centigrays to point A (2 cm lateral and 2 cm superior to the external cervical os) and point B (3 cm lateral to point A, representing

Table 22–7. FIGO staging for uterine cervix cancer.[1]

Stage	Clinical Findings
Preinvasive Carcinoma	
0	Carcinoma in situ, intraepithelial carcinoma (cases of stage 0 should not be included in therapeutic statistics).
Invasive Carcinoma	
I	Carcinoma strictly confined to the cervix (extension to the corpus should be disregarded).
Ia	Preclinical carcinomas of the cervix, ie, those diagnosed only by microscopy.
Ia1	Minimal microscopically evident stromal invasion.
Ia2	Lesions detected microscopically that can be measured. The upper limit of the measurement should not show a depth of invasion of more than 5 mm taken from the base of the epithelium, either surface or glandular, from which it originates, and a second dimension, the horizontal spread, must not exceed 7 mm. Larger lesions should be staged as Ib.
Ib	Lesions of greater dimensions than stage Ia2 whether seen clinically or not. Preformed space involvement should not alter the staging but should be specifically recorded to determine whether it should affect treatment decisions in the future.
II	The carcinoma extends beyond the cervix but has not extended on to the wall. The carcinoma involves the vagina but not the lower third.
IIa	No obvious parametrial involvement.
IIb	Obvious parametrial involvement.
III	The carcinoma has extended on to the pelvic wall (on rectal examination, there is no cancer-free space between the tumor and the pelvic wall) or the tumor involves the lower third of the vagina. All cases with hydronephrosis or non-functioning kidney.
IIIa	No extension to the pelvic wall.
IIIb	Extension on to the pelvic wall and/or hydronephrosis or nonfunctioning kidney.
IV	The carcinoma has extended beyond the true pelvis or has clinically involved the mucosa of the bladder or rectum. A bullous edema as such does not permit a case to be allotted to stage IV.
IVa	Spread of the growth to adjacent organs.
IVb	Spread to distant organs.

[1]Modified and reproduced, with permission, from Bearhs OH et al (editors): *Manual for Staging of Cancer,* 4th ed. Lippincott, 1992.

the pelvic sidewall). The optimal dose is thought to be 3500–8500 cGy to point A and 4500–6500 cGy to point B.

Transvaginal radiation may be delivered via a cone inserted into the vagina for control of a bleeding tumor. Extended field radiation, including microscopically involved positive para-aortic lymph nodes, has been proposed as effective therapy. Pelvic radiotherapy following hysterectomy is common for patients with adverse factors such as pelvic lymph node involvement and lymphatic vascular involvement. Complications of pelvic radiotherapy include severe radiation cystitis, enteritis, and proctitis. Complications result in bleeding, obstruction, and visceral perforation in less than 15% of cases. Radiotherapy has a clear role in the palliation of metastatic lesions.

C. Chemotherapy: Chemotherapy has a limited role in treatment. Drug activity is thought to be compromised by poor tumor vascularity due to previous surgery and radiation. Obstructive uropathy compromises drug dosing. Pelvic recurrences cause infection and inanition that lower patient performance status and tolerance to therapy. Single-agent activity has been observed with mitomycin, melphalan, fluorouracil, chlorambucil, doxorubicin, bleomycin, methotrexate, carboplatin, and ifosfamide. Cisplatin has been extensively studied and shows response rates of 20–50%. The optimal dose is 50 mg/m² with no survival advantage for higher doses. Response lasts approximately 4–6 months with patient survival of about 9 months. Combination therapy has not proved superior to single agents. Single-agent cisplatin or a combination (Table 22–9) are reasonable alternatives. The duration of treatments is unclear, but no advantage has been seen with prolonged chemotherapy. Often the disease is difficult to objectively measure, particularly in the irradiated pelvis. One often has to rely on subjective indicators such as pain relief, improvement in performance status, and increase in sense of well-being as a guide to the efficacy of therapy. Responses usually are seen with two cycles, uncommonly occur in previously irradiated sites, and

Table 22–8. Surgical management of early invasive cancer of the cervix.[1]

Stage	Clinical Findings	Surgical Procedure
Ia1	Early stromal invasion (<1mm)	Conization or simple hysterectomy
Ia2	1–3 mm invasion With lymph-vascular space invasion	Modified radical hysterectomy with or without pelvic lymph node dissection.
	3–5 mm invasion <1 cm width	Modified radical hysterectomy with pelvic lymphadenectomy.
	>1 cm width	Radical hysterectomy with pelvic lymphadenectomy.
Ib	>5 mm invasion ≤3 cm diameter	

[1]Modified and reproduced, with permission, from Hatch KD: Cervical cancer, In: *Practical Gynecologic Oncology.* Berek JS, Hacker NF (editors). Williams & Wilkins, 1989.

Table 22–9. Chemotherapy regimens for cervical carcinoma.

Tumor Type	Drug	Dose (mg/m²)	Frequency (weekly)
Squamous cell	Mitomycin	10	8
	Bleomycin	10	4
	Cisplatin[1]	50	4
Adenocarci-noma	Fluorouracil	500 over 24 hours[2]	
	Doxorubicin[3]	40–50 over 48 hours	4
	Cisplatin	50 over 4 hours	
Small cell	Etoposide	100 daily for 3 days	
	Doxorubicin[3]	40–50	4
	Cisplatin	50	

[1]May be given as a single agent.
[2]Continuous intravenous infusion sequentially.
[3]Patients who have had prior pelvic radiotherapy should have lower initial doses of doxorubicin.

rarely result in complete remission of several years' duration. Four to six courses of chemotherapy probably are adequate treatment.

Numerous radiation sensitizers have been tried. Hydroxyurea given concomitantly with radiotherapy has resulted in increase in response rates compared to radiotherapy alone in a randomized trial. However, long-term survival in both groups is the same. Chemotherapy either intravenously or arterially prior to radiotherapy has demonstrated high response rates but no survival prolongation. Concomitant radiotherapy and systemic chemotherapy show the same phenomena. Mature survival data and large randomized trials are presently lacking to support such multimodality therapies. Recent work has shown the combination of interferon alpha and 13-cis-retinoic acid produce objective responses in 40–50% of previously untreated patients with advanced cervical cancer.

D. Recurrent or Persistent Cervical Cancer: The treatment of localized pelvic tumor following primary treatment failure involves either radiotherapy or surgery. For patients failing surgery, standard radiotherapy techniques may be used. However, the dosimetric advantage of brachytherapy is lost. Special techniques involving the interstitial implantation of radioactive sources into the tumor area are considered essential. Survival in these cases is approximately 15–40% depending on the volume of tumor. Patients failing radiotherapy and not having pelvic wall fixation of tumor or distant metastases should undergo pelvic exenteration. Total exenteration results in removal of the bladder, cervix, uterus, vagina, and rectum, followed by urinary conduit, colostomy, and vaginal reconstruction. Anterior exenteration spares the rectum, and posterior exenteration spares the bladder. Major surgical morbidity is common with a mortality rate of approximately 3–7%. Five-year survival is 40–60%. Data concerning quality of life are lacking. Sexual function even with vaginal reconstruction is compromised.

E. Special Situations: Patients who have had a supracervical hysterectomy may develop cancer in the residual cervix (cervical stump cancer). A first consideration is radical trachelectomy (cervicectomy) to remove the parametrial tissues and dissect pelvic lymph nodes. For larger lesions, radiotherapy is utilized. Survival rates are excellent for early stages and analogous to those for other cervical cancers.

Inadvertent simple hysterectomy ("cut-through" hysterectomy) in a case of invasive cancer is problematic. Management depends on extent of residual disease. Usually radiotherapy is utilized. Patients with disease-free margins following surgery have a survival rate of 80% or better. Patients with gross residual disease have an approximate 20% survival.

Cervical cancer in pregnancy requires definition of extent of invasion. However, cone biopsies present a major risk to the fetus, particularly during the first trimester. Patients with >5 mm invasion should be treated definitively with minimal delay. Less invasive disease is not as urgent, and treatment can be delayed to allow gestation to proceed without interruption.

Prognosis

Survival rates of patients at the authors' institution are as follows:

Stage	Five-year Survival
I	92%
IIA	84%
IIB	67%
IIIA	45%
IIIB	36%
IV	14%

Most recurrences are within the first year. Relapse sites are pelvis alone in approximately 20%, distant metastases in 50%, and combined sites in 25%. Pelvic relapse rates are higher in patients presenting with bulky advanced disease. The survival of patients with refractory or metastatic disease is 9–12 months.

Supportive Care

The patient with refractory cervical cancer is difficult to palliate. A rectovaginal fistula should usually be surgically corrected. A vesicovaginal fistula may be handled as for any patient with urinary incontinence, including the use of an indwelling Foley catheter. Ureteral diversion is reserved for patients with reasonable longevity. Inanition may be slightly ameliorated by low-dose androgens. Pain particularly from pelvic recurrences requires careful management. In difficult cases, continuous subcutaneous infusion of hydromorphone with low doses of haloperidol and metoclopramide is useful.

VULVAR CANCER

Essentials of Diagnosis
- Older woman with chronic pruritus.
- Bleeding, discharge, or pain in advanced disease.

Epidemiology & Etiology
Vulvar cancer is uncommon and accounts for 0.3% of all female cancer and 4% of gynecologic cancer with an annual incidence of 1.5:100,000 women. Incidence increases with age, peaking at the seventh decade. No etiologic agent has been identified. Vulvar dystrophy, a broad term for a condition associated with chronic vulvar itching, variable gross skin changes, and microscopic hyperplasia or atrophy, is not usually premalignant. Only those with microscopic atypia or medically uncontrolled disease are at risk for cancer. Approximately 20% of patients have a second neoplastic process, usually invasive or in situ cervical carcinoma. The disease is more common in the obese and those with a prior history of syphilis and other granulomatous sexually transmitted diseases.

Pathogenesis
The cancer begins in the squamous epithelium of the vulva. There may be a precursor vulvar intraepithelial neoplasia (VIN), which is graded 1, 2, or 3 similarly to its cervical counterpart. After the cancer penetrates the basement membrane, direct extension follows, particularly to the urethra, clitoris, and anus. Lymphatic involvement may be early to the superficial inguinal, femoral, and other pelvic lymph nodes. Lesions >2 cm or invasion >3 mm has a minimum of 25% lymph node metastases. Hematogenous spread is late and is usually accompanied by lymph node involvement. Pulmonary and bone metastases are common with advanced disease. Local dermal infiltration, nodularity, and ulceration evolve with uncontrolled local disease. Major vessels may be involved.

Pathology
Over 90% of cases are **squamous cell** carcinoma. Well-differentiated microinvasive lesions rarely metastasize. **Adenocarcinoma** represents less than 5%, usually arises from Bartholin's gland, and occurs in younger women. Carcinoma of Bartholin's gland may also be of squamous or transitional origin. **Melanoma,** usually of the labia minora or clitoris, rarely occurs and is associated with a 30% survival rate. **Verrucous** carcinoma of the vulva requires surgical excision and has an indolent, locally destructive course. **Vulvar sarcoma** usually is leiomyosarcoma, and prognosis depends on tumor size and histologic

grade. **Adenosquamous** carcinoma is an aggressive tumor with a poor prognosis.

VIN represents squamous cell carcinoma in situ and includes erythroplasia of Queyrat, Bowen's disease, and carcinoma simplex in situ. Paget's disease of the vulva is adenocarcinoma in situ. About 20–30% have associated invasive adenocarcinoma in the immediate anatomic vicinity or a distant primary. Surgical excision with wide surgical margins is indicated.

Clinical Findings
A. Symptoms and Signs: Complaints of pruritus of long standing are common. Patients will often palpate the mass. As disease advances, there is bleeding, discharge, and pain. Groin discomfort may indicate lymph node involvement.

The gross appearance of the lesion is usually an elevated mass that is pale appearing, wartlike, or ulcerative. The labia majora are the usual site. A small percentage have multiple primary sites. Examination may suggest urethral, bladder, or rectal involvement in larger lesions. Palpable groin nodes may indicate metastatic involvement.

B. Laboratory Findings: There are no specific laboratory abnormalities. A serologic test for syphilis should be obtained.

C. X-Ray and Other Studies: In early cases, no routine tests are required. A chest x-ray and pelvic/abdominal CT scan may demonstrate metastases in advanced disease.

Patients should have a cervical cytologic smear and vaginal-cervical colposcopic examination. If clinically indicated, sigmoidoscopy and cystoscopy should be done to rule out local invasion.

The biopsy should be excisional in a small lesion and a wedge that includes surrounding skin in larger masses to allow evaluation of stromal depth of malignant invasion.

Differential Diagnosis
The differential usually is that of vulvar dystrophy, granulomatous inflammation, and condylomatous lesions.

Staging
Staging is based on clinical examination with additional information obtained from a chest x-ray, cystoscopy, proctoscopy, and bone radiographs (Table 22–10). The error rate is approximately 25% in examination of groin nodes.

Treatment
A. Surgery and Radiation: The principles of treatment are governed by en bloc surgical resection appropriate to disease extent, preservation of urinary and sexual function, and minimalization of the long-term morbidity of leg lymphedema with recurrent infection and ambulatory disability. Stage I lesions

Table 22–10. FIGO staging of vulvar cancer.[1]

Stage	Clinical Findings
0	Carcinoma in situ.
I	Tumor confined to the vulva or perineum; ≤2 cm in greatest dimension; no nodal metastasis.
II	Tumor confined to the vulva or perineum; >2 cm in greatest dimension; no nodal metastasis.
III	Tumor of any size with adjacent spread to the urethra, vagina, or the anus or with unilateral regional lymph node metastasis.
IVA	Tumor invades upper urethra, bladder mucosa, rectal mucosa, pelvic bone, or bilateral regional node metastases.
IVB	Any distant metastasis, including pelvic lymph nodes.

[1]Adopted at FIGO meeting in Rio de Janeiro, 1988.

with <1 mm invasion in an otherwise normal-appearing vulva are amenable to conservative but complete local excision without groin lymph node dissection. If lesions have >1 mm invasion, ipsilateral groin dissection is recommended. If groin dissection uncovers two or more positive nodes, ipsilateral groin radiation therapy is appropriate. Patients with stage II or III disease usually require radical vulvectomy and bilateral inguinal and femoral lymphadenectomy. This involves total removal of the vulva and may create large skin defects requiring grafts. Postoperative mortality is about 2%. The major complication is breakdown of the groin and vulva wounds with tissue necrosis, infection, and groin lymphocysts. Late complications include chronic leg lymphedema with episodic lymphangitis, urinary stress incontinence, vaginal prolapse, and stenosis of the lower vagina.

Some investigators advocate pelvic node dissection if groin nodes are positive or the lesion involves the clitoris or Bartholin's gland. Patients with more than one position groin node should receive postoperative pelvic and groin radiation. Postsurgical radiotherapy may be useful in patients with positive surgical margins or large primaries. Patients with advanced disease involving the proximal urethra, bladder, or rectum present a difficult problem. Pelvic exenteration may be considered if the nodes are clinically negative and the patient is sufficiently medically stable to tolerate the procedure. Carefully individualized radiotherapy including precisely planned brachytherapy may be a more reasonable primary treatment. Surgical resection of the residual tumor upon completion of radiotherapy may be indicated.

Local recurrences following primary therapy are usually in lesions >4 cm in size. Repeat surgical resection, radiotherapy, or both may salvage a patient. Groin recurrences are difficult problems associated with higher mortality. Again, radiation and surgical excision are attempted.

B. Chemotherapy: The literature is sparse with few patients per trial. Limited activity has been reported with methotrexate, bleomycin, fluorouracil,

and cisplatin. Usually patients are treated similarly to cervical cancer patients. Combined modality trials are under way in advanced diseases.

Prognosis

Prognosis depends on stage and lymph node status. Stage I and II patients have a 90% and 80% 5-year survival, respectively. Stage III cancers are associated with a 50% mortality. Only about 20% of patients with stage IV disease survive. Patients with clinically suspicious groin nodes have a 50% survival. Fixed or ulcerated nodes carry a 33% survival. Positive pelvic lymph nodes or more than three pathologically positive lymph nodes carry a very poor prognosis.

VAGINAL CANCER

Essentials of Diagnosis

- Asymptomatic in a minority of patients.
- Vaginal bleeding or discharge, especially postcoital.

Epidemiology & Etiology

Vaginal cancer represents 2% of gynecologic neoplasms. The age-adjusted incidence is 0.6:100,000. Malignant involvement of the vagina is usually metastatic from the cervix, vulva, or endometrium. Trophoblastic disease uncommonly involves the vagina. Direct extension also occurs from bladder or rectal cancer. The disease is diagnosed after 50 years of age. The cause is unknown; however, the human papillomavirus has been implicated. About one-third of patients have a history of in situ or invasive cervical carcinoma.

Pathogenesis

Early events are poorly understood. Vaginal intraepithelial neoplasia (VAIN) progressing to invasive cancer has been observed in a small percentage of cases. After invading the basement membrane, the tumor metastasizes by the lymphatic and hematogenous routes. Lower vaginal lesions involve inguinal femoral nodes. Direct extension to adjacent pelvic tissues is common as disease progresses.

Pathology

Over 90% are **squamous cell** carcinomas. **Verrucous** carcinoma is an uncommon variant with a pale, wartlike appearance and little tendency to metastasize. The histologic pattern is characteristic, and wide surgical excision is recommended. Vaginal **melanoma** rarely occurs and usually presents with deep invasion; radical surgery is advocated. **Vaginal sar-**

comas are usually fibrosarcomas and leiomyosarcomas. Surgery is primary treatment. **Sarcoma botryoides** (embryonal rhabdomyosarcoma) is a vaginal tumor of infancy and childhood. Conservative surgery and chemotherapy are recommended. Endodermal sinus tumor (yolk sac tumor) of the vagina also occurs during infancy. Chemotherapy combined with surgery or radiotherapy may be curative. **Adenocarcinomas** represent 5% of cases. They may arise from foci of adenosis, endometriosis, wolffian cell rests, and periurethral glands. In utero exposure to diethylstilbestrol is associated with tumor development in adolescence. Treatment is similar to that of squamous cell carcinoma.

Clinical Findings

A. Symptoms and Signs: The most common complaint is vaginal bleeding or discharge that may be provoked by sexual intercourse. Other symptoms are related to location and size of the tumor. The minority are found as asymptomatic lesions on pelvic examination.

Usually the lesions are polypoid or ulcerative masses. Submucosal thickening and firmness may be a primary lesion or extension from another mass. Vaginal cancer is usually in the posterior third of the vagina, often on the posterior wall. This location makes detection difficult, since the speculum covers this area during routine examination.

B. Laboratory Findings: In early vaginal carcinoma, there are no laboratory abnormalities. With persistent vaginal bleeding, anemia may occur.

C. X-Ray and Other Studies: A chest x-ray to rule out metastatic disease is usually obtained. With advanced disease, CT scans of the pelvis may be useful in treatment planning.

Cystoscopy and proctoscopy are recommended to determine local invasion.

Differential Diagnosis

The differential diagnosis is limited and includes metastatic and contiguous spread of cancer from surrounding pelvic organs. Vaginal endometriosis, foreign body reactions, and benign tumors are also noted.

Staging

The malignancy is clinically difficult to stage because of occult submucosal spread of disease. Staging is based on physical examination, cystoscopy, and proctoscopy (Table 22–11). Most patients present with disease beyond the vagina.

Treatment

Radiotherapy is the usual mode of therapy and combines external irradiation with interstitial or intracavitary treatment. Thicker lesions usually require interstitial techniques. Lower vaginal lesions may require surgical or radiotherapeutic treatment of groin

Table 22–11. FIGO staging of vaginal cancer.[1]

Stage	Clinical Findings
0	Carcinoma in situ.
I	Tumor confined to vaginal mucosa.
II	Tumor invading submucosa but not extending to the pelvic wall.
III	Tumor extension to the pelvic wall.
IVA	Tumor invades the bladder or rectal mucosa or extends outside the true pelvis.
IVB	Distant metastasis.

[1]Modified and reproduced, with permission, from Beahrs OH et al (editors): *Manual for Staging of Cancer,* 4th ed. Lippincott, 1992.

nodes. Complications are the development of pelvic fistulae and tissue reactions with inflammation and bleeding. Vaginal stricture is common, and attention must be paid to maintenance of vaginal caliber by sexual intercourse or use of a dilator. Surgery has a limited role. Radical hysterectomy or upper vaginectomy may be suitable for smaller lesions high in the vagina. Pelvic exenteration is an option for recurrences following radiation therapy or lesions presenting with pelvic fistulae. Chemotherapy has a palliative role, and regimens usually mimic the treatment of cervical cancer.

Prognosis

Prognosis correlates with stage. Five-year survival rates are approximately 70% for stage I, 50% for stage II, 30% for stage III, and 15% for stage IV. The relatively low survival for the early stage represents the difficulty of clinically defining submucosal extravaginal extent of disease.

GESTATIONAL TROPHOBLASTIC NEOPLASIA

Essentials of Diagnosis

- Gestational event.
- Vaginal bleeding and anemia.
- Hyperemesis gravidarum, preeclampsia-eclampsia.
- Excessive uterine and theca lutein cyst enlargement.
- Abnormal uterine contents on pelvic sonogram.
- β-hCG levels proportionate to body tumor burden.
- Dyspnea secondary to trophoblastic emboli.
- Hyperthyroidism, serologic or clinical.
- Lung metastasis on chest x-ray.
- Stroke or coma syndrome secondary to hemorrhagic brain metastasis.

The term gestational trophoblastic neoplasia encompasses the spectrum of trophoblastic abnormalities resulting from an aberrant gestational event, ie, partial mole, complete or hydatidiform mole, chorioadenoma destruens, choriocarcinoma, and placental site tumor.

Epidemiology & Etiology

In the USA this disease is uncommon, occurring in 1:1700 pregnancies and representing less than 1% of neoplasia in women. Asia and Latin America have an incidence of approximately 1:200 pregnancies. There is a higher incidence in lower socioeconomic classes, at extremes of reproductive age (under 20, over 40), in twin pregnancy, and for the paired blood types of female A and male O. Women with a history of molar pregnancy are at greater risk for subsequent moles. High-meat diets may have a protective effect in Asians. The cause of molar pregnancy is not known, and no specific preventive measures are available.

Pathogenesis

The pathologic trophoblast results from the abnormal union of sperm and egg. This "blighted" ovum usually excludes the female genetic material and is androgenic. However, occasionally exclusion is incomplete and triploidy results in a partial mole. The partial mole has a mixture of normal placental or embryonic components and the typical grapelike molar tissue. Complete spontaneous resolution is the rule. The complete or classic molar pregnancy consists of a grapelike cluster of tissue that grows within the cavity and myometrium of the uterus. Histologically there are vesiculated cavitated villi and trophoblastic hyperplasia. Spontaneous resolution usually occurs, including that of tissue deported to the lungs.

This phenomenon is poorly understood. Immunologic mechanisms such as cytoxic lymphocytes have been implicated. Production of β-hCG parallels the growth of tumor and is proportionate to the number of viable cells. About 20% of moles persist, with continued growth resulting in distention of the uterine cavity, penetration of the uterine serosa into parametrial tissue, tubal ovarian extension, and submucosal vaginal metastases. Hematogenous metastases develop, with pulmonary lesions a common clinical presentation. Liver metastases occur with advancing disease. Brain involvement is found at presentation in about 10% of patients requiring chemotherapy. Lesions in the gastrointestinal tract are infrequent but cause bleeding. Unusual or end stage disease occurs in subcutaneous tissues, kidney, and the eye. The bone, bone marrow, and epidural space are usually spared. The cause of death is usually pulmonary insufficiency or cerebral herniation caused by bleeding or mass effect.

Pathology

In a generous tissue sample, hydropic villi and trophoblastic hyperplasia lend themselves to the diagnosis of molar tissue. However, mole (classic or partial) should be distinguished from trophoblastic hyperplasia at an early implantation site. Differentiation may be difficult with the limited tissue available from uterine evacuation of early-stage abnormalities. In doubtful cases, postevacuation surveillance and serial β-hCG measurements are mandatory. Attempts at grading molar tissue have been unsuccessful. The distinction between hydatidiform mole, chorioadenoma destruens, and choriocarcinoma should be considered historical, and the biologic behavior of the tumor should determine therapy.

Placental site trophoblastic tumor is a rare malignancy of varying gross appearance, disproportionately low serum β-hCG to tumor bulk, and insensitivity to chemotherapy. It is composed predominantly of cytotrophoblasts that stain immunohistochemically for human placental lactogen (hPL). They may resemble decidual cells. Surgical extirpation including metastatic lesions is the principle of treatment.

Sometimes no tissue sample is available. In its place is a woman of reproductive age with a history compatible with an interrupted gestational event and an elevated β-hCG level.

Clinical Findings

A. Symptoms and Signs: Molar pregnancy is characterized by vaginal bleeding and anemia. Preeclampsia-eclampsia and hyperemesis gravidarum may occur. On pelvic examination, there is excessive uterine enlargement, and large theca lutein cysts may be present as disease progresses. Uncommonly there is the picture of hyperthyroidism due to the thyroid-stimulating effect of β-hCG. Tissue deportation to the lungs occasionally causes pulmonary embolism and pulmonary hypertension. Parenchymal involvement causes cough, shortness of breath, and hemoptysis. Involvement of the liver is usually asymptomatic. Brain metastases may present catastrophically owing to hemorrhage. Vaginal tumors appear as raised dark pink or purple areas and cause irregular bleeding or discharge. A woman who has symptoms of pregnancy or persistent vaginal bleeding following an observed or suspected abortive event may harbor trophoblastic disease.

B. Laboratory Findings: The measurement of serum β-hCG is the cornerstone of diagnosis, treatment, and surveillance. Quantitative techniques by immunoradiometric or enzyme immunometric methods are preferred. Urinary measurements are not useful. Cross-reactivity with FSH and LH is minimal and causes only modest elevations of β-hCG. Current efforts are aimed at defining unique segments of the carboxyterminal peptides of the beta subunit to further refine the assay. The secretory product has a half-life of 24 hours. The hemoglobin should be checked for anemia. Coagulopathies are observed, and these parameters should be elevated. If clinically warranted, thyroid functions should be obtained.

C. Imaging Studies: The extent of the radiologic evaluation depends on the clinical presentation. Ultrasound of the uterus is an excellent diagnostic study. For patients with a persistent molar pregnancy, a normal chest x-ray will suffice for staging. Radiographic patterns of metastatic pulmonary disease are protean, and any abnormalities must be viewed with suspicion. If there is pulmonary metastatic disease or any clinical indication of an adverse prognostic factor, then the liver, spleen, kidney, and brain should undergo evaluation. Ultrasound and CT scan with contrast are the preferred methods. Careful attention should be directed to the cerebellum and brain stem. MRI is useful in patients with contrast allergy, aids in defining questionable lesions found by other methods, and may be useful in detecting residual uterine disease. This technique is particularly valuable with central nervous system lesions. Occasionally arteriography is necessary to define questionable abnormalities. Nuclear medicine studies are not recommended for staging purposes.

D. Special Test: Some authorities recommend sampling cerebrospinal fluid (CSF) for measurement of β-hCG as part of the staging evaluation. A ratio of serum:CSF of < 60:1 is considered indicative of cerebral tumor involvement. The value of this data with a completely normal CT scan or MRI of the brain is questionable.

Differential Diagnosis

The differential diagnosis is that of conditions causing a persistently elevated β-hCG with inadequate or equivocal uterine pathology. These conditions include ectopic pregnancy, trophoblastic hyperplasia at an early implantation site, missed or incomplete abortion, placental site tumor, and nongestational ovarian choriocarcinoma. Nontrophoblastic β-hCG–producing tumors such as gastric, colon, and small-cell lung cancers are rare. Usually the clinical picture, serial measurements of β-hCG, and careful attention to pathologic studies will resolve these issues.

Staging & Treatment

Treatment is based on recurrence risk of disease (Table 22–12 and Figure 22–1. The foundation of therapy is adequate evacuation of uterine contents. Patients with a normal chest x-ray following evacuation of a molar pregnancy require observation and weekly measurement of β-hCG. Approximately 80% will spontaneously resolve. Normalization of the titer usually occurs within 10 weeks, but 25% of patients will require 16 weeks.

Indications for chemotherapy are a plateau or increase in the β-hCG level on consecutive measurements, failure to reach normal titer by 16 weeks, or development of metastatic disease. Such patients are usually at low risk, and methotrexate suffices (Table 22–13). Therapy is continued for 1–2 courses after a negative titer is achieved.

In the USA, prophylactic chemotherapy following uterine evacuation for molar pregnancy is not considered useful. However, in patient populations where surveillance is difficult or impractical, prophylactic therapy may have a role. Significant vaginal bleeding during resolution of the mole may require chemotherapy. Life-threatening uterine bleeding may be treated by arterial embolization, chemotherapy, or hysterectomy. The medium or higher risk patient requires more intensive therapy. The underlying strategy is frequent treatment with the maximum tolerated methotrexate-based regimen. The addition of etoposide is helpful in advanced disease. Chemotherapy is continued for 2–3 cycles or 12–16 weeks beyond achievement of normal titer.

Multiple criteria exist for categorizing the high-

Table 22–12. World Health Organization (WHO) prognostic index score for gestational trophoblastic disease.[1]

Prognostic Factor	Score[2]			
	0	1	2	4
Age (yr)	≤39	>39		
Antecedent pregnancy	Mole	Abortion	Term	
Interval[3]	<4	4–6	7–12	>12
hCG (IU/L)	$<10^3$	$<10^3$–10^4	10^4–10^5	$>10^5$
ABO groups (female x male)		O x A	B x Any[4]	
		A x O	AB x Any[4]	
Largest tumor, including uterine tumor (cm)		3–5	≥5	
Site of metastases		Spleen, kidney	Gastrointestinal tract, liver	Brain
Number of metastases identified		1–3	4–8	>8
Prior chemotherapy			1 drug	≥2 drugs

[1]Modified and reproduced, with permission, from Bagshawe KD: Treatment of high-risk choriocarcinoma. J Reprod Med 1984;29:813.

[2]The total score for a patient is obtained by adding the individual scores for each prognostic factor. Total score 0–4, low risk; 5–7, intermediate risk; ≥8, high risk.

[3]The number of months between the end of an antecedent pregnancy and the start of chemotherapy.

[4]Any = any blood group.

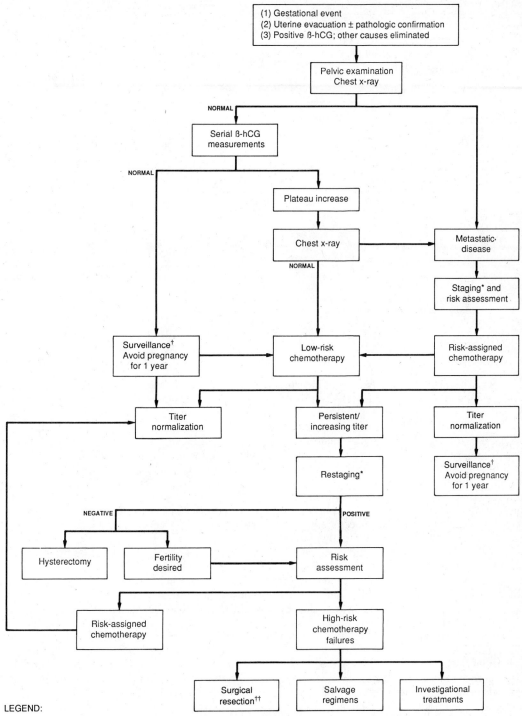

Figure 22–1. Treatment schema for trophoblastic disease.

The diagram contains the following text:

(1) Gestational event
(2) Uterine evacuation ± pathologic confirmation
(3) Positive ß-hCG; other causes eliminated

Pelvic examination
Chest x-ray

NORMAL

Serial ß-hCG measurements

NORMAL

Plateau increase

Chest x-ray

NORMAL

Metastatic disease

Staging* and risk assessment

Surveillance†
Avoid pregnancy for 1 year

Low-risk chemotherapy

Risk-assigned chemotherapy

Titer normalization

Persistent/ increasing titer

Titer normalization

Restaging*

Surveillance†
Avoid pregnancy for 1 year

NEGATIVE

POSITIVE

Hysterectomy

Fertility desired

Risk assessment

Risk-assigned chemotherapy

High-risk chemotherapy failures

Surgical resection††

Salvage regimens

Investigational treatments

LEGEND:
*Includes radiologic evaluation of brain, liver, spleen, kidney, and lungs.
†ß-hCG titers every month for 1 year, then every 4 months for 1 year, then yearly for 2 years.
††Restaging of prior or suspected disease sites, including uterus.

Table 22–13. Chemotherapy regimens for gestational trophoblastic disease.[1]

Low risk (WHO Prognostic Index Score ≤4)			
MFA			
Day 1,3,5,7	Methotrexate	1 mg/kg (maximum 70 mg)	IM injection every 48 hours
Day 2,4,6,8	Folinic acid	0.1 mg/kg	IM injection 30 hours after each methotrexate injection
Non–low risk (WHO Prognostic Index Score ≥5)			
EMA-CO			
Course A			
Day 1	Dactinomycin	500 μg	IV bolus
	Etoposide	100 mg/m^2	IV infusion over 30 minutes
	Methotrexate[1]	100 mg/m^2	IV bolus
		200 mg/m^2	IV infusion over 12 hours
Day 2	Dactinomycin	500 μg	IV bolus
	Etoposide	100 mg/m^2	IV infusion over 30 minutes
	Folinic acid	15 mg	IM/PO every 12 hours for 4 doses beginning 24 hours after methotrexate infusion started
Course B			
Day 8	Vincristine	1 mg/m^2 (maximum 2 mg)	IV bolus
	Cyclophosphamide	600 mg/m^2	IV infusion
Day 15	Start day 1 of the next cycle of EMA-CO		

[1]Modified and reproduced, with permission, from Berkowitz RS, Goldstein DP: Gestational trophoblastic disease. In: *Practical Gynecologic Oncology.* Berek JS, Hacker NF (editors). Williams & Wilkins, 1989.
[2]In patients with central nervous system metastases, increase methotrexate to 1 g/m^2 as 24-hour IV infusion. Increase folinic acid to 15 mg IM/PO every 8 hours for 9 doses beginning 24 hours after methotrexate infusion started. IM = intramuscular; IV = intravenous; PO = oral.

risk patient. The main adverse factors influencing outcome are brain metastases (40–80% survival), liver metastases (40–80% survival), full-term pregnancy (25–70% survival), prior chemotherapy (30–80% survival), and disease duration >4 months prior to therapy (60–90% survival). The overall disease-free survival of high-risk patients treated with chemotherapy ranges from 50% to 85%.

Brain metastases are usually treated with corticosteroids, whole-brain radiotherapy, and concomitant chemotherapy. If higher doses of methotrexate are employed, doses should be reduced initially to avoid catastrophic intracerebral hemorrhage. This applies to extensive pulmonary metastases as well. Patients may require urgent neurosurgical resection of expanding life-threatening brain lesions. Some authorities recommend cautious initial methotrexate therapy without whole-brain irradiation. Liver metastases are treated with chemotherapy, and radiotherapy is not recommended.

Hysterectomy is indicated as primary therapy for molar pregnancy in the patient unable or unwilling to undergo chemotherapy. Surgery is also indicated for removal of combination chemotherapy–resistant disease or persistent disease. Unfortunately, trophoblastic disease leaves radiographically measurable masses despite tumor sterilization. No radioimmunoimaging studies are effective for localizing metabolically active trophoblasts. The clinician is thus faced with persistent disease that may be anywhere in the patient's body. As a rule, complete restaging is in order, with particular attention paid to the brain, lungs, liver, and uterus. Consideration is given first to hysterectomy in the hope of finding a persistent uterine neoplasm. Then sites of bulky residual disease may be proposed as worthy of removal. These difficult decisions require a multidisciplinary effort and collective clinical experience. It should be noted that extirpation of persistent disease may result in greater sensitivity of the remaining disease to chemotherapy.

Other than for the treatment of brain metastases, radiation therapy has almost no role.

Prognosis & Posttreatment Management

Patients with low-risk disease are generally cured. High-risk patients have survival rates generally above 50% depending on adverse factors present.

In all cases of trophoblastic disease achieving normal β-hCG titers, monthly measurements should be continued for 1 year. Patients requiring prolonged or combination therapy should have titers every 4 months for a second year and yearly thereafter for 3 years. The patient is advised not to become pregnant for at least 1 year following titer normalization. Subsequent pregnancies including those following chemotherapy are normal with normal fetal outcomes although the chance of another molar pregnancy is slightly higher than normal. Late relapse of the disease beyond 2 years is uncommon. There usually are no long-term sequelae of the disease or its treatment assuming no intercurrent event resulting in permanent organ dysfunction.

REFERENCES

General

Berek JS, Greer BE (editors): *Gynecologic Oncology: Treatment Rationale and Techniques.* Elsevier, 1991.

Berek JS, Hacker NF (editors): *Practical Gynecologic Oncology.* Williams & Wilkins, 1989.

Boring CC, Squires TS, Tong T: Cancer statistics, 1992. *CA* 1992;**42:**19.

Coppleson M (editor): *Gynecologic Oncology.* Churchill Livingstone, 1992.

Deppe G (editor): *Chemotherapy of Gynecologic Cancer.* Liss, 1990.

Hoskins WJ, Perez CA, Young RC (editors): *Principles and Practice of Gynecologic Oncology.* Lippincott, 1992.

Kurman RJ (ed): *Blaustein's Pathology of the Female Genital Tract.* Springer-Verlag, 1987.

Nash JD, Young RC: Gynecologic malignancies. In: Pinedo HM, Longo DL, Chabner BA (eds), *Cancer Chemotherapy and Biological Response Modifiers,* Annual 12. Pinedo HM, Longo DL, Chabner BA (editors). Elsevier, 1991.

Thigpen JT: Chemotherapy of cancers of the female genital tract. Pages 1039–1067 in: *The Chemotherapy Source Book.* Perry MC (editor). Williams & Wilkins, 1992.

Ovarian & Uterine Tube Cancer

Albert DS et al: Improved therapeutic index of carboplatin plus cyclophosphamide versus cisplatin plus cyclophosphamide: Final report by the Southwest Oncology Group of a phase III randomized trial in stages III and IV ovarian cancer. *J Clin Oncol* 1992;**10:**706.

Bjorkholm E, Pettersson F: Granulosa-cell and theca-cell tumors: The clinical picture and long term outcome for the Radiumhemmet series. *Acta Obstet Gynecol Scand* 1975;**59:**278.

Bostwick DG et al: Ovarian epithelial tumors of borderline malignancy: A clinical and pathologic study of 109 cases. *Cancer* 1986;**58:**2052.

Calvert AH et al: Carboplatin dosage: Prospective evaluation of a simple formula based on renal function. *J Clin Oncol* 1989;**17:**1748.

Hacker NF et al: Primary cytoreductive surgery for epithelial ovarian cancer. *Obstet Gynecol* 1983;**61:**413.

McGuire WP et al: Taxol: A unique antineoplastic agent with significant activity in advanced ovarian epithelial neoplasms. *Ann Intern Med* 1989;**111:**273.

Rowinsky EK, Cazenave LA, Donehower RC: Taxol: A novel investigational antimicrotubule agent. *JNCI* 1990;**82:**1247.

Rowinsky EK, McGuire WP: Taxol and its current status in cancers of the ovary and breast. *Principles and Practice of Gynecologic Oncology Updates* 1992;**1:**1.

Sevelda P et al: Goserelin, a GnRH analogue as third-line therapy of refractory epithelial ovarian cancer. *Int J Gynecol Cancer* 1992;**2:**119.

Swenerton K et al: Cisplatin-cyclophosphamide versus carboplatin-cyclophosphamide in advanced ovarian cancer: A randomized phase III study of the National Cancer Institute of Canada Clinical Trials Group. *J Clin Oncol* 1992;**10:**718.

Uterine Cancer

Jeffrey JF, Krepart GV, Lotocki RJ: Papillary serous adenocarcinoma of the endometrium. *Obstet Gynecol* 1986;**67:**670.

Tiitinen A et al: Endometrial adenocarcinoma: Clinical outcome in 881 patients and analysis of 146 patients whose deaths were due to endometrial cancer. *Gynecol Oncol* 1986;**25:**11.

Cervical Cancer

Lippman SM et al: 13-*cis*-retinoic acid plus interferon α-2a: Highly active systematic therapy for squamous cell carcinoma of the cervix. *JNCI* 1992;**84:**241.

Palefsky J: Human papillomavirus infection among HIV-infected individuals: Implication for development of malignant tumors. In: *Hematology/Oncology Clinics of North America.* Mitsuyasu RT, Golde DW (editors). Saunders.

Rutledge FN et al: Pelvic exenteration: An analysis of 296 patients. *Am J Obstet Gynecol* 1977;**129:**881.

Shingleton HM et al: Adenocarcinoma of the cervix: Clinical evaluation and pathologic features. *Am J Obstet Gynecol* 1981;**139:**799.

Werness BA, Munger K, Howley PM: The role of human papillomavirus oncoproteins in transformation and carcinogenic progression. In: *Important Advances in Oncology.* DeVita VT Jr, Hellman S, Rosenberg SA (editors). Lippincott, 1991.

Trophoblastic Disease

Bagshawe KD: Trophoblastic tumors: Diagnostic methods, epidemiology, clinical features and management. In: *Gynecologic Oncology.* Coppleson M (editor). Churchill Livingstone, 1992.

Rustin GJS: Trophoblastic tumours. Third Biennial Meeting of the International Gynecologic Cancer Society, 1991, p. 100. [Abstract.]

23

Head & Neck Cancer

G. Richard Holt, MD, MPH, & William W. Shockley, MD

Tumors of the head and neck are diverse in size and spread at the time of presentation. At most major medical centers where large numbers of cancer patients are seen, Head and Neck Tumor Boards provide the format to discuss each patient's case and to plan a treatment course based on input from each specialist involved with some aspect of cancer care. A comprehensive plan is developed from the point of staging the tumor (through dental extractions if needed) to the definitive combination of chemotherapy, surgery, or radiation therapy.

Most physicians caring for the head and neck cancer patient have been trained under the Tumor Board concept and use it to some degree in private practice. In the absence of a formal board, the head and neck surgeon usually coordinates and directs the care of the cancer patient.

Throughout the past five decades, surgery has been the mainstay of treatment for head and neck tumors. With increasing technologic sophistication in radiation therapy, more combined therapy is being used, resulting in less morbidity for the patient. New cancer chemotherapy drug development has led to increasingly effective drugs when used as adjuncts to surgery or irradiation. Most cancer treatment centers are members of a large regional oncology group that offers statistical evaluations of treatment plans and develops randomized treatment protocols to better understand the response of cancers to these various modalities. It is through wide-scale participation in these treatment protocols that advancements in therapy can be obtained. Since the protocols are based on the same tumor staging systems, comparison between protocols can be readily made.

Generally speaking, squamous cell carcinoma is the most common histopathologic type in the upper aerodigestive system. Smaller tumors are usually treated by wide surgical excision, although the patient should be informed of the possible primary use of radiation therapy in order to make an informed decision. Additionally, radiation therapy may be the treatment of choice in some cases. In large tumors, a combination of therapy is almost always agreed upon. For bulky, fixed tumors in the oral cavity and neck, the use of initial chemotherapy will often de-

crease the tumor bulk significantly, allowing for surgical resection and subsequent radiation therapy. Additionally, in some intermediate tumors with a good response to chemotherapy, the use of radiation therapy as the primary modality therapy is adequate, with surgical excision utilized for salvage of recurrent cases. With the use of the CT scans and MRI for following deep-seated tumors, unobserved spread or recurrence may be detected earlier and salvage therapy initiated.

Close follow-up is critical to detecting recurrent disease at an early stage. A common schedule for follow-up examinations is monthly for the first year, every 2 months for the second, 3 months for the third, 4 months for the fourth, and 6 months for the fifth year after primary therapy. After 5 years, the follow-up visits can be yearly. The schedule reverts to another one if new therapy is initiated. The common use of this schedule facilitates the scheduling of appointments with multiple treating physicians.

In recent years, the surgical approach to tumor resection has become more aggressive owing to improvement in reconstructive and rehabilitative techniques. Most defects in the head and neck region can be anatomically restored using pedicled musculocutaneous or muscular flaps or free microanastomotic flaps. Additionally, improved techniques in base of skull surgery now allow the possibility of resection of previously unresectable tumors with less morbidity and mortality. Many cases require combined intracranial and extracranial approaches.

TNM Staging System

Under the TNM staging system (T, tumor; N, node; M, metastasis), the T stage is variable from one head and neck region to another. In the oral cavity, oropharynx, and salivary glands, the T stage is defined primarily by size. In the larynx, hypopharynx, and nasopharynx, the definition varies with tumor extent and structures involved. In all regions, T_1 is an early localized tumor, while T_4 indicates massive invasion with involvement of surrounding structures (such as bone, soft tissues of the neck, skull base, and skin).

The N stage describes the status of the regional

lymph nodes. The definitions are homogeneous for all regions and are as follows:

N_0: No clinically involved nodes.
N_1: Single ipsilateral node ≤3 cm in diameter.
N_2: Single ipsilateral node, 3–6 cm in diameter.
N_{2b}: Multiple ipsilateral nodes, none >6 cm.
N_{2c}: Bilateral or contralateral lymph nodes, none >6 cm.
N_3: Lymph node metastasis >6 cm in diameter.

M categories are defined as follows:

M_0: No distant metastases.
M_1: Distant metastases present.

Once a clinical TNM classification is determined, the patient's disease status can be further classified using a tumor stage grouping I–IV. Again, patients with stage I disease have early lesions, while those with stage III and IV have advanced disease (Figure 23–1).

The approximate 5-year survival for each stage is as follows: stage I, 75–95%; stage II, 50–75%; stage III, 25–50%; and stage IV, <25%

Nodal Involvement

In general, head and neck cancers spread to regional nodes in highly predictable patterns (Table 23–1). For example, tumors of the floor of mouth tend to spread to the submandibular and subdigastric nodes, whereas nasopharyngeal carcinoma spreads not only to the nodes along the jugular vein but also to the posterior triangle nodes. In order to classify the nodes by their location, Lindberg uses a simplified

Table 23–1. Risk of occult lymph node metastasis associated with primary tumor site.

Tumor Site	Risk of Occult Lymph Node Metastasis (%)
Glottis	<5
Floor of mouth	30
Epiglottis	35
Oral tongue	40
Tongue base	60
Hypopharynx	60

system in which nodes are classified into 10 locations (Figure 23–2).

Clinicians and pathologists find it useful to divide the neck into different levels when discussing nodal involvement (Figure 23–3). Multiple nodes, nodes at multiple levels, larger nodes, and soft tissue invasion are all indicative of a worse prognosis. Once metastatic tumor deposits breach the lymph node capsule, they are much less curable than those in which the tumor remains confined to the node. This phenomenon, known as extracapsular spread (ECS), is associated with a higher rate of recurrence and a lower survival rate.

The prognostic factors related to cervical metastasis are size and number of nodes, levels of involvement, soft tissue invasion, and extracapsular spread. The larger the node and the more nodes involved, the worse the prognosis. Nodal involvement in the lower portion of the neck is a more ominous sign then when lymph nodes at a more superior level are involved. Soft tissue invasion causes marked fall-off in survival statistics. The most dreaded features of tumor involvement are direct extension of the primary tumor into the neck, invasion of the skull base, carotid involvement, and invasion of the deep neck muscles. Any of these factors signals a dismal outcome.

Biopsy Techniques

In the case of mucosal surface lesions, biopsy forceps are used to obtain tissue, normally under topical or injectable anesthesia. Only those easily accessible biopsy sites are closed with chromic catgut sutures—the rest are left open to heal secondarily. Lesions in the nasopharynx, hypopharynx, and larynx are best biopsied under operating room conditions because of their decreased accessibility.

For skin lesions, the biopsies can be shave, punch, incisional, or excisional. Shave biopsies do not always give adequate tissue at the base for the pathologist to identify invasive carcinoma. Punch biopsies are easy to perform and give adequate depth of tissue but require longer to heal. When performing an excisional biopsy, include a transitional zone (ie, part abnormal and part normal tissue), which may yield evidence of frank invasion. To obtain such a specimen, perform an elliptical or fusiform excision and

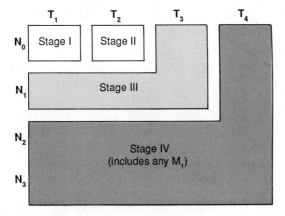

Figure 23–1. Staging of oral squamous carcinoma. (American Joint Committee, 1988.) (Reproduced, with permission, from Strong EW, Spiro RH: Cancer of the oral cavity. Page 310 in: *Cancer of the Head and Neck.* Suen JY, Myers EN [editors]. Churchill Livingstone, 1981.)

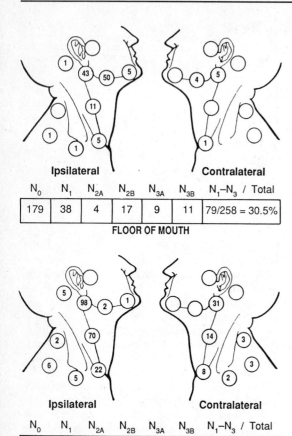

N$_0$	N$_1$	N$_{2A}$	N$_{2B}$	N$_{3A}$	N$_{3B}$	N$_1$–N$_3$ / Total
179	38	4	17	9	11	79/258 = 30.5%

FLOOR OF MOUTH

N$_0$	N$_1$	N$_{2A}$	N$_{2B}$	N$_{3A}$	N$_{3B}$	N$_1$–N$_3$ / Total
120	49	15	29	11	43	147/267 = 55%

SUPRAGLOTTIC LARYNX

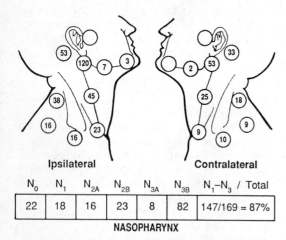

N$_0$	N$_1$	N$_{2A}$	N$_{2B}$	N$_{3A}$	N$_{3B}$	N$_1$–N$_3$ / Total
22	18	16	23	8	82	147/169 = 87%

NASOPHARYNX

Figure 23–2. Lymph node groups represented, from upper to lower neck, are the preauricular, upper posterior cervical, subdigastric, submaxillary triangle, submental, midjugular, midposterior cervical, low posterior cervical, low jugular, and supraclavicular. (Modified and reproduced, with permission, from Lindberg R: Distribution of cervical lymph node metastases from squamous cell carcinoma of the upper respiratory and digestive tracts. *Cancer* 1972;**29:**1448.)

close the wound with one or two sutures. If the lesion is malignant and requires wide local excision, the sites of the biopsy sutures should be generously included in the excision. In many cases, the lesion will be small enough (2–5 mm) that a narrow field total excision can be performed. If the tumor is benign, the treatment is completed; if malignant, the scar must be reexcised with appropriate margins. If a negative biopsy is obtained from a highly suspicious area, then another biopsy from an adjacent or deeper site is indicated. Keep in mind that on deeper mucosal surfaces, the reparative process after a biopsy (pseudoepitheliomatous hyperplasia) may be misinterpreted as squamous cell carcinoma; thus, several weeks should elapse before another biopsy is made to allow for this temporary surface change.

The fine-needle aspiration (FNA) technique has gained increasing acceptance in diagnosing head and neck malignancies. A fine-gauge (23 or 25) needle is introduced into a soft tissue mass and the mass suction aspirated with a 5-mL syringe, yielding clumps of cells for histologic evaluation. This technique is most helpful for diagnosing the cellular content of cervical neck nodes, which are metastatic from some primary site. Greater difficulty in histologic interpretation comes from masses in the salivary glands and thyroid. If positive, the FNA is helpful preoperatively, but a negative sample has essentially no bearing on therapy or diagnosis. FNA is readily available and can be mastered with practice. Its importance in the evaluation is heightened by increased mastery.

Surgery

Four basic types of neck dissections are performed at present: radical, modified radical, modified, and regional.

Radical neck dissection (RND): The lymph nodes are removed en bloc with the submandibular gland, sternocleidomastoid muscle, internal jugular vein, and spinal accessory nerve. This operation is generally performed as therapeutic dissection.

Modified radical or nerve-sparing neck dissection (MRND): This procedure is virtually the same as the RND except that the spinal accessory nerve is preserved. It can be used as either an elective or therapeutic operation depending on extent and location of disease. Nerve preservation diminishes problems related to the shoulder pain and disability often seen after RND.

Modified neck dissection (MND): Only the lymph nodes and fascia are removed, while the sternocleidomastoid muscle, internal jugular vein, and spinal accessory nerve are left intact. This surgery is most often performed as an elective dissection.

Regional or selective neck dissection: Only those nodes at greatest risk are removed along with the primary tumor. Thus, different regions of the neck may be addressed for specific tumor sites.

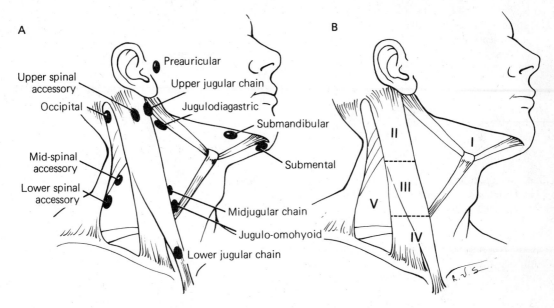

Figure 23–3. *A:* Major lymph node areas of the head and neck. *B:* Levels of cervical lymph nodes used in descriptions of clinical findings, operations, and pathology specimens. I = submandibular, II = upper jugular chain, III = midjugular chain, IV = lower jugular chain, V = posterior cervical triangle. (Reproduced, with permission, from Urist MM, O'Brien CJ: Head and neck tumors. In: *Current Surgical Diagnosis & Treatment,* 9th ed. Way LW [editor]. Appleton & Lange, 1991.)

FACIAL SKIN CANCER

Essential of Diagnosis

- Changes in growth pattern and appearance of sun-exposed skin in susceptible individual.

General Considerations

Most skin cancers of the head and neck region are localized to exposed areas. Therefore, early diagnosis and treatment are possible if medical attention is sought. Nearly 90% of all skin cancers are found in the head and neck region as well as 20% of all malignant melanomas. Most head and neck skin cancers are preventable by adequate protection against sun exposure.

Etiology

Solar and ionizing radiation are the two most common causative agents for facial skin cancers. Men have at least twice as many facial skin malignancies as women, and this finding probably relates to both occupational and recreational exposure to etiologic agents. In the southern USA, many people receive a high degree of sun exposure in out-of-doors occupations such as ranching, farming, and oil field work. In addition, the summer is longer and weather better for outdoor recreational activities, resulting in increased sun exposure. Exposure to inorganic arsenic is a known carcinogen for skin cancers but is no longer common in the USA. In the northern USA, basal cell

carcinoma outnumbers squamous cell carcinoma by 30:1, but in the southern USA, especially Texas, basal cell carcinoma is only twice as common as squamous cell carcinoma. Approximately 1:200 inhabitants of Texas will at some time have a malignancy of the facial skin. However, dark-skinned individuals have fewer skin cancers than the fair skinned. Burn scars carry a high risk of squamous cell carcinoma forming at the margins, and this is associated with increased aggressiveness of the tumor.

Pathogenesis

Fair-skinned, blue-eyed individuals with light hair have more facial skin malignancies than darker skinned individuals. The lack of pigment probably increases the risk of melanin absorption, leading to DNA alterations from ultraviolet energy. Additionally, some hereditary susceptibility or predisposition to the effects of solar radiation is likely. Other cocarcinogens may come into play in certain individuals. Once initiated, the neoplasm is no longer dependent on the original causative agent but continues to become neoplastic even in the absence of further exposure to that agent. Further irritation of an injured site or irritation of a benign nevus may give rise to malignant degeneration, although this finding is not well documented.

Pathology & Staging

Facial skin malignancies have a histologic classification and a behavioral classification. The behavior of some tumors is clinically benign and has a low aggressive tendency. Other tumors that carry the same histologic diagnosis may have a rapid growth spread and a high incidence of lymph node metastases. This is probably due to a combined effect of the biologic behavior of the tumor cells and an alteration in the immune status of the host.

Basal cell carcinomas are more common than squamous cell carcinomas, although the ratio approaches 2:1, basal to squamous, in the southern USA. Actinic, or solar, keratoses are considered premalignant and should be considered a warning sign when found on a biopsy. They indicate that an area of skin damage is undergoing dysplasia, and a frank neoplasm may occur from further exposure. Some actinic keratoses become firm and develop cutaneous horns. Not only can Bowen's disease (carcinoma in situ) occur at the base of cutaneous horns but frank invasive squamous cell carcinoma can also be present. Therefore, these lesions should be excised and carefully evaluated histologically. Basal cell carcinomas occur on sun-exposed areas and are seen as small cells with regular cytoplasmic size and local invasiveness. The superficial spreading and nodular basal cell carcinomas generally carry a reduced risk of metastasis and recurrence. However, morpheaforme basal cell carcinoma is the most bothersome type and has a high rate of inapparent spread to adjacent tissues.

Squamous cell carcinoma may arise in solar keratoses and at the base of a keratoacanthoma. It may be associated with reduced immune system response. Squamous cell carcinomas metastasize more commonly than basal cell carcinomas and follow the expected spread of lymphatic tumor cells to the regional lymph nodes of the head and neck. The so-called basosquamous carcinoma appears to be an intermediate carcinoma and is considered more similar to the squamous than the basal cell variety.

Malignant melanoma is seen on the skin and mucous membranes of the head and neck region. The most common form is superficial spreading melanoma, which is seen in approximately 60% of patients. It has an intermediate prognosis among the three types of malignant melanoma. The most favorable and least common type is the malignant lentigo, which is found in 10% of cases and usually in older patients. It is also known as Hutchinson's freckle and is seen as a flat, diffuse brown spot on the cheek and forehead in elderly patients. The third type, which is the most invasive and worrisome, is the nodular malignant melanoma found in approximately 30% of patients. Malignant melanoma is generally classified according to its depth of penetration, and both the Clark and Breslow system are employed for diagnostic and prognostic histologic classification (Table 23–2).

Adnexal tumors are seen in the head and neck re-

Table 23–2. Histologic staging of malignant melanoma (MM).

Clark's Levels		Breslow's System	American Joint Committee System (1988)
I	Confined to epidermis	. . .	
II	Invasion into papillary dermis	0.75 MM	T_1
III	Complete invasion of papillary dermis	0.76–1.5 MM	T_2
IV	Invasion into reticular dermis	1.51–3.0 MM	T_3
V	Invasion into subdermal tissues	3.0 MM	T_4

gion but most commonly in the ear canal and on the nose. Several of these, including the adenoid cystic and the ceruminoma of the external canal, are uncommon but require surgical extirpation for long-term survival. Most adnexal tumors that are malignant carry a high rate of neck metastases. Kaposi's sarcoma is being seen with greater frequency in patients with AIDS and should be a primary consideration in any patient having AIDS and a skin abnormality. It presents as a smooth or crusty purplish lesion on the face.

Clinical Findings

A. Symptoms and Signs: Most patients with a facial skin malignancy will complain of an area of roughness, redness, or irritation that may get better and then worsen. Occasionally the lesion is associated with bleeding or frank infection but usually is indolent. In cases of malignant melanoma, there may be a history of a change in a skin lesion with respect to size, coloration, margins, or behavior. If a lump in the neck occurs in association with a change in a skin lesion or the appearance of a new skin lesion, it carries a graver prognostic significance.

Every area of the scalp, face, and neck including the external auditory canal, the nasal vestibule, and the postauricular skin should be examined. In patients with thick hair, it is important to mount a careful examination from the back of the neck forward to the hairline so that no area of scalp is missed. The most common sites for development of facial skin malignancy are the cheeks, ear, and preauricular regions, the lower lip, forehead, neck, and nose. Of these the nose is perhaps the most common site for cancer. Although metastases are rare, the neck and also the pre- and postauricular areas, posterior neck, and buccal region should be palpated. Both direct and angled lighting are helpful to differentiate the nodular from superficial appearance. Classically a nodular basal cell carcinoma has a pearly margin and a center crater. A magnifying loupe allows the physician to closely examine the lesion from several angles and become familiar with its magnified appearance.

B. Laboratory Findings: If metastases to the liver are considered, liver function tests may be abnormal. In malignant melanoma, which can metastasize to the bone, the calcium and alkaline phosphatase levels will be occasionally elevated. Additionally, urinary melanogen may be in disseminated malignant melanoma. Hepatic metastases and alcoholic cirrhosis may lead to a prolonged prothrombin time.

C. X-Ray Findings: In malignant melanoma, a chest x-ray is mandatory to evaluate for pulmonary metastases. In the rare nevoid basal cell carcinoma syndrome, look for jaw cysts in the mandible and other characteristic skeletal abnormalities.

D. Special Examinations: CT scans and MRI are helpful in areas of suspected regional lymph node metastases to identify the size and number of the nodes. In malignant melanoma, when nodal disease is not palpable it may be seen on fine-cut CT scan and MRI through the region of greatest suspicion. CT scans of the lung and abdomen also may demonstrate metastases to the lung and liver.

Differential Diagnosis

Skin lesions of the face, scalp, and neck are common, and most are not neoplastic. One type, the keratoacanthoma, is widely misdiagnosed as a squamous cell carcinoma because of its rapid growth rate and elevated appearance. Keratoacanthomas are commonly seen on the cheek, eyelid, lip, and ear and have a history of a rapid growth over several months. They usually spontaneously regress. However, in a patient with sun-damaged skin and other suspicious lesions, it is wise to excise the area to rule out a carcinoma at the base or frank carcinoma.

Senile sebaceous hyperplasia and seborrheic keratosis may commonly be misdiagnosed as cancer. A biopsy should be used to rule out frank carcinoma. Pigmented basal cell carcinomas can look like melanomas, and amelanotic melanomas can be misdiagnosed as small basal cell carcinomas,. In children, spindle cell nevi, which are flat and brown lesions, may look like melanomas and may require removal for diagnosis. Giant hairy nevi in children carry a worse prognosis and should be evaluated for the possibility of malignant degeneration. The clinical differentiation of these lesions between benign and malignant is 80–90% accurate; when in doubt, perform a biopsy.

Prevention

Early detection is one way to prevent further spread and growth of facial skin malignancies. The public should be educated about the risks of exposure to ultraviolet radiation in the natural environment as well as the "unnatural" setting of tanning parlors. The use of a sunscreen with a high filtration factor generally is protective in susceptible individuals when coupled with decreased exposure to the sun and the use of a broad-brimmed hat. A patient who has a family history of skin cancers should be apprised of the risks and encouraged to use sunscreen protection at all times. Topical retinoic acid may reduce conversion of metaplasia from sun-damaged skin to a frank malignancy.

Treatment

Surgery is the mainstay of therapy. Essentially, the lesion, whether it be a squamous or basal cell carcinoma, is excised with adequate margins or frozen section evaluation. A small lesion can be excised in an outpatient setting, the tissue submitted for permanent section, and the wound left closed or unclosed. If the permanent sections are negative, an unclosed wound can be either closed or allowed to heal by secondary intent. Surgical excision in the operating room utilizing frozen section guidance is preferred. One-half to 1-cm margins of normal tissue are left around the lesion with a narrower strip of normal skin being included in the specimen when basal cell carcinoma is suspected. Frozen sections are performed on the entire margin as well as the base. Any remaining tumor or any area of tumor close to the margin should be reexcised and resubmitted for frozen section diagnosis. When the frozen sections are said to be negative, the wound may be closed. In the case of a recurrent or morpheaforme basal cell carcinoma, consideration should be given to utilizing Mohs' fresh tissue preparation excision. This is also helpful in areas of tissue plane cleavage such as the nasal ala, medial canthus, and temporal and preauricular areas. The wound is appropriately reconstructed later.

Radiation therapy normally is not utilized for facial skin malignancies except in patients who are at high risk for a surgical procedure or in areas where reconstruction would be very difficult. It is generally reserved for very aggressive tumors that carry with them a high chance of nodal metastases or those which are not surgically controllable.

Electrodesiccation and curettage as well as cryosurgery are commonly employed for small premalignant or malignant lesions of the face and neck. However, there is no record of the tissue margins, and there is some increased risk of recurrence, particularly of more aggressive lesions. Topical fluorouracil can be used for premalignant lesions once they have been identified clinically or histologically. Topical treatment may retard further carcinoma development.

Resection of a malignant melanoma carries a higher chance of recurrence, and therefore the margins must be expanded. In general, 3–5 cm of normal skin around the area is the norm. The best therapy may be the fresh tissue preparation of Mohs because of its ability to "track" the tumor without excessive margins. Around the orbit, ears, and scalp, the fresh tissue preparation appears to be a favorable excision technique. If the depth of tumor penetration is 1.5 mm or greater and there is no evidence of distal metastases, an elective neck dissection may be performed in the area of risk. If clinically positive lymph nodes are present, a neck dissection should be carried out with excision of the lesion itself.

Reconstruction of the defect created by excising a facial skin malignancy may range from primary closure of the small wound through the use of local advancement or rotational flaps to the use of a large regional musculocutaneous flap or free flap attached through microvascular anastamoses. In areas of recurrent or morpheaforme carcinoma, a split-thickness skin graft may be used in the area of excision so that further residual disease would be noticed earlier. It is generally not wise to use flap reconstruction in a dangerously high-grade or aggressive lesion after excision and healing by secondary intent. Full-thickness skin grafts are occasionally used to reconstruct small defects of the face.

When carcinomas are found on the eyelids, it is important to completely reconstruct the skin, muscular, and skeletal components of the eyelid to protect the globe from exposure and loss of vision. Carcinomas of the external ear canal are generally aggressive and usually result in some form of temporal bone resection in addition to excision of the skin element. These lesions are worrisome and deserve extensive preoperative evaluation by CT scan to determine the depth of the invasion. In some cases, a parotidectomy is required in conjunction with the surgical extirpation of cancers of the scalp, forehead, and auricle because of the presence of lymph nodes beneath the parotid fascia itself. Neck dissection should be carried out for high-grade and aggressive lesions overlying regional nodal areas or where palpable nodes are present.

When extensive skin cancers result in the loss of the ear, nose, or orbital contents, the use of a prosthetic device anchored by osseointegrated titanium implants is preferred. This technology enables the prosthetic device to be firmly anchored by means of rare-metal magnets and has resulted in significant improvement in the quality and appearance of the prosthetic device.

Course & Prognosis

The prognosis for small basal and squamous cell carcinomas of the head and neck is good. Recurrent lesions and aggressive lesions found in facial cleavage planes carry a higher risk of deep invasion and nodal metastases. Basal cell carcinomas have less than a 5% risk for nodal metastases, whereas squamous cell carcinomas may have up to 25% cervical metastases in the head and neck region. If distant metastases occur, they are usually found in the lung, liver, or bone.

They are usually treated with radiation, chemotherapy, or both and have a poor prognosis. Malignant melanomas have widely ranging prognoses from 90% 5-year survival in small favorable lesions to less than 10% in large lesions with metastases. Radiation and chemotherapy are also utilized in disseminated malignant melanoma but are rarely curative. A small incidence of spontaneous remission occurs in melanoma and probably is an immune system response. In Kaposi's sarcoma, treatment is limited to palliation. The prognosis of melanoma 5-year survival diminishes with increasing depth of invasion and presence of lymph node disease. Therefore, the arbitrary decision to perform elective nodal dissection for lesions that invade deeper than 1.5 mm (stage T_3 or T_4) is relatively well founded. However, the performance of the neck dissection does not appear to have a significant impact on the survival of the patient with disseminated melanoma.

SALIVARY GLAND TUMORS

Essentials of Diagnosis
- Major salivary gland tumors usually benign.
- Minor salivary gland tumors usually malignant.
- Tumors associated with pain and neural dysfunction more likely malignant.
- Positive fine-needle aspiration cytologic specimen.

General Considerations

The salivary glands are classified as major and minor. The major salivary glands include the parotid, submandibular, and sublingual glands. The minor salivary glands, numbering up to 1000, can be found anywhere in the upper aerodigestive tract, including the paranasal sinuses. As many as 750 glands can be found in the oral cavity. Tumors of the major and minor salivary glands are relatively uncommon. They account for only about 5% of all head and neck tumors. The incidence of occurrence as well as the chance of malignancy varies with the site of origin.

Approximately 85% of salivary gland tumors arise in the parotid gland. About 10% occur in the submandibular gland, and most of the remaining 5% occur in the minor salivary glands. Tumors rarely occur in the sublingual glands. These neoplasms encompass a wide variety of histopathologic diagnoses and show marked variability in tumor behavior and prognosis. Taken as a group they are more often benign than malignant, they can involve multiple structures in the head and neck, and they are generally treated with surgery.

Etiology

Few major risk factors have been identified in the development of salivary gland tumors. There may be an increased incidence in patients who have received prior radiotherapy for treatment of benign disorders.

Pathogenesis

Two theories have arisen concerning the histogenesis of salivary tumors. Both theories share the concept that there are two major groups of tumors. Some arise from the distal excretory duct and result in an epithelial malignancy, whereas others arise from acinar cells or proximal ductal structures and result in a glandular type malignancy.

Pathology

Of the parotid neoplasms, approximately 80% are benign, while tumors of the submandibular gland are benign in 50–60% of the cases. From 25% to 50% of minor salivary gland tumors are benign.

The most commonly accepted nomenclature for salivary gland tumors is shown in Table 23–3. The most common tumor of the parotid gland is the pleomorphic adenoma or "benign mixed" tumor. The most common malignancy of the parotid is mucoepidermoid carcinoma. In both submandibular and minor salivary glands, the most common benign tumor is pleomorphic adenoma and adenoid cystic carcinoma is the predominant malignancy.

Clinical Findings

A. Symptoms and Signs: Tumors of salivary gland origin generally present as a painless slow-growing mass. Most tumors occur in the tail of the parotid gland. This corresponds to the region immediately behind the angle of the mandible and just below the ear lobe. Tumors involving the deep lobe of the parotid may involve the parapharyngeal space and are manifested as a bulge into the lateral pharyngeal wall. Facial paralysis in association with a parotid mass is an ominous sign and usually indicates cancer. Pain is not commonly associated with salivary neoplasms.

Tumors of submandibular gland origin present as lateral submandibular masses. They become more evident upon bimanual palpation. Minor salivary gland tumors are usually located in the oral cavity and typically are smooth submucosal tumors. The hard palate is the site of predominance.

B. Laboratory Findings: Laboratory tests are generally not helpful.

C. Imaging Studies and Other Tests: CT scan and MRI are generally not helpful in diagnosis but can be of benefit in delineating tumor extent. Sialography is of limited use.

Once the diagnosis of neoplasm is entertained, a biopsy is necessary. If the tumor is accessible to fine-needle aspiration, a cytologic specimen can be taken. Although this may provide useful information in treatment planning, its overall accuracy in salivary gland tumors is only about 75%.

Differential Diagnosis

A painless slow growing mass in the parotid gland, submandibular gland, or oral cavity should be considered a neoplasm. Differential diagnosis includes chronic sialadenitis, granulomatous disease (eg, sarcoidosis, tuberculosis, actinomycosis, cat-scratch fever), Sjögren's syndrome, and lymphoma.

Treatment

Treatment for all resectable tumors is surgical excision. For most parotid tumors, this will usually entail a superficial parotidectomy, removing the tumor en bloc with all the parotid tissue superficial to the facial nerve. For malignancies that involve the facial nerve, a radical parotidectomy (with sacrifice of the nerve) is required. Neural repair can be undertaken by using nerve grafts, most commonly from the greater auricular or sural nerves.

Submandibular gland tumors necessitate removal of the gland. If malignancy is encountered, adjacent structures may have be to be resected to ensure tumor-free margins. Benign tumors of minor salivary gland origin can usually be excised with conservative margins because of the capsule encompassing the tumor. Malignancies must be resected with a cuff of normal tissue and may require removal of the underlying bone.

The lymphatic spread of these salivary malignancies must be considered. Depending on the tumor stage and histologic features, a neck dissection may be appropriate. In most malignant tumors of the major salivary glands, postoperative radiation therapy is appropriate to minimize local or regional recurrence. Chemotherapy is not standard treatment at this time. It may be useful for palliation of recurrent, unresectable tumors.

Course & Prognosis

The recurrence rate for benign tumors is extremely low. Malignant tumors are associated with a wide range of prognoses (Table 23–4). Some neoplasms are known for their aggressive, life-threatening nature, whereas others behave in an indolent fashion and may pose no threat to survival. Still others affect mortality rates 10–20 years after initial therapy.

CANCER OF THE NASOPHARYNX

Essentials of Diagnosis

• High risk in native Orientals, followed by American Orientals.

Table 23–3. Parotid tumors.

Benign	Malignant
Pleomorphic adenoma (mixed tumor)	Mucoepidermoid carcinoma
	Low grade
	High grade
Warthin's tumor (papillary cystadenolymphoma)	Adenoid cystic carcinoma
Oncocytoma	Adenocarcinoma
Monomorphic adenomas	Acinic cell carcinoma
Benign lymphoepithelial lesion	Carcinoma ex–pleomorphic adenoma
	Undifferentiated carcinoma
	Squamous cell carcinoma

Table 23–4. Prognosis of parotid cancer.

Histologic Type	Five-year Survival (%)	Ten-year Survival (%)
Mucoepidermoid		
Low grade	95	92
High grade	50	45
Acinic cell	90	80
Adenoid cystic	75	60
Adenocarcinoma	75	60
Carcinoma ex–pleomorphic		
adenoma	50	30
Squamous cell	50	50
Undifferentiated	30	25

- Serous otitis media, nasal obstruction or discharge, or neck mass.

General Considerations

Nasopharyngeal carcinoma is one of the least commonly occurring carcinomas of the upper aerodigestive tract in the USA. It is characterized by late appearance of symptoms and signs and a dismal prognosis. The most prevalent rates are found in mainland China, particularly around the Canton region. It appears to be of low incidence in whites but has a rising incidence in blacks and other dark-skinned individuals. It appears at the mean age of 40, which is considerably younger than the mean age for other head and neck carcinomas. It may remain undetected for a considerable amount of time because of its location deep within the nasopharynx and base of skull region, although it often presents with a neck mass as the first sign of disease. Staging of the primary tumor is according to the location of the disease, and the neck staging is commensurate with the general staging of neck disease. Primary practitioners need to have a high index of suspicion for the presence of such a carcinoma in high-risk groups (eg, individuals of Chinese heritage) and to encourage early referral for diagnostic studies if clinical suspicions so warrant.

Etiology

Many etiologic factors have been proposed but discarded. Individuals of Chinese heritage have an overwhelming predisposition to this disease. Mainland Chinese have approximately a 40-fold risk over Caucasians of developing nasopharyngeal carcinoma, and while this drops to a 20-fold increase in Chinese-Americans born in the USA, it is still a significantly high risk. Thus, not only hereditary but also environmental factors may be involved in the development of this carcinoma. It is still commonly held that the high incidence in China may be related to deficiencies in vitamins A and D, poor balance of dietary elements, chronic rhinoadenitis, and exposure to the Epstein-Barr virus. Although smoking may contribute to disease development in blacks and whites, it is less likely to do so in those of Chinese origin.

Pathogenesis

The disease begins as a neoplasia in the high recesses of the nasopharynx, particularly the area of the fossa of Rosenmüller. This recess, which is posterior and lateral to the auditory tube orifices, has a variety of epithelial surfaces that appear to be capable of rapid transition to be neoplastic state. Bone invasion is common because of the proximity to the base of the skull. Because of the rich periauditory lymphatic drainage, the incidence of cervical metastases approaches 70%. The fascial planes of the nasopharynx allow for rapid transit of the tumor to the peripharyngeal space laterally, to the intracranial contents via the foramen lacerum superiorly, and inferiorly into the oropharynx. Sixty percent of nasopharynx epithelium is squamous, while the rest is some form of respiratory epithelium. In adults, acanthosis and keratinization are common. A third or "intermediate" epithelium characterized by cuboidal cells and absence of cilia is found in random patches in the nasopharynx. These patches occasionally separate respiratory and squamous epithelia, thus providing areas where three epithelial surfaces are concomitantly present. Because of the open modes of spread, cranial nerve abnormalities are not uncommon and should cause a high index of suspicion for nasopharyngeal cancer.

Pathology & Staging

The most common carcinoma in the nasopharynx is squamous cell carcinoma. It accounts for approximately 80% of all nasopharyngeal tumors. The keratinizing type is the most common. Next are the nonkeratinizing tumors, which include both undifferentiated squamous cell carcinomas and lymphoepitheliomas (formerly called transitional carcinomas). The lymphoepithelioma appears to be associated with the highest titers for Epstein-Barr virus. Squamous cell carcinomas can arise from any of the epithelia present in the nasopharynx. Approximately 20% of tumors of the nasopharynx are nonsquamous. These include adenocarcinomas, malignant melanoma, and lymphoma. It is difficult with small punch biopsies to distinguish pathologic cells of an undifferentiated squamous cell carcinoma from normal reticuloendothelial cells that have undergone some distortion in the biopsy process. Therefore, multiple, large biopsies should be obtained for histologic evaluation. Tumor staging is related to site of involvement and tumor extension (Table 23–5).

Most tumors arise in the lateral or posterosuperior walls of the nasopharynx. These tumors are associated with a high incidence of metastases, both nonpalpable and palpable, to the upper jugulodigastric region. Because of the rich lymphatic and blood supply, distant metastases as well as lymph-borne metastases are possible.

Table 23–5. Tumor staging of the nasopharynx (American Joint Committee, 1988).

Stage	Clinical Findings
T_{1s}	Carcinoma in situ
T_1	Tumor confined to one site of nasopharynx or no tumor visible (positive biopsy only)
T_2	Tumor involving two sites (both posterosuperior and lateral walls)
T_3	Extension of tumor into nasal cavity or oropharynx
T_4	Tumor invasion of skull or cranial nerve involvement or both

Clinical Findings

A. Symptoms and Signs: The most common presenting symptom is a mass in the neck (up to 70% of patients). Patients will often recall a period of increased nasal irritation and mucous production that may or may not have led to nasal obstruction and epistaxis. Deep pain in the vertex of the head and periorbital region is a late finding. Cranial nerve abnormalities cause the symptoms of pain and diplopia and indicate disease that has progressed out of the nasopharynx. In nearly half of cases, patients will relate a fullness or stuffiness in the ear associated with a mild hearing loss. This is usually due to a blocked auditory tube with the development of a middle ear effusion.

The most consistent sign is a mass in the upper jugulodigastric cervical chain, but the submandibular area is also a common site. These nodes can be readily palpated; however, the very high nodes of Ranvier cannot be palpated and may represent early nodal disease seen only on scans. When these particular nodes found at the base of the skull are markedly enlarged, other cranial nerves, eg, IX, X, and XI, can be compromised because of the pressure effect at their exit from the jugular foramen. With cranial nerve involvement, diminished sensation in the second and third divisions of the trigeminal nerve can be elicited on examination. This will correlate well with the deep-seated pain that the patient often describes secondary to trigeminal nerve involvement. The second most common nerve involved is the abducens (sixth) cranial nerve, which leads to palsy of the lateral rectus muscle, giving rise to diplopia. Thus, the common presentation is a patient with mild nasal obstruction, mild epistaxis, a mass in the neck, pain in the face, and an ipsilateral sixth cranial nerve palsy.

B. Laboratory Findings: Most laboratory findings are normal except for the high number of antibodies to the viral capsid antigen of Epstein-Barr virus. These antibody levels correlate well with a high tumor load and can be used to follow the regression or recurrence of a nasopharynx tumor.

C. Imaging Studies: Plain x-rays of the paranasal sinuses and nasopharynx are not helpful. A CT scan with fine cuts through the region of the nasopharynx or MRI will show the presence of a soft tissue mass in the nasopharynx itself. If bone invasion from the skull base is suspected, the CT scan is usually confirmatory. Intracranial involvement may be seen on MRI, but results are variable. MRI can indicate deep-seated but nonpalpable nodes at the base of the skull. This finding is important because of the need to treat the base of the skull by irradiation.

D. Special Examinations: In the past, the primary method of inspecting the nasopharynx in the office setting was the indirect mirror examination. The flexible fiberoptic nasopharyngoscope now allows for the opportunity to visualize the entire nasopharynx and to identify slight abnormalities as well as gross tumor. Biopsies are usually taken in the operating room under general anesthesia. Here complete triple endoscopy with nasopharyngoscopy can be performed, and areas previously identified by the flexible scope can be serially biopsied. Because of the chance of nasopharyngeal bleeding following biopsy, general anesthesia is required.

Differential Diagnosis

With any deep-seated base of skull pain, the diagnosis of sphenoid sinusitis must be entertained. Additionally, such diseases as Wegener's granulomatosis, midline lethal granuloma, and eosinophilic granuloma should be considered. Chronic nonallergic rhinitis, adenoiditis, and lymphoid hypoplasia secondary to chronic posterior rhinorrhea can also cause some of the same signs and symptoms as nasopharyngeal carcinoma. A mass in the nasopharynx that is mucosally lined could be a chordoma. Any large obstructing mass in the nasopharynx might be normal adenoid tissue or antral-choanal polyps.

Prevention

No preventive measures are currently identified.

Treatment

The mainstay of treatment is radiation therapy. High-dose megavoltage radiation therapy with the use of the electron beam has resulted in a high incidence of palliation of symptoms, but the disease still defies a high long-term cure rate. Certain histologic types may have a better response to irradiation. In particular, the undifferentiated carcinoma and lymphoepithelioma respond well, whereas keratinizing squamous cell carcinoma shows a poor response. An adenocystic carcinoma of the nasopharynx responds poorly to radiation therapy over the long term because of the high risk for cranial nerve involvement and late recurrence. Node biopsies are not routinely performed in diagnosing nasopharyngeal carcinoma, but fine-needle aspiration of the node can be obtained to correlate with the nasopharyngeal biopsy. Radiation therapy should be directed toward the primary tumor, the potential spread at the base of the skull, and the treatment of both sides of the neck. Radical neck dissection is generally reserved for patients in whom the primary has been controlled and in whom there is residual neck disease after radiation therapy. Primary radical neck dissection for nodal disease is not recommended prior to radiation therapy. The N_0 neck should be treated with radiation therapy because of the high incidence of deep, nonpalpable nodal involvement.

Complications of radiation therapy to the nasopharynx include myelitis of the spinal cord, bone necrosis, trismus, cataract, and chronic otitis media. Surgical approaches to the nasopharynx for control of residual disease at the primary site have been described, but the trials are too small to give any predictive value to their efficacy. These surgical approaches are extensive and often result in significant morbidity to the patient through other cranial nerve injuries. At this time, surgical excision of the nasopharyngeal primary is not widely advocated.

Course & Prognosis

Since most nasopharyngeal carcinomas are diagnosed late in their progress, the prognosis and outcome are generally dismal. With a high index of suspicion and early diagnosis, radiation therapy with surgical salvage of residual disease could result in over a 50% 5-year survival. Salvage in general is related to stage of disease, presence of metastases, and histologic type of the primary, with lymphoepithelioma demonstrating the highest survival rate. Invasion of the base of the skull and cranial nerve involvement is ominous and rarely results in significant 5-year survival. Salvage appears to be better with lesions of the posterior wall and in younger or female patients. However, those who present with significant nasal obstruction, bilateral neck disease, and base of skull invasion have essentially no demonstrable 5-year survival. If metastases are present in the primary control, the survival rate is approximately 25% for 5 years, and for those with intracranial invasion, it is 10% or less.

No survivors are likely at 5 years if distant metastases are present or occur during the course of treatment. There appears to be at least a 30% increase in survival of those patients with lymphoepithelioma as opposed to keratinizing squamous cell carcinoma. When present, distant metastases occur to the lung, liver, and bone and are associated with pain and rapid demise of the patient. Diagnostic use of the flexible nasopharyngeal scope, MRI, and CT scan help follow the progress of the primary tumor's response to radiation therapy. New modalities of treatment including chemotherapy are being identified as possible adjuvant therapies. However, at present, the cure rate for nasopharyngeal carcinoma is probably less than 10%.

CANCER OF THE NASAL CAVITY & PARANASAL SINUSES

Essentials of Diagnosis

- Nasal obstruction and bleeding.
- History of smoking or exposure to occupational carcinogens.

General Considerations

Cancers of the nasal cavity and paranasal sinuses are often mistaken for a chronic inflammatory disease or remain undiscovered until they present late with a nonresectable tumor. There is an average delay from symptoms to diagnosis of 6–12 months. Anatomy of the nasal cavity and paranasal sinuses is complex and difficult for non–head and neck surgeons to appreciate. Radiographic findings may be read as inflammatory disease or polyps, and a high index of suspicion must be held by the primary care physician as well as the radiologist. Since bone destruction is present in greater than 80% of cases, it is wise to use radiography as an initial screen for tumor. In general, tumors of the nasal cavity and paranasal sinuses are serious because they may erode to the base of the skull or travel through foramina or along nerves to the intracranial contents. Additionally, there is a high incidence of regional and distant metastases, which may be present at the time of diagnosis. The orbit may be involved in up to half of late cases, requiring orbital exenteration. If the pterygoid plates and muscles are invaded, leading to trismus, the cranial nerves likely are also involved at the base of the skull.

This area is difficult for primary care physicians to visualize and usually requires direct visualization using fiberoptic or direct nasal endoscopes or indirect visualization by CT scan. Seventy-five percent of sinus cancers are found in the maxillary sinus, and the rest are essentially located in the ethmoid sinus. The incidence of nasal cavity carcinoma is less than one-third that of paranasal sinuses, but a high index of suspicion must be held for both areas. These tumors are characterized more by local invasion than by nodal disease, and death usually occurs from complications of local recurrence. Carcinoma of the sinuses may be less frequent than in the past, and there may be a slight increase in nasal cavity carcinomas, particularly neuroendocrine tumors.

Etiology

Smoking is less commonly associated with carcinoma of the nasal cavity and paranasal sinuses than other occupational hazards. Workers who are exposed to certain dyes and woodworking dust products classically are at risk for developing adenocarcinoma of the nasal cavity and ethmoids sinus. Exposure to nickel has caused squamous cell carcinoma of the nasal cavity but is decreasing with improvements in material processing. Tumors in these regions may be related to chronic irritations and infections, with the inciting carcinogens being nicotine and environmental hazards.

Pathogenesis

Seventy-five percent of patients with nasal cavity cancer are males over 50 years of age. Approximately 5% of cancers are bilateral, and the lateral walls of the nasal cavity are most often involved; septal carcinoma is quite rare. Primary carcinoma of the sphenoid and frontal sinuses is extremely rare; tumors in these regions usually are involved by contiguous spread from the nasal cavity or ethmoid sinus. The majority of sinus primaries originate in the maxillary antrum, suggesting a possible relationship to chronic sinusitis. Maxillary sinus and nasal cavity cancer both behave like an oral cavity cancer once they erode through the palate, giving rise to an increased risk of cervical metastases. Ethmoid sinus cancers may extend into the intracranial fossa via the cribiform plate and are at great risk for nonresectability. On the other hand, tumors arising on the nasal septum are common in the nasal vestibule and usually more amenable to surgical therapy.

Pathology & Staging

Squamous cell carcinoma makes up 80–85% of tumors in the nasal cavity and paranasal sinuses. The rest are adenocystic carcinomas and mucoepidermoid carcinomas (usually high grade), all from mucosal elements in minor salivary glands. Less well differentiated squamous carcinoma is found posteriorly in the nasal cavity, whereas differentiated squamous carcinoma is more common in the anterior septum or nasal vestibule.

The tumor staging of the maxillary sinus is given in Table 23–6. If adenocystic carcinoma is found, it is usually related to minor salivary gland involvement.

Lymphatic drainage anteriorly is to the facial and submandibular nodes initially and then to the midjugulodigastric nodes. Posterior drainage is in the auditory tube region, and retropharyngeal and high jugulodigastric nodes are commonly involved.

Table 23–6. Tumor staging of the maxillary sinus (American Joint Committee, 1988).

Stage	Clinical Findings
T_{1s}	Carcinoma in situ
T_1	Tumor limited to the antral mucosa with no erosion or destruction of bone
T_2	Tumor with erosion or destruction of the infrastructure (anteroinferior portion), including the hard palate and/or the middle nasal meatus
T_3	Tumor invading any of the following: skin of cheek, posterior wall of maxillary sinus, floor or medial wall of orbit, anterior ethmoid sinus
T_4	Tumor invading orbital contents and/or any of the following: cribiform plate, posterior ethmoid or sphenoid sinuses, nasopharynx, soft palate, pterygomaxillary or temporal fossa, or base of skull

Other tumors in this region include spindle cell carcinoma, malignant melanoma, lymphoepithelial carcinoma, and metastatic carcinoma. Breast and renal cell carcinoma commonly metastasize to the maxilla when metastases are found above the clavicle. Neuroesthesioblastoma and neuroendocrine tumors are being seen more commonly, and their identification and classification is becoming more precise.

Wegener's granulomatosis and malignant histiocytosis are rarely found in the midfacial region, but a high index of suspicion should be held when lesions involve considerable pain, crusting, and irritation, with pain far out of proportion to clinical findings.

Clinical Findings

A. Symptoms and Signs: Most patients with carcinoma of the nasal cavity will present with unilateral nasal obstruction with or without epistaxis. Chronic sinusitis and nasal polyps may be associated with paranasal sinus carcinoma in approximately half of cases. Patients with maxillary sinus carcinoma commonly present with pain in the cheek, dental crowding or dental looseness, and a mass in the palate or the cheek. In the case of ethmoid sinus carcinoma, epiphora and a mass in the nasolacrimal sac region combined with proptosis and anosmia complete the usual symptom complex. Pain in the maxillary region should lead to suspicion of carcinoma of the nasal cavity or paranasal sinus. Neck nodes are seen infrequently in the initial presentation but subsequently develop in a high percentage of patients during or following treatment.

Epiphora, a mass in the nasal lacrimal sac, proptosis, and widening of the intercanthal region all point to a space-occupying lesion in the ethmoid or high nasal cavity. The nasal septum may be irritated, and the turbinate may be swollen or eroded. There may be bloody mucus in the nasal cavity and hypoesthesia of teeth or the cheek. The palate and cheek should be palpated to elicit tenderness or a mass in these regions as well as the area of the pterygoid fossa. Lymph nodes may be present in the upper jugulodigastric area in posteriorly located cancers or in the submandibular or buccal space for anterior cancers. Since there is drainage of the tumor potentially to the peritubal area, otitis media with effusion may be seen in the ipsilateral side. This is an ominous sign because of the extension directly to the nasopharynx or through nodal involvement at the base of skull.

B. Laboratory Findings: Most laboratory findings are pertinent only to the general medical condition of the patient. They will help decide whether the patient is a candidate for large exenterative surgery or whether there is a need for presurgical hyperalimentation. If the lesion is located at the anterior base of the skull, pituitary function tests should be performed to see if there is pituitary dysfunction or hypofunction from direct extension.

C. Imaging and Other Studies: When a screening sinus series or CT scan of the face and head reveals a mass or opacity, the clinician must have a high index of suspicion for a tumor. If the mass does not clear with conservative therapy, consideration should be given to endoscopic or transantral biopsy as appropriate. The mass in the maxillary sinus seen on the lateral view should be evaluated by drawing Ohngren's line on the film. This line runs from the medial canthus to the angle of the mandible and divides the maxillary sinus into a posterosuperior segment and an anteroinferior segment. The importance of this line lies in prognosis because tumors located in the posterosuperior element of the maxillary sinus are more likely to have base of skull and orbital invasion, and successful management is diminished in comparison to that of anteroinferior presentation.

Differential Diagnosis

A tumor of the nasal cavity or paranasal sinuses must be differentiated from chronic and recurrent rhinosinusitis. Nasal polyps, chronic irritation, and early nasal septal perforations from illicit drug use all can mimic a tumor. Since inflammatory and allergic diseases are more common than tumors, one must maintain a high index of suspicion to diagnose tumors when they occur. Other considerations in the differential diagnosis include benign tumors, adenoma, dermoid tumors, papilloma, polyps, osseous lesions, cysts, inverting papilloma, plasmocytoma, and angiofibroma. Endoscopic examination and CT scan will differentiate many of these benign or intermediate lesions from invasive carcinomas.

Prevention

Except for workers exposed to the dye, nickel, and wood processing industries, there are no known preventive measures to take against carcinoma of the nasal cavity and paranasal sinuses. For the few individuals who develop carcinoma of the interior nasal septum and nasal vestibule from smoking, cessation of smoking is an important measure.

Treatment

Firstly, inverted papilloma as an intermediate lesion needs to be dealt with by wide surgical resection, usually a medial maxillectomy or septal resection. These lesions are often difficult to diagnose and may require multiple pathologists' opinions. Since there is a high incidence of local recurrence with inadequate excision, wider than normal excisions should be considered.

Most treatment modalities for nasal cavity and paranasal sinus carcinomas are decided upon relative to histologic type, extent of disease (stage), and the patient's general health. There is no definite staging of the primary tumor for the nasal cavity, but the size of the primary tumor can be used to gauge its stage. Criteria guiding maxillary sinus tumors do exist and can be loosely applied to primary staging for ethmoid sinus tumors. CT scans and MRI help determine the extent of resection necessary to encompass the tumor. In many cases, this is far too great for functional reconstruction, and the patient is at great risk for postoperative mortality. Thus, a decision may be made not to perform exenterative surgery.

Intracranial extension by direct spread through the cribiform plate or base of skull in the past was a contraindication to surgical excision. However, with improved surgical approaches to the base of the skull and refinement of combined intracranial and extracranial resections, more lesions are being approached surgically with greater success. There is a need for immediate reconstruction of the defect, generally using pericranial tissue and microvascular flaps. In this region, functional considerations are usually limited to the area of the orbit and globe, although with exenteration this is not a possibility. When the frontal lobe or brain stem are involved, surgery is not anticipated to be helpful and palliation with chemotherapy and irradiation are normally elected.

For cancers of the nasal vestibule and anterior septum, wide local excision with or without postoperative radiation therapy to regional nodes is selected. This area of nodal irradiation is controversial because of the small number of cases constituting long-term studies. If the patient is definitely reliable, node-bearing regions can be followed closely and treatment initiated if metastases occur after the wide local excision.

Cancers of the lateral nasal wall usually require a wide maxillectomy with or without orbital exenteration. Normally, orbital exenteration is not required, since the cleavage plane of the ethmoid and maxillary sinus is a barrier for tumor progression. Radiation therapy to node-bearing areas is usually indicated.

Cancer of the maxillary sinus can usually be approached with a maxillectomy, either radical or with orbital preservation. The decision to preserve the orbit can be made at the time of surgery guided by coronal and axial CT scans indicating freedom of the orbit from bone erosion as well as the absence of tumor on the periosteum of the orbit clinically. If the tumor is highly aggressive and is found in a young individual, it is probably wise to consider orbital exenteration. Certain tumors found in elderly patients without evidence of gross invasion probably do not warrant removal of the globe because of the significant difficulties an older person has with only one eye.

Radical neck dissections are not often carried out for nasal cavity and paranasal sinus tumors because of the late occurrence of the nodal disease and because of the bilaterality of the lymphatic drainage. Usually both sides of the neck are treated with radiation therapy, and surgical dissection is reserved for those patients in whom irradiation did not sterilize the neck or who developed nodes after irradiation.

Tumors of the ethmoid sinus and the superior nasal cavity usually require combined intracranial and extracranial resection. This can be performed utilizing a coronal flap as well as a lateral rhinotomy or extended external ethmoidectomy. Orbital exenteration can be combined with resection of the anterior cranial fossa segment. Pericranial tissue for reconstruction is uniformly used to provide a dural seal.

Other approaches for nasal cavity and paranasal sinus tumors include lateral rhinotomy, rhinectomy when tumor also involves the dorsum of the nose, Weber-Ferguson incision, and midfacial degloving approach. The Weber-Ferguson incision is helpful in exposing the entire maxilla and orbit for exenteration although it is a cosmetically very unpleasing approach. Midfacial degloving involves a complete maxillolabial sulcus incision combined with circumferential intranasal incisions and allows retraction of the entire midfacial skin superiorly with exposure of the midfacial bone structures, maxillary sinuses, and nasal cavity. For small lesions that require a medial maxillectomy or septal excision, both lateral rhinotomy and midfacial degloving are acceptable.

Prosthetic rehabilitation is important, since the loss of a segment of the hard palate, orbit, or nose creates a cosmetic as well as a functional problem. For palate rehabilitation, preoperative impressions should be made and a temporary surgical prosthetic device produced for intraoperative use after tumor resection. It is important to show the maxillofacial prosthodontist the areas of probable resection on the preoperative impression mold so that the prosthetic device can be fabricated initially as closely as possible to the likely defect. Further modification of the prosthesis at the time of surgery may be necessary if the frozen sections are positive and further excision of the palate is necessary. The prosthesis can be wired to the teeth (or wired to the maxillary bone if the patient is edentulous), and packing of the cavity above the prosthetic device can be brought out the nasal opening. Following healing, a form of prosthetic obturator for the palate can be fabricated by the maxillofacial prosthodontist.

For patients who have lost the orbital contents or nose, new technology involving implantation of titanium osseointegrated implants is becoming available. The titanium screws become integrated with the bone over time, and they are magnetized for attachment of the prosthetic device. This procedure should not be performed earlier than 1 year after completion or radiation therapy to allow time for the radiation osteitis to heal and to facilitate osseointegration of the implants. With any type of prosthetic device, care must be taken not to cover the postsurgical cavity, so that the cavity may be inspected easily and recurrent disease identified early.

Course & Prognosis

The failure of early diagnosis and initiation of treatment in these cancers is the main reason for the low survival rates. The recent emphasis on functional endoscopic sinus surgery and ability to view the intranasal and sinus structures with greater ease and magnification may make it possible to identify early lesions that are amenable to surgical excision and radiation therapy.

The 5-year survival for maxillary sinus carcinoma is about 25% overall with the more advanced lesions having approximately a 15% 5-year survival and the smaller lesions having a 45% survival. Tumors that are diagnosed late in their course at an advanced stage usually require either massive surgery with postoperative radiation therapy or radiation therapy with or without chemotherapy for palliation purposes. With recurrence, the outcome is almost always fatal.

In general, small and early lesions of the accessible areas of the nasal cavity and paranasal sinuses carry a 60–70% 5-year survival rate. However, late and advanced lesions have less than a 10% survival. This low rate is usually due to local recurrence in the base of the skull and vascular triangle of the neck, the presence of brain metastases or direct invasion intracranially, or distant metastases to the lung, liver, and bone. The patient's demise is often associated with intense pain, and patient-controlled analgesia (PCA) is usually required for comfort.

Local recurrences tend to vary in rate from 30% to 60% and are usually difficult to manage. Regional neck disease is usually not the cause of death but rather meningitis, pneumonia, or catastrophic hemorrhage.

CANCER OF THE ORAL CAVITY

Essentials of Diagnosis
- Nonhealing lesion on lips up to base of tongue.
- History of smoking, chewing tobacco, or sun exposure.

General Considerations

The oral cavity is the most common region in the upper aerodigestive tract to be involved by cancer, with approximately 22,000 new cases of oral carcinoma each year. There is a male to female predominance of 3:1, reflecting a trend of increasing incidence in women.

The oral cavity is composed of seven sites: lips, tongue, floor of mouth, buccal mucosa, gingiva, retromolar trigone, and hard palate (Figure 23–4).

Etiology

Most patients with oral cancer have excessively used tobacco and alcohol. Although individually these agents are associated with a threefold increased risk of cancer, when the two are used together the risk of developing cancer is 15 times that for a non-

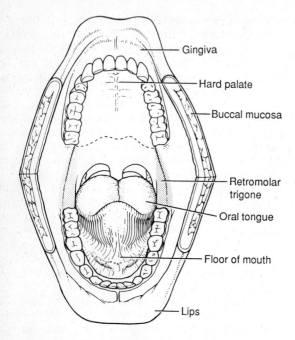

Figure 23–4. Oral cavity. (Modified and reproduced, with permission, from Strong EW, Spiro RH: Cancer of the oral cavity. Page 302 in: *Cancer of the Head and Neck.* Suen JY, Myers EN [editors]. Churchill Livingstone, 1981.)

Table 23–7. Tumor staging of the oral cavity (American Joint Committee, 1988).

Stage	Clinical Findings
T_1	Tumor ≤2 cm in greatest dimension
T_2	Tumor 2–4 cm in greatest dimension
T_3	Tumor >4 cm in greatest dimension
T_4	Tumor invades bone, deep muscles of tongue, maxillary sinus, or skin

logically these lesions are squamous cell carcinoma and can be graded using Broder's classification system (Table 23–8). Tumors that are poorly differentiated or have anaplastic features generally behave more aggressively and carry a worse prognosis. Metastasis to regional lymph nodes at the time of diagnosis is seen in at least 30% of patients.

Clinical Findings

A. Symptoms and Signs: The patient may present with a host of symptoms or a single minor complaint. Most commonly there will be some discomfort noted such as localized pain, "a sore," or odynophagia. Associated symptoms are anorexia and weight loss. Other symptoms may include bleeding, change in denture fit, feeling of fullness or a lump, trouble opening the mouth (trismus), or difficulty with tongue movement.

The physician can usually see a change in the mucosal surface of the involved structure. Most invasive carcinomas show signs of either ulceration or exophytic growth. In general, ulcerative tumors are more aggressive in behavior. Occasionally tumors present as submucosal masses, and these can be confirmed by bimanual palpation of the oral cavity. Care should be taken to document any sensory deficits, such as loss of sensation over the maxillary or mandibular division of the trigeminal nerve. Hypoglossal function testing is mandatory, and any evidence of trismus should be noted.

B. Laboratory Findings: There are no serum markers for diagnosis of oral cavity carcinoma. A complete blood count, general health profile with liver enzymes, and coagulation studies are advisable, since many patients have a history of heavy ethanol use. Baseline studies of total protein and albumin can be beneficial in assessing the extent of malnutrition.

C. X-Ray Findings: A panoramic view of the

smoker, nondrinker. Other factors implicated in the development of carcinoma include poor oral hygiene, syphilis, and chronic trauma. Chewing betel nuts is closely associated with the development of oral cancer in the Far East. Sun exposure (ultraviolet radiation) has been implicated as a cause of lip cancer.

Pathogenesis

There is a general perception that development of cancer relates to epithelial changes that result from chronic exposure to carcinogens and that there is a "time-dose" relationship. In other words, the longer and more pronounced the exposure to tobacco and alcohol, the higher the risk for cancer. This concept is manifested by the development of precancerous lesions, which may be white or red patches (leukoplakia and erythroplakia). Histologically these patches can be hyperplasia, hyperkeratosis, cellular atypia, or dysplasia. The erythroplastic lesions are generally more dangerous and more often represent premalignant or preinvasive tumors. If a lesion at this stage goes unattended, there is a significant chance that it will progress to invasive carcinoma.

Pathology & Staging

The staging for these lesions is based on tumor size and invasion of adjacent structures (Table 23–7). Approximately 90% of cancers affecting the structures of the oral cavity are of epithelial origin. Histopatho-

Table 23–8. Broder's classification of squamous cell carcinoma.

Grade	Differentiation of Tumor
I	Well differentiated
II	Moderately well differentiated
III	Moderately differentiated
IV	Poorly differentiated

mandible may be useful in evaluating tumors close to the mandible. Chest x-ray is advisable, since most patients are smokers and because the lungs are the most common site for distant metastatic disease.

D. Special Examinations: Bone scan is part of the metastatic workup in high-risk patients. It is also useful in detecting early local invasion of bone, such as tumors approaching the mandible. CT scan is used to assess skull base invasion or involvement of the paranasal sinuses. In evaluating tumor extension into soft tissue structures, such as involvement of the pterygoid muscles, MRI may be indicated.

Differential Diagnosis

Any lesion of the oral cavity must be explained or a biopsy must be made. Inflammatory processes do occur, but they are generally short-lived and more diffuse in nature. Red lesions occasionally are manifestations of histoplasmosis, pemphigus, candidiasis, lichen planus, or a systemic illness such as erythema multiforme.

Prevention

The most effective preventive measure is to minimize tobacco and alcohol use. Many programs are available to help smokers quit and to help control alcohol abuse. Teenagers who use snuff or chewing tobacco are often unaware of the dangers involved. Education and encouragement are useful tools for the health care provider to deal with an "at risk" patient. Regular dental evaluations help promote good oral hygiene as well as provide a mechanism for early cancer detection.

Treatment

Once a thorough head and neck evaluation has been completed, an outpatient biopsy can be undertaken if appropriate. Many head and neck surgeons prefer to perform a triple endoscopy. This will allow tumor assessment and biopsy under anesthesia. Proper tumor staging will be completed at that time. Once the biopsy is confirmatory of invasive carcinoma, therapeutic decisions can be made.

The treatment plan must take into account many factors, including the general health status of the patient, psychosocial status, tumor stage and prognosis, structures involved, tumor histology, availability of radiation therapy, and patient compliance. In general, early-stage tumors (T_1 and T_2) can be treated adequately with either surgery or radiation therapy. Most advanced lesions (T_3 and T_4) or those with palpable neck disease (N_1, N_2, and N_3) should be treated with combination therapy. This involves surgical resection combined with pre- or postoperative radiation therapy. In some institutions, adjuvant chemotherapy is also used in this high-risk group (stages III and IV). All general medical problems must be addressed and measures to reverse the negative nitrogen balance instituted. These commonly include oral nutritional supplements, enteral feeding by tube, and hyperalimentation.

Surgical techniques vary with tumor site and stage. A 1- to 2-cm margin is recommended for most tumor resections. Early lesions can be excised transorally with little functional deficit. Use of the laser has become more common in this setting. Advanced tumors may require sacrifice of major portions of the oral cavity. Mandibular involvement is a key issue. Techniques that preserve mandibular continuity include splitting the mandible or removing the upper or inner surface of the mandible. Partial segmental resections are necessary for some neoplasms. The lymphatic drainage of the tumor is of vital importance and must be addressed.

Reconstructive techniques in head and neck surgery have made dramatic advances over the past decade. Small defects can be left to heal by secondary intention, closed primarily, or resurfaced with skin grafting techniques. Larger defects may require the use of regional myocutaneous flaps or free flaps in which microvascular "hookups" are used to transfer tissue from another part of the body to the oral cavity. Recent advances include restoration of mandibular continuity with metal plating techniques as well as transfer of bone by way of pedicled or free flaps.

These reconstructive efforts can be tremendously enhanced with appliances created by maxillofacial prosthodontists. These specialized prosthetics can provide benefits to both cosmetic and functional rehabilitation.

A team approach to the evaluation, treatment, and rehabilitation of these patients provides maximal results. The team should include the head and neck surgeon, radiation oncologist, medical oncologist, dental professional, psychologist, social worker, nurses, dietician, physical therapist, speech therapist, and prosthondontist.

Course & Prognosis

Functional and cosmetic rehabilitation are directly dependent on extent of disease, treatment modalities involved, and extent of surgery. Tumors that are early in stage can be more readily treated and will have a better prognosis and a better functional result. Patients with more advanced tumors will have greater disabilities and a worse outcome.

The overall 5-year survival rates for T_1, T_2, T_3, and T_4 tumors are 80%, 60%, 40%, and 20%, respectively. Patients with lymph node metastasis have a significantly worse outcome. Regional node involvement roughly halves the survival for a given T stage.

CANCER OF THE OROPHARYNX & HYPOPHARYNX

Essentials of Diagnosis

- Dysphagia, odynophagia, and a neck mass.

- Characteristic muffled ("hot potato") voice.
- Hoarseness and aspiration with large lesions.

General Considerations

The oropharynx extends from the nasopharynx to the tip of the epiglottis in a vertical plane and from the circumvallate papillae to the posterior pharyngeal wall. The area includes the base of the tongue and the palatine arches as well as the soft palate. The hypopharynx extends vertically from the free margin of the tip of the epiglottis to the lower border of the cricoid cartilage and encompasses the funnel-shaped area from below the base of the tongue to the cervical esophagus including the piriform sinus. Carcinomas in this area are considered to be directly related to smoking and drinking. They are approximately four times more common in men than women although this ratio is changing owing to the increased rate of smoking in women. The average age for development of a cancer in this area is approximately 60 years although cancers in a few heavy smokers occur by age 40. Pain and dysphagia with weight loss are the hallmarks. A neck node is usually the first sign and is present in 50–75% of patients. These lesions are not commonly diagnosed in early stages. A patient who has had a sore throat for at least a month should be referred to a head and neck specialist. A sore throat persisting this long in an adult is considered cancer until proved otherwise. The most common site of cancer in the oropharynx is the tonsil and posterior trigone region and in the hypopharynx is the posterior and lateral pharyngeal wall.

Etiology

Smoking is universally considered to be the main cause of cancers in the oropharynx and hypopharynx. The most common carcinogen is excessive alcohol use. Alcohol is thought to depress the immune response and allow the hydrocarbon carcinogen in tobacco to become effective. Other cocarcinogen states include local infection and irritation, poor general nutritional status, and depressed immune status for other reasons.

Because of the flow of smoke and hydrocarbons dissolved in saliva, the areas of the tonsil, base of tongue, and pharyngeal wall are continually bathed in these irritants. In India, base of tongue carcinoma is three times greater than anterior tongue cancer, a reverse statistic from that seen in the USA, and probably reflects the fact that the population in India practices poor oral hygiene while chewing and smoking carcinogens on a daily basis.

Pathogenesis

While leukoplakia and erythroplasia both are precursors, finding erythroplasia in the oral cavity is more ominous. Erythroplasia indicates a more intense dysplastic process to which the oral mucosa has become sensitive and reactive. In general, when a carcinoma is found in the oropharynx or hypopharynx, the entire mucosa in the upper aerodigestive tract is abnormal, and many areas of dysplastic changes can be found on examination and on biopsy. Chronic irritation along the entire aerodigestive tract is known as "field cancerization" and bears with it the high risk, nearly 10% in most series, of a second or even a third primary in the mucosa-lined surface of the head and neck. The larger the primary tumor, usually greater then 2 cm, the greater the chance for regional metastases. Carcinoma of the tonsil appears to be second only to that of the larynx in frequency in upper aerodigestive tract cancers.

Pathology & Staging

Squamous cell carcinoma makes up well over 90% of all cancers of the oropharynx and hypopharynx. Lymphomas, adenocarcinomas, and rhabdomyosarcomas are found in decreasing order and are unusual. When non–squamous cell carcinomas are found in the oropharynx or hypopharynx, they are usually of salivary gland origin and are usually mucoepidermoid or adenocystic. Lymphomas are generally seen at the base of tongue, tonsil, and posterior pharyngeal wall in the region of Waldeyer's tonsillar ring.

Squamous cell carcinomas of the oropharynx and hypopharynx are usually keratinizing although nonkeratinizing undifferentiated carcinomas are being seen more frequently. The squamous cell carcinomas are generally of two varieties: (1) The infiltrative type carries the worse prognosis of the two because it is often not seen or does not cause symptoms as readily as the exophytic type. (2) The exophytic type is the most common form and is not infiltrative to the extent that it can be detected early if high index of suspicion is present. The soft palate can be a site for salivary gland tumors because of its high density of minor salivary glands. While the tonsils are a common site for squamous cell carcinoma, lymphomas can also be seen; they usually present with unilateral enlargement of one tonsil. When found in the hypopharynx, squamous cell carcinomas are usually large and fungate and have a 50–75% rate of neck metastases early in the course.

Tumor staging of the oropharynx and hypopharynx is shown in Tables 23–9 and 23–10.

Table 23–9. Tumor staging of the oropharynx (American Joint Committee, 1988).

Stage	Clinical Findings
T_{is}	Carcinoma in situ
T_1	Tumor ≤2 cm in greatest diameter
T_2	Tumor >2 cm but not >4cm in greatest diameter
T_3	Tumor >4 cm in greatest diameter
T_4	Tumor invades adjacent structures (eg, through cortical bone, soft tissue of neck, deep muscle of tongue)

Table 23–10. Tumor staging of the hypopharynx (American Joint Committee, 1988).

Stage	Clinical Findings
T_{1s}	Carcinoma in situ
T_1	Tumor confined to site of origin
T_2	Extension of tumor to adjacent site or region without fixation of hemilarynx
T_3	Extension of tumor to adjacent site or region with fixation of hemilarynx
T_4	Tumor invades adjacent structures (eg, cartilage or soft tissues of neck)

Clinical Findings

A. Symptoms and Signs: The main symptoms of carcinomas of the oropharynx and hypopharynx are sore throat, foreign body sensation, a lump in the throat, and referred pain to the ear. The referred pain route is from the internal branch of the superior laryngeal nerve, which innervates the region of the hypopharynx, to Arnold's nerve, which innervates the deep external auditory canal. It is not uncommon for patients with hypopharyngeal tumor to be treated for ear pain without thought given to the possibility of cancer at a lower anatomic level.

Cancers of the tonsil and base of the tongue often present with a muffled voice, the "hot potato" voice that can also be seen with hypopharyngeal tumors. When the tumors are exophytic, they generally cause more pain, and the patient will relate discomfort after eating acidic and rough-textured foods. Occasionally trismus is present with tumors located in the region of the tonsil and posterior trigone, and weight loss can be seen due to bulky and painful tumors in any region of the upper aerodigestive tract. Cancers of the low hypopharynx and postcricoid region can cause fixation of the vocal cords, with aspiration and hoarseness.

Special attention should be paid to inspection of the base of the tongue and tonsil region. Since the base of the tongue is very difficult to examine, the use of the indirect mirror and flexible nasopharyngoscope by the head and neck specialist constitutes an important reason for referral. Mirror examination is also helpful in examining the nasopharynx, oropharynx, and hypopharynx. Signs include a unilaterally enlarged tonsil, a mass on the palate, a firm or exophytic mass at the base of the tongue, abnormally large lingual tonsils, and ulcers on the pharyngeal wall. If no tonsil is present, there may be an ulcer in the fossa that is tender to palpation. Edema of the arytenoid cartilages may indicate a postcricoid tumor, and fixation of the vocal cord is suggestive of piriform sinus carcinoma. Additionally, pooling of saliva in the piriform sinus indicates poor flattening of the piriform sinus during swallowing and the potential for a space-occupying mass in that region.

Nodal disease in the neck is a common presentation and is usually in the midjugulodigastric area, nodal levels II and III. Low level IV paratracheal nodes can be present with piriform sinus and posterior cricoid carcinomas. With posterior pharyngeal wall and tonsil carcinomas, the nodes of Ranvier may be enlarged and although not palpable may give rise to other cranial nerve dysfunctions.

B. Laboratory Findings: Weight loss and laboratory evidence of a catabolic state are often present. Liver function and bleeding time studies should be performed in patients with a history of alcoholism. A liver-spleen scan is considered important by many clinicians to rule out the small possibility of metastases to these areas from infiltrative hypopharyngeal carcinomas.

C. Imaging Studies: A chest x-ray is needed to rule out the presence of a second primary, particularly in the heavy smoker. Cervical spine tonograms may be helpful in evaluating the area of the posterior pharyngeal wall and posterior cricoid for bone erosion or soft tissue masses, but these may be better delineated on an axial or coronal CT scan. CT scan and MRI of the base of skull down to the thoracic inlet may demonstrate nonpalpable metastatic nodal disease as well as extent of tumor invasion into surrounding soft tissues. These scans are important in staging, since staging of hypopharyngeal carcinoma depends largely on its extension into surrounding tissues.

D. Special Examinations: Outpatient fine-needle aspiration of a neck node on the initial examination can yield the diagnosis of cancer in a majority of cases. All patients require triple endoscopy with biopsies for appropriate staging, performed under general anesthesia. Multiple biopsies of the area should be taken to confirm the diagnosis although "mapping" of the region with marginal biopsies does not appear to be helpful because of the risk of submucosal spread beyond the obvious mucosal involvement.

Differential Diagnosis

Very few nonmalignant lesions present in the areas of the base of tongue or hypopharynx. In some cases, recurrent aphthous ulcers may appear as tonsillar or soft palate lesions with surrounding erythroplasia. Papillomas, mucous cysts, and benign adenomas may present as masses in the oropharynx but do not have the classical ulcerative appearance of carcinomas in this region. Hemangiomas and benign lymphoid hypoplasia are usually distinguishable from frank carcinomas. A lingual thyroid usually does not persist to adulthood.

Prevention

Cessation of smoking and drinking should effectively reduce the chance of developing a squamous cell carcinoma in these regions to practically zero. However, other nonsquamous carcinomas such as adenocarcinomas and lymphomas cannot be avoided in this manner and can potentially occur in nearly all individuals.

Treatment

Treatment protocol studies are under way in nearly all major head and neck cancer centers. However, most of these protocols utilize "up-front" chemotherapy and radiation therapy followed by surgery, whereas most surgeons prefer postoperative radiation therapy because of the edema and pain involved in preoperative irradiation and subsequent inanition of the patient.

Cancer of the tonsil and posterior trigone region is generally treated by radiation therapy when small and with combined therapy when large. With combined therapy, the surgical procedure is usually performed initially and often consists of a composite resection of the tumor and mandible with a concomitant radical neck dissection. If possible, a wide local resection of the tonsillar or trigone tumor can be performed utilizing a lateral pharyngotomy approach or a mandibular split approach, and the neck dissection is performed separately. In these cases, a pectoral muscular flap is used to reconstruct the intraoral defect and to provide protection for the carotid artery.

Base of tongue cancers are usually treated with primary radiation therapy with or without adjuvant chemotherapy. Surgery is generally reserved for salvage cases in failures of radiation therapy or in localized disease where combined surgery and radiation appears to be efficacious. It is almost always combined with at least a unilateral radical neck dissection with a possible functional neck dissection on the contralateral side. Postoperative radiation therapy is given to the primary site as well as to both sides of the neck.

Carcinoma of the soft palate is generally treated by surgical excision if the lesion is small or by radiation therapy if it is large. Radiation therapy is usually selected because resection of the soft palate in an older individual who is edentulous creates a difficult problem for prosthetic rehabilitation. In the patient has no teeth onto which to anchor the prosthetic device, a large defect will generally cause much bothersome nasal regurgitation. Small tumors of the posterior and lateral pharyngeal wall can be treated with wide local excision and irradiation to both sides of the neck if no occult nodes are present. If positive nodes are present in the neck, a concomitant radical neck dissection should be performed on one side with radiation therapy given postoperatively. If both sides of the neck are involved, a functional neck dissection can be performed on the contralateral side and postoperative radiation given.

Tumors of the posterior and lateral hypopharyngeal walls carry an intermediate prognosis in the spectrum of hypopharyngeal tumors. They tend to present late because of the inaccessibility for diagnosis, and they present more than half of the time with a mid-neck metastatic node. If a lesion is small and accessible, a pharyngotomy approach (either lateral or transhyoid) can afford a wide local excision of the primary with radiation therapy to both sides of the neck or neck dissection if palpable nodes are present. Mandibular osteotomy can be used to expose the lesion; however, this procedure is a source of considerable morbidity to the patient, and nonunion may occur in the face of postoperative radiation therapy. In larger lesions, radiation therapy is usually the treatment of choice, with surgery for salvage if possible. Combined therapy of hypopharyngeal wall tumors can be performed, but the primary must be accessible and the defect must be amenable to functional reconstruction using a myocutaneous or free flap.

Carcinomas of the piriform sinus are often mistakenly considered laryngeal tumors. In spite of the fact that they are located in the anatomic hypopharynx, they often involve the larynx and cause laryngeal hypomobility or paralysis of one or both vocal cords. If the larynx is grossly involved, a hypopharyngeal resection including laryngectomy is the treatment of choice. Usually an ipsilateral radical neck dissection is performed, and radiation therapy is given postoperatively to the primary in both sides of the neck. Some authors advocate partial laryngectomy in the face of a small piriform sinus carcinoma, but most clinicians feel that it is risky to leave the larynx behind in such a tumor. In small carcinomas of the piriform sinus, radiation therapy is probably the treatment of choice, with combined surgery followed by postoperative radiation therapy utilized in advanced stages. There is a high rate of nodal metastases with piriform sinus carcinoma, so both sides of the neck must be treated in some fashion in all cases. It is usually possible to reconstruct the remainder of the hypopharynx and esophagus into a competent swallowing passage; if not, this can be effected by the use of a pedicle myocutaneous flap or gastric pull-up procedure.

The worse disease in the hypopharynx is that of the postcricoid region; it almost always carries a dismal prognosis. It is difficult to diagnose and often is missed until it has progressed beyond the possibility of surgical management. In these cases, the only therapy is to perform a diversion or feeding esophagostomy or to insert an indwelling stent for untreatable carcinoma. However, if there is no evidence of bone erosion and if the postcricoid tumor is identified in an early stage, a total laryngopharyngectomy with cervical esophagectomy can be performed in conjunction with bilateral neck dissections. The gullet can be reconstructed, either utilizing a gastric pull-up procedure or a colon-interposition procedure. The gastric pull-up procedure is more physiologic and results in less morbidity and mortality for the patient. Because of the difficulties associated with abnormal motility in the colon segment that is interposed, the second procedure appears not to be as effective as the gastric pull-up procedure. These procedures are fraught with a high likelihood or catastrophe, and the patient often develops recurrent disease before completion of the rehabilitation process. Recurrence is usually due to unsuspected submucosal spread of the tumor as well as uncontrollable regional or distant metastases.

In the surgical resection of all these tumors, frozen section margins at the time of surgery are mandatory. It is difficult, however, for the pathologist to identify every margin perfectly, and for this reason, there is an inherent error in the use of frozen sections. If positive or close margins are found on permanent sections, postoperative radiation therapy affords the opportunity to sterilize the microscopic disease; however, this is not always possible, and such patients tend to die of local recurrent disease as well as distant metastases. All advanced stage cancers of the oropharynx and hypopharynx have a high morbidity rate as well as a high chance for recurrent disease. In many cases, because of the long-term reconstruction attempts, a percutaneous gastrostomy tube is placed to feed the patient and put the patient in a positive anabolic state during the time of healing from the multiple surgical procedures and radiation therapy. Adjuvant chemotherapy has not been significantly successful in influencing the course of the outcome of the serious cancers.

Course & Prognosis

Nearly all larger tumors of the oropharynx and hypopharynx present with regional node metastases. Only small stage I and possibly stage II lesions without nodal metastases appear to have a chance for cure. Cure is extremely rare in stages III and IV when nodal metastases have occurred. If small T_1 and T_2 lesions are diagnosed early, surgery and radiation therapy are equally efficacious treatment. While radiation therapy usually allows better rehabilitation, the surgical procedure allows for margin identification and the possibility of postoperative radiation therapy if margins are positive. Surgical salvage after radiation therapy is not highly successful.

All of the procedures tend to require flap reconstruction of the defect, which also protects the great vessels in the neck from salivary contamination. Most reconstruction in this case utilizes the musculocutaneous flaps of the pectoral and latissimus muscles. These flaps are highly successful and have greatly improved the functional rehabilitation of patients with these serious deformities.

Approximately 10% of cancers in the oropharynx and hypopharynx will present at some time with distant metastases, and these are usually rapidly fatal. The disease tends to occur in older patients who exhibit poor healing and other medical disorders and whose general response to major surgical procedures and radiation therapy is poor. Five-year survival rates for oropharyngeal tumors are slightly better than those for hypopharyngeal tumors. They range from approximately 60% to 65% for early lesions in the oropharynx to 10% to 20% in large lesions in the oropharynx with metastases. By comparison, hypopharyngeal tumors have approximately 40–50% 5-year survival with early lesions and only a 10–15% survival with large tumors and multiple metastases. Overall survival for these lesions for over 5 years is 30–40%.

Early detection and initiation of multiple modality therapy give the best chances for long-term survival. Reconstruction of defects by means of musculocutaneous flaps and gastric pull-up procedures has improved the success rate of functional rehabilitation. However, as patients continue to smoke and drink, these serious tumors will continue to pose challenges for the head and neck oncologic surgeon.

CANCER OF THE LARYNX

Essentials of Diagnosis

- Hoarseness of >1 month duration.
- Stridor indicating involvement or fixation of the vocal cord or a bulky tumor.
- Neck mass (supraglottic and subglottic tumors).

General Considerations

Cancer of the larynx is the second most common malignancy of the upper aerodigestive tract. It makes up about 2% of all malignancies and accounts for approximately 12,000 cases annually. As in other head and neck tumors there is a male predominance (5:1), with recent studies reflecting a trend of increasing incidence in females. The peak incidence is in the seventh decade.

In order to better stage neoplastic disease, the larynx is considered to be composed of three regions: the supraglottis, glottis, and subglottis (Figure 23–5). The supraglottis occupies the area above the apex of the ventricles and is composed of the epiglottis, arytenoepiglottic folds, arytenoid cartilages, and false vocal cords. The true vocal cords make up the glottis. The subglottis is the region extending from the lower boundary of the vocal cords to the margin of the cricoid cartilage.

Etiology

There is a definite relationship between laryngeal carcinoma and the use of tobacco and alcohol. A "dose-related" correlation exists between the risk of disease and the number of cigarettes smoked per day. Laryngeal malignancy in nonsmokers accounts for only about 5% cases.

Pathogenesis

The polynuclear hydrocarbons and nitroso- compounds are suspected as primary carcinogenic agents in cigarette smoke. Chronic exposure leads to continuum of histologic findings. Early changes are represented as hyperplasia, keratosis, mild dysplasia, or cellular atypia. Continued exposure causes progression of disease leading to moderate to severe dysplasia, carcinoma in situ, microinvasive carcinoma, and

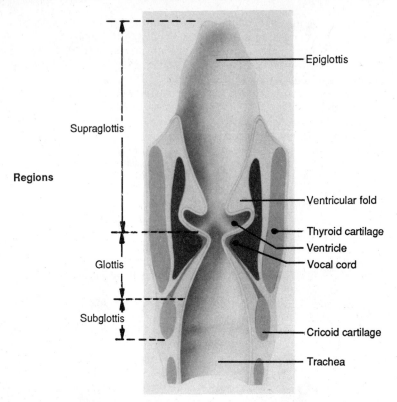

Regions

Supraglottis

Glottis

Subglottis

Epiglottis

Ventricular fold

Thyroid cartilage

Ventricle

Vocal cord

Cricoid cartilage

Trachea

Figure 23–5. Larynx. (Modified and reproduced, with permission, from Lehmann W, Widmann JJ: *Larynx: Microlaryngoscopy and Histopathology*. Franceschinis R, Lualdi P [editors]. Inpharzam Medical Publications, 1981.)

finally invasive squamous cell carcinoma (Figure 23–6).

Pathology

Over 90% of malignancies of the larynx are squamous cell carcinomas. Tumors tend to stay confined to the "compartments" of the larynx until more advanced stages. Epiglottic tumors tend not to traverse the ventricle; glottic tumors tend not to invade supraglottic structures and do not spread past the midline until advanced stages. Of course, more aggressive lesions do not "play by the rules." Tumors that affect cord mobility are associated with a worse prognosis. An immobile or "fixed" cord is staged as a T_3 lesion in all three sites of the larynx. Limitation of motion is most often due to muscle invasion but can be secondary to tumor bulk, cricoarytenoid joint involvement, or impairment of the recurrent (laryngeal) nerve.

Tumors that cross the ventricle are called transglottic tumors and by definition involve the glottis and supraglottis. These lesions can metastasize to regional nodes in up to 50% of cases. Lesions confined to the glottis have a low incidence of lymphatic spread (<5%). Supraglottic carcinoma is associated with regional lymphatic spread in 30–40% of cases.

The metastatic rate for subglottic carcinoma is 10–20%.

Clinical Findings

A. Symptoms and Signs: The cardinal symptom of carcinoma of the larynx is hoarseness. Tumors involving the supraglottic region may produce a "muffled" voice. Airway obstruction may be a presenting symptom in tumors of the subglottis or in more advanced lesions of the glottis and supraglottis. Other symptoms may include pain, a sensation of a lump in the throat, dysphagia, odynophagia, and hemoptysis. In some patients, the cervical metastasis (neck mass) may provide the impetus to seek medical attention.

Physical findings for the experienced examiner are seldom subtle. Evaluation of the larynx can generally be accomplished by mirror examination (indirect laryngoscopy). A fiberoptic flexible laryngoscope can also be used to visualize lesions in patients who are difficult to examine or to better assess the laryngeal structures and the pathologic features.

Tumors involving the glottic region are the most common. Typically, early lesions present as white or red patches on the vocal cords. More advanced tu-

Benign modifications of squamous epithelium

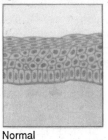 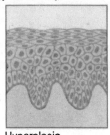 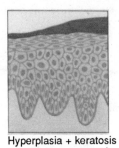

LEGEND:

Atypical cells + mitoses

Keratosis (facultative)

Normal   Hyperplasia   Hyperplasia + keratosis

Malignant transformation of precancerous epithelial lesions

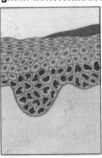 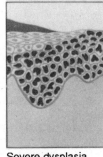 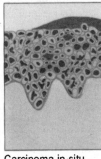 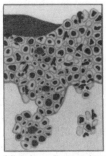

Moderate dysplasia   Severe dysplasia   Carcinoma in situ   Microinvasive carcinoma

Figure 23–6. States of differentiation of squamous epithelium. (Modified and reproduced, with permission, from Lehmann W, Widmann JJ: *Larynx: Microlaryngoscopy and Histopathology.* Franceschinis R, Lualdi P [editors]. Inpharzam Medical Publications, 1981.)

mors are usually exophytic and irregular. Prognosis is dramatically affected once tumor involvement is associated with impaired mobility of the vocal cord.

Supraglottic tumors generally arise on the epiglottis but may involve the false vocal cords, arytenoepiglottic folds, and arytenoid cartilages. Lesions involving the vallecula and tongue base are the most lethal. Clinically they are usually exophytic masses but can also appear as ulcerative lesions. Supraglottic tumors are associated with a rich lymphatic network and are the most likely to metastasize to regional nodes.

Subglottic neoplasms are the least common. They often present with hoarseness and airway obstruction and generally are "silent" until advanced stages. They are recognized on examination as a bulge or tumor mass immediately below the vocal cords. Often by the time of diagnosis the glottis is involved as well (ie, invasion from below to the adjacent vocal cord). Associated lymphadenopathy is uncommon.

B. Laboratory Findings: Laboratory tests are generally not helpful in diagnosis.

C. Imaging studies: The presumptive diagnosis of neoplasm is made based on clinical examination. Soft tissue neck x-rays, CT scan, and MRI can be helpful on occasion in determining tumor extent. Some centers use the CT scan as a survey for lymphadenopathy.

Differential Diagnosis

The features of malignancy are usually characteristic, but occasionally rare conditions can mimic these findings. These conditions include fungal diseases, mycobacterial infections, syphilis, and granulomatous disorders. A biopsy is mandatory before definitive therapy is undertaken.

Prevention

Nonsmokers rarely are affected by laryngeal carcinoma, although alcohol abuse can be associated with supraglottic cancers. In the absence of these agents, the chance of developing a carcinoma is remote. Smokers who quit can lower their risk to the level of a nonsmoker in 10 years.

Treatment

Preliminary treatment includes direct laryngoscopy under anesthesia. At this time, biopsies are obtained, tumor extent is "mapped out," and tumor stage is determined. Tumors thought to be preinvasive can be removed using microsurgical techniques. This is referred to as microlaryngoscopy with vocal cord stripping. This technique is reserved for benign or preinvasive lesions (eg, dysplasia, carcinoma in situ).

Treatment of invasive squamous cell carcinoma of the larynx depends on tumor site, tumor stage, and patient status. Early cancers (stage T_1 or T_2) of the glottis can be effectively treated with surgery or radiation therapy. Selected tumors can be removed endoscopically by microsurgical excision. Many surgeons use the CO_2 laser for this procedure. Other early glottic cancers are best treated with a vertical frontolateral laryngectomy (hemilaryngectomy). In this procedure, the involved vocal cord is removed with a portion of the thyroid cartilage. This results in a husky, sometimes breathy voice, but the patient breaths and swallows normally.

Cancer of the supraglottis generally behaves more aggressively than cancer of the glottis. Again, stage T_1 and T_2 lesions can be effectively treated with surgery or radiation therapy. Patients with carcinoma of the epiglottis are ideal candidates for a supraglottic laryngectomy. In this operation, the upper half of the larynx is removed en bloc with the tumor. This entails resection of the epiglottis, arytenoepiglottic folds, and false cords. The vocal cords remain in their normal position. After rehabilitation during the immediate postoperative period, the patient is able to breathe, swallow, and speak normally.

Most subglottic cancers as well as advanced (stage T_3 or T_4) cancers of the glottis and supraglottis require removal of the entire larynx. This procedure is known as total laryngectomy. The pharynx is reconstructed, and the patient swallows normally but breathes through a permanent tracheostoma.

In locally advance tumors such as those with involvement of the hypopharynx and those invading the thyroid cartilage, adjuvant radiation therapy is recommended. Elective neck irradiation may be appropriate if the patient is at risk of having subclinical involvement of the regional lymph nodes. Chemotherapy protocols are being used in stage III and IV disease. At this time, however, chemotherapy does not have a role in standard therapy of laryngeal tumors.

Course & Prognosis

The patient who has had a total laryngectomy must master a new method of speech. The most common methods include use of an artificial larynx (electrolarynx), esophageal speech, and prosthetic speech. Esophageal speech is created by swallowing air and using the mucosal vibrations caused by this escape of air as a sound source. In prosthetic speech, a small appliance is placed in the back wall of the tracheostoma, allowing air from the lungs to be temporarily diverted to the pharyngeal lumen. The passage of air creates a low pitched sound that can be used as an alternate voice. The articulation mechanism remains the same in all three types of postlaryngectomy speech.

The overall 5-year survival for laryngeal carcinoma is 67%. The 5-year survival for T_3 lesions (ie, those having a fixed cord) is 60–70% when surgery is employed as the primary treatment modality. Prognosis is related to tumor site, with glottic tumors having the best prognosis, followed by supraglottic and then subglottic lesions. Tumors treated at the T_1 stage can usually be cured in 80–90% of patients. As for other head and neck tumors, the presence of regional lymphatic spread profoundly affects survival.

REFERENCES

American Joint Committee for Cancer Staging and End Results Reporting: *Manual for Staging of Cancer,* 3rd ed. Lippincott, 1988.

Baden E: Prevention of cancer of the oral cavity and pharynx. *CA* 1987;**37**:49.

Bailey BJ, Biller HE (editors): *Surgery of the Larynx.* Saunders, 1985.

Baker SR: Malignant neoplasms of the oral cavity. In: *Otolaryngology—Head and Neck Surgery.* Vol 2. Cummings CW (editor). Mosby, 1986.

Batsakis JG (editor): *Tumors of the Head and Neck: Clinical and Pathological Considerations,* 2nd ed. Williams & Wilkins, 1979.

Berg HM et al: Correlation of fine needle biopsy and CT scanning of parotid masses. *Laryngoscope* 1986;**96:** 1357.

Byrne MN, Spector JG: Parotid masses: Evaluation, analysis and current management. *Laryngoscope* 1988;**98**:99.

Collins SL: Controversies in management of cancer of the neck. In: *Comprehensive Management of Head and Neck Tumors.* Thawley SE, Panje WR (editors). Saunders, 1987.

DeSanto LW et al: Neck dissection: Is it worthwhile? *Laryngoscope* 1982;**92:**502.

Headington T: Epidermal Carcinoma of the Integument of the Nose and Ear. In: *Tumors of the Head and Neck—Clinical and Pathological Considerations.* Batsakis JG (editor). Williams & Wilkins, 1974.

Holt GR, Parel SM: Prosthetics in nasal rehabilitation. *Facial Plast Surg J* 1984;**2**:74.

Holt GR, Carlson, E, Davis WE: Malignant melanoma of the nasopharynx. *Arch Otolaryngol* (June) 1975;**102:** 380.

Holt GR, Holt JE, Venturi LM: Mohs' Surgical Treatment and Reconstruction of Lesions in the Medial Orbit. *Facial Plast Surg J* 1987;**5(1):**49.

Jansen GT, Westbrook KC: Cancer of the Skin. In: *Cancer of the Head and Neck.* Suen JY, Myers EN (editors). Churchill Livingstone, 1981.

Johns ME, Kaplan MJ: Salivary gland: Malignant neoplasms. In: *Otolaryngology—Head and Neck Surgery.* Vol 2. Cummings CW (editor). Mosby, 1986.

Johnson JT el al: Cervical lymph node metastasis: Incidence

and implications of extracapsular carcinoma. *Arch Otolaryngol* 1985;**111**:534.

Lehman W, Pidoux J-M, Widmann J-J: *Larynx: Microlaryngoscopy and Histopathology.* Inpharzam Medical Publications, 1981.

Leipzig B et al: The role of endoscopy in evaluating patients with head and neck cancer. *Arch Otolaryngol* 1985;**111**:59.

Lindberg R: Distribution of cervical lymph node metastases from squamous cell carcinoma of the upper respiratory and digestive tracts. *Cancer*1972;**29**:1446.

McGuirt WF: Panendoscopy as a screening examination for simultaneous primary tumors in head and neck cancer: A prospective sequential study and review of the literature. *Laryngoscope* 1982;**92**:569.

Million RR, Cassisi NJ: General principles for treatment of cancers in the head and neck: Selection of treatment for the primary site and for the neck. In: *Management of Head and Neck Cancer: A Multidisciplinary Approach.* Million RR, Cassisi NJ (editors). Lippincott, 1984.

O'Brien CJ et al: Neck dissection with and without radio-therapy: Prognostic factors, patterns of recurrence, and survival. *AM J Surg* 1986;**152**:456.

Parel SM et al: Osseointegration and facial prosthetics. *Int J Oral Maxillofac Surg* 1986;**1**:27.

Rice DH, Spiro RH: *Current Concepts in Head and Neck Cancer.* American Cancer Society, 1989.

Rothman KJ: The effect of alcohol consumption on risk of cancer of the head and neck. *Laryngoscope* 1978;(**Suppl 8**):51.

Sasaki CT, Carlson RD: Malignant neoplasms of the larynx. In: *Otolaryngology—Head and Neck Surgery.* Cummings CW (editor). Mosby, 1986.

Schuller DE, Batley F: *Management of Epidermoid Cancer of the Oral Cavity.* American Academy of Otolaryngology—Head and Neck Surgery, 1980.

Smith JL Jr: Pathology of Skin Tumors of the Head and Neck. In: *Comprehensive Management of Head and Neck.* Thawley SE, Panje WR (editors). Saunders, 1987.

Spiro RH: Salivary neoplasms: Overview of a 35-year experience with 2,807 patients. *Head Neck Surg* 1986;**8**:177.

Strong EW, Spiro RH: Cancer of the Oral Cavity. In: *Cancer of the Head and Neck.* Suen JY, Myers EN (editors). Churchill Livingstone, 1981.

Urist MM, O'Brien CJ: Head and Neck Tumors: In: *Current Surgical Diagnosis & Treatment,* 9th ed. Way LW (editor). Appleton & Lange, 1991.

Wynder EL: The epidemiology of cancers of the upper alimentary and upper respiratory tracts. *Laryngoscope* 1978;**88(Suppl 8)**:50.

Lung Cancer

Daniel D. Von Hoff, MD

Incidence & Epidemiology

Lung cancer is the most common cause of cancer death in the USA. The incidence is increasing and the number of deaths doubling every 12–15 years (Figure 24–1). In 1992, approximately 93,000 deaths were caused by lung cancer in men and 53,000 in women.

Several agents have been associated with the causation of lung cancer. Tobacco smoking is by far the most common etiologic factor. It is implicated in every type of lung cancer with the exception of bronchoalveolar lung cancer. The specific materials responsible in tobacco smoking that produce lung cancer have not been identified. However, there is a clear dose-response relationship between the number of cigarettes smoked and the development of lung cancer. The risk of developing lung cancer declines if an individual stops smoking. Of even greater interest is the finding that patients who already have lung cancer may have a longer survival if they stop smoking at the time of diagnosis.

Other possible etiologic agents include asbestos, chloromethyl-methyl ether, nickel, radon, vinyl chloride, chromate, and arsenicals. Evidence indicates that the above factors can be synergistic (eg, the risk of developing lung cancer in smokers exposed to asbestos can be 8–9 times that of smokers not exposed to asbestos). Other risk factors for lung cancer include pulmonary fibrosis from scleroderma, bronchiectasis, scar from pulmonary infarctions, mycobacterial disease, and lung abscess.

There is increasing evidence that lung cancer may be, in part, a genetic disease. Deletion of a portion of the short arm of chromosome 3 (a 3p21 deletion) has been associated with small-cell and other types of lung cancer. Loss of DNA from chromosomes 13, 17, and 11 has also been described. These deletions fit the recessive oncogene or tumor suppressor gene hypothesis whereby a deletion uncovers an oncogene that can initiate carcinogenesis when present in only one copy. There is also evidence that 40% of patients with adenocarcinoma of the lung have some abnormality (deletion) in the *ras* proto-oncogene.

The natural history for the development of lung cancer includes exposure to carcinogens with eventual changes from the common ciliated columnar epithelial cell and the less common mucus-producing cell (or goblet cell) lining the tracheobronchial tree to a metaplastic stratified squamous epithelium with atypia. These changes eventually progress to carcinoma in situ and then on to frank invasion by the tumor.

Pathology

The most frequently used histologic classification for lung cancer is that of the World Health Organization (WHO) (Table 24–1).

The first four histologic types listed in Table 24–2 represent the majority of lung cancers. Epidermoid represents 33–71% of cases (depending on the reporting institution); adenocarcinoma, 16–29%; large cell, 9–20%; small cell, 19–25%; and others (eg, bronchoalveolar and mixed types), 1–3%.

Epidermoid (squamous cell) carcinomas appear to arise in columnar epithelial cells, produce a more centrally located lesion, and do not often have metastases at presentation. Patients with epidermoid cancer have a better survival rate and may benefit from adjuvant chemotherapy (see below).

In contrast to epidermoid carcinomas, adenocarcinomas of the lung more commonly arise in peripheral locations. Pleural effusions are more commonly seen with adenocarcinomas than with any other cell type. The tumor frequently arises in an area of pulmonary scar or fibrosis.

Patients with small-cell carcinomas commonly present with a hilar mass. The tumors are thought to arise from the Kulchitsky cells and thus were thought to be of possible neuroectodermal origin, but recent observations cast doubt on that hypothesis. Small-cell carcinomas are the histologic type most likely to have distant metastases (particularly to bone marrow, brain, and adrenal glands). In addition, small-cell carcinomas are the most common histologic type associated with paraneoplastic syndromes at the time of diagnosis. Most patients (95%) with small-cell lung cancer do not have resectable tumors. Thus, surgery is precluded for these patients, although the use of surgery to resect residual disease after the tumor has regressed following chemotherapy plus radiation therapy is an area of clinical investigation.

Large-cell carcinomas of the lung are usually large peripheral lesions that may be necrotic or cavitary

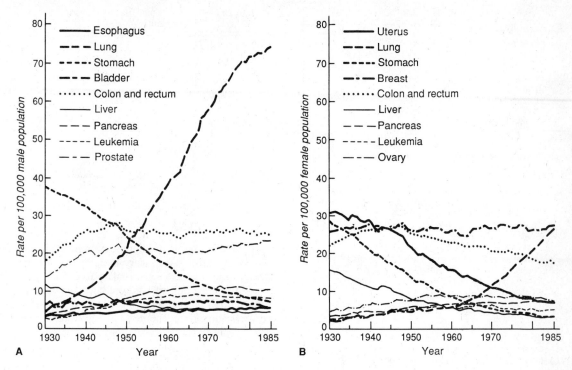

Figure 24–1. Cancer death rates (age-adjusted) for males (left) and females (right) in the USA (1970–1988). (Modified and reproduced, with permission, from Silverberg E: Cancer statistics. *CA* 1988;**38:**5, and the American Cancer Society, Inc.)

and invade the pleura. Microscopically they are poorly differentiated. Patients with large-cell carcinomas have 5-year survivals equal to those of patients with adenocarcinoma of the lung.

One histologic subtype of adenocarcinoma that deserves mention is bronchoalveolar carcinoma. This histologic type is not associated with smoking. Bronchoalveolar carcinoma is frequently multicentric and often interstitial, and patients can present with copious sputum production (bronchorrhea). Bronchoalveolar carcinoma may arise from the Clara cells (also known as type II pneumonocytes or uncil-

iated bronchoalveolar cells). The tumor commonly forms in pulmonary scar tissue.

It is becoming increasingly common to identify two different histologic types of lung cancer in the same lung cancer specimen. This finding has prompted some investigators to speculate that the various histologic types of lung cancer really arise from some common (stem) cell. The different histologic types may simply represent different stages in differentiation of the tumor cells.

Staging

Each patient's disease must be carefully staged according to the International Staging System. Table 24–2 defines the TNM classifications for lung cancer, and Table 24–3 shows the details of the International Staging System using the TNM classifications. Figure 24–2 is provided to help visualize the TNM classifications.

Clinical Findings

A. Symptoms and Signs: The appearance of signs and symptoms of lung cancer (Table 24–4) early enough to make a difference in patient survival is a rare phenomenon.

One or more episodes of pneumonia in a patient with other risk factors (eg, smoking) should raise the suspicion of lung cancer. Hoarseness usually is sec-

Table 24–1. Histologic classification of lung cancer (WHO).

I	Epidermoid (squamous cell) carcinoma
II	Small-cell carcinoma
III	Adenocarcinomas (bronchogenic and bronochoalveolar)
IV	Large-cell carcinomas
V	Combined epidermoid and adenocarcinomas
VI	Carcinoid tumors
VII	Bronchial gland tumors
VIII	Papillary tumors of the surface epithelium
IX	Mixed tumors and carcinosarcomas
X	Sarcomas
XI	Unclassified
XII	Mesotheliomas
XIII	Metastatic

Table 24–2. TNM classification for lung cancer.

Primary Tumors (T)

T_0 No evidence of primary tumor.

T_X Tumor proved by presence of malignant cells in bronchopulmonary secretions but not visualized radiographically or bronchoscopically.

T_1 Tumor that is 3 cm or less in greatest diameter surrounded by lung or visceral pleura and without evidence of invasion proximal to a lobar bronchus at bronchoscopy.

T_2 Tumor more than 3 cm in greatest diameter or tumor of any size that with associated atelectasis or obstructive pneumonitis extends to the hilar region. At bronchoscopy, the proximal extent of demonstrable tumor must be at least 2 cm distal to the carina. Any associated atelectasis or obstructive pneumonitis must involve less than an entire lung, and there must be no pleural effusion.

T_3 Tumor with circumscribed extrapulmonary extension which is of any size, which has extension into the chest wall, mediastinal pleura, or pericardium, but which does not involve the heart, great vessels, trachea, esophagus, or vertebral bodies. It may also be a main bronchus tumor within 2 cm of the carina but not involving it.

T_4 Tumor of any size wiht invasion of the structures excluded in the T_3 classification. Also, any kind of malignant pleural effusion.

Regional lymph nodes (N)

N_0 No demonstrable metastasis to lymph nodes.

N_1 Metastasis to lymph nodes in the ipsilateral lung and/or hilar region (including direct extension).

N_2 Involvement of only the ipsilateral, mediastinal, or subcarinal nodes.

N_3 Metastasis to contralateral mediastinal lymph nodes, contralateral hilar lymph nodes, and ipsilateral or contralateral scalene or supraclavicular nodes.

Distant metastases (M)

M_0 No distant metastasis.

M_1 All metastases beyond the regional lymph nodes and contralateral hilar lymph nodes. Metastases in the contralateral lung are considered M_1.

Table 24–3. International Staging Classification for lung cancer.

Stage I	$T_1N_0M_0$
	$T_2N_0M_0$
Stage II	$T_1N_1M_0$
	$T_2N_1M_0$
Stage IIIA	$T_1N_2M_0$
	$T_2N_2M_0$
	$T_3N_2M_0$
Stage IIIB	$T_4N_0M_0$
	$T_4N_1M_0$
	$T_4N_2M_0$
	$T_4N_3M_0$
Stage IV	$T_XN_XM_1$

neuropathies, corticocerebellar degeneration, gynecomastia (secondary to ectopic human chorionic gonadotropin [hCG] production), syndrome of inappropriate secretion of antidiuretic hormone (SIADH) with hyponatremia (secondary to ectopic ADH production), hypercalcemia (secondary to ectopic parathyroid hormone or a parathyroid hormone–like factor most often seen with non–small-cell lung cancer), and a cushingoid appearance (secondary to ectopic corticotropin [ACTH] production). Rarely, acanthosis nigricans, fever, scleroderma, and marantic endocarditis can also be seen.

By the time a sign or symptom occurs or a lesion is noted on the chest x-ray, it is unlikely that the disease is localized. In one study of patients who had autopsies performed after dying within 30 days of undergoing a supposed curative resection for their lung cancer, 14–63% (depending on histologic subtype of their lung cancer) already had silent distant metastases. A review of all Lung Cancer Study Group data indicates that 50% of all patients with lung cancer have obvious disseminated disease beyond the thorax at the time of presentation. Local, potentially curable modalities such as surgery and radiation therapy produce overall 5-year survival rates of only about 10%.

Screening & Prevention

Several approaches have been undertaken to screen large populations in the hope of detecting disease at an earlier stage. Mass screening programs involving men who are heavy smokers using chest x-rays performed 2–3 times per year as well as sputum cytologic specimens have been performed by several groups. Screening this high-risk population enabled detection of lung cancers that were at a more resectable stage than were found in populations in which no screening was performed. However, survival was the same in both groups. For this reason, at present there is no justification for large-scale screening, even of patients at high risk for developing lung cancer. However, new evidence indicates that use of monoclonal antibodies to various histologic types of lung cancer may enable detection of tumor cells in the sputum as early as 3 years before a histologic diagnosis. More testing is required.

ondary to vocal cord paralysis caused by invasion of the recurrent (laryngeal) nerve. Other modes of presentation include hemoptysis (actually reported as a presenting symptom in only 10–20% of patients), dyspnea or wheezing (caused by tumor obstructing the bronchi or lymphangitic spread), Horner's syndrome (meiosis, ptosis, anhidrosis, and enophthalmos due to invasion of cervical sympathetic chain), superior vena cava syndrome (edema of face, neck, and arms with or without conjunctival suffusion), brachial plexus compression, elevated hemidiaphragm (secondary to phrenic nerve paralysis), pleurisy (invasion of the pleura), cardiac arrhythmias, cardiac tamponade (secondary to local invasion by the tumor with effusion), and dysphagia (secondary to invasion of the esophagus).

Other presenting signs and symptoms are often produced by endocrine (ectopic hormone production by the tumor) and nonendocrine effects of the tumor. Systemic effects include weight loss, clubbing, hypertrophic osteoarthropathy, thrombophlebitis, carcinomatous myopathies (Eaton-Lambert syndrome),

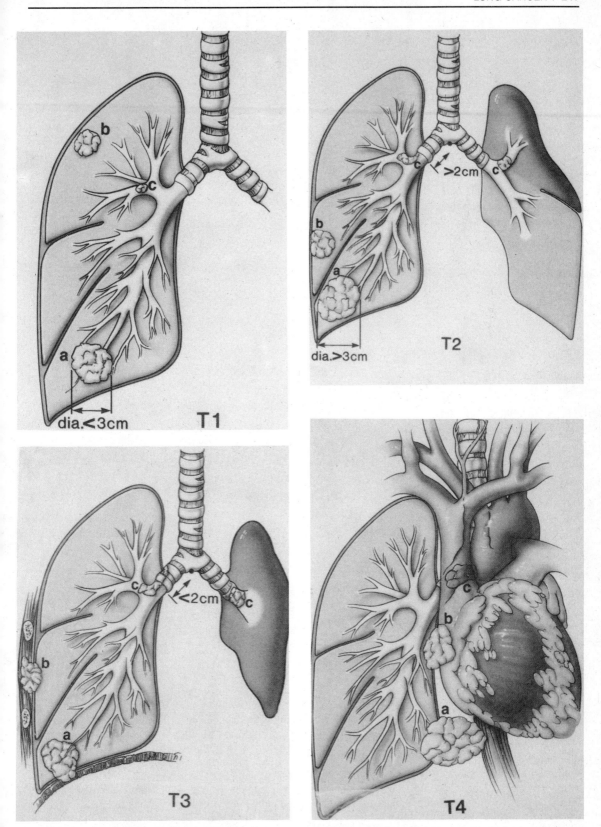

Figure 24–2. Illustrations of the various T and N classifications. (Modified and reproduced, with permission, from Rice TW: Staging and treatment of bronchogenic carcinoma. *J Respir Dis* 1988;**9**:77.)

(continued)

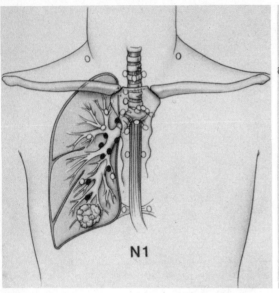

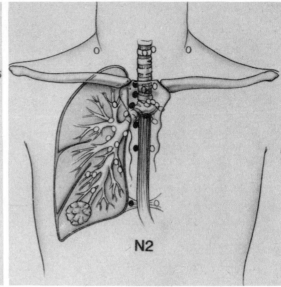

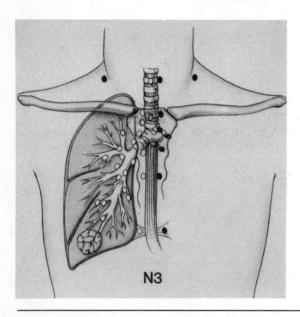

Figure 24–2. (cont.)

B. Diagnostic Studies: Cytologic or histologic proof of the diagnosis may be achieved by examination of sputum cytologic specimens (note that head and neck tumors can also give positive results), bronchoscopy with biopsy (for central lesions), transthoracic needle aspiration, mediastinoscopy, biopsy of a metastatic lesion or enlarged lymph node, or even thoracotomy.

Flexible fiberoptic bronchoscopy has become one of the most useful procedures. When forceps biopsy, bronchial brushings, and washings are done for an endoscopically visible lesion, the diagnostic yield is 94% for a central lesion and 86% for a peripheral tumor. For the peripheral lesion that cannot be seen, brushings and washings can still give a high diagnostic yield.

After the histologic diagnosis is confirmed, it is important to determine whether the patient has a tumor that is amenable to surgical resection. For patients with non–small-cell lung cancer, the workup should include a thorough history and physical examination, chest x-ray, CT scan or MRI of the chest (to assess mediastinal involvement), and complete blood count and chemistries with attention to liver function tests and bone alkaline phosphatase levels. A radionuclide bone scan with additional spot films of any abnormal areas is sometimes indicated. Any involve-

Table 24–4. Modes of presentation of patients with lung cancer.

Cough (most frequent but nonspecific symptom)	Cardiac tamponade
	Dysphagia
One or more episodes of pneumonia	Weight loss
	Clubbing
Hoarseness	Hypertrophic osteoarthropathy
Hemoptysis	
Dyspnea or wheezing	Myopathies and neuropathies
Horner's syndrome	
Superior vena cava syndrome	Corticocerebellar degeneration
Brachial plexus compression	
Elevation of hemidiaphragm	Gynecomastia
Pleurisy	Syndrome of inappropriate secretion of ADH
Cardiac arrhythmia	
	Hypercalcemia
	Cushing's syndrome

ment of the mediastinum revealed by any imaging technique should be confirmed by mediastinoscopy.

For the patient with histologically documented small-cell carcinoma, it is important to determine whether the disease is limited (confined to one hemithorax, mediastinum, and regional lymph nodes, including contralateral hilar and supraclavicular) or extensive (disease beyond limited). (If the tumor site can be included in a radiation therapy port, the disease is limited.) This determination is a more important prognostic factor than is the total tumor bulk (as determined by the TNM classification). Staging procedures for patients with small-cell lung cancer should include a history and physical examination, chest x-ray, CT scan or MRI of the chest (with or without the liver), liver-spleen scan (if CT scan was not performed), bone scan with spot films of any ab-

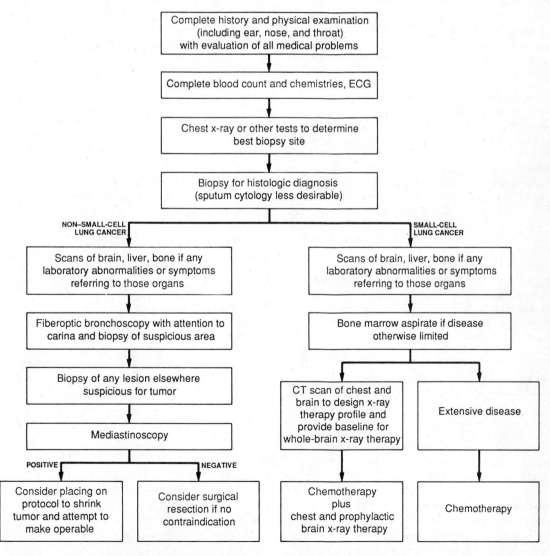

Figure 24–3. Algorithm for workup of a patient with suspected lung cancer.

normal areas, CT scan of the brain, complete blood count and chemistries, and bone marrow aspirate and biopsy. The latter is performed because 30% of patients with small-cell lung cancer will have tumor cells found in the bone marrow. Approximately 5% of patients will have bone marrow involvement as the only indication of metastic disease.

Treatment

A. Non–Small-Cell Lung Cancer, Stages I and II: For patients with stage I or II disease, the treatment of choice is surgical resection. However, certain physiologic considerations may preclude a surgical approach. It is not always possible to predict ahead of time whether a lobectomy or pneumonectomy will be required. Therefore, it is best to determine whether a patient can tolerate a pneumonectomy, should one be required. Considerations include the patient's performance status (fully ambulatory patients tolerate surgery better than those who are not fully ambulatory) and pulmonary function. The patient should stop smoking and have pulmonary function tests and radionuclide ventilation scans performed. Patients with maximal breathing capacities >40% predicted are acceptable surgical risks as are those with a forced expiratory volume (FEV_1) >2.5 L. If a patient has an FEV_1 <1 L, a Pco_2 >45 mm Hg, dyspnea at rest, pulmonary hypertension, or cor pulmonale, the patient is not a candidate for pulmonary resection. Nor is a patient who has had a myocardial infarction within the last 3 months a candidate for surgical resection. Patients with active angina should have the appropriate cardiac workup, and consideration should be given to concomitant bypass grafting with the pulmonary resection (4.6% mortality). In addition to the above contraindications, patients with signs of more advanced disease are not eligible for surgical resection (ipsilateral mediastinal lymph nodes proved by mediastinoscopy or phrenic nerve paralysis).

For patients with stage I or II disease who are not candidates for a surgical resection, radiation therapy offers an alternative treatment.

The 5-year survival rate for patients with stage I disease who have undergone potentially curative resections is 65–89% overall. It is about 34% for patients with stage II disease. Within the classification of stage I disease, patients with T_1N_0 disease who have an epidermoid carcinoma will do the best (approximately a 90% 5-year survival). The Lung Cancer Study Group is currently evaluating whether patients with $T_1N_0M_0$ can be treated with a wedge or segmental resection rather than a lobectomy. The results will be important for patients who have stage I disease but limited pulmonary reserve. Patients who have stage I or II disease but who receive radiation therapy because of their poor general condition have a 5-year survival rate of about 20% Since neither surgery nor radiotherapy alone will cure all patients with stage II disease, combining the two modalities has been tried but is controversial. A study of postoperative mediastinal radiation therapy for patients with completely resected stage II disease performed by the Lung Cancer Study Group showed that postoperative radiation therapy reduced local recurrences after resection of epidermoid lung cancer but did not increase survival rates. Other smaller studies have indicated that postoperative radiation therapy does improve survival.

The use of combined surgery plus radiation therapy plus chemotherapy remains an area of active investigation. Clinical trials employing the more active drug regimens against non–small-cell lung cancer (eg, platinum plus etoposide) have begun to be used both preoperatively and postoperatively in prospective clinical trials for patients with stage I and II disease. In addition, the use of immunotherapy with tumor vaccines is being pursued. To date, no immunotherapeutic approach has proved beneficial to patients with stage I or II non–small-cell lung cancer.

B. Non–Small-Cell Lung Cancer, Stage III: Reports of therapeutic approaches for patients with this stage of disease are difficult to interpret because of difficulties in staging the disease. For patients with stage IIIA disease with T_3N_0 or T_3N_1 disease, surgery is a possibility. For patients in these categories who have residual disease after resection, if radiation therapy and chemotherapy (with cyclophosphamide plus doxorubicin plus platinum) are also given a significantly longer disease-free survival can be achieved than with postoperative radiation therapy alone. For patients with N_2 disease in the stage IIIA category, the best choice is to enter the patient on a study to determine whether therapy (chemotherapy, radiation therapy, or chemotherapy plus radiation therapy) can be given to convert the patient from unresectable to resectable. Initial reports indicate that as many as 70% of unresectable patients may be able to be converted into resectable patients, with 2-year survivals of 34% (versus historical controls of 10–15% of patients with 2-year survivals). The real impact of these approaches on survival of patients remains to be determined.

C. Non–Small-Cell Lung Cancer, Stages IIIB and IV: Treatment is largely confined to chemotherapy. A large number of conventional and investigational single agents have been used to treat patients with this stage of disease. The agents with the greatest response rates include cisplatin (10–30% response rate), etoposide (9–18%), vindesine (8–22%), doxorubicin (9–18%), mitomycin-C (15–27%), ifosfamide (15–26%), and vinblastine (10–22%). Almost all the reported responses have been partial responses, and none of the agents has had an impact on patient survival. Combination chemotherapy regimens also have been devised. The most active combination regimens include CAP (cyclophosphamide plus doxorubicin plus platinum), with overall response rates of 4–48%; MVP (mitomycin-C plus either vinblastine or vindesine plus platinum), with response rates of 31–60%; and VP (platinum plus etoposide [VP-16]), with response rates of 21–38%. Again, most of the responses are partial responses, and the impact of the combination regimens on patient survival is uncertain. Two major trials were performed that randomized patients to treatment with a combination chemotherapy regimen versus a supportive care regimen. One study showed a positive effect of the chemotherapeutic regimen on survival, while the other could not document such a benefit. Overall, even with treatment, median survival of patients is 5–6 months in most large series testing combination chemotherapy regimens.

D. Small-Cell Lung Cancer, Limited Disease: In contrast to non–small-cell lung cancer, small-cell lung cancer is very responsive to chemotherapy. Single agents such as doxorubicin, etoposide, cisplatin, methotrexate, cyclophosphamide, and carmustine can produce response rates of greater than 30%. However, the greatest advances in the treatment of patients with limited small-cell lung cancer have been through the use of combination chemotherapy regimens given in an aggressive manner with maximization of dose intensity. Some of the most active combination chemotherapy regimens include CAV (cyclophosphamide plus doxorubicin plus vincristine), VP (etoposide [VP-16] plus platinum), and CMC (cyclophosphamide plus methotrexate plus lomustine [CCNU]). All these regimens can give response rates in the 70% range with approximately one-half of those responses being complete responses. The median survival in patients with limited disease ranges from 12 to 16 months with the 2-year survival ranging from 10% to 25%. Of great interest is that women with small-cell lung cancer have significantly better survival than men. (When comparing results of various treatment regimens, keep in mind the percentage of female patients in the various regimens.)

Radiation therapy also has a role in the management of patients with limited small-cell lung cancer. There is clear evidence that radiation therapy improves local control of the disease and also improves survival. In addition, prophylactic whole-brain radiotherapy has been used to prevent central nervous system recurrence. Although this approach decreases the incidence of brain recurrence, patients who receive whole-brain radiation therapy at the time they are receiving chemotherapy may have an increased incidence of dementia, ataxia, and optic atrophy.

E. Small-Cell Lung Cancer, Extensive Disease: Use of the same combination chemotherapy regimens discussed above for patients with limited small-cell lung cancer gives responses rates of 70%, but only 15–30% of those responses are complete responses. The median survival for patients is 7–11 months, with a 0–3% 2-year survival rate. Clearly, more innovative approaches are needed.

F. Pancoast's Tumor: Pancoast's tumor is usually an epidermoid tumor (50% of histologic types) that grows in the apex of the lung and presents with shoulder pain radiating in the C8 distribution. It can also be associated with Horner's syndrome. It is a rare entity, and little systematic study has been undertaken. However, surprisingly good results have been reported (40% 3-year survival) in patients who have preoperative radiation therapy followed by extensive resection.

G. Superior Vena Cava Syndrome: This syndrome, which is due to obstruction of the superior vena cava by tumor, presents with facial swelling, conjunctival suffusion, dyspnea, and prominent venous patterns on the neck and anterior chest. Several tumors as well as a rare benign condition can cause superior vena cava obstruction. In attempting to obtain a histologic diagnosis, remember that the vessels in the area are all now a "high-pressure system" and severe bleeding can occur during a biopsy procedure. The most effective therapy for superior vena cava syndrome secondary to small-cell lung cancer is either combination chemotherapy or radiation therapy. If the syndrome is due to non–small-cell lung cancer, the most effective therapy is irradiation.

H. Brachytherapy and Laser Therapy: Radioactive implant of ^{125}I, ^{198}Au, or ^{192}Ir has been used to treat patients who have bronchial obstruction, who are refractory to external beam radiation therapy or other therapy, or who are inoperable (medically) or unresectable (eg, tumor involves great vessels). The procedure is well tolerated, morbidity low, and local control rate rather high. The method provides palliation but has no impact on survival. Recurrent endobronchial lesions can also be treated with an Nd: YAG laser through a bronchoscope, which provides excellent palliation.

REFERENCES

Dillman RV et al: A randomized trial of indiction chemotherapy plus high-dose radiation versus radiation alone in stage III non–small cell lung cancer. *N Engl J Med* 1990;**323**:940.

Johnston-Early A et al: Smoking abstinence and small cell lung cancer survival. *JAMA* 1980;**244**:2175.

Klastersky J, Sculier JP: Chemotherapy of non–small cell lung cancer. *Semin Oncol* 1985;**12**:38.

Kris MG et al: Trail of the combination of mitomycin, vindesine, and cisplatin in patients with advanced non–small cell lung cancer. *Cancer Treat Rep* 1986;**70:**1091.

Lad T, Rubinstein L, Sadeghi A: The benefit of adjuvant treatment for resected locally advanced non–small cell lung cancer. *J Clin Oncol* 1988;**6:**9.

LeChevalier TL et al: Radiotherapy alone versus combined chemotherapy and radiotherapy in non-resectable non–small-cell lung cancer: First analysis of a randomized trial in 353 patients. *J Natl Cancer Inst* 1991;**83:**417.

Lin AY, Ihde DC: Recent developments in the treatment of lung cancer. *JAMA* 1992;**267:**1661.

Lung cancer mortality appears unaffected by roentgenographic and sputum screening in asymptomatic persons: Report from the NIH. *JAMA* 1979;**241:**1582.

Matthews MJ et al: Frequency of residual and metastatic tumors in patients undergoing curative surgical resection of lung cancer. *Cancer Chemother Rep* 1973;**3:**63.

Matthews MJ: Morphologic classifications of bronchogenic carcinoma. *Cancer Chemother Rep* 1973;**3:**2291.

Mountain CF: The new international staging system for lung cancer. *Surg Clin North Am* 1987;**67:**925.

Naylor SL et al: Loss of heterozygosity of chromosome 3p markers in small cell lung cancer. *Nature* 1987;**329:**451.

Olsen GN et al: Pulmonary function evaluation of the lung resection candidate: A prospective study. *Am Rev Respir Dis* 1975;**111:**379.

Paulson DL: Superior sulcus tumors: Results of combined therapy. *NY State J Med* 1971;**71:**2050.

Rapp E et al: Chemotherapy can prolong survival in patients with advanced non–small cell lung cancer: Report of a Canadian Multicenter Randomized Trial. *J Clin Oncol* 1988;**6:**633.

Ruckdeschel JC et al: A randomized trial of the four most active regimens for metastatic non–small cell lung cancer. *J Clin Oncol* 1986;**4:**14.

Schaake-Koning C et al: Effects of concomitant cisplatin and radiotherapy on inoperable non–small cell lung cancer. *N Engl J Med* 1992;**326:**524.

Silverberg E. Cancer statistics, 1988. *CA* 1988;**38:**5.

Tockman MJ et al: Sensitive and specific monoclonal antibody recognition of human lung cancer antigen on preserved sputum cells: A new approach to early lung cancer determination. *J Clin Oncol* 1988;**6:**1685.

Vena JE et al: Occupation and lung cancer: An analysis by histologic subtype. *Cancer* 1985;**56:**9110.

Weisenburger TH, Gail M: Effects of postoperative mediastinal radiation on completely resected stage II and stage II epidermoid cancer of the lung: The Lung Cancer Study Group. *N Engl J Med* 1986;**315:**1377.

Wynder EL, Hoffman D: Tobacco and tobacco smoke. *Semin Oncol* 1976;**3:**5.

Malignant Melanoma

25

Theresa A. Shouse, MD, & Calvin L. Day, Jr., MD

Nonmelanoma skin cancer is by far the most common type of cancer in the USA, with an estimated 600,000 new cases annually. Of all new cases of cancer, about one-third will be skin cancer. There will be an estimated 480,000 new cases of basal cell carcinoma, 120,000 new cases of squamous cell carcinoma, and 32,000 new cases of malignant melanoma in the USA in 1992. Skin cancer will kill approximately 8900 people in the USA in 1992, and three-fourths of the deaths will be due to malignant melanoma.

Cutaneous melanoma is a malignant neoplasm arising from melanocytes. Melanocytes synthesize and transport melanin pigment, which is the primary determinant of skin pigmentation.

Although the survival rate for malignant melanoma increased from 41% to 83% between 1940 and 1983 (Figure 25–1), the number of deaths due to melanoma increased 2½-fold (Figure 25–2). The number of newly diagnosed melanomas has increased faster than the population rise (Figure 25–3). The rate of increase in the incidence of melanoma since 1930 is over 1000%. A Caucasian born today has a projected lifetime risk of developing malignant melanoma of 1 in 135 (Figure 25–4). By the year 2000, this risk is projected to be 1 in 90. The reasons for this melanoma "epidemic" are unclear.

Essentials of Diagnosis

- Pigmented skin lesion with the following clinical characteristics (ABCDs): *a*symmetric, *b*order irregularity, *c*olor variegation, *d*iameter ≥6 mm.
- Changing "mole" without any "classic" features of melanoma.

Etiology & Risk Factors
(See Table 25–1.)

A. Precursor Lesions:

1. Changing mole–A persistently changed or changing mole may be the most important risk factor for the development of cutaneous melanoma. Early melanomas may not have any of the clinical features associated with "classic" malignant melanoma, and the physician should consider a biopsy of any pigmented lesion that is changing.

2. Congenital nevi–Nevi present at birth occur in approximately 1% of Caucasians. Congenital nevi that are greater than 20 cm in greatest diameter occur in less than 1 in 20,000 births and carry a lifetime risk of malignant degeneration of 6.3–8.5%. Two-thirds of the melanomas that arise in these large congenital nevi have a nonepidermal origin, making early recognition difficult. Large congenital nevi are melanoma precursors, and excision should begin before the child's first birthday. Smaller congenital nevi probably are also precursors for malignant melanoma and should be removed prophylactically. Malignant degeneration of these smaller congenital nevi is rare before puberty and removal need not be accomplished until just before puberty unless the lesion is clinically suspicious.

3. Lentigo maligna–Lentigo maligna is an irregular pigmented lesion, rather like a brown shoe polish stain, that usually occurs on the sun-exposed skin of elderly persons. Histologically, this lesion is malignant melanoma in situ. Progression to invasive melanoma with resultant metastatic disease and death occurs in approximately 5% of cases.

4. Dysplastic nevi–Dysplastic nevi are clinically and histologically "abnormal moles" that occupy the spectrum between "normal moles" and malignant melanomas. They occur in 2–7% of the normal population and in 30–34% of patients with malignant melanoma. Dysplastic nevi are markers for patients at risk for developing malignant melanoma. The lesions themselves have been documented to spawn malignant melanoma.

B. Sun Exposure: The following observations imply that there is not a simple causal relationship between sun exposure and malignant melanoma. (1) Other skin cancers that are generally believed to be caused mainly by sunlight are more common in men than women (perhaps because men work more often out of doors). Malignant melanoma, in contrast, occurs as commonly in women as in men. (2) Other skin cancers increase exponentially in incidence with age as would be expected from lifelong exposure to an agent that can initiate cancer, ie, sunlight. Malignant melanoma, in contrast, shows a relative peak incidence in middle life. (3) Other skin cancers occur most commonly on the head, neck, and hands, areas that are more or less continually exposed to sunlight. Malignant melanoma, in contrast, occurs most commonly on the back in men and on the legs in women.

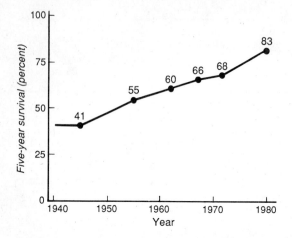

Figure 25–1. Average 5-year survival of patients with melanomas in the USA (1940–1983). (Reproduced, with permission, from Rigel DS et al: The rate of malignant melanoma in the United States: Are we making an impact? (Editorial.) *J Am Acad Dermatol* 1987;**17**:1050.)

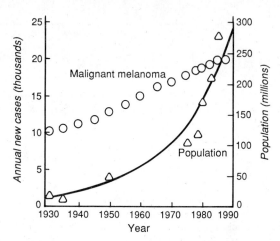

Figure 25–3. Malignant melanoma cases in the USA compared with the population rise. (Reproduced, with permission, from Rigel DS et al: The rate of malignant melanoma in the United States: Are we making an impact? (Editorial.) *J Am Acad Dermatol* 1987;**17**:1050.)

(4) Other skin cancers are more common in outdoor than indoor workers. The opposite is true for malignant melanoma. (5) There is an anomalous relationship between latitude and melanoma in Europe. A minimum incidence in melanoma is seen in those residing at about latitude 50 degrees. From this point, incidence tends to rise both with increasing proximity and increasing distance from the equator.

However, case-control studies have conclusively demonstrated that intermittent (recreational) sun exposure and in particular sunburn are major contributing factors in the etiology of melanoma. There is no general agreement among investigators concerning

lifetime total exposure, recent total exposure, and occupational exposure to sunlight.

C. Genetics:

1. Caucasian race–The incidence of cutaneous melanoma is 12 times greater in whites than in blacks and seven times greater in whites than in Hispanics. Melanoma occurring in nonwhites is more likely to be located on the palms, soles, nail beds, or mucous membranes.

2. Family history of malignant melanoma– Two to 10% of patients with malignant melanoma have a parent, sibling, or child who has or has had a

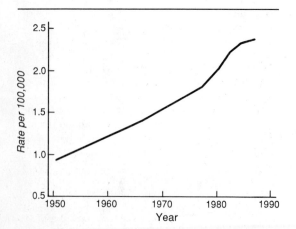

Figure 25–2. Death rate from malignant melanoma in the USA (1950–1987). (Reproduced, with permission, from Rigel DS et al: The rate of malignant melanoma in the United States: Are we making an impact? (Editorial.) *J Am Acad Dermatol* 1987;**17**:1050.)

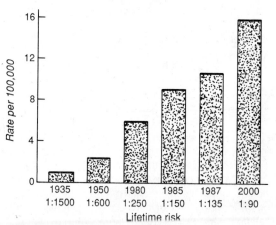

Figure 25–4. Past, current, and projected lifetime risk for an individual in the USA of developing malignant melanoma. (Reproduced, with permission, from Rigel DS et al: The rate of malignant melanoma in the United States: Are we making an impact? (Editorial.) *J Am Acad Dermatol* 1987;**17**:1050.)

Table 25–1. Risk factors for cutaneous malignant melanoma.[1]

Risk Factor	Relative Risk
Precursor lesions	
Changing mole	>400
Dysplatic/no familial melanoma	27
Congenital mole	21
Lantigo maligna	10
Sun exposure	
Excessive exposure	3
Occupational exposure	2
Vacation exposure	2
Recreational exposure	2
Genetics	
Caucasian race	12
Dysplastic/familial melanoma	148
Previous melanoma in first-degree relative	8
Phenotypic factors	
Freckles	4
Hair color: Red versus all others	3
Hair color: Fair/blond versus all others	2
Eye color: Blue versus all others	2
Complexion: Fair/pale versus all others	2
Nevocytic nevi: Upper extremities	15
Nevocytic nevi: Total body	8
Reaction pattern to sun experience: Sunburn	2
Reaction pattern to sun experience: Tanning	2
Age	
Adulthood	88
Socioeconomic Status	
Higher socioeconomic status	2
Immune system	
Immunosuppressed	4
Prior history of skin cancer	
Previous melanoma	9
Nonmelanoma skin cancer/precancer	4

[1]Data from Rhodes et al and from Evans et al.

Table 25–2. Annual age-specific incidence rate of cutaneous malignant melanoma.

Age (years)	Annual Age-specific Incidence Rate per 100,000 Population
0–4	0.1
5–9	0.1
10–14	0.2
15–19	1.4
20–24	3.6
25–29	6.8
30–34	9.9
35–39	11.7
40–44	13.9
45–49	15.9
50–54	17.0
55–59	17.9
60–64	20.2
65–69	19.4
70–74	20.9
75–79	20.7
80–84	20.6
≥85	25.0

that of the risk for unskilled workers. It remains to be determined whether socioeconomic status per se is a risk factor or whether people of higher socioeconomic status are more likely to have greater intermittent sun exposure and sunburn.

F. Immunosuppression: Renal transplant recipients and patients with leukemia and lymphoma are at increased risk for developing melanoma. Many of the melanomas in these cases have arisen in association with dysplastic nevi.

G. Prior History of Skin Cancer:

1. Previous melanoma–Approximately 3% of patients who have had a primary malignant melanoma will subsequently develop a second primary malignant melanoma. Approximately one-third of second primaries are present when the first primary is diagnosed, one-half appear in the first 5 years after diagnosis, and the remaining one-sixth appear more than 5 years after diagnosis. Therefore, patients with malignant melanoma should have a head-to-toe skin examination at the time of initial diagnosis and be examined periodically thereafter.

2. Nonmelanoma skin cancer–A history of prior skin cancer or precancer carries a significant relative risk for malignant melanoma. For this reason, patients with nonmelanoma skin cancer should periodically have a complete cutaneous examination.

Differential Diagnosis

Pigmented skin lesions often mistaken for malignant melanoma include nevocellular nevi, dysplastic nevi, seborrheic keratoses, blue nevi, lentigines, infarcted acrochordons, pigmented basal cell carcinomas, pigmented Bowen's disease (squamous cell carcinoma in situ), darkly violaceous hemangiomas, and venous lakes.

malignant melanoma. For this reason, all first-order relatives of patients with malignant melanoma should have a head-to-toe skin examination and be advised that they are at increased risk for developing malignant melanoma.

3. Phenotypic factors–A significantly increased relative risk factor for malignant melanoma is associated with the following phenotypic factors: freckles, red hair, blond or fair hair color, blue eyes, fair or pale complexion, multiple nevi, and tendency to sunburn easily.

D. Age: Individuals aged 15 years and older have an 88-fold increased risk for malignant melanoma compared with younger individuals. Although the peak incidence is between age 30 and 60, the annual age-specific incidence increases with increasing age (Table 25–2). The reason for the relative peak incidence in middle age is simply that more 50-year-olds are alive than 80-year-olds.

E. Socioeconomic Status: The risk of developing melanoma for males who have completed graduate school level education is twice that of males who have completed high school or trade school. The risk of melanoma for professionals is almost three times

Nonpigmented melanomas are often confused with solar keratoses, basal cell carcinomas, squamous cell carcinomas, and pyogenic granulomas.

Staging & Clinical Features

The most widely accepted clinicopathologic classification system for extraocular malignant melanoma is that of Clark et al. In this system, malignant melanomas have 11 subtypes. The following four primary subtypes represent over 95% of all primary cutaneous malignant melanoma: (1) lentigo maligna melanoma, (2) superficial spreading melanoma, (3) nodular melanoma, and (4) acral-lentiginous melanoma. The clinical and histologic features of each of these four subtypes are summarized in Table 25–3.

The basis of the Clark system is that melanomas can be divided into two groups based on their patterns of growth: (1) biphasic or (2) monophasic. In the biphasic pattern, a proliferation of atypical melanocytes grow in a more or less horizontal fashion in the epidermis and papillary dermis for variable periods of time before a vertical growth phase occurs. During the vertical growth phase, melanocytes invade the dermis vertical to the long axis of the dermis. In the monophasic pattern, there is no initial horizontal growth phase. The subtypes with a biphasic pattern are lentigo maligna melanoma, superficial spreading melanoma, and acral-lentiginous melanoma. Nodular melanoma is the only subtype with a monophasic growth pattern.

An alternative classification based solely on gross morphologic features of malignant melanoma is dis-

Table 25–3. Clark's clinicopathologic classification of malignant melanoma.

Melanoma Subtype	Clinical Features	Histologic Features
Lentigo maligna melanoma	5% of all cases of melanoma Sun-exposed skin of elderly patients. Large, flat freckle with irregular borders and variegation in color. Dark-brown to black papules or nodules may be present.	Atypical melanocytes that form the radial growth phase are confined to the dermoepidermal junction. Atypical melanocytes show marked variation in size and shape. Atypical melanocytes extend downward along skin appendage structures. Epidermis is usually atrophic. Dermis usually has solar elastotic changes. Vertical growth phase is usually composed of spindle-shaped melanocytes.
Superficial spreading melanoma	Most common type of melanoma; accounts for 70% of cases. Occurs at an earlier age than does lentigo maligna melanoma. Affects males and females equally. More common on legs of women and on the back of men and women. Appears initially as an irregularly colored, slightly raised plaque that gradually spreads centrifugally over months to years. Kaleidoscopic combination of colors. May eventually give rise to a nodular excrescence that correlates with the vertical phase of growth.	Radial phase of growth is characterized by a proliferation of atypical malignant melanocytes spreading throughout the epidermis in nests and in single cell array (pagetoid spread). Cells are usually epithelioid and contain a prominent nucleolus. Cytoplasm is usually pink-tan and contains coarse melanin granules in various stages of melanization. Regression is usually present.
Nodular melanoma	Second most common growth pattern; accounts for 15% of cases. Radial growth phase absent. Presents as a rapidly growing elevated mass. It is already a well-circumscribed nodule by the time it can be identified clinically as melanoma. Often ulcerated. May be pedunculated. May be amelanotic.	All the intraepidermal growth has associated underlying dermal invasion. Intraepidermal melanocytic proliferation must extend no more than 3 rete ridges lateral to the dermal invasion to qualify as a nodular melanoma. Often there is little to no inflammatory reaction. Most commonly the cells are epithelioid, but small-cell and spindle-cell nodular melanomas are frequently observed.
Acral-lentiginous melanoma	Most common type in blacks and Asians. Affects the palms, soles, ungual and periungual skin, mucosa and perimucosa. Usually begins as a flat, irregularly shaped pigmented macule that spreads centrifugally over months to years. Onset of the vertical growth phase is apparent clinically as a palpable area. However, invasion is often observed in flat lesions on plantar surfaces. Subungual malignant melanoma may present as an area of pigmentation in the nail bed. On mucosal surfaces presents as an irregularly pigmented macule with irregular borders and an irregular surface.	Atypical melanocytic hyperplasia at the dermoepidermal junction. Hypertrophied melanocytes with prominent dendritic processes filled with melanin granules that extend into the upper epidermis. Epidermal hyperplasia with retention of the rete ridge pattern.

played in Table 25–4. The Day et al system is clinically and prognostically useful and when combined with histopathologic parameters produces a prognostic model that is superior to other prognostic models (Table 25–5).

Prognosis

The simplest approach is to classify patients on clinical grounds as having (1) localized disease, (2) metastases to regional lymph nodes, or (3) metastases to distant sites.

A. Localized Melanoma: More than three-quarters of patients are diagnosed with localized disease without any clinical evidence of metastases.

The best determinant of prognosis for patients with localized disease is the vertical height of the primary melanoma measured in millimeters under the microscope by means of an ocular micrometer. This vertical height is referred to as Breslow's thickness measurement. The risk of metastases and death increase with increasing thickness. Patients with malignant melanomas <0.76 mm in thickness have a 99% 5-year survival, whereas those with melanomas >3 mm thick have only a 46% survival.

Since the treatment for clinically localized melanoma is tailored according to the thickness measurement, other prognostic factors are not used. The reason for this is evident from the data in Table 25–6, in which are displayed survival rates associated with various histologic and clinical factors after first stratifying by primary tumor thickness.

Clark et al devised a method of determining prognosis using the depth of penetration of the melanoma into various levels of the skin (Table 25–7). The likelihood that the melanoma has metastasized increases with an increasing level of penetration, but this is really an indirect method of measuring thickness. Although Clark's levels add only a moderate amount of prognostic information to some thickness categories, the initial dissemination of information about level of invasion was much greater than it was for thickness.

Table 25–5. Clinical features of dysplastic and common nevi.[1]

Dysplastic	Common
Ill-defined border	Well-defined border
Irregularly distributed pigmentation	Regular, even pigmentation
Maximum diameter often >5 mm	Diameter usually <5 mm
	No erythema
Erythema	Skin markings normal or no skin markings
Accentuated skin markings	Tan/brown pigment without black foci
Irregular border	
Foci of black pigmentation	

[1]Modified from Kelly, Crutcher, and Sagebiel.

For this reason, levels of invasion continue to be reported by pathologists and physicians need to be familiar with both Breslow's thickness measurement and Clark's levels of invasion.

B. Metastases to Regional Lymph Nodes: Approximately 80% of melanoma first metastases are to the regional lymph nodes. The following two groups of patients must be recognized: (1) Many patients who have lymph node metastases are clinical stage I, ie, their regional lymph nodes are not enlarged to palpation. These patients undergo elective regional node dissection and are found on histologic examination of the removed nodes to harbor microscopic metastases (clinical stage I, pathologic stage II). (2) The second group of patients have suspiciously enlarged regional lymph nodes. They undergo therapeutic node dissection, and microscopic examination confirms regional node metastasis (clinical stage II, pathologic stage II).

The importance of this distinction is demonstrated by survival statistics. Clinical stage I, pathologic stage II patients have a 5-year survival of 45%, whereas clinical stage II, pathologic stage II patients have a 31% 5-year survival.

1. Clinical stage I, pathologic stage II patients–The most important prognostic factors are thickness of the primary malignancy and percentage of positive lymph nodes. Patients whose primary lesion is <3.5 mm thick and who have <20% of regional lymph nodes involved with metastases have an 80% 5-year survival despite having had metastases in regional lymph nodes. In another study, patients whose primary lesion was <2 mm thick had a 5-year survival of 65%.

2. Clinical stage II, pathologic stage II patients–In four studies, the number of positive nodes or the extent of nodal involvement was a significant prognostic factor. The investigators did not agree on other significant factors. However, in 3 studies, features of the primary tumor (eg, ulceration, thickness, or growth pattern) were still significant despite the presence of metastases to regional lymph nodes.

C. Metastases to Distant Sites: Inasmuch as

Table 25–4. Proposed classification for malignant melanoma based on gross morphology.

TNM Stage	Gross Morphology	Metastatic Rate (%)
T_1	Plaque <2 cm in largest diameter with no associated nodule.	6
T_2	Plaque ≥2 cm in largest diameter with no associated nodule.	19
T_3	Single nodule located completely within the borders of its associated plaque.	33
T_4	Single nodule abutting normal skin or multiple nodules; nodule diameter ≤15 mm and ulceration absent.	57
T_5	Single nodule abutting normal skin or multiple nodules; nodule either >15 mm or ulcerated.	87
T_5	Four-fifths of surface ulcerated.	85

Table 25–6. Five-year disease-free survival rates for patients with stage I melanoma when stratified by primary tumor thickness.

Variable	Thickness Range (mm)		
	0.76–1.69 (%)	1.51–3.99 (%)	≥3.65 (%)
Lymphocyte response			
Nearly absent	93	71	16
Minimal	93	71	16
Moderate	93	71	59
Marked	96	87	59
Location			
Forearm	. . .	100	. . .
Leg	—	79	—
Arm	—	79	—
Thigh	—	76	—
Hands or feet	—	66	0
Trunk	—	74	23
Head and neck	—	46	64
Extremities (excluding hands and feet)	—	—	78
BANS[1] location	84	—	—
Non-BANS location	99	—	—
Microscopic satellites			
Absent	94	79	61
Present	90	54	26
Pathologic stage			
Negative nodes	95	77	56
Positive nodes	80	53	21
Node dissection not done	94	66	34
Level of invasion			
Level II	96	77	—
Level III	97	77	46
Level IV	88	72	46
Level V	—	72	25
Histologic type			
Superficial spreading	94	79	57
Lentigo maligna	100	50	33
Nodular	89.5	71	27
Acral lentiginous	100	74	0
Unclassified centrifugal growth phase	—	—	0
Indeterminate	89	—	0
Sex			
Female	96	81	47
Male	92	68	29
Surgical treatment			
Wide local excision only	94	66	34
Wide local excision plus elective regional node dissection	94	73	39
Ulceration width			
None or <3 mm wide	—	79	49
>3 mm	—	52	34
Received adjuvant therapy			
No	95	77	41
Yes	87	49	21
Type of adjuvant therapy received			
Bacillus Calmette-Guérin (BCG)	—	—	25
Dacarbazine (DTIC)	—	—	20
BCG and DTIC	—	—	25
Mitoses			
<6/mm^2	94	81	41
>6/mm^2	100	40	31
Age			
<40 years	95	75	27
40–60 years	94	71	47
>60 years	93	78	26
Thickness			
0.76–1.25 mm	94	—	—
1.26–1.65 mm	95	—	—
1.51–2 mm	—	85	—
2.01–2.5 mm	—	74	—
2.51–3 mm	—	71	—
3.01–3.99 mm	—	54	—
3.61–5 mm	—	—	41
>5 mm	—	—	35
Histologic regression			
Absent	97	79	37
Present	92	68	39

[1]B = upper back, A = posterior aspect of the arm, N = posterior and lateral aspect of the neck, S = the scalp posterior to the ears.

Table 25–7. Five-year survival rate for malignant melanoma by level of invasion.

Level	Description	Five-Year Survival %
I	Malignant melanoma in situ Atypical melanocytes confined to the epidermis	100
II	Tumor invading, but not filling, the papillary dermis	99
III	Tumor filling the papillary layer but not invading the reticular dermis	91
IV	Tumor invading the reticular dermis	69
V	Tumor penetrating into the subcutaneous fat	34

long-term survival is rare following distant metastases from primary malignant melanoma, patients in this category are usually the first to be subjected to experimental therapeutic protocols. Therapies causing a rather meager lengthening of survival may possibly result in greater length of survival when administered at earlier stages in the natural history of malignant melanoma.

1. Prognostic factors–See Table 25–8.

(a) Surgical resectability–Patients are classified as having stage IVA melanoma if they have one or more distant metastases, all of which are removed surgically leaving no evidence of disease elsewhere as judged clinically and by laboratory and radiologic tests. Stage IVA also includes patients who have resected nodal disease distant from the regional lymph nodes. Patients with inoperable distant metastases and those who undergo debulking surgery leaving residual disease behind are classified as having stage IVB melanoma. The median survival is 18 months for stage IVA and 4.7 months for stage IVB disease.

(b) Initial site of metastasis–Patients with skin and lymph node metastases have the best prognosis, and those with metastases to multiple sites have the poorest prognosis. No liver involvement has been found to be a favorable independent prognostic indictor, second only to performance status. However,

Table 25–8. Summary of prognostic factors for patients with distant metastases.[1]

Major favorable prognostic factors
  Surgical resectability
  Metastasis location
    Skin and lymph nodes only
    No liver involvement
  Single rather than multiple sites
  Karnofsky performance status ≥80%
  Interval of ≥6 months from time of primary melanoma
    diagnosis to distant metastasis
Factors having minimal or no effect
  Location of the primary melanoma
  Age
  Sex

[1]Data from Day and Lew.

this analysis did not group skin and nodes together and did not test multiple sites as a variable.

(c) Performance status–Patients having a Karnofsky performance status (PS) of 80% or more and no liver involvement by metastases had a median survival rate of 6 months, compared with 3 months for a PS less than 80%.

(d) Interval between diagnosis and onset of distant metastases–In one study, patients who had a disease-free interval of more than 6 months prior to the onset of distant metastases had a median survival duration of 7.1 months, compared with 3 months for patients with a shorter disease-free interval between diagnosis and first evidence of dissemination.

(e) Number of metastatic sites–The number of metastatic sites was found to be the most important prognostic factor in one study.

(f) Age–Age has not been found to be a significant prognostic factor.

(g) Location of the primary melanoma–Survival is equally poor once the disease becomes disseminated regardless of the primary site.

(h) Sex–Females survive slightly longer than males.

2. Survival following stage IVA disease–In one series, the median time from initial diagnosis to stage IVA disease was 33 months, and the most common site of metastasis was the skin beyond the regional lymph nodes. Although the length of survival following metastases to skin and lymph nodes was longer than the length of survival following metastases to other sites, this difference was not statistically significant. This study found no difference in the median survival time by sex. Rather surprisingly, patients who achieved a IVA status more than once had a median survival of 36 months. In addition, the length of survival once stage IVB was finally reached was 8 months, compared with 4.7 months if the patient bypassed stage IVA and went directly to stage IVB.

Treatment

A. Suspicious Pigmented Lesions: Surgery is still the only effective modality for cure of malignant melanoma. Early excision of suspicious pigmented lesions can be lifesaving.

Suspicious pigmented lesions should have a total excisional biopsy with a 3-mm skin margin and underlying subcutaneous fat. Lesions that are too large and lesions that are located in areas that are cosmetically too sensitive to warrant complete excision without prior histologic proof of malignancy are best managed by incisional or punch biopsy. Care must be taken to sample the most nodular appearing, raised, or elevated component of the lesion. For lesions lacking this type of component, the biopsy sample should be taken from the darkest portion of the lesion. Management and follow-up of patients with dysplastic nevi are summarized in Table 25–9.

Table 25–9. Management of dysplastic nevi.

Take biopsy of at least one lesion for documentation.
Examine entire integument.
Take detailed family history.
Examine first-degree relatives.
Teach self-examination.
Follow up every 3–6 months.,
Advise patient to avoid sun exposure.
Advise patient to use sunscreens.
Excise or photograph to document for future excision.

B. Stage I Malignant Melanoma:
1. Excision of the primary lesion–
(a) Thin melanomas (<0.85 mm Thick)–These lesions can be safely excised with a 1-cm margin. The local recurrence rate is 2% or less.

(b) Thick melanomas (≥0.85 mm Thick)– Thicker melanomas should be excised with a 3-cm margin. This recommendation is based on findings that local recurrence rate increases from 3–4% up to 12% as the excision margin decreases from 3 cm to 1 cm. Furthermore, although three groups of investigators found that there was no adverse effect of decreasing margins on the length of survival, one study demonstrated that patients with melanomas ≥2 mm thick had a lower survival rate if their melanoma was excised with less than a 2-cm margin. Although the local recurrence rate decreases as the margin increases from 1 cm to 3 cm, there is no advantage to excision with a margin >3 cm. Regarding the depth of excision, there are no data. It is customary to extend the excision in depth to underlying fascia. Inasmuch as only one of four studies showed an adverse effect on survival of a narrow margin on excision, one should not remove an eye or transect the facial nerve in order to achieve a 3-cm margin. Judgment is required for melanomas located in cosmetically important areas and near important structures.

2. Elective removal of regional lymph nodes–Regional lymph nodes of patients with stage I cutaneous malignant melanoma may harbor clinically occult microscopic metastases despite feeling normal to palpation. These clinically occult metastases are discovered when the lymph nodes are removed electively and then examined microscopi-

cally. The probability that these clinically occult regional lymph node metastases exist increases with increasing primary tumor thickness.

(a) Thin melanomas (<0.85 mm thick)–Clinical stage I patients with melanomas measuring less than 0.85 mm almost never have occult metastases in the regional nodes. Therefore, elective regional node dissection is not indicated for these patients.

(b) Thick melanomas (≥0.85 mm thick)–Because occult regional lymph node metastases often exist without coexistent distant metastases, some investigators have advocated elective regional lymph node dissections to save lives. However, the available data show that this hypothesis is incorrect (Table 25–10). Every prospective study published to date, whether randomized or nonrandomized, shows that the survival rate for patients with clinical stage I melanoma is the same whether or not patients have elective lymph node dissection. Other investigators have advocated elective node dissection as necessary to properly stage the patient, but the data in Table 25–6 refute this idea. Within each thickness category are other factors that are equally good in determining prognosis, and a major surgical procedure is not needed to obtain these other factors. Therefore, at this time, clinical stage I patients with thick melanomas should not have elective regional node dissection.

3. Adjuvant therapy–There is no proved beneficial adjuvant therapy regimen for high-risk stage I patients. High-risk patients should be encouraged to enter investigational protocols.

4. Initial evaluation of the stage I patient–
(a) Head-to-Toe skin examination–Approximately 1% of patients with primary cutaneous malignant melanoma will have a second primary melanoma synchronous with diagnosis of the first primary. Thus, a thorough examination of the entire integument and mucous membranes is mandatory.

(b) Routine periodic follow-up–An additional 2% of patients will have an asynchronous second primary. Three-fourths of these asynchronous second primaries will occur within 5 years after diagnosis of the first primary, and one-fourth will occur more than 5 years after diagnosis. Thus, patients should be advised to have periodic follow-up examinations.

(c) Examination of first-order relatives–Ap-

Table 25–10. Efficacy of elective lymph node dissection in (ELND) in stage I cutaneous melanoma.[1]

Study Group	Year	Was the Study Prospective?	Was the Study Randomized?	Did the Study Show a Benefit for ELND?
World Health Organization	1977, 1982	Yes	Yes	No
Mayo Clinic	1978	Yes	Yes	No
University of Alabama	1979, 1983	No	No	Yes
Melanoma Clinical Cooperative Group	1981–1983	Yes	No	No
New South Wales, Australia	1982	No	No	Yes
University of California, San Francisco	1983	Yes	No	No
Duke University	1983	No	No	Yes

[1]Limited to studies that stratified data by primary tumor thickness and sophisticated statistical techniques.

proximately 2–10% of first-order relatives of patients with malignant melanoma have, have had, or will have malignant melanoma. Therefore, patients should be advised to have their parents, siblings, and children examined by a dermatologist.

(d) Sun avoidance and sunscreen use–Patients should be advised to adhere to strict sun avoidance and the daily use of sunscreens. Such advice may prolong their longevity more than any of the currently available chemotherapeutic or immunotherapeutic agents.

(e) Skin and lymph node examination–Since approximately 80% of the first metastases from clinical stage I melanoma occur near the primary site or in the regional lymph nodes, it is important to carefully inspect and palpate the skin surrounding the primary melanoma and the regional lymph node area. There are no laboratory or radiographic tests to detect subclinical local-regional metastases.

(f) Baseline chest x-ray–Of the remaining 20% of initial metastases, one-half, or 10%, of all initial metastases occur in the lung. For this reason, a baseline chest x-ray is indicated.

(g) Radiologic restraint–The remaining initial metastases can occur in almost any organ. A distant metastasis is rarely found by radiologic means in an asymptomatic, newly diagnosed clinical stage I patient. With the exception of a chest x-ray, radiologic studies are not indicated in newly diagnosed, asymptomatic, high-risk stage I patients.

C. Clinical stage II melanoma: The outcome for patients with stage II melanoma is far from hopeless. If only a single node is positive, the 10-year survival with surgical resection alone is 40–43%. Therefore, clinically enlarged regional lymph nodes should be resected without delay. Radiotherapy using high doses per fraction should be considered for patients judged to have a high morbidity or mortality risk from therapeutic node dissection. Overall response rates approaching 100% and complete response rates of 60% or better can be expected with radiation therapy used in this fashion. There is no effective chemotherapy or immunotherapy. Patients with stage II melanoma should be referred to investigational protocols.

D. Clinical stage III melanoma: Systemic therapeutic interventions for patients with distant metastases have been conspicuously ineffective. Patients with complete responses to various agents have the same survival as patients who do not respond to these same agents. Therefore, all patients with stage III melanoma should be referred to investigational protocols. High dose per fraction radiotherapy offers excellent palliation, particularly for patients who have central nervous system metastases, bony metastases, massive lymph node metastases, or other symptomatic metastases. Aggressive surgery is indicated, since prolonged survivals have been observed in patients rendered clinically disease-free by resection of distant metastases.

Single anticancer agents that have been administered to patients with stage III malignant melanoma include dacarbazine, cisplatin, and the nitrosoureas (carmustine, lomustine). Alpha-interferon and interleukin-2 also have modest antitumor activity against advanced malignant melanoma. High-dose chemotherapy and autologous bone marrow transplantation remain unproved as treatment for advanced malignant melanoma. Interesting avenues of clinical research include tumor vaccines, tumor infiltrating lymphocytes, and monoclonal antibodies conjugated to radionuclides or cellular toxins. Combination therapies have shown slight gains in response against advanced disease but remain of unproved value in most patients with malignant melanoma.

REFERENCES

Ackerman AB: Disagreements with the current classification of malignant melanomas. *Am J Surg Pathol* 1982;**6**:733.

Ackerman AB: Macular and patch lesions of malignant melanoma: Malignant melanoma in situ. *J Dermatol Surg Oncol* 1983;**9**:615.

Ackerman AB: Malignant melanoma, A unifying concept. *Am J Dermatopathol* 1980;**2**:309.

Ackerman AB: Malignant melanoma in situ: The flat, curable stage of malignant melanoma. *Pathology* 1985;**17**:298.

Blois MS et al: Judging prognosis in malignant melanoma of the skin. *Ann Surg* 1983;**198**:200.

Breslow A: Thickness, cross-sectional areas and depth of invasion in the prognosis of cutaneous melanoma. *Ann Surg* 1970;**172**:902.

Breslow A, Macht SD: Optimal size of resection margin for thin cutaneous melanoma. *Surg Gynecol Obstet* 1977;**145**:691.

Cascinelli N et al: Prognosis of skin melanoma with regional node metastases (stage II). *J Surg Oncol* 1984;**25**:240.

Cascinelli et al: Stage I melanoma of the skin: The problem of resection margins. *Eur J Cancer* 1980;**16**:1079.

Clark WH et al: The developmental biology of primary human malignant melanomas. *Semin Oncol* 1975;**2**:83.

Clark WH Jr et al: The histogenesis and biologic behavior of primary human malignant melanomas of the skin. *Cancer Res* 1969;**29**:705.

Clark WH Jr et al: Origin of familial malignant melanomas from heritable melanocytic lesions. *Arch Dermatol* 1978;**114**:732.

Day CL Jr, Lew RA: Malignant Melanoma Prognostic Factors 3: Surgical margins. *J Dermatol Surg Oncol* 1983;**9**:797.

Day CL Jr et al: Classification of melanoma according to the histologic morphology of melanocytes in the nodules. *J Dermatol Surg Oncol* 1982;**6**:874.

Day CL Jr et al: Malignant melanoma patients with positive nodes and relatively good prognosis: Microstaging retains prognostic significance in clinical stage I melanoma patients with metastases to regional nodes. *Cancer* 1981;**47**:955.

Day CL Jr, Lew RA: Malignant melanoma prognostic factors 6: Distant metastases and length of survival. *J Dermatol Surg Oncol* 1984;**10**:686.

Day CL Jr et al: A multivariate analysis of prognostic factors for melanoma patients with lesions 3.65 mm in thickness. *Ann Surg* 1982;**195**:44.

Day CL Jr et al: A multivariate analysis of prognostic factors for melanoma patients with lesions > or = 3.65 mm in thickness. *Ann Surg* 1982;**195**:44.

Day CL Jr et al: Prognostic factors for melanoma patients with lesions 0.76–1.68 mm in thickness. *Ann Surg* 1982;**195**:30.

Day CL Jr et al: Prognostic factors for melanoma patients with lesions 0.76–1.69 mm in thickness, an appraisal of "thin" level IV lesions. *Ann Surg* 1982;**195**:30.

Day CL Jr et al: Prognostic factors for patients with clinical stage I melanoma of intermediate thickness (1.51–3.99 mm), a conceptual model for tumor growth and metastasis. *Ann Surg* 1982;**195**:35.

Day CL Jr et al: A prognostic model for clinical Stage I melanoma of the lower extremity. *Ann Surg* 1981;**89**:599.

Day CL Jr et al: A prognostic model for clinical stage I melanoma of the lower extremity, location on foot as independent risk factor for recurrent disease. *Surgery* 1981;**89**:599.

Day CL Jr et al: A prognostic model for clinical Stage I melanoma of the trunk. *Am J Surg* 1981;**142**:247.

Day CL Jr et al: A prognostic model for clinical stage melanoma of the trunk, location near the midline is not an independent risk factor for recurrent disease. *Am J Surg* 1981;**142**:247.

Day CL Jr et al: A prognostic model for clinical Stage I melanoma of the upper extremity. *Ann Surg* 1981;**193**:436.

Day CL Jr et al: A prognostic model for clinical stage melanoma of the upper extremity, the importance of anatomic subsite in predicting recurrent disease. *Ann Surg* 1981;**4**:436.

Evans RD et al: Risk factors for the development of malignant melanoma—I: Review of case-control studies. *J Dermatol Surg Oncol* 1988;**14**:393.

Harrist TJ et al: "Microscopic satellites" are more highly associated with regional lymph node metastases than is primary melanoma thickness. *Cancer* 1984;**53**:2183.

Kelly J, Crutcher W, Sagebiel R: Clinical diagnosis of dysplastic melanocytic nevi: A clinicopathologic correlation. *J Am Acad Dermatol* 1986;**14**:1044.

Rhodes AR et al: Risk factors for cutaneous melanoma: A practical method for recognizing predisposed individuals. *JAMA* 1987;**258**:3146.

Veronesi R et al: Delayed lymph node dissection in stage I melanoma of the skin of the lower extremities. *Cancer* 1982;**49**:2420.

Veronesi R et al: Inefficacy of immediate node dissection in stage I melanoma of the limbs. *N Engl J Med* 1977;**297**:627.

Plasma Cell Myeloma

Lon Shelby Smith, MD

Essentials of Diagnosis
- Bone marrow plasmacytosis >10%.
- Presence of monoclonal immunoglobulin in serum or excretion of monoclonal light chains in urine, or both, associated with a depression in normal serum immunoglobulins.
- Radiologic evidence of osteolytic lesions. Generalized osteoporosis may serve as a criterion if the marrow contains >30% plasma cells.
- Anemia, renal impairment, and hypercalcemia often associated.

Epidemiology
Multiple myeloma is characterized by the uncontrolled expression of a clone of plasma cells or their precursors. Accounting for about 1% of all malignant tumors, this disease causes the death of about 7000 individuals in the USA each year. The frequency of diagnosis has increased over the past 20 years, probably because of the wider diagnostic use of screening chemistries, protein electrophoresis, and bone marrow aspiration. The disease has been reported in people throughout the world. In the USA, the incidence in blacks is twice that in whites. The disease occurs predominantly in the 50- to 70-year age group. Fewer than 2% of patients are under the age of 40.

Etiology
The cause of plasma cell dyscrasias is obscure. Genetic factors may play a role. Plasma cell dyscrasias have been reported to occur in siblings and other close relations. In specific strains of mice, plasma cell dyscrasias can be induced by mineral oil injection and similar means.

For many years, chronic stimulation of the reticuloendothelial system has been thought to play a major role in the development of myeloma. In Balb/C mice, myeloma can be induced following injection of Freund's adjuvants, mineral oil, and plastics. After initial injection, granulomatous lesions develop at the site of injection. A diffuse polyclonal hypergammaglobulinemia also develops. Six to 12 months later, about two-thirds of these mice develop plasmacytomas that produce serum M-component and Bence Jones protein.

In other animal models such as the Aleutian mink and New Zealand black mouse, the development of monoclonal plasma cell dyscrasias is preceded by an autoimmune disease and polyclonal hypergammaglobulinemia. In all these models, genetic factors associated with prolonged stimulation of the lymphoreticular system seems to lead to the development of plasma cell tumors.

Clinical observations in humans suggest a link between chronic stimulation of the immune system and development of plasma cell dyscrasias. Perhaps the best known instance is the association of chronic infection and amyloidosis. Plasma cell dyscrasias occur in association with chronic osteomyelitis, pyelonephritis, tuberculosis, and chronic hepatitis. While these associations are of interest, a molecular basis for the development of myeloma remains to be elucidated.

Pathogenesis
One of the most fruitful research efforts to contribute to understanding of the biology of myeloma has been the application of flow cytometry to the study of myeloma plasma cells. This technique can be used to evaluate the DNA, RNA, and monoclonal immunoglobulin content of myeloma cells.

Myeloma plasma cells are typically hyperdiploid with a DNA content 10–15% higher than that of normal diploid cells. Since about 80% of patients have abnormal amounts of DNA in their tumor cells, this serves as an excellent tumor marker. Generally, the tumor cells found in the marrow have the same DNA content as those found in extramedullary disease. In about 10–20% of patients, however, at least two clones of cells are present. Serial studies in the same patient indicate that only rarely will the DNA stem line change with disease progression. Hypodiploid tumor cells have been associated with drug resistance.

Myeloma cells have long been known to have a high RNA content, presumably because of a substantial commitment to protein production. Flow cytometry has permitted quantitation of RNA content. In general, the RNA content is four to six times greater than that of peripheral blood lymphocytes. The RNA content remains stable in the tumor cells of most individual patients throughout the course of their disease. A lower RNA content is often associated with IgA myeloma and high tumor mass. Drug sensitivity increases with plasma cell RNA content.

The monoclonal immunoglobulin produced by myeloma cells has been demonstrated by flow cytometry using anti–heavy and anti–light chain antibodies. About 15% of patients show coexpression of kappa and lambda light chains. These cells are usually aneuploid, supporting their malignant nature.

Since plasma cells have low proliferative activity, it has been thought for many years that a stem cell exists which directly influences tumor growth. According to this view, plasma cells would primarily accumulate as an end cell without true self-renewal capacity. Since clinical observation supports the view that the major expansion and proliferation of tumor cells in myeloma occurs in cells that are already committed to the production of an idiotype-specific monoclonal protein, the stem cell has been assumed to be a B cell. Several studies have indicated the presence of B cells that produce a specific idiotypic protein. Reports have suggested the presence of a common acute lymphocytic leukemic antigen (CALLA)–positive precursor population in the peripheral blood and bone marrow of myeloma patients. In one series, aneuploid tumor cells expressed CALLA in more than half the cases. This antigen was often coexpressed with mature B cell markers such as cytoplasmic immunoglobulin, indicating the presence of unusual tumor cell phenotypes without normal B cell counterparts. Recent observations suggest that other subpopulations of cells exist that express T and even myelomonocytic features. While these changes may be due simply to malignancy related aberrations, they may indicate that myeloma arises from a far distant primordial stem cell.

Phenotypic studies in patients with myeloma have increased awareness that subpopulations of cells express many cytokines and associated receptors. Progression of myeloma may reflect escape from this regulatory network.

Identification of a committed B lymphocyte representing the predominant stem cell in myeloma has led to the hope that idiotype-specific regulation by T lymphocytes, macrophages, or both, might exist at this stage. Further, progression of myeloma may reflect a population of cells that have escaped from this idiotype-specific regulation. An important factor in this maturation escape may be the production of interleukin-6 (IL-6) by the macrophage.

Because plasma cells have low proliferative activity, cytogenetic studies in myeloma have been less comprehensive than those in related lymphoid tumors.

At one institution, a significant correlation was found between structural chromosome abnormalities involving chromosome 6q, the presence of extensive bone lesions, and the presence of tumor necrosis factor beta (TNF-β) and supernatants from myeloma cell cultures. Since the genetic (DNA) material coding for TNF-β is located on chromosome 6 just below the centromere, these changes in chromosome 6q may relate to the enhanced secretion of lymphotoxin in myeloma patients.

Of further interest are the abnormalities found on chromosome 7. The presence of the 7q abnormality occurs with the acquisition of multidrug resistance. The doxorubicin resistance subline (8226/DOX) both acquires the 7q abnormality and also expresses high levels of messenger RNA for the P glycoprotein and contains high levels of P glycoprotein in the cell membrane. The screening of tumor specimens in this way may one day permit selection of patients for treatment with calcium channel blockers in an effort to reverse drug resistance to doxorubicin.

Conventional karyotypic analysis has shown cytogenetic abnormalities in about one-fourth of patients. Patients with DNA aneuploidy and greater than 10% plasmacytosis have a higher incidence of karyotypic abnormalities. The chromosomal abnormalities consist mainly of numeric changes, with the addition of chromosomes 3, 5, 7, 9, 11, 15, 19, and 21 and losses of chromosomes 8, 13, 16, and 22. Structural aberrations involving chromosomes 1, 6, 8, 11, and 14 were also seen. An association was also noted between light chain disease and hypodiploid karyotypes. In addition, an association between IgA myeloma and translocations involving chromosome 8 was described.

The observation of translocations in chromosomes 8 and 14, and between chromosomes 11 and 14, implicates involvement of the c-*myc* and VCL-1 oncogenes. These are associated with B cell neoplasms.

Research also has been devoted to host-tumor and tumor-host interactions that occur in myeloma in the hope of elucidating immunologic regulatory mechanisms. The hypogammaglobulinemia that occurs in patients with myeloma is perhaps the best known example of a tumor-host interaction. This immunosuppressive effect occurs at relatively low tumor loads and is believed to be specific for the malignancy. Its cause, however, is unknown.

Some evidence also suggests that the host's immunologic mechanisms may modulate tumor growth. Many patients are found to have a tumor mass that remains stable for many years. The duration of this plateau is not influenced by continuing chemotherapy. This phase is associated with suppression of peripheral blood lymphocytes bearing the same light chain isotype as that of the malignant paraprotein. This phenomenon has been termed light chain isotype suppression (LCIS). The presence of LCIS in one series of patients was found to confer a favorable prognosis and to be a marker of stable disease at presentation. LCIS occurs in plasma cells and peripheral blood lymphocytes but not in bone marrow lymphocytes, suggesting that the suppression process may act at the site of egress of bone marrow cells to the periphery. The presence of precursor cells that are CALLA positive in patients with myeloma inversely correlates with the presence of LCIS. The presence of these cells in the peripheral blood is a marker of progressive disease and suggests that their appearance results from a breakdown of immunoregulatory mechanisms.

Staging of Generalized Myeloma

Myeloma offers a model of disease that lends itself to quantitative measurement. Studies in the mouse demonstrated the quantitative relationship between serum myeloma protein concentration and tumor weight. These studies permitted the development of techniques for calculating myeloma cell mass in patients with IgG myeloma from measurements of monoclonal immunoglobulin synthesis in metabolism. In another set of experiments, a correlation was demonstrated between the weights of subcutaneously implanted MOPC-104 plasmacytomas in mice and the weights derived from measurement of M-component synthesis in metabolism. Using similar techniques, it was possible under carefully controlled circumstances to measure M-component synthesis in metabolism in humans and obtain estimates of myeloma cell burden. These data were later correlated with presenting clinical features, response to treatment, and survival. Information gained from serial measurements of tumor burden in patients has been of great importance in designing optimal chemotherapy schedules and in managing individual patients.

Clinical features that correlate with measured tumor mass and survival have been used to define a clinical staging system for multiple myeloma (Table 26–1). This system has been refined to make the staging of patients more quantitative and relevant to clinical outcome. This system recognizes that factors other than tumor load may contribute to anemia and hypercalcemia. Less emphasis is placed on defining the extent of lytic lesions and bone demineralization, since this subjective variable often leads to overstaging of individual patients. The degree of marrow plasmacytosis, level of serum β_2-microglobulin, and levels of normal immunoglobulins also contribute to more consistent staging of individuals.

Treatment

A. Approach: Before chemotherapy is begun, optimal control of reversible medical complications such as overt infection is desirable. Treatment should not be delayed owing to hypercalcemia, particularly since the therapeutic regimen always includes corticosteroids. For patients with severe vertebral fracture pain, at least one course of chemotherapy is useful before local radiation is considered unless radiation therapy is required for spinal cord compression.

The effectiveness of chemotherapy should be monitored by means of serial measurements of serum my-

Table 26–1. Staging of plasma cell myeloma by tumor mass.[1]

High tumor mass
  Hemoglobin <8.5 g/L without renal failure or hypoferremia
  Calcium >11.5 mg/L[2] or without bedridden status
  Supporting features often present
    Marrow plasmacytosis >40% on flow cytometry or suspension smears in most patients
    IgM <20 mg/L or IgA <40 mg/L or IgG <400 mg/L in about half of patients
    Serum β_2-microglobulin >8.0 mg/L without creatinine >1.8 mg/L in about half of patients
Low tumor mass
  Hemoglobin >10.5 g/L unless other factors causing anemia present
  + Calcium <11.0 mg/L[2]
  + IgG or IgA peak <5.0 g/L
  + Serum β_2-microglobulin <4.5 mg/L
  Supporting features often present
  Marrow plamacytosis <20% on flow cytometry or suspension smears in most patients
    IgM >50 mg/L and IgA >100 mg/L and IgG >750 mg/L in about half of patients
Intermediate tumor mass
  All other patients

[1]Slightly modified and reproduced, with permission, from Smith L, Alexanian R: Treatment strategies for plasma cell myeloma. *CA* 1985;**35:**214.
[2]Corrected calcium (mg/L) = serum calcium (mg/L) – serum albumin (g/L) + 4.0.

eloma protein concentration, Bence Jones protein excretion, or both. The true degree of tumor reduction will be underestimated if consideration is not given to the changing catabolic rate for different IgG levels, reduction of plasma volume with therapy, and possible effect of normal background globulin in the calculation of tumor mass change. When the data are corrected for these factors, a reduction in monoclonal IgG peak from 4 g/dL to 2 g/dL conforms more closely to a 75% reduction in tumor mass.

While it is possible to assess low monoclonal IgG peaks from routine serum electrophoresis, low monoclonal IgA globulins are frequently obscured by normal globulins. For this reason, IgA peaks below 2000 mg/dL should be evaluated serially from direct quantitations. The tumor burden can then be inferred using a simple computer program that includes serum myeloma protein component, albumin, hemoglobin, and body weight. Monthly changes in tumor mass can be calculated from these data (an arbitrary value of 100% is assigned at the start of therapy). The serial changes in each patient's tumor mass can be plotted and, when viewed in the context of sequential therapies or no treatment follow-up, serve as an invaluable aid to management.

Definitions of response vary, but for patients undergoing initial treatment, response is usually defined by a 75% reduction in calculated tumor mass, disappearance of Bence Jones protein, or both. Less strict criteria, such as a 50% reduction in tumor mass, will result in a 20% higher response rate. Thus, it is important to be aware of the response criteria used when evaluating reports of various therapies. For patients responding to various combination therapies, eg, vincristine-doxorubicin and corticosteroids, the onset of remission is usually rapid so that the tumor halving time is less than 4 months. Therefore, a stable serum peak during the first few months usually indicates that remission will never occur. When Bence Jones protein is present, either as the only abnormality or in combination with a serum peak, conclusions can be reached even earlier. In one study, Bence Jones protein excretion was reduced by 50% within 2 months in all patients who achieved a 75% reduction in tumor mass as defined by change in serum peak. Failure to reduce Bence Jones protein excretion by 50% within this period identified resistant patients.

The reason Bence Jones protein excretion is such a sensitive indicator of therapy is due to the fact that the kidneys metabolize far more Bence Jones protein than they excrete. Thus, a small decrease in Bence Jones protein production results in a marked decrease in excretion of the protein, assuming kidney metabolism remains constant.

A 1969 study reported that 4-day courses of melphalan and prednisone given at 6-week intervals reduced myeloma tumor mass by 75% in about 45% of patients. Since this report, further progress in controlling the disease has been limited. The main drug combinations that have been evaluated include combinations of different alkylating agents with or without a nitrosourea compound and combinations of doxorubicin, vincristine, and corticosteroids with or without an alkylating agent.

Combinations of different alkylating agents with or without a nitrosourea, such as carmustine, have been evaluated for use in patients resistant to melphalan, but use of these combinations did not consistently improve the results in comparison with melphalan-prednisone.

In contrast, a favorable experience was reported with a combination of vincristine-melphalan-cyclophosphasmide-carmustine and prednisone (the M-2 protocol). The authors reported a 78% response in 81 patients using this regimen, compared with a 33% response rate in 46 patients in a historical control group treated with either melphalan or melphalan-prednisone. The median survival for patients in this group was significantly longer (38 months) than the median survival in the control group (15 months). A 50% reduction in myeloma protein was used as a criterion for response. The apparent superiority of the M-2 protocol when compared with other trials using similar drugs at different doses is unexplained. Considering the conflicting results, no convincing and reproducible gain seems evident from combinations of different alkylating agents with or without a nitrosourea.

Slightly superior results have been obtained when vincristine-doxorubicin and prednisone with either an alkylating agent or nitrosourea were used. Among 256 patients so treated, the response rate was 58% for patients who received combinations containing both vincristine and doxorubicin, compared with 42% for patients for whom one or both of these drugs were omitted.

Of further importance, the onset of remission occurred more rapidly among patients receiving the vincristine-doxorubicin combinations. This is of practical import in treating patients with high tumor mass who are at risk for early death or the development of renal failure.

Most patients resistant to melphalan and prednisone receive doxorubicin-containing combinations later in their course and many respond to this regimen. These data suggest that the outcome of patients with low tumor mass not at risk for early death due to progressive disease or renal failure may be the same when the initial treatment consists of melphalan-prednisone only, provided that vincristine, doxorubicin, and high-dose corticosteroids are used later in the disease course. Since many patients treated initially with melphalan and prednisone never receive doxorubicin later when their disease is progressing, there is some support for the use of a doxorubicin-containing combination in the initial treatment of all patients because of the higher response rate and the opportunity to stop or change therapy after maximum tumor reduction.

B. Localized Myeloma: About 5% of patients with plasma cell myeloma have a solitary lesion that is defined by one area of bone destruction with no bone marrow plasmacytosis and no complications such as anemia or hypercalcemia. At the author's institution, only about half of these patients have a serum or urine myeloma protein. In all patients, the IgG or IgA serum peak is less than 1.6 g/dL. The Bence Jones protein excretion is less than 500 mg/d, and normal immunoglobulin levels are preserved. These patients showed a marked diminution of the myeloma protein level when irradiated with 4000 cGy to the local site of disease. About two-thirds of patients presenting with a solitary bone lesion eventually progress to overt myeloma; the remaining third have probably been cured.

C. Indolent Myeloma: About 5% of patients can be described as having indolent myeloma. These patients are asymptomatic but show changes typical of generalized myeloma, including marrow plasmacytosis, monoclonal globulin peaks above 4 g/L, and occasionally lytic bone lesions. Often diagnosis is made following detection of an elevated serum protein on a routine chemical profile. There is no necessity to treat these patients immediately after diagnosis. They may be followed without treatment provided that serial electrophoretic studies are obtained every 2–3 months. Treatment should be initiated when there is a clear upward trend in the myeloma protein concentration and calculated tumor mass. Chemotherapy has been deferred for more than 2 years in about half of patients. The delay in treatment has not affected long-term outcome (this is also true for patients with indolent lymphoma).

D. Practical Recommendations: Patients with myeloma should be encouraged to drink fluids. A high fluid intake may decrease the risk of renal insufficiency due to hypercalcemia, protein casts in the proximal and distal tubules, and hyperuricemia. In one report, a fluid intake ≥3 L/d reduced renal failure in 39 of 49 patients with myeloma and renal insufficiency. Dehydration, especially when preparing patients for studies such as barium enemas, should be avoided. Patients with myeloma are at high risk for nephrotoxicity due to iodine-containing contrast media used in such procedures as intravenous pyelograms and CT scans.

Hypercalcemia eventually occurs in about one-third of patients with myeloma and should be suspected when patients present with nausea, vomiting, polyuria, increased constipation, confusion, stupor, or coma. Because dehydration is a consequence of hypercalcemia, patients should be hydrated. Isotonic saline is the fluid of choice because sodium promotes the renal excretion of calcium. After hydration is achieved, additional treatment with furosemide may further enhance the excretion of calcium. Calcitonin, corticosteroids, and bisphosphonates are often useful in the management of hypercalcemia.

Patients with myeloma who present with weakness of the legs or difficulty in voiding or defecating should be evaluated for spinal cord compression. The sudden onset of severe thoracic pain or abdominal pain may also raise the question of acute spinal cord compression. Patients with this problem are probably best evaluated by MRI and prompt neurosurgical consultation. Radiation therapy in a dose of approximately 3000 cGy can usually control this complication if it is detected early.

Patients with severe back pain may benefit from use of a brace. Physical activity should be encouraged because it tends to decrease decalcification in bone. When anemia is present in patients with myeloma, erythropoietin levels should be obtained and exogenous administration of recombinant erythropoietin should be considered.

E. Remission Maintenance: After a patient responds to therapy, a decision must be made about length of treatment. Early studies showed no advantage for maintenance therapy in patients who enjoyed a 75% reduction in tumor mass over no treatment until relapse. The median duration of remission in recent trials has been 18 months in those who achieved disappearance of their abnormal protein, and about 6 months in those with a persistent serum peak. When relapse occurs in either group, about half will achieve a 50% or greater reduction in tumor mass when therapy is resumed. In those who fail to respond by these criteria, the myeloma protein either remains stable or rises slowly for many months. Thus, unmaintained remission follow-up is appropriate for those responding patients in whom the myeloma protein has disappeared (20% of the total patient population) or in whom a markedly reduced serum myeloma protein remains stable following 24 months of treatment (10% of the total patient population). This approach is not recommended for patients with less than a 75% reduction in tumor mass or for whom regular follow-up is not possible.

In addition to the obvious reduction in costs associated with a policy of no treatment during remission, the incidence of acute leukemia is greatly reduced in this population. About 6% of responding patients treated indefinitely with alkylating agents will ultimately develop acute leukemia. With the reduced use of melphalan in patients followed on no therapy, this frequency has been reduced to about 1–2%. Interferon suppresses progression of myeloma in 20–30% of newly diagnosed patients with low tumor burden and seems to prolong periods of remission in patients induced with standard regimens.

F. Remission Relapse: All patients who achieve remission eventually relapse if they do not die of another cause. Occasionally, the pattern of relapse involves a rising Bence Jones protein level or progressive bone lesions and soft tissue tumors, even with no change in the myeloma protein level. Such occurrences often presage the development of a more aggressive disease course, possibly associated with new clones apparent in flow cytometry studies. For this reason, patients in remission should be followed by periodic measurement of Bence Jones protein and by bone films in addition to regular assessments of their abnormal globulin. The onset of relapse is followed by a median survival time of only 9 months unless remission is achieved.

Until recently, few effective chemotherapeutic regimens were available for patients with melphalan-resistant myeloma. Response rates were about 25% in patients treated with nitrosourea-doxorubicin combinations. More recent experience suggests a role for more intensive courses of glucocorticoids. One group reported responses in about 25% of patients with refractory myeloma who received weekly courses of vindesine and prednisone. In further trials, no patient responded to vindesine alone, pointing to a significant effect due to frequent pulses of prednisone, either alone or in combination with vindesine. About half the patients then responded with a 50% reduction in tumor mass to pulses of prednisone combined with vincristine and doxorubicin.

These encouraging results prompted the design of a vincristine–doxorubicin (Adriamycin)–dexamethasone (VAD) regimen. Dexamethasone was substituted for prednisone in a dose that provided a fourfold increase in glucocorticoid effect. Vincristine and doxorubicin were given over 4 days by continuous infusion to provide slowly cycling cells with prolonged exposure to cytotoxic agents. About two-thirds of relapsing patients and about one-third of unresponsive patients achieved a 75% reduction in tumor mass. These results were superior to those described for any other group of patients with myeloma refractory to alkylating agents.

In a subsequent study, the response to VAD chemotherapy was compared with the activity of high-dose dexamethasone alone, both in resistant and relapsing patients. With a greater than 75% reduction in M-protein synthesis used as the criterion for response, the VAD regimen and high-dose dexamethasone alone had a similar response rate of approximately 30% for patients initially resistant to chemotherapy, but the VAD regimen was more effective in relapsing patients than was dexamethasone alone. Numerous trials have corroborated the effectiveness of VAD therapy, which is one of the most active combinations for patients with relapsing or resistant myeloma reported to date.

The major toxicity associated with the VAD regimen is the increased likelihood of infection. In the initial series, 11 of 29 patients had episodes of fever. The infectious agent was identified in eight: four cases of pneumonia, two cases of gram-positive bacteremia probably related to an indwelling catheter, and two cases of gram-negative sepsis. Viral infections were common including herpetic esophagitis in two patients, herpes zoster infection in one patient, and cytomegalovirus infection with hepatitis in one patient. Although the VAD regimen results in moderate to severe toxicity in about one-third of patients treated, it remains the treatment of choice in patients with relapsing myeloma at the present time.

For patients who are truly resistant to doxorubicin-containing regimens, treatment with a glucocorticoid alone in high doses may be as effective as the VAD regimen. Dexamethasone, 40 mg orally for 4 days starting on days 1, 9, and 17, every 28 days, is probably the least toxic schedule of high-dose glucocorticoid treatment.

In patients who do not respond to glucocorticoids or the VAD regimen, systemic radiotherapy is worth consideration. The technique most commonly used involves sequential hemibody irradiation starting with the more symptomatic half. Objective responses are observed in about one-third of patients. The duration of these responses is not clear, but since the median survival after completion of radiotherapy is in the range of 6–7 months, the response durations were probably short-lived. The major benefit of this treatment is significant relief of bone pain, which is probably obtained in more than 75% of patients. Common side effects of this treatment include myelosuppression, pneumonitis, nausea, vomiting, diarrhea, and stomatitis. Treatment-related deaths, however, are uncommon.

High-dose chemotherapy, either alone in combination with bone marrow transplantation, has been attempted in an effort to overcome drug resistance in myeloma cells. High-dose chemotherapy has yielded a high response rate, but in most cases, these responses were short-lived. The toxicity of these regimens is significant, similar to that observed for induction therapy in acute leukemia. At present the role of high-dose chemotherapy and bone marrow transplantation is not well defined, but the use of this technique should at least be considered in the planning strategy for patients with this disease.

Prognosis

The frequency of response is similar for patients regardless of the initial tumor burden. Flow cytometric measurements have indicated that patients with a high RNA content in plasma cells have a greater likelihood of response than those with a lower content. High serum LDH levels at initiation of therapy has been associated with resistance to VAD. The most important predictor of prolonged survival is the occurrence of a response. The pretreatment tumor mass at time of presentation is a secondary factor. In evaluating response, serial measurements of the serum β_2-microglobulin during the induction phase is helpful in addition to a careful evaluation of the serum M-component values. β_2-Microglobulin represents the light chain of the major histocompatibility complex of the cell membrane. Increased β_2-microglobulin is present in the serum of patients with tumors with a high growth fraction and increased cell turnover. Because the β_2-microglobulin is a small protein that is excreted largely in urine, renal failure can lead to elevations in serum levels. In patients with normal renal function and increased cell turnover associated with disease progression, β_2-microglobulin will increase, indicating a lack of response to therapy.

Longevity is clearly determined by the residual number of tumor cells after an optimal program of chemotherapy. For this reason, projections of prognosis should be deferred for several months after the start of chemotherapy.

REFERENCES

Alexanian R, Dreicer R: Chemotherapy for multiple myeloma. *Cancer* 1984;**53**:583.

Alexanian R, Barlogie B, Dixon D: High-dose glucocorticoid treatment of resistant myeloma. *Ann Intern Med* 1986;**105**:8.

Barlogie B, Epstein J, Alexanian R: Genotypic and phenotypic characteristics of multiple myeloma. *Hematol Oncol* 1988;**6**:99.

Barlogie B, Smith L, Alexanian R: Effective treatment of

advanced multiple myeloma refractory to alkylating agents. *N Engl J Med* 1984;**310:**1353.

Barlogie B et al: Cytoplasmic immunoglobulin content in multiple myeloma. *J Clin Invest* 1985;**76:**765.

Barlogie B et al: High-dose melphalan with autologous bone marrow transplantation for multiple myeloma. *Blood* 1986;**67:**1298.

Bergsagel DE: Use a gentle approach for refractory myeloma patients. (Editorial.) *Clin Oncol* 1988;**6:**757.

Durie BG: The biology of multiple myeloma. *Hematol Oncol* 1988;**6:**77.

Durie BG, Salmon SE: A clinical staging system for multiple myeloma: correlation of measured myeloma cell mass with presenting clinical features, response to treatment, and survival. *Cancer* 1975;**36:**842.

Grogan T et al: Delineation of a novel pre-B cell component in plasma cell myeloma: Immunochemical, immuno-phenotypic, genotypic, cytological, cell culture, and kinetic features. *Blood* 1987;**70:**932.

Jaffe JP, Bosch A, Raich PC: Sequential hemibody radiotherapy in advanced multiple myeloma. *Cancer* 1979;**43:**124.

Joshua PE: Biology of multiple myeloma—host/tumor interactions and immune regulation of disease activity. *Hematol Oncol* 1988;**6:**83.

McElwain TJ, Powles RL: High-dose intravenous melphalan for plasma cell leukemia and myeloma. *Lancet* 1983;**2:**822.

McLaughlin P, Alexanian R: Myeloma protein kinetics following chemotherapy. *Blood* 1982;**60:**851.

Waldenstrom J: Some reflections on myeloma. *Scand J Haematol* 1985;**35:**4.

27 Sarcomas of Soft Tissue & Bone

Kathleen A. Havlin, MD

Essentials of Diagnosis

- Abnormal growth in any soft tissue or bone.
- Symptoms often referable to affected body part (eg, back pain from retroperitoneal sarcoma, gastrointestinal bleeding from leiomyosarcoma of gastrointestinal tract, vaginal bleeding from uterine sarcoma).
- Predisposing conditions (eg, Paget's disease of bone, chronic lymphedema of an extremity, previous radiation therapy, von Recklinghausen's disease, previous or family history of retinoblastoma, asbestosis).

Sarcomas are malignant tumors of the musculoskeletal system that arise predominantly from mesodermal structures. Other sarcomas arise from ectodermal structures (Schwann cells), and still others arise from mesodermal epithelium (endothelium of blood vessels and lymphatic channels; mesothelium of body cavities and visceral organs). In general, these latter tumors behave similarly to tumors arising from connective tissue cells and are included in the category of sarcomas.

Approximately 7000 new sarcomas are diagnosed each year and account for 1–2% of all solid tumors in adults and 15% of pediatric solid tumors. Sarcomas account for 2% of all cancer deaths in adults. The average annual age-adjusted incidence rate is approximately 2:100,000. Peak incidence in adults occurs in the fifth decade. There is no sexual or racial predilection. No proved genetic predisposition in the development of sarcomas has been confirmed although soft tissue sarcomas are thought to occur with slightly increased frequency in a variety of genetically transmitted diseases such as basal cell nevus syndrome, tuberous sclerosis, Werner's syndrome, intestinal polyposis, Gardner's syndrome, and von Recklinghausen's disease. The most common sites (with approximate percentages) are the lower extremities (40%), trunk (30%), upper extremities (15%), and head and neck (15%).

Because of the relative rarity of these tumors, patients should be referred to and evaluated at centers experienced in treatment of these patients and with established multidisciplinary tumor boards. Pathologic specimens should be reviewed by a pathologist experienced in diagnosis of sarcoma. Through referral to such centers, these patients can be entered on existing clinical protocols in the attempt to answer the many remaining questions regarding optimal therapy.

Etiology

A. Trauma: The etiologic relationship with trauma is unclear but likely may draw attention to an underlying abnormality. There are rare reports of sarcomas arising in scar tissue from burns, surgery, fracture sites, and in the vicinity of plastic or metal implants.

B. Chemical Carcinogens:

1. Exposure to vinyl chloride (used in preparation of synthetic rubber) or thorium dioxide (Thorotrast), previously used as a radiopaque medium, and arsenic-based insecticides have established associations with the development of angiosarcoma of the liver.

2. Exposure to phenoxyacetic acids (herbicides) and chlorophenols (wood preservatives) in some studies is associated with a six-fold increase in soft tissue sarcomas. However, conflicting evidence regarding this association exists in other studies. Occupational exposure to these chemicals occurs in forestry workers, farmers, and those employed in wood-working occupations.

3. Agent Orange (dioxin), a phenoxyherbicide used during the Vietnam War, has been previously associated with an increased risk of developing soft tissue sarcomas. A recent study from the Centers for Disease Control revealed no association after 15–25 years of follow-up.

C. Previous Radiation Therapy: Previous radiation therapy is associated with an increased incidence of sarcomas, particularly fibrosarcoma, osteosarcoma, and malignant fibrous histiocytoma. The latent period can be as short as 4 years and as long as 24 years.

D. Radium Exposure: Exposure to radium (eg, watch dials) is associated with an increased incidence of osteosarcoma.

E. Asbestos Exposure: There is a definite association between asbestos exposure and the development of mesothelioma. Asbestos miners and workers in occupations involving the processing, installation, or repair of electrical and thermal insulation, brake linings, cement tiles, and pipes are at increased risk of asbestos exposure. The tumor can develop 10–30 years after exposure.

F. Predisposing Medical Conditions:

1. Prolonged lymphedema, usually following a radical mastectomy, can lead to lymphangiosarcoma (Stewart-Treves syndrome).

2. von Recklinghausen's disease is associated with a 10% lifetime risk of developing neurofibrosarcoma.

3. Paget's disease of bone is associated with a 0.2% incidence of osteosarcoma.

4. Asbestosis, particularly the accumulation of fibers >8 μm and <1.5 μm in diameter, is associated with the development of mesothelioma.

5. Previous or family history of retinoblastoma is associated with 7% incidence of osteosarcoma. Cytogenetic analysis of these osteosarcomas reveals homozygous 13q deletion, which is also present in retinoblastoma.

Pathology

A. Histologic Classification: Current classifications are based on the cell or tissue of origin (eg, Schwannoma, fibrosarcoma, osteosarcoma, rhabdomyosarcoma). The tendency of these tumors to dedifferentiate with the appearance of several histologic elements in the same tumor often makes a definitive diagnosis difficult. There are some sarcomas without an identifiable cell of origin, such as extraskeletal Ewing's sarcoma, alveolar soft part sarcoma, epithelioid sarcoma, and Kaposi's sarcoma.

B. Histologic Grade: Histologic grade often may predict clinical behavior. Histologic grade is usually based on mitotic rate; nuclear morphology; degree of cellularity; cellular anaplasia, or pleomorphism; and the presence of necrosis. In general, low-grade tumors are more indolent and remain localized; high-grade tumors are aggressive and metastasize early.

C. Natural History

1. Soft tissue sarcomas–See Table 27–1.

2. Bone sarcomas–

a. Classic osteosarcoma–This high-grade malignancy is characteristically recognized by formation of tumor osteoid. It has a male predominance and occurs most commonly under the age of 20. Occurrence over age 40 is usually associated with underlying bony abnormalities (Paget's disease, fibrous dysplasia, hereditary exostoses, irradiated bone). The most common sites include the humerus, femur, and tibia. The presence of "skip" metastases (tumor not in continuity with primary tumor) correlates with higher recurrence and lower survival rates. There has been a recent improvement in survival with combined modality therapy.

b. Parosteal osteosarcoma–This tumor arises in the cortex of bone rather than being intramedullary, as seen in classic osteosarcoma. It occurs in older age groups. The most frequent site is the distal posterior femur. It is an indolent tumor with late metastases.

c. Periosteal osteosarcoma–This rare tumor also arises from the cortex. Characteristic "scooped out" lesions with intact cortex are seen on radiographs. The most common site is the proximal humerus and tibia. It can be aggressive with a high metastatic rate.

d. Chondrosarcoma–This tumor arises from cartilage. The most common sites are the pelvis, femur, sternum, and shoulder girdle. It occurs in older age groups. It can arise from benign cartilage tumors by malignant transformation, and it has a broad spectrum of metastatic potential dependent on histologic grade. The histologic variants include

(1) Medullary chondrosarcoma–

(a) Arises within cancellous bone or medullary cavity.

(b) Mean age of 40.

(c) Most common in large tubular bones.

(2) Exostotic Chondrosarcoma–

(a) Arises from surface of bone.

(b) Rare tumor.

(c) Wide age range.

(d) Most common in pelvis.

(3) Dedifferentiated Chondrosarcoma–

(a) 10% of chondrosarcomas.

(b) Peak incidence in sixth decade.

(c) Aggressive lesion.

e. Giant cell sarcoma–This rare tumor arises de novo and is not to be confused with secondary transformation of recurrent benign giant cell tumors. It most commonly occurs around the knee joint.

f. Malignant fibrous histiocytoma of bone– This is a highly aggressive tumor with early metastasis. It commonly occurs at metaphyseal ends of long bones. It may arise in previous bone infarcts, sickle cell disease, or Paget's disease. It can be confused with sarcomatoid renal cell carcinoma.

g. Fibrosarcoma of bone–Long bones are the most common site. This rare tumor can arise from underlying abnormal bone such as in Paget's disease, fibrous dysplasia, bone infarcts, osteomyelitis, postirradiation bone, and giant cell tumors. The metastatic rate correlates with histologic grade.

h. Chordoma–This rare tumor arises from notochordal remnants. The most common sites are base of skull (35%) and sacrococcyx (50%). It is an aggressive tumor with a high rate of local recurrence.

i. Ewing's sarcoma of bone–This is the second most common bone tumor in children. The cell of origin is unknown. The most common sites are femur and pelvis. It is a highly malignant tumor with recent improved survival and disease-free interval due to combined modality therapy.

j. Lymphoma of bone–This rare tumor was

Table 27-1. Soft tissue sarcomas.

Tumor Type	Comments
Liposarcoma	Arises from adipose tissue. Most common soft tissue tumor of adults. Median age 53. Most common site extremities. High-grade lesions metastasize.
Fibrosarcoma	Arises from fibrous tissue. Peak age 30–55 years. Most common site thigh and knee. Can arise in previous radiation field. Most well-differentiated (desmoid) tumors.
Leiomyosarcoma	Tumor of smooth muscle. Median age 60. Most common sites gastrointestinal tract, uterus, and retroperitoneum. Predominantly aggressive tumors.

Rhabdomyosarcoma	Tumor of striated muscle.
	Most common soft tissue tumor in childhood and adolescence.
	Sites: paratesticular (20%);
	      orbit, eye, skull (19%);
	      naso-, oropharnyx (13%);
	      neck, sinuses (8%);
	      trunk (7%);
	      extremities (7%).
	Three histologic variants:
	  (1) Embryonal—genitourinary tract, orbit common sites.
	  (2) Alveolar—more common in adolescence.
	  (3) Pleomorphic—more common in >40 age group.
	Combined modality therapy can be curative.
	Without chemotherapy, 80% relapse at distant sites.
	Orbital and paratesticular tumors have more favorable prognosis.

Embryonal	Median age 8 years. Botryoid-type (mucosa-lined hollow organs), eg, vagina, urinary bladder
Alveolar	Median age 16. Higher incidence in extremities.
Pleomorphic "classical"	Median age 53. Most common site thigh.
Malignant fibrous histiocytoma	Pleomorphic, high-grade malignancy. Most common sarcoma in late adult life. Can arise in previous radiation field. Most common sites extremities, trunk, and retroperitoneum.
Neurofibrosarcoma	Arises from neural sheath. Median age (with von Recklinghausen's) 28, (without von Recklinghausen's) 41. Most develop in regions of major nerve trunks. 10% incidence over lifetime in patients with von Recklinghausen's.
Synovial sarcoma	Tumor of tendosynovial tissue. Peak age 15–35 years. Median age 26. Most common sites lower extremity, popliteal space.
Alveolar soft parts (clear cell sarcoma)	Peak age 15–35 years. Common sites extremities, head and neck. Can be an indolent tumor. Unknown tissue/cell of origin.
Epithelioid sarcoma	Peak age 15–30 years. Most common site extremity. Can resemble necrotizing, granulomatous process or be confused with carcinoma. Unknown tissue/cell of origin.
Extraosseous Ewing's	Peak age 15–30 years. Most common sites paravertebral and intercostal regions. Unknown tissue/cell of origin.

Angiosarcoma	Arises in blood vessels.
	33% arise in skin, 24% arise in soft tissue.
	Stewart-Treves syndrome—lymphangiosarcoma arising in the setting of lymphedema
	    following mastectomy (<1% incidence).
	Hepatic angiosarcoma associated with chemical exposure (thorium dioxide, insecticides,
	    vinyl chloride).

(continued)

Table 27–1. Soft tissue sarcomas. (continued)

Tumor Type	Comments
Hemangiopericytoma	Rare; arises in smooth muscle of blood vessels. Median age 45. Most common sites lower extremities, retroperitoneum. Associated with telangectasia, increased warmth, pulsation, audible bruit in area of tumor.
Glomus tumors	Peak age 20–40 years. Most common site subungual region of finger.
Kaposi's sarcoma Non–AIDS-related	Unknown cell of origin (?blood vessel versus endothelial cell). Peak incidence sixth and seventh decades. Prolonged disease course (8–10 years). 25% die of second malignancy. 0.4% incidence in renal transplant patients; may respond to a decrease in immunosuppressive therapy.
AIDS-related	HIV positive 30% have gastrointestinal lesions.
Mesothelioma	Tumor arises from the mesothelium in pleural, pericardial, or peritoneal surfaces. Confirmed relationship with asbestos exposure.

previously termed reticulum cell sarcoma. Half the patients will have disease other than the primary solitary lesion.

3. Postirradiation sarcomas–These sarcomas are defined as histologically documented sarcomas arising in a previous radiation field after an asymptomatic latent period. The latent period between initial treatment and secondary malignancy varies from as early as 4 years to over 20 years in some series. The median latency period in most studies is 10–13 years. The reported incidence ranges from 0.1% to 1.5%. Patients with Hodgkin's disease surviving over 8 years have an incidence of 1%. Patients receiving radiation for a diagnosis of breast cancer who survive greater than 5 years have a reported incidence of 0.2%. The use of a megavoltage energy source has not resulted in a decrease in the incidence of postirradiation sarcomas. There is some evidence that subcutaneous and cutaneous sarcomas are fewer in the megavoltage group. In addition, the latency period appears to be shorter (3.4 years) in patients treated with megavoltage than in those treated with orthovoltage (11.3 years). The most common histologic types are fibrosarcoma, osteosarcoma, and malignant fibrous histiocytoma, but all histologic types have been reported. The most common tumors preceding the second malignancy are retinoblastoma, female gynecologic malignancies, breast cancer, and Hodgkin's disease. Case reports of a variety of other tumors including prostate, germ cell and Wilms' tumors have been published. The overall prognosis is worse than for similar stages of primary soft tissue and bone sarcomas. In a recent review, the median survival was 12 months with a 2-year survival of 22% and a 5-year survival of 11%.

4. Metastatic Disease–

a. Lymph node metastases–Most sarcomas at diagnosis have not metastasized to lymph nodes. The overall incidence of lymph node metastases in soft tissue sarcomas ranges from 5% to 39% and is dependent on histologic type. The histologic types that more frequently metastasize early to lymph nodes are angiosarcoma, rhabdomyosarcoma, synovial cell sarcoma, hemangiopericytoma, and malignant fibrous histiocytoma.

b. Lung metastases–The lung is the most common site of metastatic disease in both soft tissue sarcomas and bone sarcomas. Surgical resection of pulmonary nodules has become accepted salvage therapy. Studies evaluating the administration of chemotherapy prior to resection have not clearly shown a survival advantage over resection alone. Median survivals range from 18 to 56 months. In general, disease recurrence from initial diagnosis to discovery of pulmonary metastases is longer for soft tissue sarcomas than for osteosarcomas or other bone sarcomas. Most relapses occur within 2 years in patients with osteosarcomas. Five-year actuarial survivals after pulmonary resection of metastatic disease have ranged from 22% to 35% and 10-year survivals from 18% to 21%. With additional pulmonary resections, further improvement in survival has been reported in the range of 37% to 47% at 5 years postresection. Several factors may predict a more favorable outcome following resection: a disease-free interval greater than 12 months, fewer than 5 pulmonary nodules, and a tumor doubling time greater than 20 days.

c. Brain metastases–The occurrence of brain metastases is rare with a reported incidence of 1.6% to 9.6% for all types of sarcoma. Increasing numbers are being reported, possibly owing to more aggressive treatment with chemotherapy. Fibrosarcoma, alveolar soft part sarcoma, and leiomyosarcomas are among the more common histologic types to metastasize to the brain.

d. Bone metastases–These occur not infrequently with both soft tissue and bone sarcomas.

e. Criteria for resection of metastatic disease–See Table 27–2.

Clinical Findings

A. Symptoms and Signs: A slowly growing

mass in an extremity or other body part is typical. The mass may be painless unless nerves or blood vessels are compromised by the mass. The lack of complete resolution of a muscle pull or extremity hematoma within 3–4 weeks should be viewed with suspicion for a malignancy. Patients with osteosarcoma may present with pathologic fractures through a lytic lesion. Any unexplained bone or joint pain, especially in young males, should be evaluated. Many symptoms and signs of sarcoma are dependent on the body part affected. Retroperitoneal sarcomas may present with back pain, obstructive uropathy, or lower extremity edema. Head and neck sarcomas may present with a variety of cranial nerve defects, proptosis, or headache. Gastrointestinal or genitourinary hemorrhage may herald a sarcoma of gastrointestinal or genitourinary origin.

B. Laboratory Findings: These findings may be nonspecific. Anemia may reflect chronic illness or blood loss depending on the site of disease. Alkaline phosphatase values are not reliably elevated in all osteosarcomas; marked elevation is noted in approximately half of cases. Hypoglycemia may be seen with retroperitoneal sarcomas and is thought to be a component of a paraneoplastic syndrome with production of an insulinlike factor. Hypercalcemia has also been described with extremity sarcomas. These paraneoplastic syndromes are rare, occurring in only 1% of all sarcomas.

C. X-ray Findings: Plain films of the affected extremity may reveal lytic or blastic lesions in osteosarcoma. In addition, elevation of the periosteum forming a triangular appearing abnormality with the bony cortex termed "Codman's triangle" is a diagnostic radiologic finding in osteogenic sarcoma. Bone spiculations may be present. Ewing's sarcoma of bone may have a typical "onionskin" appearance with elevation of the periosteum and mottling of underlying bone. Involvement of bone cortex by soft tissue sarcomas is identified by scalloping of the cortex. Scattered calcifications may be present in the soft tissue surrounding a sarcoma on plain film and are the result of new bone formation by the tumor.

D. Pretreatment Evaluation: The evaluation consists of laboratory tests including a complete blood count and chemistry profile and diagnostic imaging studies including a chest radiograph, CT scans, or MRI of the affected area. These studies accomplish more precise definition of the anatomic extent of tumor invasion. At present, MRI is preferred in the evaluation of extremity and spine lesions, and CT

scans are preferred for evaluation of thoracic and abdominal disease. Other studies that may be indicated depending on the patient's symptoms or site of disease include bone scans, lymphangiograms, and arteriograms. An arteriogram is essential in establishing the extent of vascular involvement by tumor prior to a decision regarding limb-sparing surgery.

Essential to establishing a diagnosis of sarcoma is obtaining a tissue diagnosis from biopsy. Incisional biopsy is the most common method of biopsy of a suspected soft tissue sarcoma (large, deep-seated mass). The biopsy should be performed so that the biopsy scar can be totally removed at the time of the definitive procedure along with the primary mass. Biopsies of suspected osteosarcomas can be accomplished with a core biopsy or biopsy with a Tru-cut needle. Either technique should provide adequate tissue for diagnosis. Ideally, the biopsy is done by the same surgeon who will perform the definitive operative procedure. Wound seeding by incompletely excised tumors or by poorly performed biopsies does occur and commonly results in amputation. Needle aspirate biopsies often do not provide adequate information regarding cell type and surrounding stroma for diagnosis and are not recommended when establishing the initial diagnosis. Excisional biopsies of deep-seated masses should not be done. With large tumors, fascial planes are disturbed, interfering with wound healing and complicating plans for subsequent definitive surgery.

Staging

A. Soft Tissue Sarcoma: Soft Tissue sarcoma is determined by histologic grade 1–3 (well-differentiated to poorly differentiated), size, and the presence of regional or distant metastases.

Stage IA	Grade 1 tumor < 5 cm.
IB	Grade 1 tumor > 5 cm.
Stage IIA	Grade 2 tumor < 5 cm.
IIB	Grade 2 tumor > 5 cm.
Stage IIIA	Grade 3 tumor < 5 cm.
IIIB	Grade 3 tumor > 5 cm.
IIIC	Any grade or size tumor with regional lymph node metastases but without distant metastases.
Stage IVA	Any grade or size tumor that grossly invades bone, major vessels, or major nerves with or without regional lymph node metastases but without distant metastases.
IVB	Any tumor with distant metastases.

B. Bone Sarcoma: Bone sarcoma is determined by histologic grade and anatomic confines of the lesion (penetration beyond bone compartment).

Table 27–2. Criteria for resection of metastatic disease.

1. Primary disease controlled.
2. Patient medically fit to undergo surgery.
3. One site of metastatic disease.
4. Disease-free interval >1 year.

Stage IA	Low-grade tumor, intracompartmental.
IB	Low-grade tumor, extracompartmental.
Stage IIA	High-grade tumor, intracompartmental.
IIB	High-grade tumor, extracompartmental.
Stage III	Any grade tumor with regional or distant metastases.

Treatment

A. Surgery: The major goals of surgery for sarcomas are to control the primary lesion, maintain function of the extremity or body part, and provide long-term survival.

1. Surgical procedures and margins–The type of surgery depends on the site of the tumor. Most extremity soft tissue sarcomas can be resected without amputation. Wide local excision with removal of the tumor together with surrounding reactive tissue and a cuff of grossly normal tissue is the procedure of choice. Lesions that are close to joints in distal extremities or that overlie the shoulder or pelvic girdles usually require amputation to obtain adequate margins. Muscle tumors are removed along with the entire muscle group from origin to insertion. In osteosarcomas, the surgical margin is at least 7.5 cm proximal to the known intramedullary extent of tumor.

2. Limb-sparing surgery–This surgery provides local control rates of 90% with disease-free survival of approximately 60% for both osteosarcoma and soft tissue sarcoma. Functional results are excellent in 60–75% of cases; 1–2% eventually require amputation owing to complications or local recurrence. Not all patients are candidates for limb-sparing surgery. Contraindications to such surgery with soft tissue sarcomas include (**a**) inability to achieve adequate surgical margins, (**b**) inability to deliver adequate postoperative radiation therapy owing to concerns regarding complications of radiation therapy to the area, and (**c**) involvement of major vessels and nerves that will compromise an adequate functional result. In addition to the above criteria, in cases of osteosarcoma, the operative procedure should provide limb function equal or superior to the function of a prosthetic device. Metastatic disease is not an absolute contraindication to limb-sparing surgery. Preoperative chemotherapy, either intra-arterial or systemic, or radiation therapy may render a patient eligible for limb-sparing surgery if there is a response to preoperative therapy. All patients undergoing limb-sparing procedures for soft tissue sarcoma should receive postoperative radiation therapy; patients with osteosarcoma should receive adjuvant chemotherapy.

B. Chemotherapy:

1. Adjuvant Chemotherapy for Soft Tissue Sarcoma–Chemotherapy in the adjuvant setting for soft tissue sarcoma remains controversial. More than one dozen randomized controlled trials have examined the benefit of adjuvant chemotherapy in soft tissue sarcomas. Only one study with a relatively short follow-up period of 2 years has shown a significant survival advantage, notably for patients with extremity lesions receiving doxorubicin-based combination chemotherapy. The initial report of an earlier randomized study of soft tissue sarcomas conducted at the NCI revealed a significant survival and disease-free survival in the subset of patients with extremity lesions. However, with longer follow-up, the survival advantage was no longer present. Adjuvant chemotherapy in soft tissue sarcoma currently is recommended only within a randomized, prospective trial. Treatment of rhabdomyosarcomas and Ewing's sarcoma in children and young adults are the exceptions. Combined modality treatment with multiagent chemotherapy and radiation therapy has resulted in improved disease-free survival in these cases.

2. Adjuvant chemotherapy for osteosarcomas–In contrast to the case for soft tissue sarcomas, adjuvant chemotherapy in osteosarcomas significantly improved disease-free and overall survival in several studies (Table 27–3). The most effective combinations and doses are yet to be identified. In general, cisplatin-based multiagent regimens appear to have the highest response rates and to show significant improvement in disease-free and overall survival.

Currently under study is the concept of preoperative (neoadjuvant) chemotherapy. Theoretical advantages to preoperative treatment include (**a**) prompt treatment with early eradication of microscopic metastases, (**b**) increased feasibility of limb-sparing surgery in responders, and (**c**) histologic evaluation of response with the opportunity to modify treatment in nonresponders. Tumor necrosis greater than 90% in surgical specimens has been associated with improved survival and local control in several studies. The major risk of preoperative chemotherapy is the possibility of increased local and distant failure in patients who are poor responders. Final recommendations regarding neoadjuvant chemotherapy await completion of randomized trials comparing preoperative and postoperative chemotherapy.

3. Chemotherapy for metastatic disease–Chemotherapy for metastatic disease is palliative. In patients with osteosarcoma, if multiagent adjuvant chemotherapy is given more than 6 months from the time of diagnosis of metastatic disease, repeating the adjuvant regimen may provide palliation. Most single agents offer response rates of 15–40% in metastatic sarcoma. Single agents used in the treatment of metastatic osteosarcoma include doxorubicin, high-dose methotrexate with leucovorin rescue, cisplatin, dacarbazine, and ifosfamide. Doxorubicin, dacarbazine, and ifosfamide are the most common single

Table 27–3. Randomized multiagent adjuvant studies for treatment of osteosarcoma.

Author	Regimen[1]	No. of Patients	Disease-Free Survival %	Surgery %	p Value
Link et al (1986)	Surgery versus HDMTX, BCD, ADR CDDP	18 18	17 66	. . . . . .	<0.001 (DFS)
Eilber et al (1987)	Surgery versus ADR, HDMTX, BCD	27 32	20 55	48 80	<0.01 (DFS, S)

[1]HDMTX, high-dose methotrexate; ADR, doxorubicin (Adriamycin); CDDP, cisplatin; BCD, bleomycin, cyclophosphamide, dactinomycin; DFS, disease free survival; S, overall survival.

agents used in treatment of metastatic soft tissue sarcoma. Although initial studies of combinations reported higher overall response rates (36–55%), randomized studies completed to date have not shown significant advantages of the combinations over single-agent doxorubicin in either response or overall survival. At this time, treatment with single-agent doxorubicin remains the standard to which new agents or combinations should be compared. Current areas of exploration in clinical research in metastatic sarcoma include evaluation of doxorubicin and methotrexate analogs in phase II new agent trials and dose-escalation studies with growth factor support of agents known to be effective in sarcoma.

C. Radiation Therapy: Radiation therapy has a prime role in the adjuvant treatment of soft tissue sarcomas following limb-sparing procedures. In addition, some studies have shown that its use preoperatively has resulted in the subsequent ability to perform limb-sparing surgery rather than amputation.

Randomized studies comparing the benefits of preoperative radiation therapy to postoperative treatment are being completed. Most centers recommend a dose of 6000 cGy for local control and eradication of microscopic disease. The local failure rates reported in most studies are 16–18%. Wound complications of infection and delayed healing occur in a minority of patients.

In addition to its role in combined modality approaches to soft tissue sarcomas, radiation therapy offers excellent palliation in the control of painful bony and soft tissue lesions. The treatment of bulky retroperitoneal lesions is often limited by tissue toxicity to the surrounding viscera.

The control of occult metastatic disease continues to be the main determinant in overall survival and focus of continued investigation in patients with sarcomas with adequate local control from previous surgery and radiation therapy.

REFERENCES

Antman KH, Elias AD: Chemotherapy of advanced soft-tissue sarcomas. *Semin Surg Oncol* 1988;**4**:53.

Benedict WF, Fung YT, Murphee AL: The gene responsible for the development of retinoblastoma and osteosarcoma. *Cancer* 1988;**62**:1691.

Eilber FR et al: Adjuvant chemotherapy for osteosarcoma: A randomized prospective trial. *J Clin Oncol* 1987;**5**:21.

Enzinger FM, Weiss SW: *Soft Tissue Tumors*, 2nd ed. Mosby, 1983.

Fingerhut MA et al: Cancer mortality in workers exposed to 2,3,7,8-tetrachlorodibenzo-p-dioxin. *N Engl J Med* 1991;**324**:212.

Lewis AJ: Sarcoma metastatic to the brain. *Cancer* 1988;**61**:593.

Link MP et al: The effect of adjuvant chemotherapy on relapse-free survival in patients with osteosarcoma of the extremity. *N Engl J Med* 1986;**314**:1600.

Lynge E, Storm HH, Jensen OM: The evaluation of trends in soft tissue sarcoma according to diagnostic criteria and consumption of phenoxy herbicides. *Cancer* 1987;**60**:1896.

Mazanet R, Antman KH: Adjuvant therapy for sarcomas. *Semin Oncol* 1991;**18**:603.

NIH Consensus Conference: Limb-sparing treatment of adult soft-tissue sarcomas and osteosarcomas. *JAMA* 1985;**254**:1791.

Pao WJ, Pilepich MV: Postoperative radiotherapy in the treatment of extremity soft tissue sarcomas. *Int J Radiat Oncol Biol Phys* 1990;**19**:907.

Roth JA et al: Differing determinants of prognosis following resection of pulmonary metastases from osteogenic and soft tissue sarcoma patients. *Cancer* 1985;**55**:1361.

Schwartz MB, Burgess PA, Fee WE: Postirradiation sarcoma in retinoblastoma: Induction or predisposition? *Arch Otolaryngol Head Neck Surg* 1988;**114**:640.

Scully JM et al: Radiation-induced prostatic sarcoma: A case report. *J Urol* 1990;**144**:746.

Selected Cancers Cooperative Study Group: The association of selected cancers with service in the US military in Vietnam. 2. Soft-tissue and other sarcomas. *Arch Intern Med* 1990;**150**:2485.

Suit HD et al: Preoperative, intraoperative, and postoperative radiation in the treatment of primary soft tissue sarcoma. *Cancer* 1985;**55**:2659.

Taghian A et al: Long-term risk of sarcoma following radiation treatment for breast cancer. *Int J Radiat Oncol Biol Phys* 1991;**21**:361.

Wiklund TA et al: Postirradiation sarcoma. Analysis of a nationwide cancer registry material. *Cancer* 1991; **68**:524.

Wingren G et al: Soft tissue sarcoma and occupational exposures. *Cancer* 1990;**66**:806.

Winkler K, et al: Neoadjuvant chemotherapy of osteosarcoma: Results of a randomized cooperative trial (COSS-82) with salvage chemotherapy based on histologic tumor response. *J Clin Oncol* 1988;**6**:329.

28

Leukemia

Timothy J. O'Rourke, MD, & Steven P. Kalter, MD

ACUTE LEUKEMIA

Essentials of Diagnosis

- Failure of normal hematopoiesis.
- Bone marrow replacement by clonal proliferation of immature hematopoietic stem cells.
- Organ infiltration and failure.

Acute leukemia (AL) is a neoplastic condition of hematopoietic stem cells that results in bone marrow failure and organ infiltration by malignant leukemic cells. The leukemic cells are termed **blasts** and are classified as having either lymphoid or myeloid differentiation. Thus, there are two types of leukemia corresponding to the presumed ontogeny of the leukemic blasts: **acute lymphocytic leukemia** (ALL) and **acute myelogenous leukemia** (AML). In some cases, the blasts may be undifferentiated or may have both lymphoid and myeloid features. Although the two types cause similar clinical problems, their demographics and treatment are different.

The mechanism of marrow failure may be the physical exclusion of normal cells or the production of factors that suppress normal hematopoiesis. In addition to their detrimental effect on hematopoiesis, blasts can infiltrate other organs, eg, the central nervous system, skin, liver, spleen, or gastrointestinal tract, leading to local symptoms or organ failure.

Acute leukemia occurs in approximately 11,000 individuals in the USA each year. This translates to an annual incidence of 3–4 per 100,000 persons. In all age groups, the disease is more common in men than in women. Acute lymphocytic leukemia has a peak incidence in the 3- to 5-year age group and accounts for 80% of acute leukemia in children. There is a smaller, gradual rise in the incidence of ALL in adults over the age of 55. Acute myelogenous leukemia is primarily a disease of adults with an increase in incidence with advancing age.

Etiology

Most cases are idiopathic. Nevertheless, certain factors may increase risk or have a role in pathogenesis.

A. Genetic Factors:

1. Family history–There is an increased risk of developing leukemia for siblings of children with leukemia. In monozygotic twins, this risk is very high; there is an approximately 20–25% chance that if one twin develops leukemia, the other will also. This pattern is usually seen in children with ALL. There have also been reports of families with multiple cases of leukemia. Because leukemia is a rare disease, these clusters quite probably are not due to random chance. Whether genetic or environmental factors (or both) are dominant is not clear.

2. Hereditary syndromes–

a. Down's syndrome (trisomy 21) is associated with an increased risk of both AML and ALL. In addition, an increased incidence of Down's syndrome occurs in siblings of patients with leukemia.

b. Fanconi's anemia is a hereditary aplastic anemia that is often associated with skeletal deformities, mental and sexual retardation, hypoplasia of the kidneys, and patchy pigmentation of the skin. This condition often terminates in AML.

c. Bloom's syndrome is a recessive disorder found in Ashkenazic Jews, consisting of growth retardation, photosensitivity, and facial erythema. Affected individuals are more likely to develop cancer, particularly leukemias or lymphomas. This risk includes both AML and ALL. Individuals with this condition have extreme chromosomal fragility, which is thought to be the factor responsible for neoplastic transformation.

d. Other conditions associated with leukemia include chromosomal disorders such as Klinefelter's syndrome and trisomy D, immunodeficiency states such as ataxia-telangiectasia and Wiskott-Aldrich syndrome, and other inherited disorders of the bone marrow such as congenital agranulocytosis.

B. Radiation:

1. Nuclear weapons exposure–Exposure to nuclear weapons is a well-established leukemogen. There has been an excess risk in survivors of the atomic bomb explosions at Hiroshima and Nagasaki. All types of leukemia other than chronic lymphocytic leukemia have been associated with irradiation.

There does not appear to be a threshold dose; cases have been observed in individuals with 25–50 cGy exposure.

2. Medical radiation–Medical radiation has also been associated with an increased incidence of leukemia. This is seen in older studies of radiologists and patients treated with radiation for ankylosing spondylitis.

C. Chemicals:

1. Benzene–Benzene exposure has been associated with aplastic anemia and the development of AML. The risk is dose dependent with higher concentrations in the environment resulting in a greater risk of development of both conditions.

2. Alkylating agents–Alkylating agents used in the treatment of both solid and liquid tumors have been associated with an increased risk of development of AML. AML in these cases is often preceded by a myelodysplastic syndrome.

3. Other drugs–Chloramphenicol has been implicated as a cause of marrow damage and as a risk of the development of AML. Other drugs associated with marrow damage are also capable of causing leukemia, eg, phenylbutazone and arsenicals.

D. Viruses: Viruses are well established as a cause of leukemia in animal species but, with the exception of HTLV-I infection, have not yet been proved to be an etiologic agent in humans. HTLV-I (human T cell lymphotropic virus type I) has been shown to cause an acute or chronic lymphoproliferative disease having features of both leukemia and lymphoma. It is the most common hematopoietic neoplasm in endemic areas of Japan and the Caribbean but is rare in the USA. The leukemia it causes is distinct clinically from typical AML and ALL. It is also suspected that other C-type RNA viruses cause leukemia in humans.

E. Hematologic Diseases:

1. Natural history–Certain conditions such as myeloproliferative disorders, aplastic anemia, and paroxysmal nocturnal hemoglobinuria may have acute leukemia as part of their natural history. Chronic myelogenous leukemia (see below) typically eventuates in a blast crisis if the patient survives long enough. This blast crisis is clinically similar to acute leukemia. It can be either myeloid or lymphoid in differentiation and does not respond well to conventional antileukemic therapy.

2. Alkylating agent therapy–As mentioned above, alkylating agent therapy of both solid and liquid tumors is associated with the development of acute leukemia. This has been described in Hodgkin's disease, multiple myeloma, polycythemia vera, ovarian carcinoma, breast cancer, and colon cancer. It appears from Hodgkin's disease studies that combination treatment with radiation bears a higher risk than chemotherapy used alone.

3. Germ cell tumors–Some patients with germ cell tumors have developed acute leukemia. These cases have not been thought to be treatment related, since they occurred very close to the time of treatment, but they might be due to a transforming event within the germ cell tumor itself.

F. Myelodysplastic syndromes: Myelodysplastic syndromes may precede the development of AML, either when it develops de novo or as a consequence of alkylating agent therapy. ALL is almost never preceded by a myelodysplastic phase.

1. Diagnostic features–Myelodysplastic syndromes are characterized by the presence of pancytopenia and abnormal bone marrow (always). Drug toxicity should be ruled out, especially due to chemotherapy. Nutritional anemias such as vitamin B_{12} or folate deficiency should be excluded also. Patients with myelodysplastic syndromes do not necessarily develop overt acute leukemia prior to death from other causes. They may become transfusion dependent. Leukopenia and thrombocytopenia cause morbidity such as infection or bleeding. Various cytogenetic abnormalities have been associated with the myelodysplastic syndromes, including 5q–, –5, –7, +8, 11q–, and 12p–, and these are different from those seen in de novo AML.

2. Classification–The FAB (French, American, British) classification is most often used (Table 28–1). Examination of both bone marrow and peripheral blood is required for classification.

3. Treatment–

a. Supportive care–Supportive care is provided by treatment of infections and administration of transfusions for anemia and thrombocytopenia as needed.

b. Specific therapy–The following agents have marginal utility: pyridoxine, corticosteroids, androgens, retinoic acid, low-dose cytarabine, conventional antileukemia treatment, bone marrow transplantation, and colony-stimulating factors. Results have been disappointing except that some patients have experienced long-term remissions after undergoing allogeneic bone marrow transplantation.

Pathogenesis

Acute leukemia results from the malignant transformation of a hematopoietic stem cell. This results in a clone of cells that have a selective advantage over normal cells and eventually supplant them in the bone marrow. This clone is characterized by disordered growth and maturation. These cells do not respond normally to the usual controls on stem cell proliferation. Differentiation is limited, and those cells that do mature may be morphologically and functionally abnormal. Maturation may thus appear "frozen" at an early stage of development, with normal hematopoiesis replaced by a mechanism making a product that is both quantitatively and qualitatively deficient.

A. Acute Lymphocytic Leukemia:

1. Lymphocyte ontogeny–Mature lymphocytes are classified as T or B cells. B cells are respon-

Table 28–1. FAB classification of myelodysplastic syndromes.

	Peripheral Blood	Bone Marrow	Comment
Refractory anemia (RA)	<1%	<5%	Usually present in anemia but patients rarely may only have neutropenia, thrombocytopenia, or both.
Refractory anemia with ringed sideroblasts (acquired idiopathic sideroblastic anemia)	<1%	<5%	>15% of nucleated cells in the bone marrow are ringed sideroblasts.
Refractory anemia with excess of blasts (RAEB)	<5%	5–20%	
Chronic myelomonocytic leukemia (CMmL)	<5%	<20%	Absolute leukemic monocytosis (>1 × 10^9 cells/L), otherwise like refractory anemia with excess of blasts (RAEB), sometimes with promonocytes.
RAEB "in transformation" (RAEB-T)	>5%	20–30%	Presence of Auer rods is sufficient to make diagnosis in cases with lower percentages of blasts in the bone marrow.

sible for humoral immunity. T cells have a variety of functions associated with cellular immunity and regulation of the immune response. These two groups have a common progenitor that is derived from a pluripotent stem cell.

2. Leukemia ontogeny–ALL occurs when cells are blocked in some phase of this developmental process. Surface markers and other techniques result in the typing of ALL blasts into three classes:

a. T cell ALL–15–20% of cases.

b. B cell ALL–<5% of cases. Surface membrane immunoglobulin identifies these cells as relatively mature B cells.

c. Common ALL antigen (CALLA)–positive ALL–70% of cases. These cells have CALLA on their surface and represent an earlier stage of B cell development (pre–B cell).

d. Null ALL–Cell does not type clearly as T, B, or pre-B.

B. Acute Myelogenous Leukemia:

1. Myeloid ontogeny–Like lymphocytes myeloid cells are derived from a pluripotent stem cell that gives rise to a multipotent stem cell which is correlated with an in vitro culture equivalent (CFU-GEMM). This multipotent stem cell gives rise to committed stem cells for each of the myeloid lines. These include CFU-GM (colony-forming unit, granulocyte and monocyte), BFU-E (burst-forming unit, erythroid), CFU-E (colony-forming unit, erythroid), and CFU-Mega (colony-forming unit, megakaryocyte).

2. Leukemia ontogeny–In AML there is a block in differentiation somewhere in the scheme of myeloid cell development. The location of the derangement and its nature determines the characteristics of the leukemia.

C. Clonal origin of leukemia: A population of leukemic cells is derived from a single precursor cell. For this reason, the blasts have the property of "clonality." This means that although a population of normal cells is heterogeneous for a given characteristic, the leukemic cell population will tend to be uniform for that characteristic.

1. Glucose-6-phosphate dehydrogenase (G6PD) isozymes– If a female with leukemia is heterozygous for this X-linked enzyme, it can be shown that her blasts will express a single isozyme, implying derivation from a single clone.

2. Gene rearrangement–In some lymphocytic leukemias the blasts demonstrate a single pattern of gene rearrangement for the immunoglobulin gene or the T cell receptor gene. Since this reflects a somatic mutation, it also implies a clonal origin. In addition, it gives an indication of the cell type of origin.

Pathology

Acute leukemia is broadly characterized as lymphoid or myeloid. This remains the most important distinction for treatment purposes. Some cases have features of both lineages or are undifferentiated. The most commonly used classification system for acute leukemia is the FAB (Tables 28–2 and 28–3). Classification of leukemias in this system is made on the basis of Wright's-stained smears of peripheral blood and bone marrow along with cytochemical stains. With newer techniques, eg, surface markers and cytogenetics, classification has become more ambiguous because of cases that are found to have markers of both lymphoid and myeloid lineages. Recognized entities undefined by the FAB include acute undifferentiated leukemia, eosinophilic leukemia, and basophilic leukemia.

Pathologic Physiology

Three techniques for examining the biology of leukemia are discussed. Additional tests likely will become available in the near future.

A. Cytogenetics: With improvement in cytogenetic techniques, particularly banding, chromosomal abnormalities have been more frequently identified in patients with AML and have been associated with particular clinical syndromes.

1. inv 16 (p13;q22)–Acute myelomonocytic leukemia with abnormal eosinophils (M4). Patients with this syndrome enter remission 80% of the time and have a prolonged median duration of remission.

Table 28–2. FAB classification of AML.

Subtype	Description	Comment
M1	AML without maturation	Blasts must account for 90% of nonerythroid cells. At least 3% of blast cells will be Sudan-black-positive.
M2	AML with maturation	Blasts must account for 30–89% of nonerythroid cells. Monocytes should be less than 20% of cells.
M3	Acute promyelocytic leukemia (APL)	At least 30% of cells are promyelocytes. Some may have fine dustlike granules ("microgranular" APL).
M4	Acute myelomonocytic leukemia (AMmL)	Blasts must be 30% of nonerythroid cells. At least 20% of the remainder should be monocytic. Usually there is also peripheral monocytosis (>5000/µL)
M5	Acute monocytic leukemia	At least 80% of nonerythroid cells are of monocytic origin. For M5a, 80% of monocytic cells are blasts; for M5b, less than 80% are blasts.
M6	Erythroleukemia	At least 30% of nonerythroid cells should be myeloblasts. Greater than 50% of all nucleoloid cells will be erythroblasts, and there are prominent megaloblastic and dyspoietic changes.
M7	Acute megakaryoblastic leukemia	At least 30% of cells are blasts identified as megakaryocytic by electron microscopy or monoclonal antibody marking with factor VIII antigen or platelet glycoprotein IIb/IIIa.

2. t (8;21)–Acute myelogenous leukemia (M2). Patients have a good response to therapy with a high remission rate.

3. t (5;17) (q22;q21.1)–Acute promyelocytic leukemia (M3). Patients frequently develop disseminated intravascular coagulation (see below) and have abnormal promyelocytes. Some cases are a so-called microgranular variant for which electron microscopy is necessary to identify the granules. Interestingly, this translocation involves the retinoic acid receptor gene on chromosome 17, and it has recently been found that acute promyelocytic leukemia responds to treatment with all-*trans*-retinoic acid.

4. t (9;11)–Acute monocytic leukemia (M5). Skin and gums are often infiltrated with leukemic cells.

5. t (4;11)–Biphenotypic leukemia with features of both lymphoid and myeloid lineages. Patients tend to have a high white cell count, splenomegaly, and a poor outcome.

6. Rearrangement of 3q21 or q26–Thrombocytosis occurs along with abnormal megakaryocytes and a leukemia that often resembles M4. Prognosis is poor.

Table 28–3. FAB classification of all.

Subtype	Comment
L1	Homogeneous population of small cells with scanty cytoplasm and uniform nuclei with inconspicuous nucleoli. Corresponds to common childhood ALL often (CALLA+).
L2	Blasts are larger and polymorphic with heterogeneous nuclear chromatins, irregular nuclear shape, and one or more nucleoli. Cytoplasm is variable in quantity and basophilia. This type is more common in adults and has a poorer prognosis.
L3	Blasts are larger and homogeneous. Nuclei are regular with prominent nucleoli. Cytoplasm is moderately abundant, deeply basophilic, and often has prominent vacuolation. This corresponds to Burkitt's lymphoma.

7. t (6;9)–Acute myelogenous leukemia with increased basophils. This rare abnormality affects less than 1% of patients.

8. t (9;21)–The Philadelphia chromosome seen in CML but also found in some cases of ALL. In ALL, it confers a poor prognosis in both adults and children.

B. Cell Surface Markers: Monoclonal antibodies and antisera have been developed that permit the identification of antigenic determinants on the surface of leukemic cells. These are useful in classifying leukemias as lymphoid or myeloid and also in making some subclassifications. These markers are not all absolutely specific for the cell line identified. As an example, some T cell leukemias mark with CALLA, a pre–B cell marker. Markers may also be useful in assessing prognosis. An an example, the identification of certain myeloid markers in patients with ALL indicates a worse prognosis.

C. Cytochemistry: These are tests for enzymes or macromolecules unique to certain cell lines that help identify the origin of the blast cell.

1. Terminal deoxynucleotidyltransferase (TdT)–This enzyme is characteristic of primitive lymphocytes. It is seen in ALL and some CML blast crises. It has been rarely described in patients with AML and when seen indicates a worse prognosis.

2. Acid phosphatase–This lysosomal enzyme is usually seen in high concentrations within T cells.

3. Adenosine deaminase (ADA)–This is a T cell enzyme.

4. Myeloperoxidase–This granulocyte marker is contained in primary granules.

5. Nonspecific esterase–This monocyte marker is inhibited by addition of sodium fluoride in monocytes but not in lymphocytes or polymorphonuclear leukocytes.

6. Periodic acid–Schiff (PAS)–This stain marks intracellular carbohydrates and is present in ALL blasts as well as erythroid precursors.

7. Sudan-black–This stains lipid and has the

same significance as a peroxidase but is often preferred in the laboratory because the reagents are safer to handle.

8. Specific esterase–This granulocyte marker is also called chloracetate esterase.

Clinical Findings

A. Symptoms and Signs: On presentation the dominant symptoms are often constitutional. Patients may have fever, pallor, malaise, and weight loss. There may also be bacterial infections or hemorrhagic complications of thrombocytopenia.

Organ infiltration can be present. There can be enlargement of lymph nodes, liver, and spleen owing to infiltration with leukemic cells. Soft tissues can also be affected, especially the gingiva or skin. In AML, tumors in any soft tissue can result in localized proliferation of myeloblasts. These are often green in color from myeloperoxidase and are called a chloroma. Interestingly, chloromas may precede the diagnosis of AML by months.

B. Laboratory Findings: Patients are generally anemic and thrombocytopenic. White cell counts may be low, normal, or high. Peripheral blood smears are almost always abnormal with evidence of abnormal red cell forms as well as circulating blasts. When circulating blasts are not present, a so-called aleukemic leukemia is present. Platelets will usually be decreased. There is sometimes evidence of disseminated intravascular coagulation (see below) with prolonged clotting studies and depressed fibrinogen, especially with the M3 variant of AML.

C. Special Studies: Serum and urine lysozyme are elevated in patients with acute monocytic leukemia.

Bone marrow aspirate and biopsy are essential. The bone marrow is hypercellular. At least 30% of the nucleated cells should be blasts in order to make a diagnosis of acute leukemia. For myeloid leukemia, blasts are type 1 or type 2; type 1 have no granules, and type 2 have a few granules.

Cytogenetic, cytochemical, and surface marker studies should be done.

Differential Diagnosis

Myelodysplastic syndromes may have many clinical features of acute leukemia but should be distinguished on the basis of bone marrow examination. Vitamin B_{12} and folate deficiency can cause severe abnormalities of both the bone marrow and peripheral blood counts but should be excluded on the basis of blood levels as well as on clinical grounds. Other agents that cause diminished blood counts, such as drug therapy or aplastic anemia, should be ruled out as well as other malignancies and infections that can involve the bone marrow and cause alterations in the peripheral blood.

Treatment

Treatment consists of supportive measures to control the effects of the leukemia and its therapy as well as chemotherapy to eliminate the leukemic cell population.

A. Supportive Treatment:

1. General–

a. Reverse isolation should be maintained with particular attention to hand washing on the part of all those in contact with the patient in order to limit exposure to nosocomial pathogens.

b. Nutritional support including hyperalimentation should be considered, since patients often limit oral intake because of nausea, mucositis, and other toxicity.

c. Psychological support is essential so that the patient will be able to cooperate with all required treatment measures.

d. Intravenous access should be ensured with an implantable system.

2. Anemia–Anemia is corrected by transfusion of packed red blood cells. Because patients are severely immunosuppressed, blood products should be irradiated to avoid graft-versus-host disease.

3. Thrombocytopenia–Spontaneous bleeding occurs in individuals with platelet counts <10,000–20,000/μL. Prophylactic platelet transfusions are given when the patient's platelet count is <20,000/μL. When an active hemorrhage is present, the platelet count should be maintained at the 50,000–100,000/μL level. The response to each platelet transfusion should be monitored by obtaining a platelet count 1 hour after the transfusion. Poor responses may be seen when platelet survival is decreased, such as with platelet alloimmunization, fever, sepsis, and disseminated intravascular coagulation.

Eventually, half the patients develop platelet alloimmunization and become resistant to platelet transfusions owing to development of antibodies to HLA antigens on the surface of the platelets. Alloimmunization can sometimes be overcome by single donor donations from family members of HLA-matched community donors. Platelets with HLA phenotypes similar to the recipient's are more likely to have normal survival.

It might also be possible to delay alloimmunization by using only leukocyte-poor blood products. However, this policy has not proved to be practical, probably because it is difficult to achieve complete elimination of leukocytes from the product.

4. Infection–The predominant cause of death during chemotherapy of leukemia is infection. The infections are most commonly due to bacteria that are part of the normal flora present on body surfaces or in the gastrointestinal tract. Patients may also be infected by fungi, eg, *Candida* and *Aspergillus;* viruses, eg, cytomegalovirus, herpes simplex, and herpes zoster; and protozoa, eg, *Toxoplasma,*

Pneumocystis, and *Strongyloides.* Some centers treat patients prophylactically with antibiotics such as trimethoprim-sulfamethoxazole or antifungals such as ketoconazole. However, this practice may promote the development of resistant organisms and is of marginal effectiveness.

When leukemic patients are neutropenic and have fever, they should be treated with a broad-spectrum antibiotic combination. At a minimum this should include an aminoglycoside and a broad-spectrum penicillin such as amikacin or piperacillin. Vancomycin may also be included especially if a patient becomes febrile while taking broad-spectrum antibiotics. If fever persists, there should be careful scrutiny for unusual pathogens or a nidus of infection resistant to antibiotics (eg, abscess, colonized foreign body). Consideration should be given to the addition of empiric amphotericin B. Surveillance cultures of fungus are not necessarily positive in patients with documented systemic fungal infection.

Sites that are commonly infected include the lung, indwelling catheters, rectum, oropharynx, sinuses, and skin. These areas should be monitored closely, but because of the patient's neutropenia, the usual signs and symptoms of infection may be absent, since clinical evidence of infection depends on the inflammatory response generated by neutrophils.

Granulocyte transfusions are of limited efficacy, and their only proved benefit is in patients with documented gram-negative infection unresponsive to appropriate antibiotics.

Growth factors such as filgrastim (G-CSF) and sargramostim (GM-CSF) have been used to prevent neutropenia in patients with solid tumors, but their use in leukemias remains investigational because of concerns about their effect on leukemic blasts.

B. Chemotherapy: Most patients with acute leukemia undergo an immediate attempt at treatment, since the prognosis of untreated disease is so poor. Two exceptions are patients whose medical condition precludes treatment, usually the elderly, and patients whose leukemia behaves in an indolent fashion. This latter group includes patients with hypocellular acute leukemia and those with a myelodysplastic syndrome. The goal of therapy is eradication of the leukemic clone replacing the bone marrow, allowing repopulation by normal stem cells. For this to happen, the patient must go through a period of marrow aplasia. Chemotherapy has two phases: remission induction therapy and postremission therapy.

1. AML–
a. Remission induction–Single agents having activity in AML include, in order of importance, daunorubicin, cytarabine (Ara-C), doxorubicin, amsacrine, mitoxantrone, etoposide (VP-16), thioguanine, mercaptopurine, and azacytidine. Cytarabine and daunorubicin are the mainstays of treatment and are usually combined. Most regimens include a combination of cytarabine, 7–10 days, and daunorubicin,

1–3 days, eg, daunorubicin, 45 mg/m^2 intravenously on days 1–3, cytarabine, 100 mg/m^2 continuous intravenous infusion over 24 hours on days 1–7, and thioguanine, 100 mg/m^2 orally twice daily on days 1–7.

b. Postremission therapy–Consolidation is the administration of the same drugs, less frequently or in lower doses. One or two cycles of consolidation following attainment of remission are recommended.

Maintenance is long-term, lower dose chemotherapy and in AML is of unproved benefit although it may delay relapse. Maintenance has not so far been shown to improve survival.

Intensification is treatment with different drugs in high doses either shortly after remission (early intensification) or after the patient has been in remission a year or more (late intensification). The hypothesis is that high-dose treatment is necessary to eliminate clinically inapparent leukemia cells during remission in order to cure. Bone marrow transplantation of patients in remission is a kind of intensification.

Central nervous system (CNS) prophylaxis is usually not given to patients with AML, since meningeal leukemia is less frequent than in ALL and most patients who develop CNS leukemia also experience a relapse in the bone marrow. Hence, there can be little impact on survival. An exception may be monocytic leukemia, which has a higher incidence of CNS involvement.

Overall 60–80% of patients enter remission, but long-term survival remains poor with only 20–40% of patients remaining in remission 2 years.

2. ALL–
a. Remission induction–Vincristine and prednisone are the core of treatment. Additional drugs including doxorubicin and asparginase are added to current protocols for treatment of standard and high-risk groups. Children attain a complete remission in 85–95% of cases.

b. Postremission therapy–Maintenance and CNS prophylaxis are of unequivocal benefit in patients with ALL who attain a complete remission. Maintenance therapy typically consists of combination mercaptopurine daily and methotrexate weekly. Other drugs are now added, sometimes as formal consolidation or intensification. Maintenance is usually continued for 2–3 years.

CNS prophylaxis is usually whole-brain irradiation and intrathecal methotrexate. Craniospinal radiation therapy is also effective but morbid especially in children. High-dose methotrexate is used routinely as prophylaxis. Prophylaxis is usually begun during induction and continued in maintenance.

The design of ALL regimens is complex. For disease in adults and in children carrying a poor prognosis, it is even more so because of the addition of drugs and consolidation/intensification. A typical adult regimen is depicted in Figure 28–1. In children, 85–95% enter remission and 50% survive 5 years. In adults, both these percentages are much lower.

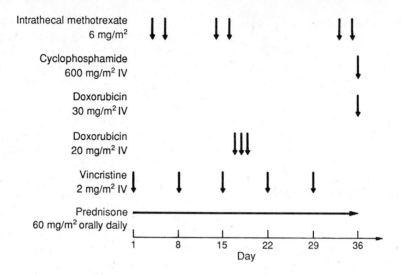

Figure 28–1. ALL treatment: L-10m induction.

3. Bone marrow transplantation–Bone marrow transplantation allows administration of high-dose chemoradiotherapy to patients with leukemia that is resistant to conventional therapy. Lethal bone marrow toxicity is circumvented by the provision of bone marrow from a donor, usually an HLA-identical sibling, which is a source of stem cells that can repopulate the recipient's bone marrow.

Toxicity is great with transplantation, primarily because of the risk of graft-versus-host disease (GVHD), which is a manifestation of immunologically competent donor T cells reacting to the recipient. This process is associated with severe immunosuppression because of both GVHD and the drugs that must routinely be given to prevent or treat it. It is a risk with all allogeneic transplants and is the major limitation of this technique. Patients undergoing transplantation experience myelosuppression comparable to that of leukemia induction treatment. In addition, the nonhematologic toxicity of preparative regimens exceeds that of those used in leukemia induction.

Autologous transplantation avoids GVHD but carries the risk of contamination of the marrow with leukemic cells. For this reason, autologous transplants in leukemia are usually done after remission has been attained (no gross tumor in the marrow) and then the marrow is "purged" by an immunologic or chemical technique.

Transplantation is considered in patients who have disease that is at high risk of relapse or is resistant to standard therapy. In AML, candidates are young patients in first remission or later. In ALL, children in second remission or later are candidates.

4. Salvage therapy–If a patient relapses, similar treatment to induction can be given with a good chance of second remission if there has been a 6- to

12-month interval from the first induction/consolidation. In patients with resistant leukemia or early relapse, alternative induction regimens or transplantation should be considered.

Treatment Complications & Sequelae
A. Hemorrhage: Because of thrombocytopenia, other derangements of coagulation, and damage to skin and mucosal barriers, hemorrhage is common. The most serious complications are massive gastrointestinal or intracranial hemorrhages. These are best avoided by prophylactic use of platelets.

B. Infection: Infection is the major cause of death during induction chemotherapy.

C. Metabolic Complications:
1. Acute tumor lysis syndrome–Effective chemotherapy is available that will cause the death of large numbers of leukemic cells in a short period of time. This can lead to the so-called acute tumor lysis syndrome, which is characterized by oliguric acute renal failure. Prior to initiation of chemotherapy, the patient should receive allopurinol, and during treatment intravenous hydration should be vigorous. Fluid input and output, weight, and laboratory measurements including uric acid, potassium, LDH, creatinine, and BUN should be monitored. Despite these measures, patients can still develop renal failure and require hemodialysis to sustain them through the period of acute renal failure.

2. Disseminated intravascular coagulation (DIC)–This is characteristic of the M3 subtype of acute myeloid leukemia and also of acute promyelocytic leukemia and will occur in 50% or more of cases. It may be present either at the time of presentation or become apparent during induction therapy. Some advocate the prophylactic use of heparin to prevent the appearance of DIC or to limit its consequences.

3. Leucostasis–With extremely high blast counts (>100,000/μL) patients can develop sludging of blood flow in capillaries with resulting neurologic changes. This is a medical emergency and requires rapid treatment to lower the blast count.

a. Hydroxyurea–Give 3 g/m^2 daily for 2 days.

b. Cranial radiation–A single dose of 600 cGy will destroy blasts trapped in cerebral capillaries.

c. Leukapheresis–This technique may lower the blast count more rapidly than cytotoxic chemotherapy.

D. Chemotherapy: Treatment aggravates many short-term problems associated with marked lowering of blood counts. To attain complete remission, the marrow generally goes through a period of aplasia. Other rapidly dividing tissues are affected, and mucositis, diarrhea, and other gastrointestinal toxicities can result. Alopecia is universal. Other unique side effects of the drugs used to treat leukemia must be kept in mind, such as the cardiotoxicity of anthracyclines and the bladder toxicity of cyclophosphamide.

E. Central Nervous System Leukemia: Central nervous system leukemia refers to the infiltration of the leptomeninges by leukemic blasts. Symptoms include those related to meningeal inflammation, cerebral dysfunction, cranial nerve findings, and radicular symptoms. In this sanctuary, blasts are not affected by the usual doses of systemic chemotherapy. Central nervous system leukemia occurs more often in ALL but can occur in AML either at diagnosis or relapse. When at relapse, it may be isolated or associated with bone marrow relapse.

Course & Prognosis

The most important factor in determining survival in leukemias is the attainment of a complete remission. Patients who do not attain a complete remission do not have long-term survival.

In AML, the following factors are adverse prognostically:

A. Age: Older patients do less well than younger patients primarily because of poor tolerance of treatment. Extremely young (ie, <1 year of age) patients also have poor outcome.

B. Previous Hematologic Disorder or Cytotoxic Chemotherapy.

C. Chromosome Abnormalities: In general, cytogenetic abnormalities are unfavorable although certain abnormalities are favorable (see above).

In ALL, the following factors are adverse prognostically:

A. Age: Individuals <2 or >10 years of age have a poor outcome.

B. Surface Markers: B cell and T cell ALL have inferior results compared with common-type ALL, which is probably of pre–B cell origin.

C. Chromosome Abnormalities: These are unfavorable, especially the Philadelphia chromosome.

An exception is hyperploidy, which is favorable compared with other cytogenetic abnormalities.

D. Leukocytosis: A white blood cell count >50,000/μL is unfavorable.

E. Race: Nonwhites do less well than whites.

F. CNS or Other Extramedullary Involvement.

CHRONIC LEUKEMIA

The chronic leukemias are differentiated from the acute leukemias by their more insidious onset and prolonged course. They often are diagnosed as part of a screening examination when a complete blood count reveals significant abnormalities in the white blood cell count. Leukocytosis is often present, with few or no symptoms. The life span of these patients after diagnosis tends to be years even when they receive only "mild" treatment as outpatients. The two main types of chronic leukemias are chronic myelogenous leukemia and chronic lymphocytic leukemia.

CHRONIC MYELOGENOUS LEUKEMIA

Essentials of Diagnosis

- Elevation of white blood cell count with appearance of full spectrum of myeloid precursors in the peripheral blood.
- Low leukocyte alkaline phosphatase score.
- Presence of the Philadelphia chromosome in the peripheral blood and bone marrow myeloid precursors.
- Hypercellular bone marrow with myeloid hyperplasia and ≤5% myeloblasts.
- Splenomegaly.

General Considerations

Chronic myelogenous leukemia (CML) is a myeloproliferative disorder diagnosed in young to middle-aged adults with a male-to-female ratio of 3:2. There has been an increased incidence in those exposed to ionizing radiation. No other obvious environmental cause has been implicated, and in the vast majority, its etiology remains unknown.

Clinical Features

A. Symptoms and Signs: Usually the patient has nonspecific malaise and fatigue at presentation. There is often a history of weight loss. Sometimes there is a complaint of sternal tenderness due to malignant cells packing the bone marrow in the sternum. Abdominal pain or fullness may be present. Splenomegaly occurs in 95% of patients and hepatomegaly in half. In a minority of patients, bleeding due to thrombocytopenia is observed in the form of petechiae or purpura. Lymphadenopathy is relatively common, yet the lymph nodes tend to be small. Fever of unknown origin is an uncommon presentation.

B. Laboratory Findings: In most cases, the white blood cell count is elevated to greater than 100 $\times 10^6/\mu L$. All stages of the myeloid series are present, with the predominant cell types being segmented neutrophils and band forms. Basophils, eosinophils, and monocytes are generally increased in absolute numbers. Over time, the number of peripheral white blood cells tends to increase although there may be some cyclic variation. The leukocyte alkaline phosphatase score will almost invariably be reduced owing to depletion of granule enzymes. Anemia is present in most patients but is usually mild and tends to be a normochromic, normocytic anemia with severity proportionate to degree of elevation of the white blood count. Nucleated red blood cells may be seen on the peripheral smear. The platelet count is elevated in most patients and may reach greater than $1000 \times 10^6/\mu L$, yet clinical thrombosis is rare.

The bone marrow tends to be "packed," with a cellularity close to 100%. A "dry" tap is not unusual and may be due to expansion of the cellular marrow or to fibrosis. Usually there are increased megakaryocytes. In the bone marrow, a marked myeloid hyperplasia exists. The myeloid precursors in the marrow tend to be more immature than in the peripheral blood and have greater percentages of myelocytes and metamyelocytes. The percentage of blasts in the marrow is less than 5% unless blastic transformation occurs.

The serum uric acid level may be elevated owing to increased cell turnover, and pseudohyperkalemia may be present owing to potassium release when blood is allowed to clot in the specimen collection tube. The lactic dehydrogenase level may be elevated, reflecting ineffective cellular production. The serum vitamin B_{12} level is usually elevated as a result of an increase in the B_{12} binding capacity in the serum.

The Philadelphia chromosome (a translocation between chromosomes 9 and 22) is present in peripheral blood and bone marrow myeloid precursors. How this cytogenetic abnormality [t(9:22)] confers a growth advantage to the leukemic clone of cells is not yet known, nor is it understood why transformation into immature blasts occurs 3 years later.

Differential Diagnosis

In the adult population, the main differential diagnoses are between a leukemoid reaction and other myeloproliferative disorders. Rarely does a leukemoid reaction show a white blood cell count ≥100 $\times 10^6/\mu L$. Usually the leukocyte alkaline phosphatase score will be normal or elevated in leukemoid reactions, whereas in stable CML, it tends to be low. The primary cause of the leukemoid reaction generally

will be apparent with fever or another malignancy, and usually the patient will not have splenomegaly, thrombocytosis, peripheral blood metamyelocytes and myelocytes, eosinophilia, or basophilia. Polycythemia rubra vera or myelofibrosis may present with white cell counts ≥100 $\times 10^6/\mu L$ and splenomegaly but will not demonstrate a low leukocyte alkaline phosphatase score or the Philadelphia chromosome.

Treatment

A. Traditional Therapies: Traditional treatment of the chronic phase of CML has been to lower the white cell count to approximately 10–40 $\times 10^6/\mu L$, thereby reducing symptoms of the disease. Until recently, the agent of choice has been busulfan (Myleran). Extremely long term remissions have been achieved with busulfan but not without significant toxicities. It can cause pulmonary interstitial fibrosis, gynecomastia, hyperpigmentation, and a wasting syndrome with addisonian symptoms and adrenal insufficiency. Its potentially life-threatening complication relates to its unpredictable duration of action and prolonged pancytopenia that may occur with indiscriminate use. Marrow aplasia may last for weeks to months and has a mortality rate of 20–90%.

More recently, hydroxyurea has been used in the chronic management of this illness. It is well tolerated. Nausea and vomiting can occur but are not common with the usual 2–3 g/d initial dose. Once the white cell count has been lowered, a maintenance dose, usually 500–1500 mg/d, is given orally. The advantage of this drug lies in its short duration of action. There is usually prompt recovery from overdosage and no prolongation of leukopenia as with busulfan. However, it may take weeks to establish the optimal dose for each patient. The patient will feel well but still experience some fatigue and malaise. This treatment does not eradicate the Philadelphia chromosome and does *not* change the natural history of the disease.

Within 4 years of the diagnosis, almost all patients will develop a transformation in the disease process. This transformation may be subtle, with a rising white cell count and relative refractoriness to oral therapy being the only signals. Usually there are a greater number of blasts in the marrow and blood and increasing basophilia, thrombocytosis, and anemia. Some patients develop fever and splenomegaly. Another Philadelphia chromosome or new chromosomal abnormality may appear. Factors predisposing to earlier blastic transformation include a high white cell count (>100,000/μL), a high percentage of precursors (blasts and promyelocytes), large spleen or liver size, and large numbers of eosinophils or basophils. Unexplained fever is a sign of imminent transformation.

Once this transformation occurs, treatment differs according to whether the blasts are lymphoblasts or myeloblasts. One-fourth of blast crises occur as a lymphoid blastic transformation. These patients can be treated for acute lymphoblastic leukemia with a combination of vincristine and prednisone. Forty percent to 70% of CALLA-positive patients will achieve a complete remission. However, remissions are brief, and the patient rarely survives longer than another 6–12 months.

For the myeloblastic type of transformation, the therapy is different and generally has been unsuccessful. Complete remission rates are 10–30% with standard cytarabine plus anthracycline induction. Combinations of high-dose cytarabine and mitoxantrone are encouraging. A study using a combination of plicamycin and hydroxyurea to treat nine patients with CML blast crisis achieved complete remission with normalization of peripheral counts in six patients.

B. Newer Therapies: In studies employing interferon, 70% of patients with chronic phase CML developed a hematologic remission. Of these complete responders, 56% lost the Philadelphia chromosome. Subsequent studies with recombinant interferon showed a 70% complete remission rate, and about half the patients had suppression of the Philadelphia chromosome. Patients treated more than 6 months to 1 year after diagnosis did not have as good a response as those treated in early phases. Gamma interferon also seems to have an antileukemic effect, and the two interferons may have a synergistic effect in the treatment of CML.

C. Bone Marrow Transplantation: Bone marrow transplantation was introduced as an intensive approach to eradicate the last malignant cell. With high doses of chemotherapy, total body irradiation, and allogeneic or syngeneic transplantation, up to 70% of patients can achieve complete remission for 3–5 years. In the chronic phase of CML, only 20% relapse, as opposed to 40–50% transplanted in the accelerated phase. Graft-versus-host disease and interstitial pneumonitis have been controlled with cyclosporine plus methotrexate along with blood products from CMV-seronegative donors and intravenous ganciclovir. However, most patients are older than 35 years of age and are poor candidates for non-autologous transplantation.

CHRONIC LYMPHOCYTIC LEUKEMIA

Essentials of Diagnosis

- Sustained and absolute lymphocytosis (>15,000 /μL) in the peripheral blood and bone marrow (>40%) that cannot be attributed to any infectious, neoplastic, or other cause.
- Possible associated lymphadenopathy, splenomegaly, anemia (hemoglobin <12 g/dL) or thrombocytopenia (platelets <100,000/μL).
- Mature-appearing B lymphocytes in the peripheral blood.

General Considerations

Chronic lymphocytic leukemia (CLL) is the most common type of leukemia seen in the USA and Europe (up to 30% of all leukemias), but it is rare among persons of East Asian ancestry. Typically this illness is seen in the elderly population (median age 60 years), with a male-to-female ratio of 2:1. There is no association with ionizing radiation, but epidemiologic studies suggest a familial tendency; however, no pattern of inheritance has been determined.

Clinical Features

Clinical manifestations depend on the stage at the time of diagnosis (see below). In early stages, there may be no significant symptoms and the illness may be diagnosed incidentally. With higher stages, lymphadenopathy, usually in multiple areas, and splenomegaly are seen in 50% of patients at diagnosis. With more advanced disease, symptoms of anemia may be present as well as bleeding due to thrombocytopenia.

Anemia or thrombocytopenia may be due to autoimmune phenomena. Autoantibodies directed against red blood cell or platelet antigens appear in up to 25% of patients with CLL and may produce autoimmune hemolytic anemia or immune thrombocytopenia.

Immune dysfunction may play additional clinical roles. Hypogammaglobulinemia is common, particularly as the illness slowly progresses. It is responsible for the high incidence of infection by encapsulated organisms (pneumococcus, meningococcus, and *Haemophilus influenzae*). Not only is B lymphocyte dysfunction seen, but T lymphocyte abnormalities are common as well. Inversion of normal T_4:T_8 ratios may been seen, associated with opportunistic infections by viruses (herpes zoster) or unusual organisms (eg, *Pneumocystis carinii, Cryptococcus*).

Staging

Not all patients with CLL have indolent disease. In 1975 Rai proposed a five-level staging system:

Stage		Median Survival (years)	Percentage of Patients
0	Lymphocytosis alone	> 10	25
I	Lymphadenopathy	> 8	50
II	Hepatosplenomegaly	< 7	50
III	Anemia	2–5	25
IV	Thrombocytopenia	< 2	25

In 1981 Binet proposed a three-stage system using discrete regions of lymph node involvement:

Stage	Involvement
A	Two or less areas of lymphoid enlargement.
B	Three or more areas of lymphoid enlargement.
C	Anemia or thrombocytopenia.

These two are the most popular and clinically useful staging systems. A poorer prognosis is predicted when the white blood cell count doubles within 6–12 months or is >50,000 at presentation, or when the bone marrow is diffusely infiltrated as opposed to nodular or interstitial.

Treatment

Treatment depends on stage of illness with certain exceptions. No therapy is recommended for patients with Rai stage 0–I disease or Binet stages A–B. Treatment should be rendered once the patient is anemic or thrombocytopenic. It is important to determine whether the cytopenia is due to immunomediated mechanisms or marrow infiltration. If it is due to immune hemolytic anemia or thrombocytopenia, prednisone, in divided doses equivalent to 1 mg/kg/d, should be administered. Most patients will respond, but if the response does not persist when the corticosteroid is slowly tapered, splenectomy should be considered. Splenectomy also may be useful if pressure symptoms arise.

Radiation therapy is mainly reserved for localized areas of tumor compression/infiltration producing painful symptoms. Rarely is whole-body irradiation used.

Once the patient has symptoms of anemia or thrombocytopenia, chemotherapy usually is initiated. Chlorambucil has been the most widely used drug. Definite activity against CLL has been observed with chlorambucil in a dose of 0.1–0.2 mg/kg/d or 0.4–0.6 mg/kg given once every 2–4 weeks. It probably has less toxicity and equal efficacy when given as a bolus rather than daily. Cyclophosphamide is probably of equal efficacy and may be less toxic to megakaryocytes. Improved response rates are achieved when prednisone is combined with the alkylating agent, eg, biweekly chlorambucil, 30 mg/m^2 for 1 day, plus prednisone, 80 mg/d for 5 days, or triweekly cyclophosphamide, 300 mg/m^2/d orally for 5 days, plus prednisone, 100 mg/m^2/d orally for 5 days with or without vincristine, 1.4 mg/m^2 intravenously on the first day.

For patients with more aggressive disease as evidenced by failure to respond to the conventional treatments, multiple drug therapy (eg, the M$_2$ protocol) or low-dose doxorubicin-containing protocols can be tried. Allogeneic bone marrow transplantation is out of the question for the usually elderly patient population.

Fludarabine monophosphate has produced responses in heavily pretreated refractory patients. This drug is given at a dose of 25 mg/m^2/d for 5 days monthly. Myelosuppression may be dose-limiting, but this drug is generally well tolerated. Two experimental nucleoside drugs, 2-chlorodeoxyadenosine and deoxycoformycin, have produced responses in patients refractory to prior therapy.

Variants of CLL

A. Prolymphocytic Leukemia: Morphologically this cell type is larger and less well differentiated than the typical CLL cell. These cells have condensed nuclear chromatin and prominent nucleoli. Typical patients have extreme leukocytosis (100 × 10^6/μL), impressive splenomegaly without prominent lymphadenopathy, and a worse outcome. Some patients (25%) with typical CLL evolve into a prolymphocytic picture, signifying a more aggressive transformation of their disease.

B. Waldenström's Macroglobulinemia: The malignant lymphocytes have a plasmacytoid appearance and secrete substantial amounts of IgM into the serum. Since this protein remains mainly in the plasma, hyperviscosity symptoms may predominate. This disease is seen in the elderly patient and often remains indolent. With disease progression, there is progressive lymphadenopathy and hepatosplenomegaly without bony disease.

C. Hairy Cell Leukemia: This disease was named when malignant lymphocytes were described that contained cytoplasmic projections. This cell probably is derived from a B lymphocyte and contains tartrate-resistant acid phosphatase granules. This illness has a marked male preponderance and is usually associated with splenomegaly and pancytopenia at diagnosis. Splenectomy often produces a beneficial response, and this malignancy shows extreme responsiveness to alpha interferon. Deoxycoformycin (Pentostatin) is used for interferon refractory patients.

D. Chronic T Cell Leukemias: These account for approximately 5% of patients. Morphologically the cells are indistinguishable from the B cell counterpart. Clinically there is a greater incidence of skin involvement. Chronic T cell lymphoproliferative disease has been described. These lymphocytes contain large numbers of cytoplasmic azurophilic granules. Patients are neutropenic and have frequent infections without lymphoadenopathy, splenomegaly, or skin infiltration. Patients may present with a combination of circulating cerebroform lymphocytes associated with a chronic cutaneous infiltration known as Sézary syndrome. This appears to be the systemic equivalent of mycosis fungoides.

E. Well-Differentiated Lymphocytic Lymphoma: Whether an illness is described as CLL or well-differentiated lymphocytic lymphoma is mainly a matter of degree. Patients may have predominantly lymph node involvement and few identifiable CLL cells. Probably these patients would be described as having more lymphoma than CLL. Additionally patients with the small cleaved-cell variety of lymphocytic lymphoma may have identifiable clefts under light microscopy.

REFERENCES

Acute Leukemia

Bennett JM et al: Proposals for the classification of the myelodysplastic syndromes. *Br J Haematol* 1982;**51:** 189.

Bennett JM et al: Proposed revised criteria for the classification of acute myeloid leukemia. *Ann Intern Med* 1985;**103:**626.

Clarkson B et al: Acute lymphoblastic leukemia in adults. *Semin Oncol* 1985;**12:**160.

Foon FA, Todd RF: Immunologic classification of leukemia and lymphoma. *Blood* 1986;**68:**1.

Gale RP, Foon KA: Therapy of acute myelogenous leukemia. *Semin Hematol* 1987;**24:**41.

Henderson ES, Lister TA: *Leukemia,* 5th ed. Saunders, 1990.

Jacobs AD, Gale RP: Recent advances in the biology and treatment of acute lymphoblastic leukemia in adults. *N Engl J Med* 1984;**311:**1219.

Koeffler HP: Syndromes of acute nonlymphocytic leukemia. *Ann Intern Med* 1987;**107:**748.

Mayer RJ: Current chemotherapeutic treatment approaches to the management of previously untreated adults with de novo acute myelogenous leukemia. *Semin Oncol* 1987;**14:**384.

Chronic Leukemia

Biret JL et al: Chronic lymphocytic leukemia: Recommendations for diagnosis, staging, and response criteria. (International workshop on CLL.) *Ann Intern Med* 1989;**110:**236.

Bolin R et al: Busulfan versus hydroxyurea in long term therapy of chronic myelogenous leukemia. *Cancer* 1982;**50:**1683.

Champlin R et al: Allogeneic bone marrow transplantation for chronic myelogenous leukemia. *Blood* 1982;**60:**1038.

Fialkow PJ, Jacobson RJ, Papayaunopoulou T: Chronic myelocytic leukemia clonal origin in a stem cell common to the granulocyte, erythrocyte platelet and monocyte/macrophage. *Am J Med* 1977;**63:**125.

French cooperative group on chronic lymphocytic leukemia: Long term results of the CHOP regimen in stage C chronic lymphocytic leukemia. *Br J Haematol* 1989;**73:**334.

Kantorjian HM et al: Chronic myelogenous leukemia: A multivariate analysis of the association of patient characteristics and therapy with survival. *Blood* 1985;**66:**1326.

Keating MJ et al: Fludarabine: A new agent with major activity against chronic lymphocytic leukemia. *Blood* 1989;**74:**19.

Rai KR et al: Clinical staging of chronic lymphocytic leukemia. *Blood* 1975;**46:**219.

Sauitsky A et al: Comparison of daily versus intermittent chlorambucil and prednisone therapy in the treatment of patients with chronic lymphocytic leukemia. *Blood* 1977;**50:**1049.

Talpaz M et al: Clinical investigation of human alpha interferon in chronic myelogenous leukemia. *Blood* 1987;**69:**1280.

Lymphomas

Margaret C. Sunderland, MD, & Charles A. Coltman, MD

HODGKIN'S DISEASE

Essentials of Diagnosis

- Enlarged, nontender lymph nodes.
- Cervical lymphadenopathy common.
- Mediastinal lymphadenopathy (50% of patients).
- Fever, weight loss, night sweats (40% of patients).
- Reed-Sternberg cells and mononuclear variants among inflammatory lymphocytes, eosinophils, histiocytes, and plasma cells.

Epidemiology & Etiology

Between 7000 and 8000 patients are diagnosed with Hodgkin's disease (HD) each year in the USA. While the incidence has increased modestly since 1950, advances in therapy have dramatically decreased mortality. With prompt evaluation and aggressive treatment, the majority of patients can be cured.

The incidence of HD follows a bimodal curve; a peak occurs in young adulthood, ages 20–25, followed by a plateau until age 55 when the incidence increases with age. The bimodal distribution is due primarily to the decline in incidence for women after age 30. For men, disease occurs at a constant rate after the initial rise in young adults. HD is uncommon in childhood; less than 15% of all cases appear in patients younger than 16 years. Except for the histologic subtype known as nodular sclerosis, HD is more common in males than in females for all age groups. Among blacks in the USA, the incidence of HD is half that of whites.

The cause of HD remains obscure, although considerable epidemiologic evidence suggests an infectious etiology. HD appearing in young adults is associated with several socioeconomic characteristics: middle- to upper-class family life, advanced educational status, and small family size. One common element shared by these risk factors appears to be minimal exposure to common environmental pathogens at an early age. Delayed exposure to an infectious agent may favor the development of HD. In older patients, social class characteristics are similar to those of population controls, and there is little evidence of an infectious etiology.

Although the association is weak, the Epstein-Barr virus (EBV) is the most likely pathogenic agent. About 20% of patients with HD have EBV DNA detected in involved tissue as well as in the genome of malignant cells. In some patients, elevated titers of IgG antibodies against the capsid antigen and the early antigen suggesting enhanced viral activation precede the development of HD. Finally, there is a slight increase in incidence of HD after infectious mononucleosis.

Genetic factors may play a role in the etiology of HD; certain HLA phenotypes are associated with increased susceptibility, and there are several examples of multiple family occurrences. A sibling of a patient with HD has a five- to nine-fold increase in risk for developing the disease.

Clinical Findings

A. Symptoms and Signs: Most patients request medical evaluation for painless, superficial adenopathy. Enlarged lymph nodes usually are located in the neck and supraclavicular areas but occasionally are felt in the axillary or inguinofemoral region. Mediastinal lymphadenopathy, which occurs in over 50% of patients, often is detected by chest x-ray before symptoms are manifest. Involved lymph nodes tend to occur in central or axial nodal areas, and disease in epitrochlear, popliteal, or mesenteric nodes is rare. The duration of adenopathy is extremely variable. Several weeks to months may elapse from the onset of symptoms to the time of diagnosis.

Constitutional symptoms of fever, night sweats, and weight loss, termed "B" symptoms, may be present and debilitating in up to 40% of patients. For some patients, the fever is cyclic with febrile episodes lasting several days to weeks alternating with periods of normal body temperature. On few occasions, "B" symptoms may be the sole manifestation of disease. In these cases, adenopathy is minimal or occult. These patients tend to be older men with the histologic types of mixed cellularity or lymphocyte-depleted (see below).

Severe generalized pruritus was removed as a "B" symptom in the staging system because objective measurement proved difficult. The cause of pruritus is unknown. Another peculiar symptom of HD is the occurrence of pain in lymphoid tissue shortly after drinking alcoholic beverages. The mechanism is not clear.

In contrast to non-Hodgkin's lymphoma, disease progression in HD follows an orderly pattern (Table 29–1). Initially, tumor extends to anatomically adjacent lymph nodes and viscera. Only in the advanced stages does hematogenous spread occur, with dissemination to the liver, bone marrow, and other organs. In some patients, hematogeneous spread to the spleen may occur early.

B. Immunologic Dysfunction: Patients with HD frequently have immunologic abnormalities that appear simultaneously with the onset of illness. Progressive loss of cell-mediated (T cell) immunity is manifested as cutaneous anergy, decreased T cell antigen responses, and a decrease in the ratio of T helper cells to T suppressor cells (CD4+:CD8+). As the disease progresses, lymphocytopenia, polymorphonuclear leukocyte dysfunction, and increased susceptibility to infections may develop. Disseminated infections with various fungi, the mycobacterial species, and DNA-viral infections appear with increased frequency in patients with advanced disease. Dermatomal or disseminated herpes zoster is especially prevalent, appearing in more than 25% of patients, even in young and relatively healthy individuals. Treatment with chemotherapy and radiotherapy may intensify the T cell defects and compound the immunologic deficiency by depressing humoral (B cell) immunity.

Currently, HD is not included in the diagnostic criteria for the acquired immunodeficiency syndrome (AIDS). The populations at risk for AIDS and for HD overlap substantially.

C. Laboratory Findings and Special Tests: Routine laboratory tests should include a complete blood count, serum alkaline phosphatase and calcium levels, and evaluation of liver and renal function. Radiologic studies should include chest x-rays and CT scan of the abdomen and pelvis.

The abdominal CT scan is a sensitive tool to assess nodes in the celiac, para-aortic, and mesenteric nodal areas and to visualize tumor nodules in the liver and spleen. If disease is not detected by CT scan, bilateral lower extremity lymphangiograms are advised. The lymphangiogram allows assessment of nodal architecture and may indicate defects indicative of HD in nodes of normal size. In addition, because radiopaque material is excreted slowly through lymphatic channels, the lymphangiogram can be used during staging laparotomy to ensure removal of any abnormal lymph nodes, and it provides a convenient way to monitor abdominal disease during therapy. In some centers, if chemotherapy is planned, laparoscopy-directed biopsies of the liver are done to establish the presence or absence of hepatic involvement, especially if liver function tests are abnormal.

The specificity of these radiographic studies is limited. In selected patients, the next step in staging evaluation includes a laparotomy and splenectomy (see below).

Differential Diagnosis

Superficial lymphadenopathy is a manifestation of many benign disorders, and enlarged cervical lymph nodes are common among young patients. Cervical and supraclavicular nodes especially may be a result of local pharyngeal infections or a manifestation of generalized adenopathy associated with infectious mononucleosis, cytomegalovirus infections, and AIDS. In the elderly, cervical lymph nodes are more often due to other tumors including nasopharyngeal, thyroid, and breast cancer, rather than infection. HD presenting as mediastinal lymphadenopathy can be confused with other benign or malignant masses arising in mediastinal structures, eg, non-Hodgkin's lymphoma, germ cell tumors, and thymomas.

Histopathology

The histologic diagnosis of HD is based on recognition of the characteristic Reed-Sternberg (RS) cells in the appropriate cellular and architectural setting. When involved with HD, lymph node architecture is effaced by a cellular infiltrate composed of normal lymphocytes, eosinophils, histiocytes, and plasma cells. The enigmatic RS cell, the malignant cell of HD, and its mononuclear variants are scattered throughout this background of inflammatory cells. The accompanying lymphocytes are primarily host-response, polyclonal T and B cells; most of the T cell population belongs to the T helper subset.

The RS cell is large, with two or more nuclei, each

Table 29–1. Comparison of Hodgkin's disease and non-Hodgkin's lymphoma.

| | | Non-Hodgkin's | |
Characteristic	Hodgkin's	Low-grade	Intermediate- and high-grade
Site of origin	Nodal	Extranodal in 10%	Extranodal in 25–40%
Node distribution	Central	Peripheral	Peripheral
Disease spread	Contiguous	Noncontiguous	Noncontiguous
Organ involvement			
Mediastinum	50–60%	Rare	Rare (except lymphoblastic lymphoma)
Central nervous system	Rare	Rare	10–15%
Bone marrow	<10%	70–90%	10–30%
"B" symptoms	30–40%	15–20%	20–30%
Stage I or II at diagnosis	60%	10–25%	30–40%

containing a single prominent nucleolus. A clear zone surrounding the nucleolus is a distinctive feature. RS cells may vary considerably in number and in their morphologic appearance among the histologic subtypes. The lineage of the RS cell remains unknown. The presence of RS cells is not pathognomonic for HD; cells of similar morphology can be detected in lymphoid hyperplasia associated with phenytoin therapy, in other lymphomas and solid tumors, and in infectious mononucleosis.

The Rye system classifies HD into four histopathologic categories: lymphocyte-predominant, mixed cellularity, lymphocyte-depleted, and nodular sclerosis (Table 29–2). The first three categories differ primarily in the relative proportion of RS cells, their mononuclear variants, and reactive lymphocytes. The fourth category, nodular sclerosis, has broad collagen bands that divide lymphoid tissue into circumscribed nodules. Nodular sclerosis HD also has distinctive clinical features. It is the only HD subtype more common in women than in men, and it has a propensity to involve lower cervical, supraclavicular, and mediastinal lymph nodes.

In lymphocyte-predominant HD, two variants— diffuse and nodular—are recognized. While the diffuse form is associated with a good prognosis, patients with the nodal variant have an increased risk of relapse after completion of therapy. This form may be related to B cell malignancies of non-Hodgkin's lymphoma.

The prevalence of histologic subtypes of HD varies widely by age. For patients below age 35, the majority, 70%, have nodular sclerosis HD and less than 20% have the mixed cellularity form. In contrast, HD in the older age group is classified as nodular sclerosis in 20% and mixed cellularity in 40%. Histologic subtype also correlates with stage. The proportion of patients with early-stage disease is highest in lymphocyte-predominant disease and progressively decreases through nodular sclerosis, mixed cellularity, and lymphocyte-depleted subtypes.

Table 29–2. Histologic subtypes of Hodgkin's disease.

Subtype	Frequency (%)	Clinical Features
Lymphocyte-predominant	5–10	Presents at stage I or II Diffuse pattern-good prognosis Nodular pattern-indolent, frequent relapses
Nodular sclerosis	40–60	Common in patients < age 40 Female predominance Mediastinum often involved
Mixed cellularity	20–30	Older patients Intermediate prognosis
Lymphocyte-depleted	<5	Older patients Poor prognosis

Staging

A. Ann Arbor System: There are four categories (Table 29–3). Patients are classified by extent of lymph node involvement for stages I, II, and III. Stage IV includes patients with disseminated disease outside the lymph node system. The subscripts E and S denote direct extension outside a lymph nodal area and involvement of the spleen, respectively. Patients are further classified as either A or B on the basis of the absence or presence of constitutional symptoms.

Approximately 60% of patients with HD in the USA are stages I and II at the time of diagnosis. The occurrence of "B" symptoms correlates with stage. Fewer than 10% of stage I patients are symptomatic at diagnosis, whereas over 80% of those with stage IV have one or more "B" symptoms. The percentage of patients with stages III and IV is generally higher in developing countries and in lower socioeconomic groups.

Clinical stage should be distinguished from pathologic stage. Clinical stage is assigned after the initial tissue biopsy studies, physical examination, bone marrow biopsy, and radiographic evaluations, including CT scan and lymphangiogram, are completed. Pathologic stage is determined by additional invasive surgical procedures such as a liver biopsy, laparoscopy-directed tissue biopsy, or staging laparotomy and splenectomy. Owing to the frequent occurrence of occult abdominal disease and limitations of radiographic studies, pathologic staging may be required before appropriate treatment can be devised.

B. Staging Laparotomy: Exploratory laparotomy and splenectomy are used to identify occult dis-

Table 29–3. Staging system for Hodgkin's disease.

Stage[1]	Clinical Features
I	Involvement of a single lymph node region (I) or a single extralymphatic organ or site (Ie).
II	Involvement limited to one side of the diaphragm, either of two or more lymph node regions (II), or localized involvement of an extralymphatic organ or site and one or more lymph node regions (IIe).
III	Involvement of lymph node regions on both sides of the diaphragm (III), which may include localized, contiguous involvement of an extralymphatic organ or site (IIIe), or involvement of the spleen (IIIs), or both (IIIes).
III$_1$	Involvement of *upper* abdominal lymphatic structures: spleen, porta hepatis, celiac, or splenic hilar nodes.
III$_2$	Involvement of *lower* abdominal nodes: para-aortic, iliac, mesenteric, or inguinal with or without upper abdominal involvement.
IV	Diffuse or disseminated involvement of one or more extralymphatic organs or tissues with or without associated lymph node involvement.

[1]"A" denotes absence of systemic symptoms. "B" is added to the stage when any of the following systemic symptoms are present: weight loss in excess of 10% of body weight, night sweats, unexplained fever >38 °C.

ease in retroperitoneal nodes, spleen, and liver and to confirm the presence of HD in abnormal nodes visualized by CT scan or lymphangiogram. The justification for surgery is to identify which patients are suitable for primary curative radiotherapy or alternatively who should receive more intensive therapy for advanced disease. Staging laparotomy should be done by an experienced and skilled surgeon.

Although staging laparotomy is an aggressive evaluative procedure, the information gained is extremely valuable for treatment planning. Clinical staging may be inaccurate for many patients. Restaging from clinical stages I and II to pathologic stages III and IV occurs in about 25% of patients. Conversely, clinical stages III and IV are determined to be pathologic stages I or II for nearly half the patients undergoing laparotomy. When performed at experienced centers, operative mortality and perioperative morbidity are less than 1% and 5%, respectively. Surgery should be avoided in the elderly, young children less than 5 years of age, and patients with pulmonary or cardiac disease for whom surgery poses major risks.

Treatment

A. Radiation Therapy: Effective tumoricidal radiotherapy of HD involves total doses of 3500–4500 cGy, with higher doses administered to involved nodal sites and lower doses administered to occult disease. Fewer than 5% of patients have disease recurrence within the treatment field. Lymphoid radiation is contained within a few large treatment fields: mantle, para-aortic, and pelvic. Mantle field encompasses the cervical, supraclavicular, infraclavicular, axillary, hilar, and mediastinal lymph nodes to the level of the diaphragm. Preauricular nodes are added for patients with high cervical lymphadenopathy. Whole-lung irradiation with partial shielding frequently is used when the ipsilateral hilum is involved with tumor. The para-aortic field covers the spleen or splenic pedicle, celiac, and para-aortic nodes to the level of the aortic bifurcation. The lower para-aortic and, iliofemoral nodes are encompassed by pelvic field radiation. Each field is shaped to the contours of nodal groups, and extranodal tumor and lead shields are placed to protect vital organs. A small gap between the inferior border of the mantle field and superior border of the para-aortic field minimizes the risk of spinal cord injury caused by overlap.

Minor adverse effects of mantle radiotherapy include xerostomia, esophagitis, and dysphagia. Another side effect, Lhermitte's sign, in which brief shocklike sensations are felt down the extremities, may be particularly disconcerting. These symptoms disappear after a few months. Laboratory evidence of thyroid dysfunction develops in 90% of patients, but overt hypothyroidism is uncommon. Rare severe and irreversible neurologic symptoms resulting from transverse myelitis usually are due to overlapping radiation fields or inadequate treatment.

Radiographic abnormalities can be detected in most patients after mantle field irradiation, but only a few patients have any clinical impairment. In rare cases, acute radiation pneumonitis develops and may be life-threatening. Patients present with a nonproductuve cough, mild to moderate dyspnea, and fever. Radiation pericarditis is usually asymptomatic but occasionally may progress to cardiac tamponade or constrictive pericarditis.

B. Chemotherapy: The first successful chemotherapy regimen, MOPP (Table 29–4), resulted in an 84% complete response rate and a 15-year overall survival rate of 54%.

The most widely used alternative regimen is ABVD (Table 29–4). In clinical trials, MOPP and ABVD appear to be comparable with no significant difference in number of patients achieving a long-term survival. The choice of initial regimen is influenced, in part, by the anticipated toxicity of each. The acute toxicity of MOPP includes nausea, vomiting,

Table 29–4. Chemotherapy regimens for advanced Hodgkin's disease.

	Agents	Dosage[1]	Schedule[2]
MOPP	**M**echlorethamine	6 mg/m^2 on days 1 and 8	Every 28 days
	Vincristine (**O**ncovin)	1.4 mg/m^2 on days 1 and 8	
	Procarbazine	100 mg/m^2 orally on days 1–14	
	Prednisone	40 mg/m^2 orally on days 1–14, cycle 1 and 4 only	
BCVPP	Carmustine (**BCNU**)	100 mg/m^2 on day 1	Every 28 days
	Cyclophosphamide	600 mg/m^2 on day 1	
	Vinblastine	5 mg/m^2 on day 1	
	Procarbazine	100 mg/m^2 orally on days 1–10	
	Prednisone	60 mg/m^2 orally on days 1–10	
ABVD	Doxorubicin (**A**driamycin)	25 mg/m^2 on days 1 and 15	Every 28 days
	Bleomycin	10 mg/m^2 on days 1 and 15	
	Vinblastine	6 mg/m^2 on days 1 and 15	
	Dacarbazine	375 mg/m^2 on days 1 and 15	

[1]All drugs are given intravenously unless otherwise stated.
[2]Regimens are repeated for a minimum of 6 cycles, or for 2 cycles beyond a complete remission.

alopecia, and myelosuppression. Peripheral neuropathy associated with vincristine may be particularly troublesome. Other more significant problems include the risk of delayed second malignancies due to nitrogen mustard and the high incidence of infertility after MOPP. Although ABVD does not appear to be leukemogenic, there are other concerns when this combination is given to young adults or when given concurrently with radiotherapy. For some patients, cardiomyopathy or pulmonary dysfunction may limit its use. In addition, the irreversible toxicities of doxorubicin and bleomycin may not be apparent until many years after completion of therapy. Prior irradiation to the pericardium may increase the risk of doxorubicin-induced cardiac toxicity, and pulmonary fibrosis may develop with the use of bleomycin in patients previously treated with lung irradiation.

C. Recommended Therapy by Stage: (See Table 29–5.) For patients with stages IA, IIA, IIIB and IV, treatment is fairly standardized and well accepted. Radiation therapy is the usual mode for the first two stages, and combination chemotherapy is used for stages IIIB and IV. Management of stages IIB and IIIA remains controversial.

1. Stages I and II–Patients with stage IA or IIA supradiaphragmatic disease without large mediastinal masses should be treated with mantle and para-aortic (subtotal lymphoid) radiation. Customarily, patients are treated with mantle radiation first, followed in 2–3 weeks with para-aortic and splenic pedicle therapy. Because the risk of relapse in the pelvis is less than 3%, pelvic irradiation can be avoided, thus minimizing long-term effects on fertility. With subtotal lymphoid radiation, the overall survival for stages IA and IIA disease is excellent. The small number of patients with disease recurrence after primary radiotherapy often are cured by subsequent chemotherapy.

Clinical stages I and II patients with large mediastinal masses exceeding one-third the chest diameter have an increased risk for relapse when treated with primary radiotherapy. More than 50% will relapse within 5 years; relapses occur within the treated field, in adjacent lymph nodes, and in nonmediastinal sites. Combined chemotherapy and radiation improve the outcome for patients with bulky mediastinal disease.

Although the presence of "B" symptoms confers an unfavorable response to therapy, subtotal lymphoid radiation often provides high response rates for stages IB and IIB patients with nonbulky disease. For subsets of patients with negative prognostic factors, however, combined modality therapy should be considered. For example, less than 50% of patients with stage II disease who have lymphocyte-depleted histologic features and all three constitutional symptoms are successfully treated with radiation. In addition, combined modality therapy should be given to patients with stage I or IIB who are not evaluated by laparotomy.

2. Stages III and IV–Radiation therapy alone is not indicated for most stage III patients except possibly stage IIIA patients having only minimal splenic or upper abdominal involvement (stage III_1A). After treatment with total lymphoid radiation, some centers show a survival rate for stage III_1A patients comparable to that attained for patients with supradiaphragmatic disease.

Most patients with stage IIIB disease have extensive nodal disease above and below the diaphragm. Combined modality therapy with MOPP (or alternating MOPP with ABVD) followed by low-dose radiotherapy to sites of bulky disease provides optimal control of the disease. Stages IVA and IVB patients generally are treated with intensive, full-dose combination chemotherapy. Low-dose radiation to bulky sites of involvement may be a useful adjunct.

D. Salvage Therapy:

1. Chemotherapy and radiotherapy–Patients

Table 29–5. Recommended therapy for Hodgkin's disease by stage.

Stage of Disease[1]	Management[2]	Complete Remission Rate (%)	Ten-year Overall Survival (%)
Stage IA Stage IB Stage IIA with nonbulky mediastinal disease	Subtotal lymphoid RT	85–90	85–95[3]
Stage IIA with bulky mediastinal disease Stage IIB	Chemotherapy for three cycles followed by subtotal lymphoid RT	85–90	80–85
Stage III_1A	Subtotal or total nodal irradiation or combined modality	95	90
Stage III_2A	Chemotherapy followed by total nodal irradiation	85	75–85
Stage IIIB	Full-dose chemotherapy with or without RT	80–85	60–65
Stage IV (A and B)	Full-dose chemotherapy with or without RT to bulky sites of disease	80–85	55–60

[1]Bulky disease = mediastinal mass that exceeds one-third the diameter of the thoracic cavity.
[2]RT = radiation therapy.
[3]Survival rate includes patients receiving salvage chemotherapy after relapse from RT.

who relapse after prior radiotherapy for early-stage disease respond well to chemotherapy. Often, the frequency and duration of remission attained in this group is superior to that of newly diagnosed patients with the same stage of disease. Disease recurrence around previous treatment margins occasionally can be treated with further radiotherapy.

When HD recurs after combined modality therapy or chemotherapy, treatment decisions are more problematic and depend, in part, on the duration of remission and extent of disease. Patients who relapse more than 1 year after completion of therapy often respond to re-treatment with the initial drug combinations. A second, durable remission can be attained in 70–85%. In contrast, if less than 12 months has elapsed, the potential for long-term disease-free survival diminishes. For patients previously treated with MOPP, regimens that include doxorubicin, such as ABVD, sometimes can acheive remission in as many as 50%, with a 5-year survival of 20%. Other second-line regimens have not been as successful. In selected patients with disease recurrence restricted to a pulmonary or nodal site, salvage radiotherapy may be of benefit.

2. Autologous bone marrow transplantation–Cumulative data suggest that autologous bone marrow transplantation after intensive myelosuppressive treatment may increase the number of patients cured after a disease relapse. A variety of preparative regimens have been used; the most common is cyclophosphamide, carmustine, and etoposide. Because many patients have received prior mediastinal radiation, few are given total body irradiation. Usually, radiation is delivered to sites of bulky or residual disease.

Complete response rates have been reported for about half the patients. Although 50% of these patients go on to relapse, many attain durable remissions. Those with minimal disease and fewer pretransplant chemotherapy regimens have an improved outcome. In young patients without concurrent medical complications, autologous bone marrow transplantation is the preferred treatment strategy at the time of first relapse.

Late Complications

As more patients are cured with aggressive therapy, more are at risk for late complications. These late complications range from mild hypothyroidism to fatal second malignancies.

A. Physiologic and Psychologic Effects: Cell-mediated immunodeficiency may persist for many years in long-term survivors. Splenectomy and radiation may compound the problem. Sustained suppression of humoral immunity has been noted after radiation. In addition, asplenic patients are particularly prone to infection by encapsulated pathogens such as *Haemophilus influenzae* and *Streptococcus pneumoniae*. Immunization before splenectomy with polyvalent pneumococcal vaccine and appropriate antibiotic coverage may prevent excessive morbidity.

Both chemotherapy and radiotherapy can effect gonadal function and fertility. After MOPP therapy, almost all men have azoospermia and elevated follicle-stimulating hormone (FSH) levels. Pelvic or abdominal radiotherapy also affects gonadal function. Pelvic irradiation is associated with infertility in more than 75% of treated patients. Ovarian atrophy is common among women receiving MOPP. The incidence of amenorrhea increases with the intensity of therapy and age of the patient. Women at greatest risk for ovarian failure are those treated with infradiaphragmatic radiotherapy and chemotherapy.

Delayed cardiac effects in survivors of HD may appear 6 months to 20 years after radiotherapy. These abnormalities include decreased left ventricular ejection fraction, symptomatic pericarditis, and accelerated coronary artery disease. Chronic cardiomyopathy after the administration of doxorubicin may occur as long as 7 years after therapy. The toxic effect is dose-dependent; the incidence of cardiomyopathy is 3.5% after 400 mg/m^2 and 18% after 700 mg/m^2.

Late pulmonary complications include interstitial fibrosis and pneumonitis. Fibrosis induced by bleomycin may have an associated morbidity as high as 11%. After initial radiation injury, clinical symptoms of acute pneumonitis may develop 1–3 months later. Fibrosis involving the endothelial walls may not occur until 3–6 months after radiotherapy, with most permanent damage evident by 2 years.

Little information on the psychosocial implications of surviving cancer is available. Marital stress and anxiety about job security and medical insurance are reported frequently by patients. The prolonged decrease in energy that is common after vigorous therapy for HD contributes to readjustment stress. Successful treatment of HD does not appear to precipitate major psychiatric illness.

B. Second Malignancies:

1. Leukemia and lymphoma–One of the more severe late complications is the appearance of an acute leukemia. The peak incidence of leukemia occurs 5–6 years after therapy, with few cases reported after 9 years. The risk of leukemia rises dramatically with age from less than 5% in patients under age 30 to over 30% in the elderly.

The alkylating agents incorporated into MOPP and MOPP-like regimens (cyclophosphamide or nitrogen mustard) are responsible for most acute leukemias. Survivors who receive only radiation therapy have a much lower risk, whereas those who receive both modalities have an increased risk. ABVD does not appear to be leukemogenic.

Diffuse aggressive non-Hodgkin's lymphoma also occurs with increased frequency in survivors of HD and usually is diagnosed more than 4 years after completion of therapy. The clinical course is similar to that observed in other immunosuppressed populations. Extranodal presentations and early dissemination are common. Complete remission and cure are difficult to achieve.

2. Solid tumors–While the risk of leukemia appears to decrease after 9–10 years, the risk of solid tumors continues to follow an upward trend. In one large series, the risk of solid tumors at 15 years was more than double that at 10 years. An increased risk of second cancers of the breast, thyroid, bone, and stomach is associated with radiotherapy. Other tumors with an increased incidence include melanoma, soft-tissue sarcoma, and lung cancer. Close surveillance of dysplastic nevi and careful screening of women for breast cancer may detect some cancers in an early stage.

NON-HODGKIN'S LYMPHOMA

Essentials of Diagnosis
- Enlarged, nontender lymph nodes.
- Minimally enlarged peripheral nodes to fulminant generalized lymphadenopathy.
- Malignant lymphocytes (most are B cell malignancies).
- Low-, intermediate, or high-grade subtype determined by cell morphology, nodal architecture, and immunophenotype.

Epidemiology & Etiology
In the USA, approximately 40,000 new cases of non-Hodgkin's lymphoma (NHL) and 20,000 deaths from the disease are expected annually. Over the past 40 years, the incidence of NHL has doubled, from 5.9 to 13.1 cases per 100,000 population, primarily owing to the increasing number of persons over the age of 65; incidence among younger adults has not changed significantly. At the same time, the 5-year survival rate has improved dramatically, from 28% in 1954 to 49% in 1984. The lymphomas occur more frequently among males than females. Blacks have a lower incidence of NHL, and no increase in incidence has been noted in the black population in the USA.

The cause of NHL is unknown. An incompetent immune system may favor the development of many lymphomas. For some aggressive forms of lymphoma, epidemiologic, clinical, and laboratory features suggest that viruses play a pathogenic role. A strong association between the Epstein-Barr virus (EBV) and lymphoma was first noted by Burkitt for endemic lymphoma in East Africa. NHL occurs with greater frequency in individuals with altered immune regulation. A predisposition for the development of lymphoma has been described for patients receiving immunosuppressive therapy after organ transplantation, for children with congenital immune deficiencies (eg, severe combined immunodeficiency, Wiskott-Aldrich syndrome), and for patients with autoimmune disorders (eg, rheumatoid arthritis,

Sjögren's syndrome). NHLs are also part of the spectrum of diseases afflicting patients with AIDS. The common feature shared by many of these autoimmune and malignant diseases is dysfunction of T-cell suppression and serologic evidence of EBV reactivation.

Nonrandom chromosomal deletions, translocations, and duplications are common cytogenetic abnormalities in malignant lymphocytes. The most prevalent event is reciprocal translocation of segments from two chromosomes, usually involving chromosome 14. Other karyotype anomalies occur regularly: deletion of the short arm of chromosome 3 or 6, trisomy of chromosome 7, and duplication of chromosome 2. Specific chromosome aberrations are associated with certain lymphomas. In Burkitt's lymphoma, translocation of a segment of chromosome 8 onto the long arm of chromosome 14 is a characteristic finding in more than 75% of patients. The two variants, reciprocal translocation of a chromosome 8 segment and chromosomes 2 or 22, are found in 25% of cases. Study of gene rearrangement associated with Burkitt's lymphoma suggests a potential role for oncogenes in the malignant process. How oncogenes influence the transformation and growth of the neoplastic cell is unknown.

Clinical Findings
A. Symptoms and Signs: Specific complaints at presentation depend on the type of lymphoma, the anatomic location of the tumor, whether it is nodal or extranodal, and the extent of tumor dissemination. Lymphadenopathy may range from minimally enlarged peripheral lymph nodes to fulminant generalized adenopathy. Airway compression, spinal cord compression, and superior vena cava syndrome are examples of acute medical emergencies that may occur with NHL.

Superficial lymphadenopathy is usually painless. Visceral lymphadenopathy causes symptoms only when critical structures are compromised. Extranodal lymphomas are more troublesome. Lymphomas infiltrating the gastrointestinal tract or mesentery may cause weight loss, abdominal pain, bleeding, and obstruction. Lymphomatous involvement of the tonsils and pharyngeal tissues (Waldeyer's ring) is common. Lytic bone lesions can cause pain and pathologic fractures. If the bone marrow is involved, patients may have symptoms related to anemia, thrombocytopenia, or granulocytopenia. Constitutional symptoms of fever, night sweats, and weight loss may be present and debilitating but do not have the same negative prognostic significance as for Hodgkin's disease.

B. Laboratory Findings and Special Tests: Although blood chemistries and cell counts are often normal, metabolic or hematologic abnormalities may suggest disseminated disease. Rapidly growing lymphomas or large tumors may cause elevation of serum levels of lactic dehydrogenase (LDH) and uric acid. Renal failure may be present owing to ureteral obstruction by retroperitoneal adenopathy or to intrinsic disease, eg, hyperuricemia with uric acid nephropathy. Enlargement of porta hepatis nodes may cause extrahepatic biliary obstruction and hyperbilirubinemia. An elevated serum alkaline phosphatase may result from liver or bone involvement. Hematologic abnormalities are most often the result of bone marrow infiltration with malignant cells. The peripheral destruction of blood cells that occurs with immune thrombocytopenia or autoimmune hemolytic anemia is rare. Paraprotein spikes (monoclonal immunoglobulin) may be present on serum protein electrophoresis; it is identical to the immunoglobulin expressed on the patient's malignant B cells.

Staging evaluation includes a detailed history, careful physical examination, and routine laboratory studies including a complete blood count and routine chemistries. Selected patients may require additional invasive procedures or radiographic studies. The presence or absence of fever, weight loss, night sweats, and the duration of lymphadenopathy should be recorded. On physical examination, special attention should be given to all lymph node areas including the oropharynx. Recommended radiologic studies include chest x-ray and CT scans of the abdomen and pelvis. Because marrow involvement is common, iliac crest bone marrow biopsy and aspirate should be performed regardless of the complete blood count result. Bilateral bone core biopsy increases the yield from this procedure.

Patients with Waldeyer's ring lymphoma, mesenteric node involvement, gastrointestinal bleeding, or suggestive symptoms should be evaluated for gastrointestinal involvement. Cerebrospinal fluid analysis to detect occult disease is indicated for all high-grade lymphomas and for intermediate-grade lymphomas with paranasal sinus, bone marrow, or peripheral blood involvement. In contrast to Hodgkin's disease, the presence of small abdominal nodes, retroperitoneal adenopathy, or splenic involvement not visible on CT scan rarely affects therapy. For these reasons, lymphangiography and staging laparotomy are not usually indicated.

Diagnosis of NHL requires surgical biopsy of the tumor. Fine needle aspirates of suspected tumor masses or abnormal lymph nodes rarely yield sufficient material for an accurate histopathologic diagnosis. Although aspirated cells may confirm the presence of malignant lymphocytes, treatment decisions rarely can be made without knowledge of the specific type of lymphoma. The tumor specimen should be analyzed by an experienced hematopathologist. Specimens with indeterminate or ambiguous histology should be referred to an expert.

Monoclonal antibodies directed against normal cellular antigens can identify the specific cell of origin for a malignant lymphocyte. Using these techniques, pathologists classify most NHLs as B cell malignancies and less than 5% as T cell or monocyte neoplasms. A few malignant cells have no identifiable antigens and are classified as null cells. Cell surface marker classification has uncovered a surprising tumor diversity. Among large cell lymphomas, for example, 50–60% of the malignant cells are B cells, 10–15% are T cells, and 15–25% are null cells.

Differential Diagnosis

Lymphadenopathy is a common feature of many benign disorders. Infectious diseases associated with lymph node hyperplasia include infectious mononucleosis, toxoplasmosis, cytomegalovirus infection, secondary syphilis, tuberculosis, and atypical mycobacterial infections. Generalized lymphadenopathy is a common feature of AIDS-related complex and AIDS. Bilateral hilar adenopathy suggests sarcoidosis, histoplasmosis, or coccidioidomycosis. Enlarged lymph nodes in the posterior auricular or occipital chain are usually related to infection and not malignancy.

Other malignant disorders may be confused with lymphoma owing to similar clinical presentation. Primary mediastinal tumors, germ cell tumors and thymomas, and metastatic disease to the mediastinum resemble lymphadenopathy on plain chest x-rays. Conversely, lymphomas that arise in nonlymphoid tissue may be mistaken for other primary cancers such as those of breast, thyroid, and stomach.

Histopathology

A "working formulation" recommended by an international panel has become widely accepted. It identifies 10 subgroups of NHL and, like the commonly used Rappaport system, distinguishes among low-, intermediate-, and high-grade lymphomas (Table 29–6). Low-grade lymphomas are characterized by an indolent clinical course. Because of the relatively long survival after diagnosis, they often are referred to as having "favorable" histology. In contrast, intermediate- and high-grade lymphomas, those with "unfavorable" histology, grow rapidly and are associated with a poor prognosis.

A. Low-grade Lymphomas: The follicular lymphomas are so named because of their characteristic cellular aggregates, or nodules, that resemble the normal germinal centers of lymph nodes. Although reactive lymphoid hyperplasia resembles follicular lymphoma, the malignant process is distinguished by the cytology of the malignant cells in the follicle and the disruption of normal lymph node architecture with nodular proliferation.

The most common type of low-grade lymphoma, accounting for approximately 60% of all cases, is follicular small cleaved cell (nodular poorly differentiated) lymphoma. Follicular mixed lymphoma, with small cleaved and large cells, represents approximately 30% of cases. The least common is the diffuse

Table 29–6. Lymphoma classification and clinical characteristics.[1,2]

Grade (Incidence)	Working Formulation	Rappaport Classification	Lymphocyte Lineage	Incidence (%)	Median Age	Advanced Disease (%)	Marrow Involvement (%)	10-Year Survival (%)
Low (40%)	A—Small lymphocytic	Diffuse, lymphocytic, well differentiated	B	4	60	89	71	45 (40–50)
	B—Follicular, predominantly small cleaved cell	Nodular, lymphocytic, poorly differentiated	B	26	54	82	51	
	C—Follicular, mixed, small cleaved and large cell	Nodular, mixed, lymphocytic and histiocytic	B	9	56	74	30	
Intermediate (43%)	D—Follicular, predominantly large cell	Nodular histiocytic	B	4	55	73	34	26 (22–30)
	E—Diffuse, small cleaved cell	Diffuse, lymphocytic, poorly differentiated	B	8	58	72	32	
	F—Diffuse, mixed, small cleaved, and large cell	Diffuse, mixed, lymphocytic, and histiocytic	70%B 25%T	8	58	55	14	
	G—Diffuse, large cell	Diffuse histiocytic	70%B 25%T	22	57	54	10	
High (17%)	H—Large cell, immunoblastic	Diffuse histiocytic	70%B 25%T	9	51	58	12	23 (18–30)
	I—Lymphoblastic	Lymphoblastic		5	17	74	50	
	J—Small non-cleaved cell	Diffuse, undifferentiated, Burkitt's and non-Burkitt's	B	6	30	66	14	

[1]Modified and reproduced, with permission, from Simon R et al: The NHL pathologic classification project: Long-term follow-up of 1153 patients with non-Hodgkin's lymphomas. *Ann Intern Med* 1988;**109**:939.
[2]Patients with cutaneous T cell lymphomas, adult T cell leukemia-lymphoma, and malignant histiocytosis are excluded.

small lymphocytic subtype. The malignant cells of this rare lymphoma are morphologically similar to those of chronic lymphocytic luekemia (CLL); small lymphocytic lymphoma may represent the solid tissue counterpart of CLL.

Most patients with low-grade lymphoma give a history of waxing and waning but asymptomatic lymphadenopathy. Malignant lymphocytes are limited to lymphoid tissue, and extranodal disease is uncommon. Although 50–90% of patients present with advanced disease and bone marrow involvement, systemic symptoms and hematologic abnormalities are uncommon. The overall prognosis is good, with median survival ranging from 5 to 7 years.

B. Intermediate-grade Lymphomas: Intermediate-grade lymphoma comprises three subtypes of diffuse lymphomas and follicular large cell lymphoma. Although a heterogeneous group, these lymphomas share a typical clinical presentation and natural history. Extranodal disease occurs in 25–30% of patients, and localized bulky tumors may arise in the gastrointestinal tract and Waldeyer's ring. In contrast to low-grade lymphomas, fewer patients have ad-

vanced disease or marrow involvement early in the disease. Without therapy, however, tumors grow rapidly and disseminate quickly. Almost 50% of patients with diffuse large cell lymphoma may be cured with combination chemotherapy regimens.

C. High-grade Lymphomas: The high-grade lymphomas include lymphoblastic, immunoblastic, and small non–cleaved cell lymphoma (Burkitt's and non-Burkitt's). In the Rappaport classification, immunoblastic lymphoma is grouped with other diffuse large cell tumors as an intermediate-grade lymphoma, but because of its aggressive nature, the working formulation places it among the high-grade lymphomas.

Lymphoblastic lymphoma is well defined but rare. Patients are typically young males (median age of 16), and more than half have an anterior mediastinal mass at the time of diagnosis. The disease disseminates early, especially to the bone marrow, meninges, and peripheral blood. The malignant cell has surface markers of an immature T cell, and the morphology is indistinguishable from the malignant cell of acute lymphocytic leukemia (ALL). Most patients develop ALL within 3–4 months of becoming symptomatic.

Diffuse, small non–cleaved cell lymphoma is called Burkitt's lymphoma when the cells are uniform in size and contour and is called non-Burkitt's when the cells are small but heterogeneous. Burkitt's lymphoma has a rapid rate of tumor growth. The endemic form of Burkitt's in Africa differs from sporadic cases diagnosed elsewhere. Bulky tumors of the jaw and orbit in young children (median age of 7) and a high rate of late relapse are characteristics of the endemic disease. Sporadic cases of Burkitt's occur in an older age group (median age of 12), and large abdominal masses, retroperitoneal adenopathy, and bone marrow involvement are frequent manifestations. The EBV genome is identifiable in biopsy specimens from 97% of cases with endemic Burkitt's lymphoma, whereas fewer than 20% of the sporadic form harbor virus genome. Both types exhibit the typical translocation, t(8;14), on karyotype analysis.

Staging

The standard staging system is based on the extent of disease, number of nodal sites of involvement, and presence of disease above or below the diaphragm (Table 29–7). Although the Ann Arbor system is useful for designing treatment for patients with Hodgkin's disease, it has its shortcomings when applied to NHL. No provision is made for bulky disease or for some organ-specific tumors such as primary gastric lymphoma. Localized large tumors require specific therapy not suggested by stage. In addition, the distinction between stages III and IV is unnecessary because systemic therapy is usually required for both stages.

Table 29–7. Staging system for non-Hodgkin's lymphoma.

Stage[1]	Clinical Findings
I	Involvement of a single lymph node region (I) or a single extralymphatic organ or site (Ie).
II	Involvement of two or more lymph node regions on the same side of the diaphragm (II) or localized involvement of an extralymphatic organ or site and of one or more lymph node regions on the same side of the diaphragm (IIe).
III	Involvement of lymph node regions on both sides of the diaphragm (III), which may be accompanied by localized, contiguous involvement of extralymphatic organ or site (IIIe), or involvement of the spleen (IIIs), or both (IIIes).
IV	Diffuse or disseminated involvement of one or more extralymphatic organs or tissues with or without associated lymph node involvement.

[1]"A" denotes absence of systemic symptoms. "B" is added to the stage when the following systemic symptoms are present: weight loss in excess of 10% of body weight, night sweats, unexplained fever >38 °C.

Treatment & Prognosis

The approach to treatment is determined by the tumor histology, extent of disease, and physiologic status of the patient. The histologic type is the best single predictor of clinical outcome. Chemotherapy is more successful in the treatment of tumors with unfavorable histology. Many patients with intermediate- or high-grade lymphomas can be cured with combination chemotherapy regimens. Aggressive therapy for patients with low-grade lymphomas has not improved survival; few patients are cured, and most die of advanced refractory disease.

A. Low-grade Lymphomas: Few patients with low-grade lymphomas can be cured despite the extreme sensitivity of malignant cells to cytotoxic therapy. Both radiation and chemotherapy induce disease regression in the majority of patients, and 90% complete response rates are not unusual. However, indolent lymphomas invariably relapse at a rate of 10–15% per year, and high response rates have not translated into improved survival. The goal of treatment for many patients is to palliate specific symptoms rather than attempt a cure (Table 29–8).

For certain subgroups, clinical trials suggest that a long disease-free interval, and perhaps a cure, may be possible. Patients with localized disease (stages I and II) have excellent 10-year survival rates when treated with regional or total body irradiation. Less than 20% of patients with indolent lymphomas, however, have early-stage disease at diagnosis. Because clinical staging often misses small abdominal nodes, the true frequency of stage I or II disease identification may be lower than 20%. Promising preliminary results have been reported for patients with follicular mixed lymphoma receiving aggressive chemotherapy regimens.

For stages III and IV, treatment is determined by severity of symptoms and presence or absence of visceral organ involvement. For asymptomatic patients with advanced disease, a "watch and wait" approach may be appropriate management at the time of diagnosis. Delaying initial therapy does not appear to alter the natural history of the disease.

Patients with minimal symptoms and without organ compromise should receive single-agent alkylator therapy, either cyclophosphamide or chlorambucil. Localized bulky tumors can be effectively treated with radiation alone or in combination with systemic therapy. When organ function is threatened, prompt disease control should be attempted with a combination chemotherapy regimen. Because survival is not improved by full-course chemotherapy, treatment should be stopped shortly after maximal response is attained. Radiation therapy is a useful adjunct for emergent situations such as spinal cord compression or superior vena cava syndrome.

Two characteristics of low-grade lymphomas complicate management decisions. Temporary spontaneous remission occurs in 20–30% of patients, and the

Table 29–8. Recommended therapy for low-grade lymphomas.

Disease Characteristics			Survival		
Extent	Presentation	Treatment	Median (years)	Five-Year (%)	Potential for Cure
Localized (stage I or II)	Stage I after careful evaluation.	Regional radiation therapy or deferred.	>10 5–7	80 (at 10 years) 50–70	Yes No
Advanced (stage III or IV)	Asymptomatic. Symptomatic but with no vital organ compromise. Organ compromise present or imminent.[1]	Deferred. Chlorambucil, 4–6 mg/m^2, or cyclophosphamide ± irradiation to bulky tumors. CHOP (see Table 29–10).	5–7	50–70	No

[1]Obstructive uropathy, malignant pleural effusion, airway compression, spinal cord compression, extrahepatic biliary obstruction, liver failure, advanced marrow infiltration.

low-grade lymphomas often undergo transformation to a more aggressive tumor. Histologic conversion from low-grade to high-grade occurs in 20–30% of patients, with an actuarial risk estimated to be higher—60% at 8 years. After histologic transformation, these aggressive lymphomas usually do not respond well to chemotherapy and have a poor prognosis.

B. Intermediate-grade and Large Cell Immunoblastic Lymphomas:

1. Stages I and II—Radiation therapy to an involved region is effective for many patients with early disease (Table 29–9). Long-term survival as high as 75% has been reported for patients whose stage was determined by exploratory laparotomy. Survival rates fall below 40% when patients undergo clinical nonsurgical staging. Although primary chemotherapy for localized disease also is efficacious, improved results are achieved by combined modalities. Chemotherapy with CHOP (Table 29–10) for three cycles followed by involved field radiation is well tolerated and results in complete remission in more than 90% of patients. Long-term survival and cure can be expected for the majority of patients. Meticulous staging is critical to avoid including patients with advanced disease who require more aggressive therapy.

2. Advanced disease—The first combination chemotherapy regimens to result in long-term disease-free survival for treated patients combined cyclophosphamide, vincristine, and prednisone with either procarbazine (C-MOPP) or doxorubicin (CHOP). Multiple regimens have since been evaluated (Table 29–10).

Complete response rates for CHOP vary from 40% to 60%. Although approximately 40% of these patients will relapse after remission, many patients remain free of disease after completion of therapy for more than 2 years and 35–45% of patients are considered cured.

Newer regimens attempt to improve these results by increasing the intensity of therapy; intervals between cycles are decreased, drugs are given intravenously, and central nervous system penetration is improved. Additional cytotoxic agents are administered in alternating cycles to minimize the emergence of drug-resistant tumor populations. Complete response rates of 60–75% and projected actuarial survival rates of 50–65% at 3 years have been achieved. Toxicity, however, is significant, with profound myelotoxicity, mucositis, and treatment-related deaths.

Special sites of disease require treatment in addition to systemic chemotherapy. The testes and central nervous system are "sanctuary" sites of disease owing to the physiologic barrier that prevents drug diffusion. When a testicle is involved with lymphoma, ir-

Table 29–9. Recommended therapy for intermediate-grade and immunoblastic lymphomas.

Stage of Disease	Treatment	Complete Response Rate (%)	Five-Year Survival (%)	Potential for Cure
Stage I or II with nonbulky (<10 cm) disease	CHOP for 3 cycles followed by involved field radiation therapy (3000 cGy).	85–90	75–80	Yes
Stage II with tumor >10 cm or "B" symptoms	Chemotherapy as for stages III and IV ± involved field radiation therapy.	40–65	20–30	Yes
Stage III or IV	CHOP for 8 cycles or MACOP-B for 12 weeks (see Table 29–10). Central nervous system prophylaxis with intrathecal methotrexate, 12 mg (see Table 29–10).	40–80	40–60	Yes

Table 29–10. Selected chemotherapeutic regimens for intermediate-grade and immunoblastic lymphomas.

		Agents	Dosage[1]	Schedule
First Generation	CHOP	**C**yclophosphamide	750 mg/m² on day 1	Every 21 days for 8 cycles.
		Doxorubicin (**H**ydroxydaunorubicin)	50 mg/m² on day 1	
		Vincristine (**O**ncovin)	1.4 mg/m² on day 1	
		Prednisone	100 mg/m² orally on days 1–5	
	C-MOPP	**C**yclophosphamide	650 mg/m² on days 1 and 8	Every 28 days.
		Vincristine (**O**ncovin)	1.4 mg/m² on days 1 and 14	
		Procarbazine	100 mg/m² orally on days 1–14	
		Prednisone	60 mg/m² orally on days 1–14	
Second Generation	ProMACE-MOPP	**P**rednisone	60 mg/m² orally on days 1–14	Every 28 days therapy changed to MOPP based on rate of response.
		Methotrexate with leucovorin rescue[2]	1.5 g/m² on day 15 — 15 mg/m² orally every 6 hours for 5 doses	
		Doxorubicin (**A**driamycin)	25 mg/m² on days 1 and 8	
		Cyclophosphamide	650 mg/m² on day 1	
		Etoposide	120 mg/m² on days 1 and 8	
		Mechlorethamine	6 mg/m² on days 1 and 8	
		Vincristine (**O**ncovin)	1.4 mg/m² on days 1 and 8	
		Prednisone	60 mg/m² orally on days 1–14	
		Procarbazine	100 mg/m² orally on days 1–14	
	m-BACOD	**M**ethotrexate with leucovorin rescue[2]	200 mg/m² on days 8 and 15 — 10 mg/m² orally every 6 hours for 8 doses	Every 21 days for 10 cycles.
		Bleomycin	4 mg/m² on day 1	
		Doxorubicin (**A**driamycin)	45 mg/m² on day 1	
		Cyclophosphamide	650 mg/m² on day 1	
		Vincristine (**O**ncovin)	1.0 mg/m² on day 1 (maximum of 2 mg)	
		Dexamethasone	6 mg/m² orally on days 1–5	
Third Generation	ProMACE-CytaBOM	**P**rednisone	60 mg/m² orally on days 1–14	Every 21 days for a minimum of 6 cycles. Two cycles are given after a complete remission is attained.
		Methotrexate with leucovorin rescue[2]	120 mg/m² on day 8 — 25 mg/m² orally every 6 hours for 6 doses	
		Doxorubicin (**A**driamycin)	25 mg/m² on day 1	
		Cyclophosphamide	650 mg/m² on day 1	
		Etoposide	120 mg/m² on day 1	
		Cytarabine	300 mg/m² on day 8	
		Bleomycin	5 mg/m² on day 8	
		Vincristine (**O**ncovin)	1.4 mg/m² on day 8	
	MACOP-B	**M**ethotrexate with leucovorin rescue[2]	400 mg/m² orally in weeks 2, 6, and 10 — 15 mg/m² orally every 6 hours for 6 doses	12 weeks of therapy.
		Doxorubicin (**A**driamycin)	50 mg/m² in weeks 1, 3, 5, 7, 9, and 11	
		Cyclophosphamide	250–350 mg/m² in weeks 1, 3, 5, 7, 9, and 11	
		Vincristine (**O**ncovin)	1.4 mg/m² in weeks 2, 4, 6, 8, and 10	
		Prednisone	75 mg orally daily for 12 weeks; taper to 0 in 5 mg increments over last 2 weeks.	
		Bleomycin	10 mg/m² in weeks 4, 8, and 12	

[1]All drugs are given intravenously unless otherwise stated.
[2]Leucovorin begins 24 hours after methotrexate is given.

radiation of the opposite testicle should be done. Intrathecal therapy is required from the onset of treatment when tumor nodules are present in brain parenchyma or lymphoma cells are found in cerebrospinal fluid. If a paranasal sinus or epidural lymphoma is present, prophylactic treatment should be initiated.

3. Prognostic Indicators–For the intermediate-grade lymphomas, certain clinical features are associated with outcome. Younger patients have longer disease-free survival and fewer relapses than patients over age 55–60. Widely disseminated or bulky disease is associated with a poor prognosis. Patients with a large abdominal mass (>10 cm in diameter) and bone marrow or central nervous system involvement are less likely to respond favorably to therapy. Indirect measures of disseminated disease are also predictive. Patients with a serum LDH greater than 250 IU/mL, hemoglobin less than 10 mg/dL, and high β_2-microglobulin are less likely to achieve a complete remission than patients without these abnormalities. In addition, the rate of tumor regression may determine outcome. Patients who experience rapid tumor regression with chemotherapy have fewer relapses and more durable remissions.

C. High-grade Lymphomas: For Burkitt's and non-Burkitt's (small cell, noncleaved) high-grade lymphomas, chemotherapy is the mainstay of treatment for all stages (Table 29–11). Radiation is used only as a palliative measure. Because these lymphomas are exquisitely sensitive to chemotherapy, tumor lysis syndrome is a common complication. Aggressive hydration, allopurinol, and intravenous bicarbonate should be initiated before the start of chemotherapy. During treatment, intensive monitoring of volume status, electrolytes, and renal function is mandatory. Hyperkalemia, hypocalcemia, and hyperphosphatemia should be anticipated and treated aggressively. Renal dialysis may be required.

Lymphoblastic lymphoma is treated with chemotherapy agents known to be effective for acute lymphocytic leukemia. With aggressive therapy and central nervous system prophylaxis, cure is possible for 40% of patients. Extensive marrow involvement and central nervous system disease are prognostic indicators of early relapse, and patients with these findings should be considered for high-dose chemotherapy followed by bone marrow transplantation early in remission.

D. Recurrent or Resistant Disease: The outlook for patients who do not acheive a complete remission of disease with standard chemotherapy regimens is poor. Few patients with resistant disease benefit from an additional second-line cytotoxic regimen. Median survival is less than 6 months. Patients who relapse after an initial remission are also unlikely to respond well to further treatment. Current chemotherapeutic regimens rarely produce durable second remissions, and few patients are cured.

For refractory disease and recurrent disease, the only promising "salvage" therapy is high-dose chemotherapy, with or without radiation, followed by infusion of hematopoietic stem cells. The strategy of bone marrow transplantation is to take advantage of the direct relationship between dose and response for many of the effective antilymphoma agents. In addition, very high doses of chemotherapy agents may overcome drug resistance. Reinfusion of bone marrow stem cells serves to minimize the toxicity accompanying the higher doses by decreasing the expected duration of neutropenia. The source of donor cells is usually the patient (autologous) if the marrow is not involved or if tumor cells have been "purged" from

Table 29–11. Recommended therapy for high-grade lymphomas.

Classification	Treatment	Complete Response Rate (%)	Five-Year Survival (%)	Potential for Cure
Lymphoblastic[1]	Cyclophosphamide, 400 mg/m^2 orally on days 1–3 every 3 weeks. Doxorubicin, 50 mg/m^2 intravenously on day 1 every 3 weeks. Vincristine, 2 mg intravenously weekly for 6 weeks, then every 3 weeks for 4 doses. Prednisone, 40 mg/m^2 orally daily for 6 weeks, then daily for 5 days for 3 weeks. During month 2, asparaginase, 6000 units/m^2 for 1 month (maximum of 10,000 units) for 5 doses. Central nervous system prophylaxis during month 2: whole-brain radiotherapy at 2400 cGy. Intrathecal methotrexate, 12 mg for 6 doses.	85–90	75–85[2]	Yes
Small non–cleaved cell	CHOP or m-BACOD with intrathecal methotrexate, 12 mg for 6 doses	60–90	60–70[2]	Yes
AIDS-related	CHOP or m-BACOD with or without central nervous system prophylaxis.	25–50	<5	?

[1]After 4 months, maintenance therapy with methotrexate, 30 mg/m^2 orally every week, and mercaptopurine, 75 mg/m^2 orally daily, is recommended for 7 months.
[2]Five-year survival is lower for patients with marrow or central nervous system involvement.

marrow before reinfusion. Siblings (allogeneic) or identical twins (syngeneic) may be donors although graft-versus-host disease poses significant morbidity and mortality.

Clinical trials with autologous bone marrow transplantation usually involve patients with intermediate- to high-grade lymphomas. Complete response rates and disease-free survival are superior for patients with minimal, responsive disease compared to patients with bulky, resistant, or advanced disease. Good performance status and fewer pretransplant chemotherapy regimens are associated with a favorable outcome. Treatment-associated morbidity and mortality can be substantial, with early deaths reported for 10–20%.

Most regimens use high-dose alkylating agents with or without total body irradiation. Complete response rates have ranged from 40% to 100%, and many durable remissions have been attained. With careful patient selection, autologous bone marrow transplantation offers a potential cure for close to 50% of patients in "drug-sensitive" relapse. Age, poor health, or bone marrow involvement, however, disqualifies many patients for this treatment.

OTHER LYMPHOMAS

AIDS-related Lymphoma

An increasingly common clinical dilemma is the development of an aggressive lymphoma in patients with AIDS. The majority of AIDS-related lymphomas are high-grade (70%) B cell neoplasms; intermediate-grade lymphomas account for the remainder. The natural history and clinical course are atypical; frequently, the disease is widely disseminated, extranodal disease is common, and survival is poor. Principle extranodal sites include the gastrointestinal tract, including the oropharynx and rectum; central nervous system (10%); and liver. Other unusual sites of disease, eg, conjunctiva, testes, and maxilla, are also common.

Aggressive chemotherapy achieves complete response rates of 25–50%, but responses are of short duration and patients often are unable to tolerate intensive therapy. Individuals with AIDS have an increased propensity for infection, and many exhibit delayed bone marrow recovery after myelotoxic therapy. The probability of long-term survival often depends more on the natural history of the underlying immune system disease than on the lymphoma.

Cutaneous T Cell Lymphomas

Mycosis fungoides and the Sézary syndrome are indolent T-cell lymphomas of the skin. Classically, patients with mycosis fungoides have chronic dermatitis consisting of red, scaly patches or plaquelike areas resembling eczema. With disease progression, ulcerating cutaneous lesions may develop, and tumor spreads to visceral sites. Patients with the Sézary syndrome have circulating malignant cells in addition to the skin involvement. Exposure to industrial solvents has been implicated in the pathogenesis of both diseases. A T cell retrovirus may also play a role in some cases.

Three clinical stages are recognized in these two diseases: a nonspecific or premycotic stage, a plaque stage, and a tumor stage. Prognosis is good for skin disease without involvement of visceral organs or lymph nodes; median survival is more than 10 years. The discovery of more extensive disease implies a shortened survival with a medial survival of 30 months. Total-skin electron beam radiation or repeated application of topical mechlorethamine can result in long-term remission when the disease is confined to skin. Therapy with photosensitizing methoxsalen with ultraviolent A is often beneficial. Patients with advanced disease may respond to a wide variety of chemotherapy regimens, but response durations are brief.

Adult T Cell Lymphoma-leukemia

Adult T cell leukemia-lymphoma (T-ALL) has attracted considerable interest because of the causative role of the human T cell lymphotropic virus (HTLV-I) in its pathogenesis. Although the distribution is worldwide, geographic clustering of viral infection occurs in the southwest archipelago of Japan and in areas of the Caribbean basin. Serologic studies in these endemic areas reveal a larger population segment (12%) with detectable antibody to HTLV-I core protein than in nonendemic areas (2%). Host factors are clearly important in the development of A-TLL; malignant transformation occurs in less than 1% of seropositive individuals, and disease onset is believed to occur many years after initial infection.

Most T-ALL patients in the USA are young black men (median age of 34). The disease is characterized by diffuse infiltration of visceral organs and lymphoid tissues. Lymphadenopathy and hepatosplenomegaly are common. Skin involvement is manifested as lesions that range from discrete erythrodermic patches to large confluent tumor nodules. Circulating malignant lymphocytes with the typical lobulated nuclear morphologic pattern can be detected as the disease progresses. Nearly all patients develop refractory hypercalcemia and lytic bone lesions owing in part to the synthesis and elaboration of parathyroid hormone–related protein by the malignant cells.

No effective treatment is available for T-ALL.

Histiocytic Lymphoma

Malignant histiocytosis is a rare, progressive, and usually fatal disease of the sinusoidal histiocytes of lymph nodes. Most patients develop hepatosplenomegaly, lymphadenopathy, and constitutional symptoms of fever, sweats, and malaise. Pancytopenia is common and results from phagocytosis of erythrocytes, granulocytes, and platelets by the malignant histiocytes. The disease is fatal unless treated with systemic chemotherapy. Some patients repond briefly to treatment with CHOP or a similar regimen, but results generally are poor and few cures have been reported.

REFERENCES

Hodgkin's Disease

Bonadonna G et al: Treatment strategies for Hodgkin's disease. *Semin Hematol* 1988;**25(Suppl 2)**:51.

Bookman MA, Longo DL: Concomitant illness in patients treated for Hodgkin's disease. *Cancer Treat Rev* 1986;**13**:77.

Cabanillas F et al: Results of recent salvage chemotherapy regimens for lymphoma and Hodgkin's disease. *Semin Hematol* 1988;**25(Suppl 2)**:47.

Card P et al: Clinical stages I and II Hodgkin's disease: A specifically tailored therapy according to prognostic factors. *J Clin Oncol* 1988;**6**:239.

Hancock SL et al: Intercurrent death after Hodgkin's disease therapy in radiotherapy and adjuvant MOPP trials. *Ann Intern Med* 1988;**109**:183.

Hoppe RT: Radiation therapy in the management of Hodgkin's disease. *Semin Oncol* 1990;**17**:704.

Kaldor JM et al: Leukemia following Hodgkin's disease. *N Engl J Med* 1990;**322**:7.

Klimo P et al: MOPP/ABV hybrid program. Combination chemotherapy based on early introduction of seven effective drugs for advanced Hodgkin's disease. *J Clin Oncol* 1985;**3**:74.

Liberati AM et al: Immunologic profile in patients with Hodgkin's disease in complete remission. *Cancer* 1987;**59**:1906.

Longo DL: The use of chemotherapy in the treatment of Hodgkin's disease. *Semin Oncol* 1990;**17**:716.

Prosnitz LR et al: Combined modality therapy for advanced Hodgkin's disease: A 15-year follow-up study. *J Clin Oncol* 1988;**6**:603.

Regula DP, Hoppe RT, Weiss LM: Nodular and diffuse types of lymphocyte predominant Hodgkin's disease. *N Engl J Med* 1988;**318**:214.

Tucker MA et al: Risk of second cancers after treatment for Hodgkin's disease. *N Engl J Med* 1988;**318**:76.

Urba WJ, Longo DL: Hodgkin's disease. *N Engl J Med* 1992;**326**:678.

Non-Hodgkin's Lymphoma

Acker B et al: Histologic conversion in the non-Hodgkin's lymphomas. *J Clin Oncol* 1983;**1**:11.

Armitage JO: Bone marrow transplantation in the treatment of patients with lymphoma. *J Clin Oncol* 1989;**73**:1749.

Armitage JO, Cheson BD: Chemotherapy for patients with diffuse large cell lymphoma. *J Clin Oncol* 1988;**6**:1335.

Connors JM et al: Brief chemotherapy and involved field radiation therapy for limited stage histologically aggressive lymphoma. *Ann Intern Med* 1987;**107**:25.

Fisher RI et al: Southwest oncology group clinical trials for intermediate and high grade non-Hodgkin's lymphomas. *Semin Hematol* 1987;**24**:21.

Gallagher CJ et al: Follicular lymphoma: Prognostic factors for response and survival. *J Clin Oncol* 1986;**4**:1470.

Hoppe RT: The role of radiation therapy in the management of the non-Hodgkin's lymphoma. *Cancer* 1985;**55**:2176.

Levine EG et al: Cytogenetic abnormalities predict clinical outcome in non-Hodgkin's lymphoma. *Ann Intern Med* 1988;**108**:14.

List AF et al: Non-Hodgkin's lymphoma of the gastrointestinal tract: An analysis of clinical and pathologic features affecting outcome. *J Clin Oncol* 1988;**6**:1125.

Morrison WH et al: Small lymphocytic lymphoma. *J Clin Oncol* 1989;**7**:598.

Simon R et al: The non-Hodgkin's lymphoma pathologic classification project: Long-term follow-up of 1153 patients with non-Hodgkin's lymphomas. *Ann Intern Med* 1988;**109**:939.

Slater DE et al: Lymphoblastic lymphoma in adults. *J Clin Oncol* 1986;**4**:57.

Urba WJ, Longo DL: Cytologic, immunologic, and clinical diversity in non-Hodgkin's lymphoma: Therapeutic implications. *Semin Oncol* 1985;**12**:250.

Young RC et al: The treatment of indolent lymphoma: Watchful waiting vs aggressive combined modality. *Semin Hematol* 1988;**25**:11.

Other Lymphomas

Knowles DM et al: Lymphoid neoplasia associated with the acquired immunodeficiency syndrome (AIDS). *Ann Intern Med* 1988;**108**:744.

Rosenblatt JD, Chen ISY, Wachsman W: Infection with HTLV-I and HTLV-II: Evolving concepts. *Semin Hematol* 1988;**25**:230.

Sausville EA et al: Histopathologic staging at initial diagnosis of mycosis fungoids and the Sézary syndrome: Definition of three distinctive prognostic subgroups. *Ann Intern Med* 1988;**109**:372.

Pediatric Cancer

30

Richard T. Parmley, MD

Cancer is the leading medical cause of death in children 1–14 years of age in the USA and results in a death rate of 4–5 per 100,000 children per year (Table 30–1). Of all causes of death in children over 1 year of age, it is surpassed only by accidents (20:100,00 per year). Approximately two-thirds of children with cancer can be effectively treated and cured with surgery, radiation therapy, chemotherapy, or a combination of these modalities.

Cancer in children differs from cancer in adults in a number of respects. Most cancers in children involve deep organ structures or tissues, such as the bone marrow, lymph nodes, brain, kidney, neural crest, and muscle cells, whereas cancers in adults more frequently involve surfaces exposed to chronic environmental insults, such as skin, lung, gastrointestinal epithelia, and mucous membranes. Presenting symptoms are also different in children compared with adults. The common symptoms seen in adults with cancer, such as changes in bowel habits, nonhealing sores, indigestion, or a nagging cough, are rarely seen in children, whose typical symptoms include adenopathy, anemia, bruising, weight loss, abdominal mass, limp, or persistent headache.

Many cancers in children occur with high frequency at an early age (ages 2–5), particularly acute lymphocytic leukemia, neuroblastoma, Wilms' tumor, hepatoblastoma, retinoblastoma, and rhabdomyosarcoma. This occurrence suggests a relatively brief exposure to a strong carcinogen or a mutagenic event that may occur even in utero. Some children appear to be predisposed to cancer as a result of specific genetic disorders. For example, children with Down's syndrome have an increased incidence (1:100) of leukemia. Children with Fanconi's syndrome and Bloom's syndrome (diseases with increased chromosomal breaks and ineffective repair mechanisms) have an increased incidence (1:10) of leukemia and other malignancies. Children with Beckwith-Wiedemann syndrome have an increased incidence of Wilms' tumor, hepatoblastoma, and adrenal tumors. Children with Wiskott-Aldrich syndrome, ataxia telangiectasia, Chédiak-Higashi syndrome, and a variety of other immunodeficiency syndromes have an increased incidence of malignancy, especially leukemias or lymphomas. An identical twin of a child who develops leukemia has a 20% chance of developing leukemia within 6 months of the first twin's diagnosis.

Once diagnosed, children should receive the benefits of a multidisciplinary approach to treatment that includes a team of pediatric oncologists, surgeons, radiation therapists, social workers, psychologists, and pediatric oncology nurses. The failure of some therapies and the side effects of others emphasizes the need for regimens having not only optimal therapeutic benefits but also minimal toxicity. Such studies are in progress by the Pediatric Oncology Group, Children's Cancer Study Group, and various children's cancer centers. Within these groups, phase III studies using specific combinations of chemotherapeutic agents have been conducted and have resulted in the best outcomes currently available. For patients who fail these therapies, phase II studies examining the effectiveness and toxicity of new drugs or combinations in specific malignancies are performed. Patients with multiple relapses are often eligible to participate in phase I studies for new drugs that appear promising in nonhuman studies. In some situations, significant testing in adults occurs first; however, the unique pharmacologic effects of some of these drugs in children often requires repetition of adult phase I trials. Because of the relative rarity of childhood cancer, it is important that information regarding treatment, response, and toxicity be retrieved through registration of patients in these cooperative group studies. Enrollment of patients in specific protocols after informed consent provides quality control and allows rapid identification of optimal therapies for childhood cancer. After the diagnosis has been made and therapy planned, the patient frequently can return to the primary physician or pediatrician for administration of significant components of therapy under the extended guidance of the pediatric oncologist and cancer center.

ACUTE LYMPHOCYTIC LEUKEMIA

Leukemia occurs in 1 of every 2000–3000 children under 15 years of age in the USA and accounts for one-third of childhood malignancies. The most common type is acute lymphocytic leukemia (ALL),

Table 30–1. Cancer in children.

Type	Percent of Total	Rate per Million per Year	Peak Age
Leukemia	30	42.1	. . .
Acute lymphocytic	21	. . .	5 years
Acute myeloid	8	. . .	None
Chronic myelocytic	1	. . .	Depends on type
Lymphoma	14	13.2	. . .
Non-Hodgkin's	7	. . .	None
Hodgkin's	7	. . .	Second decade
Brain tumor	18	23.9	5 years
Neuroblastoma	8	9.6	2 years
Soft tissue sarcoma	7	8.4	Bimodal (5 and 17 years)
Rhabdomyosarcoma	5	. . .	. . .
Wilms' tumor	6	7.8	3 years
Bone tumor	5	5.6	. . .
Osteosarcoma	3	. . .	15 years
Ewing's	2	. . .	12 years
Retinoblastoma	2	3.4	1 year
Liver	1	1.9	1 year
Other	9	. . .	. . .

which accounts for approximately 75% of cases and has a peak incidence at 4 years of age.

Clinical Findings

A. Symptoms and Signs: The clinical manifestations of leukemia are related to marrow replacement, tumor infiltration, and metabolic problems secondary to tumor cell lysis. The most common presenting symptoms are related to pancytopenia and include pallor, bruising or bleeding, fever, and infection. In some patients, there can be bone or joint pain, lymphadenopathy, or organomegaly. Less commonly, symptoms are related to central nervous system or renal involvement with tumor. Hemorrhages or leukemic infiltrates can occasionally be seen on retinal examination. Testicular enlargement may indicate leukemic infiltration, which is diagnosed by biopsy and requires specific therapy.

B. Laboratory Findings: The bone marrow is usually hypercellular with replacement by leukemic blasts. Generally at least 25% of the cells in the marrow must be blasts ("M3 marrow") for the diagnosis to be made. Immunologic and cytochemical tests and chromosomal analysis are performed on the marrow sample to determine the subtype of leukemia.

ALL can be distinguished from acute non-lymphocytic leukemia (ANLL) using morphologic and immunologic criteria. Lymphoblasts generally have less cytoplasm, are less granular, and lack peroxidase or Sudan black–positive lysosomes. Morphologically blasts most frequently demonstrate sparse cytoplasm, velvety nuclear chromatin, and small nucleoli (Figure 30–1). The FAB (French, American, British) classification system applies the designation L1 to this morphology. Larger blasts with coarser nuclear chromatin, prominent nucleoli, and more cytoplasm are termed L2 and L3. Vacuolated basophilic L3 blasts generally correlate with B cell immunotyping, whereas L1 and L2 morphology do not correlate

with a specific immunologic marker. Approximately 15–20% of ALL patients have T cell markers such as E rosette positivity or antibody reactivity to T cell antigens; 15–20% have pre–B cell markers demonstrated by immunostaining of cytoplasmic immunoglobulin; 5% are B cell (Burkitt type) in origin as demonstrated by the presence of surface immuno-

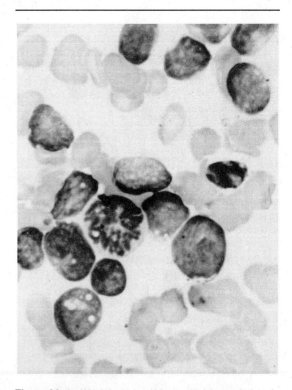

Figure 30–1. Wright's-stained blasts with L1 morphology in a child with acute lymphocytic leukemia. Note the sparse cytoplasm, fine nuclear chromatin, and inconspicuous nucleoli. A mitotic cell is centrally located in the micrograph.

globulin; the remainder (60%) lack B or T cell markers (sometimes called null cells) but frequently demonstrate immunologic reactivity for the common ALL antigen (CALLA) or contain the enzyme terminal deoxynucleotidyltransferase (TdT). Evaluation of the bone marrow should include a DNA index and chromosome analysis for hyperdiploid, hypodiploid, or specific markers, such as chromosome 14 aberrations associated with B and pre–B cell leukemias.

Spinal fluid should be sampled, since central nervous system involvement (< 5%) may be present at diagnosis and can be confirmed by demonstration of blasts in the spinal fluid. Laboratory workup should also include careful assessment of metabolic status. Where there is a large or rapidly proliferating tumor burden, metabolic problems result from cell lysis. These include hyperuricemia, hyperkalemia, hypocalcemia, and hyperphosphatemia, which may be accentuated by therapy unless precautions are taken. Chest x-ray may demonstrate a mediastinal mass particularly in cases of T cell leukemia (Figure 30–2). Similarly leukemic cells may infiltrate kidneys, which may appear enlarged on ultrasound examination, or infiltrate bones, resulting in lytic lesions on radiologic examination.

Differential Diagnosis

The signs and symptoms of leukemia are not specific. Anemia, bleeding, and infection can also occur with aplastic anemia. These symptoms may also be associated with other malignancies such as neu-

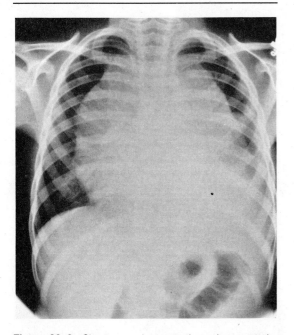

Figure 30–2. Chest x-ray demonstrating a large anterior mediastinal mass in a 7-year-old boy with T cell leukemia/lymphoma.

roblastoma or rhabdomyosarcoma, which can invade and replace the bone marrow space. Petechiae and bruises are associated with idiopathic thrombocytopenic purpura, which occurs more commonly than leukemia and frequently must be distinguished from leukemia by examination of a bone marrow aspirate. Lymphocytosis can occur with pertussis, infectious mononucleosis, or other viral diseases. Autoimmune diseases such as rheumatoid arthritis or systemic lupus erythematosus can similarly present with fever, anemia, and bone or joint pain. Laboratory studies and often bone marrow aspirate examination distinguish leukemia from these disorders.

Treatment

After assessment and initial management of secondary problems such as infection, anemia, bleeding, and metabolic disturbance (often involving the prophylactic administration of allopurinol in anticipation of tumor lysis and subsequent hyperuricemia with chemotherapy), specific combination chemotherapy can be started. Standard therapy generally involves an induction period lasting 4 weeks, a consolidation period lasting 2–4 weeks, and a maintenance period lasting 2–3 years. Induction therapy usually includes daily oral prednisone, weekly intravenous vincristine, and intramuscular asparaginase, which results in a complete remission in over 90% of children. The consolidation phase includes additional chemotherapy (eg, cytarabine, intermediate-dose methotrexate, or cyclophosphamide). Central nervous system (CNS) therapy is also given at this time and includes intrathecal medications (methotrexate or cytosine arabinoside) and occasionally cranial radiation. This is necessary to prevent relapse, which occurs in this site in 20–50% of patients not receiving prophylactic therapy. If the patient shows evidence of CNS involvement at diagnosis (cerebrospinal fluid positive for blasts), additional intrathecal medications and possibly radiation therapy are given during induction therapy. Maintenance therapy includes oral mercaptopurine and oral or intramuscular methotrexate and pulses (every 1–3 months) of vincristine and prednisone.

More intensive therapy is used for patients previously identified in clinical trials as having a poor outcome on standard therapy. Induction for these children usually includes cyclophosphamide, daunorubicin, or both, in addition to the standard agents. Induction is followed by more intensive consolidation (with or without delayed intensification) and maintenance phases. The combined phases usually utilize 6–10 chemotherapeutic agents. This intensive therapy often results in severe myelosuppression and prolonged hospitalization for management of myeloid suppression and mucositis.

Bone marrow transplantation using high-dose cyclophosphamide, total body irradiation, and infusion of marrow from an HLA-matched sibling is reserved for children who relapse while on chemotherapy and preferably are in their second remission.

Prognosis

Prognosis is influenced by multiple factors. Older children (> 10 years) and very young children (< 2 years) do worse than children between 2 and 10 years of age. Children presenting with high white cell counts, mediastinal mass, massive organomegaly, or CNS involvement have a poor outcome. Girls have a better outcome than boys. Children with hypodiploid chromosomes, the Philadelphia chromosome, or certain translocations have a poor outcome. Patients who have L2- or L3-appearing blasts or T or a B cell immunophenotype do poorly when compared with patients who lack these features. Infants with leukemia do particularly badly despite newer intensive regimens. Children who fail to achieve a remission with 4 weeks of induction therapy or who have a marrow relapse on chemotherapy have an extremely poor outcome. If marrow aspiration at 2 weeks fails to show an M1 or remission status (< 5% blasts), therapy should be intensified, since these patients have a poor outcome with standard therapy regimens.

In general, the disease-free 5-year survival for children with ALL treated with standard therapy is approximately 50% overall and as much as 80% in children with good prognostic features. For children with poor prognostic features treated with standard chemotherapy, the 5-year disease-free survival is less than 20%. More intensive regimens have resulted in a better outcome with over 60% of these children being long-term survivors. Thus, if children with leukemia are properly staged into good, intermediate, and poor prognosis categories and treated with appropriate regimens, the overall long-term survival approaches 70%.

If a child relapses on therapy, rescue chemotherapy usually is not curative. However, remission can be attained with variable frequency depending on the intensity of the previous therapy. A child who relapses more than 12 months after stopping therapy can still be successfully treated with intensive chemotherapy, although less than 40% of these children remain disease free more than 5 years from relapse. Isolated testicular and CNS relapses can be treated successfully with radiation therapy; however, the risk for subsequent marrow relapse is great, particularly if the extramedullary relapse occurs while on therapy.

ACUTE NONLYMPHOCYTIC LEUKEMIA

Acute nonlymphocytic leukemia (ANLL) accounts for approximately 25–30% of childhood leukemias and has no peak age incidence.

Clinical Findings

A. Symptoms and Signs: The presentation of children with ANLL can be very similar to that of children with ALL. The most common symptoms include pallor, bleeding, and infection related to pancytopenia. There can be variable degrees of organomegaly. Gingival hypertrophy is more common in ANLL than in ALL. Tumor lysis syndrome is less common in ANLL; however, disseminated intravascular coagulation is more common especially in patients with the promyelocytic and monocytic varieties of ANLL.

B. Laboratory Findings: The FAB classification system, using morphologic and cytochemical studies, recognizes seven types of ANLL, termed M1 to M7 corresponding to a predominance of undifferentiated myeloblasts, differentiated myeloblasts, promyelocytes, a mixture of myeloblasts and monoblasts, monoblasts, erythroblasts, and megakaryoblasts, respectively. Myeloblasts are usually larger, with abundant, often granular cytoplasm, and contain coarser nuclear chromatin and more prominent nucleoli than lymphoblasts. Frequently myeloblasts contain some peroxidase or Sudan black–positive lysosomes, which are not found in lymphoblasts. Myeloblasts and promyelocytes contain a specific chloroacetate esterase activity in their lysosomes, whereas monoblasts contain α-naphthol esterase activity (this enzyme is also present in some lymphoblasts). Specific monoclonal antibodies also are available for identification of some myeloid antigens. Factor VIII and hemoglobin stains are useful in the diagnosis of megakaryocytic and erythroblastic leukemia, respectively.

Treatment

Therapy for ANLL is more intensive and less well tolerated than therapy for ALL. Induction therapy lasting 4–6 weeks characteristically requires intensive cycles of cytosine arabinoside and daunorubicin. Total marrow aplasia usually results, and the patient frequently requires intensive support for infections and bleeding complications. Approximately 70% of patients with ANLL obtain a remission with this therapy. Previously patients had been maintained with frequent and repetitive low doses of chemotherapeutic reagents, but more recent studies indicate a better survival if induction therapy is repeated in cyclic fashion. Therapy is generally continued for 1–2 years. CNS involvement can occur, and prophylactic therapy with intrathecal medications usually is given. Etoposide and teniposide appear more effective in therapy of acute monocytic leukemia, particularly in infants. High-dose *trans*-retinoic acid appears to be useful for acute promyelocytic leukemia. Many centers recommend a marrow transplant procedure for patients with acute ANLL if a donor is available.

Prognosis

Laboratory and clinical findings in ANLL do not have as clear an impact on prognosis as in ALL. Nevertheless, infant ANLL, monocytic (M5) morphology, some chromosomal translocations, and extremely high blast counts (> 100,000) appear to more adversely affect outcome. Historically, fewer than 20% of ANLL patients have survived more than 5 years. Recent studies using more innovative chemotherapy regimens have projected as much as a 25–40% 5-year survival rate. Similarly, marrow transplantation can result in as much as a 50% 5-year disease-free survival.

CHRONIC MYELOID LEUKEMIA

Clinical Findings

Patients with chronic myeloid leukemia (CML) frequently present with massive splenomegaly and leukocytosis (> 50,000) with a predominance of band and segmented neutrophils. The bone marrow is often nondiagnostic and hypercellular, usually with less than 5% blasts (by contrast, the diagnosis of ALL or ANLL requires more than 25% blasts). CML has adult and juvenile types (Table 30–2).

Treatment & Prognosis

Adult type CML is initially controlled with minimal amounts of oral chemotherapy such as hydroxyurea or busulfan. Remissions, including cyotogenetic remissions, have been obtained in CML by the use of alpha interferon. In contrast, the juvenile type of CML rarely responds to even intensive chemotherapy and is often not treated initially. Both types of CML eventually develop a blast crisis. In juvenile CML, this is frequently associated with monoblastic proliferation, whereas in adult type CML there can be myeloblastic or less frequently lymphoblastic proliferation. When this occurs, therapy is similar to that used for acute leukemia. Neither type of CML can be cured with chemotherapy. Apparent cures have been accomplished with bone marrow transplantation.

Table 30–2. Characteristics of adult and juvenile types of chronic myeloid leukemia in childhood.

Characteristic	Adult Type	Juvenile Type
Philadelphia chromosome	Positive	Negative
Hemoglobin F	Normal	Elevated
Leukocyte alkaline phosphatase	Low	Low or normal
Platelets	Normal or increased	Low
Blood monocytosis	Not present	Present
Response to therapy	Good	Poor
Survival	3 years	6 months
Age at diagnosis	Over 3 years	1 year

HODGKIN'S DISEASE
(See also Chapter 29.)

Hodgkin's disease accounts for approximately half of childhood lymphomas. It rarely occurs before 5 years of age and steadily increases in frequency until it reaches a peak in the mid-twenties. The incidence is one-third that of leukemia, or about 1.3:100,000 children per year.

Clinical Findings & Staging

Patients with Hodgkin's disease may present with an isolated enlarged lymph node or with generalized lymphadenopathy or systemic symptoms. The most frequent symptoms are fever, weight loss, night sweats, and pruritus. Often these symptoms can be present for months before the diagnosis is made.

In patients with more advanced disease, the sedimentation rate and serum copper level are elevated; lymphopenia may be seen on peripheral smears. In addition, chest x-ray, abdominal ultrasound (or CT scan), gallium scan, and bone scan are needed to determine the extent of involvement. Many centers also utilize a lymphangiogram in staging and treatment planning. In most patients, complete staging also requires bone marrow biopsy and laparotomy with multiple lymph node biopsies, splenectomy, and liver biopsy.

The Ann Arbor clinical staging system is given in Table 29–3. The Rye classification describes four histologic subtypes: lymphocyte-predominant, nodular sclerotic, mixed cellularity, and lymphocyte-depleted. The former two are associated with a good prognosis and the latter two with a poorer prognosis. Most frequently, nodular sclerosis and mixed cellularity types are observed in children.

Treatment & Prognosis

The therapy for these patients is determined by the stage of the disease and to some extent the age of the patient. Radiation therapy to the involved lymph nodes and adjacent areas is preferred for stages IA, and IIA, and some IIIA patients, whereas chemotherapy alone or in combination with radiotherapy is used for stages IV, IIB, and IIIB. In small children, chemotherapy is preferred to extensive radiotherapy to avoid the growth arresting complications of the latter. Chemotherapy typically consists of six monthly cycles of MOPP/ABVD, or both (see Table 29–4). More than 80% of children with stage I and II disease, 60–70% of patients with stage III disease, and 50% or fewer of patients with stage IV disease are long-term (> 5 years) survivors.

NON-HODGKIN'S LYMPHOMA
(See also Chapter 29.)

Non-Hodgkin's lymphoma (NHL) occurs at a rate in children of 1–1.5:100,000 per year in the USA and accounts for approximately 10% of childhood cancer. There is no distinct peak age incidence, although the disease is rare in children less than 2 years of age.

Clinical Findings & Staging

Children with NHL may present with enlarged lymph nodes or an abdominal, jaw, or mediastinal mass. Evaluation of tumor extent and metabolic evaluation for tumor lysis syndrome (as described above for leukemia) are required. Generally, a chest x-ray, skeletal survey, gallium scan, abdominal and pelvic ultrasound (or CT scan), and often liver spleen scan are required. A gastrointestinal series may be necessary for abdominal masses, especially if presentation involves intussusception. In addition to blood counts, a bone marrow aspirate and biopsy are required to rule out marrow involvement. If 25% or greater blasts are present in the marrow (arbitrarily determined), the patient is considered to have leukemic conversion of the lymphoma. Similarly CNS involvement can occur, and examination of the cerebrospinal fluid for blasts should be performed at diagnosis. Patients with Burkitt's lymphoma often present with rapidly growing tumor resulting in a tumor lysis syndrome. The release of intracellular components results in hyperkalemia, hyperuricemia, hyperphosphatemia, and hypocalcemia.

NHL in childhood can be classified into two histologic groups: lymphoblastic and nonlymphoblastic. These are always diffuse lymphomas in children and never have the nodular pattern frequently seen in adults. In general, lymphoblastic lymphomas are tumors of thymocytes, and predominantly (70%) arise in the anterior mediastinum (Figure 30–2) or in lymph node areas usually above the diaphragm. The lymphoblasts are usually positive for terminal deoxynucleotidyltransferase (TdT) and have T cell characteristics such as E rosette positivity or T cell antibody reactivity. Nonlymphoblastic lymphomas generally have B cell characteristics and frequently (80%) are intra-abdominal. They may be subclassified as large-cell lymphomas (immunoblastic, diffuse histiocytic) or undifferentiated (Burkitt or non-Burkitt type). Burkitt type lymphomas usually contain surface immunoglobulin, which is frequently IgM. The TdT staining is negative, and reactivity with some B cell antibodies can be demonstrated. Chromosomal analysis may show a characteristic 8:14 translocation, especially in the Burkitt type; less frequently an 8:22 or 2:8 translocation can be demonstrated.

Four stages of NHL are defined in the Murphy system (Table 30–3).

Table 30–3. Murphy system for staging non-Hodgkin's lymphoma.

Stage	Clinical Findings
I	A single tumor (extranodal) or single anatomic area (nodal), with the exclusion of mediastinum or abdomen.
II	A single tumor (extranodal) with regional node involvement.
	Two or more nodal areas on the same side of the diaphragm.
	Two single (extranodal) tumors with or without regional node involvement on the same side of the diaphragm.
	A primary gastrointestinal tract tumor, usually in the ileocecal area, with or without involvement of associated mesenteric nodes only.
III	Two single tumors (extranodal) on opposite sides of the diaphragm.
	Two or more nodal areas above and below the diaphragm.
	All the primary intrathoracic tumors (mediastinal, pleural, thymic).
	All extensive primary intra-abdominal disease.
	All paraspinal or epidural tumors, regardless of other tumor site(s).
IV	Any of the above with initial central nervous system and/or bone marrow involvement.

Treatment & Prognosis

NHL in children is assumed to be disseminated at onset, even if staging shows localized disease. Consequently, surgery or radiation therapy alone is not adequate treatment, and relapses at distant sites frequently will occur if systemic therapy (chemotherapy) is not administered. Extensive surgical resection is not indicated. Radiation therapy is usually not necessary but can be helpful in local debulking of tumors affecting vital function, ie, tumors resulting in spinal cord compression, urologic obstruction, or superior vena cava obstruction. The disseminated nature of pediatric lymphomas is in contrast to adult lymphomas or Hodgkin's disease where disease is more frequently localized with less risk for dissemination.

Children with stage I or II NHL, either lymphoblastic or nonlymphoblastic, have an excellent response to chemotherapy with a better than 85% disease-free 2-year survival. Standard therapy for these patients includes 6–18 months of therapy with cyclophosphamide, vincristine, methotrexate, and prednisone. CNS prophylaxis with intrathecal medications is given to most patients with all stages of NHL to prevent recurrence of lymphoma in this site.

Children with stage III and IV lymphoblastic lymphoma have a 50–70% long-term survival if treated with intensive combination chemotherapy regimens. One such effective regimen involves the administration of multiple chemotherapeutic agents over 2–3 years with induction, consolidation, and maintenance phases. The drugs used include vincristine, prednisone, cyclophosphamide, daunorubicin, methotrexate, cytarabine, thioguanine, asparaginase, carmustine, and hydroxyurea.

Children with stage III and IV nonlymphoblastic lymphoma have the poorest outcome with standard therapies, with long-term survival rates of 50% and 20%, respectively. Intensive chemotherapy, eg, high doses of cyclophosphamide and methotrexate in addition to vincristine, prednisone, and daunorubicin, is preferred and appears to substantially improve survival. Intensive therapies employing high-dose cyclophosphamide appear to be more effective in nonlymphoblastic lymphoma, whereas the intensive use of anthracyclines is more effective in lymphoblastic lymphomas.

BRAIN TUMOR

Brain tumors are the most common type of solid tumors occurring in children and are second only to leukemia in incidence of all childhood malignancies. Brain tumors seldom metastasize outside the CNS. Consequently, the presenting symptoms and death occur as a result of the intracranial expansion of the tumor. Thus, even a benign tumor can be associated with a fatal outcome.

Clinical Findings

In children, 70% of brain tumors are infratentorial, whereas in adults the majority are supratentorial. Symptoms occur as a result of increased intracranial pressure or focal signs. Increased intracranial pressure may result in expansion of the skull in younger infants or spreading of the cranial sutures in older infants. There may be vomiting (which occurs characteristically on rising), headache, or mental changes. Papilledema may be seen. There may be focal or generalized seizures depending on the location of the tumor. Posterior fossa tumors may result in brain stem dysfunction, and cerebellar involvement may result in poor coordination, stumbling or falling toward the involved side, intention tremors, and nystagmus. Suprasellar tumors may involve the optic chiasm, hypothalamus, and pituitary gland. This group includes slow-growing optic nerve gliomas and benign craniopharyngiomas in the pituitary region. The resulting symptoms may be impaired vision, growth disturbances, personality changes, sexual precocity, and diabetes insipidus. Infants and young children with gliomas may present with the diencephalic syndrome, manifested by profound emaciation and failure to thrive.

When a brain tumor is suspected, a CT scan or MRI should be the first study performed (Figure 30–3). MRI provides more detail and is preferred if available. Lumbar puncture is contraindicated initially because of the danger of herniation.

The most common histologic types of brain tumors in children are medulloblastoma, astrocytoma, glioblastoma, and ependymoma. Medulloblastoma is thought to originate from primitive embryonic neuro-

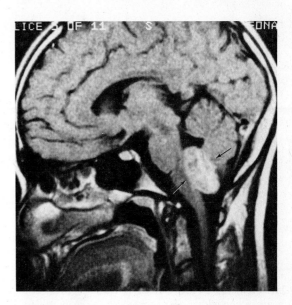

Figure 30–3. MRI of the brain in a young adolescent demonstrating a posterior fossa tumor involving the medulla and enhancing with gadolinium (arrows). The infratentorial location commonly seen in children contrasts with the more frequent supratentorial lesions seen in adults.

nal cells and is included in the broad category of primitive neuroectodermal tumors (PNET). Astrocytoma arises from transformed astrocytes, whereas glioblastoma (also termed astrocytoma grade III or IV) likely arises from a more anaplastic transformation of astrocytes or other glial cells. Ependymoma arises from another neuroglial cell, the ependymal cell, which forms the lining of the brain.

Treatment & Prognosis

If the tumor is surgically accessible, the primary treatment is surgical excision. If the tumor is incompletely resected, radiation therapy should be used. Chemotherapy has been associated with demonstrated responses in many patients; however, these are often temporary and consequently in many cases are considered palliative. The chemotherapeutic agents should be able to penetrate the blood-brain barrier and should include nitrosourea compounds (eg, carmustine, lomustine) procarbazine, cyclophosphamide, and cisplatin. For high-grade tumors, combination chemotherapy treatment regimens have included vincristine, prednisone, and lomustine; nitrogen mustard, vincristine, prednisone, and procarbazine (MOPP); and vincristine, methylprednisolone, carmustine, cytarabine, cyclophosphamide, cisplatin, procarbazine, and hydroxyurea (8 in 1). Comparative studies are under way to determine the most effective therapy. For very young children (< 2 years of age) chemotherapy may be initiated early in treatment and radiation therapy delayed for several months to 1 year to decrease radiation injury to the developing brain.

The prognosis for patients with low-grade astrocytomas that are completely resected is excellent, whereas incomplete resection followed by radiation (≥ 4500 cGy) results in an 80% survival at 1 year, 50% survival at 5 years, and 35% survival at 10 years. Few children with malignant gliomas are long-term survivors. The 5-year survival of children with medulloblastoma treated with surgery and radiation is approximately 40–50%. Surgery and irradiation are often associated with severe neuropsychologic side effects.

NEUROBLASTOMA

Neuroblastoma is the third most common malignancy of childhood (after leukemia/lymphoma and brain tumors). Over two-thirds of patients are under 5 years of age with a peak incidence at 2 years of age. Neuroblastoma arises from cells in the sympathetic nervous system, which includes the adrenal glands and paraspinal sympathetic ganglia in the pelvis, abdomen, chest, and neck and is included in the group of tumors termed primitive neuroectodermal tumors (PNET). Approximately 70% of patients with neuroblastoma have metastatic disease at diagnosis. Neuroblastoma has one of the highest spontaneous regression rates, and maturation of tumor cells to benign ganglion cells occasionally has been observed spontaneously and after treatment, especially in very young patients.

Clinical Findings

The tumor most frequently presents as an intra-abdominal mass. The mass frequently crosses the midline, x-rays frequently reveal punctate calcification, and on intravenous pyelogram or CT scan the mass appears extrarenal (ie, renal pelvis compressed or deviated but not twisted and distorted as seen in most Wilms' tumors). Frequently, patients with intra-abdominal primary lesions will have metastases to marrow, bone, distant lymph nodes, and liver. In contrast to the case for other solid tumors in children, pulmonary parenchymal metastasis almost never occurs, even with widely disseminated disease. Approximately one-third of patients with neuroblastoma present with a posterior mediastinal mass. Often the mass is asymptomatic and noted on routine chest x-ray; in other cases, there may be symptoms of spinal cord compression if the mass grows into the vertebral foramina. Such dumbbell tumors should be looked for whenever chest tumors are identified (Figure 30–4). A rare syndrome of opsoclonus in which there is cerebellar ataxia and involuntary random eye movements may be associated with neuroblastoma. The cause is unknown, but this presentation frequently is associated with a good prognosis and may not resolve

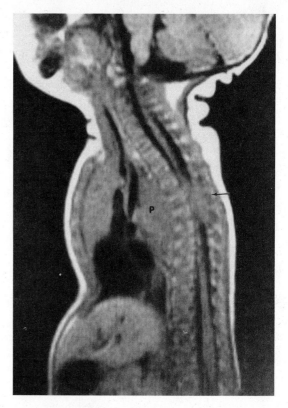

Figure 30–4. MRI illustrating a dumbbell lesion extending from a posterior mediastinal neuroblastoma (P) into the spinal canal (arrow). The anterior mediastinal mass is normal infant thymus.

with removal of the tumor. Laboratory tests should include intravenous pyelogram, abdominal CT scan, chest x-ray, skeletal survey, 24-hour urine specimen for catecholamine metabolites, bone scan, bone marrow aspirate, blood counts, and chemistry profile. Ferritin and neuronal specific enolase levels may be elevated in serum samples.

Staging

The staging system used by the Children's Cancer Study Group is as follows:

Stage I	**Tumor confined to the structure of origin.**
Stage II	**Tumor extending beyond the organ or structure of origin but not crossing the midline. Regional nodes in the ipsilateral side may be involved.**
Stage III	**Tumor extending beyond the midline. Bilateral regional nodes may be involved.**

Stage IV   Remote disease involving bone, parenchymatous organs, soft tissue, or distant lymph nodes.

Stage IV-S   Patients who would otherwise be stage I or II but have remote disease confined to liver, skin, or bone marrow (without radiologic evidence of bone metastasis).

Treatment & Prognosis

Prognosis is related to the child's age at diagnosis and the clinical stage of disease. Children at any age with localized, resectable disease are frequently cured with surgery alone or surgery and radiotherapy with or without chemotherapy (for residual disease).

Disseminated neuroblastoma is associated with a poor prognosis, especially in children over 1 year of age. Primary therapy is aggressive chemotherapy, which may include vincristine, cyclophosphamide, and other alkylating agents. Another regimen shown to be effective in inducing remission in the majority of children with this disease is cyclophosphamide and doxorubicin with or without alternating cycles of cisplatin and etoposide. Although chemotherapy has prolonged the survival of these children, it has not yet been demonstrated to have an impact on curing the disease. The 5-year survival for stage IV neuroblastoma remains less than 10%. More intensive regimens employing autologous and allogeneic bone marrow transplantation are under study.

Stage IV-S neuroblastoma frequently is observed in infants (Figure 30–5). There is a high incidence (> 50%) of spontaneous and permanent regression of this tumor. Consequently, these children are frequently observed closely with no therapy. If there is progressive disease, massive tumor involvement, or organ failure as a result of tumor infiltration, chemotherapy frequently is successful.

Molecular genetic studies have associated the N-*myc* oncogene with prognosis in neuroblastoma. Patients with tumors that amplify this gene tend to have a poor outcome, whereas patients without amplification do not. This prognostic factor appears to be independent of the stage of disease. This marker offers the potential of identifying patients who need aggressive therapy relatively early in their disease course.

WILMS' TUMOR

Wilm's tumor is the most common intra-abdominal cancer in children and is the fourth most common malignancy in childhood. The peak incidence is at 3 years of age.

Clinical Findings

A high frequency of congenital anomalies is asso-

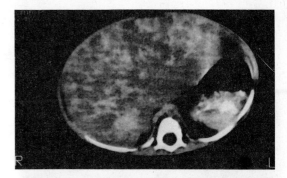
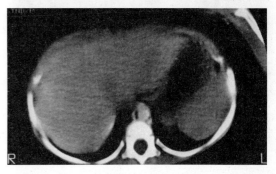

Figure 30–5. ***A:*** CT scan of the abdomen in a 7-month-old girl with stage IV-S neuroblastoma demonstrating multiple liver metastases. ***B:*** These resolved spontaneously and without treatment and could not be seen on CT scan 4 months later. Liver tumors are generally more prominent on MRI scan (not shown).

ciated with Wilms' tumor, such as genitourinary tract anomalies (abnormal collecting system or horseshoe kidney), hemihypertrophy, and aniridia. Approximately 25% of patients with Beckwith-Wiedemann syndrome will have Wilms' tumor or, less frequently, liver tumor or adrenocortical carcinoma. The syndrome can be familial and consists of gigantism, umbilical hernia (or omphalocele), macroglossia, hemihypertrophy, and visceromegaly. Wilms' tumor and aniridia also may be associated with an 11p chromosomal deletion syndrome.

Laboratory evaluation requires an intravenous pyelogram or CT scan, abdominal ultrasound, chest x-ray, skeletal survey, urinalysis, blood count, and evaluation of renal function. Imaging of the vena cava either by venogram or MRI may be useful to the surgeon so that tumor emboli (dislodged from vena cava tumor extension) can be prevented during resection. A bone marrow aspirate and biopsy are usually not performed. Characteristically the tumor distorts the caliceal system on the pyelogram or CT scan (Figure 30–6) rather than causing compression or deviation as occurs with an extrarenal mass. Radiologic evidence of calcification occurs less frequently in Wilms' tumor than in neuroblastoma but may be seen to some degree in approximately 10% of patients.

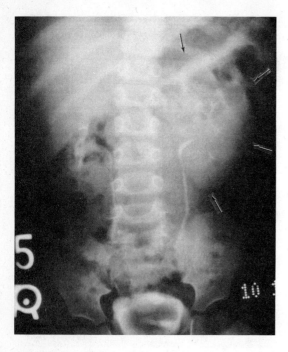

Figure 30–6. The left caliceal system is distorted by an intrarenal mass or Wilms' tumor in this intravenous pyelogram from a 3-year-old child. In contrast, extrarenal masses such as neuroblastoma would generally push an intact caliceal system either anteriorly or inferiorly. The mass also lacks calcifications more commonly seen in neuroblastoma.

Staging Wilms' tumor is staged as follows:

Stage I	Tumor limited to the kidney and completely excised.
Stage II	Tumor extending beyond the kidney (invasion of capsule) but completely excised.
Stage III	Tumor that extends beyond the kidney and/or is not completely excised; gross residual tumor in the abdomen.
Stage IV	Distant (hematogenous) metastasis (in order of frequency: lung, liver, bones, brain).
Stage V	Bilateral Wilms' tumor.

Treatment & Prognosis

The tumor is resected if possible. This should be done only after examination of the opposite kidney, which is involved in 5% of cases. If bilateral Wilms' tumor is present, every effort should be made to leave as much as possible of the least involved kidney, which may or may not be the one with the larger tumor mass.

Histologic evaluation is an important prognostic factor. The majority (90%) of patients have "favorable" histology (some evidence of differentiation). Approximately 10% of patients have "unfavorable" histology (anaplastic and sarcomatous variants). The latter group has a higher incidence of relapse and death and consequently is treated with more intensive chemotherapy. The treatment of Wilms' tumor is based on data collected by the National Wilms' Tumor Study Group. Current conventional therapy by stage and histologic characteristics is as follows:

A. Favorable Histology Stage I: Surgery plus 6 months of vincristine and actinomycin results in a 93% 3-year disease-free survival.

B. Unfavorable Histology Stage I: Surgery plus 18 months of vincristine, dactinomycin, and doxorubicin results in a 50–60% 3-year disease-free survival.

C. Favorable Histology Stage II: Surgery plus 15 months of vincristine and actinomycin results in an 82% 3-year disease-free survival.

D. Unfavorable Histology Stage II: Surgery plus radiation and 15 months of vincristine, dactinomycin, and adriamycin results in a 50–60% 3-year disease-free survival.

E. Favorable and Unfavorable Histology Stage III and IV: Radiotherapy plus 15 months of vincristine, dactinomycin, and doxorubicin. The 3-year disease-free survival for stage III favorable and unfavorable histology is 79% and 25%, respectively, and for stage IV favorable and unfavorable histology is 67% and 7%, respectively.

F. Stage V: Individualized therapy depending on extent of involvement, with an overall 3-year disease-free survival of approximately 75% for patients with favorable histology.

SOFT TISSUE SARCOMAS

The main soft tissue sarcoma is rhabdomyosarcoma, which accounts for 5–7% of childhood cancer. Rhabdomyosarcoma arises from various muscle masses, with the following frequency: nonorbital head and neck (ie, nasopharynx, middle ear), 28%; genitourinary region, 21%; extremities, 18%; orbital, 10%; trunk, 7%; retroperitoneum, 7%; intrathoracic, 3%; gastrointestinal tract and liver, 3%; perineum and anus, 2%; and other sites, 1%. The presenting symptoms vary widely depending on location of the tumor.

Clinical Findings & Staging

CT scan or MRI of the involved areas, chest x-ray, abdominal ultrasound, bone scan, skeletal survey, bone marrow aspirate, and biopsy may be required. Sites of metastasis in order of frequency include bone or bone marrow (Figure 30–7), distant lymph nodes, lung, liver, heart, and brain.

The tumor is staged as follows:

Stage I	Localized disease with complete resection.

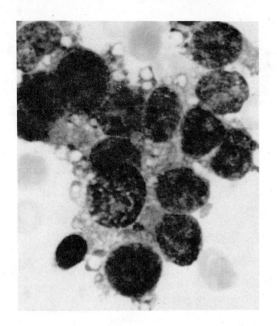

Figure 30–7. A syncytial mass of sarcoma cells is evident in this Wright's-stained preparation of bone marrow from a child with metastatic tumor. Distinct cell borders are not evident in clumped cells as seen in leukemia (see Figure 30–1).

Stage II	Localized disease with microscopic residual.
Stage III	Gross residual disease.
Stage IV	Distant metastatic disease.

Unfavorable histologic types include tumors with anaplastic, monomorphous, or alveolar appearance, whereas favorable histology includes embryonal tumors. Alveolar histology is usually present in extremity lesions. Embryonal histology is frequently associated with botryoid tumors, which resemble bunches of grapes growing into luminal spaces such as the bladder, uterus, or vagina.

Treatment & Prognosis

Treatment includes surgical resection if possible, radiotherapy to residual disease, and chemotherapy, which usually includes vincristine, dactinomycin, and cyclophosphamide. In advanced disease, doxorubicin, etoposide, and cisplatin are also used. Surgical removal or debulking should be performed, if possible, at diagnosis, or if not possible, after initial irradiation and chemotherapy. In patients with tumor localized to the bladder, vagina, uterus, prostate, and pelvis, initial tumor reduction with chemotherapy and radiotherapy is frequently attempted before complete surgical excision to preserve as much organ function as possible.

The prognosis is determined by the stage of dis-

ease, site of disease, and histologic features. The overall 5-year survival is 55%. The 3-year disease-free survival is greater than 80% for stage I patients and less than 20% for stage IV patients. Unfavorable histology carries a significantly poorer prognosis.

EWING'S SARCOMA

Ewing's sarcoma most frequently occurs in early adolescence. Its cell of origin is not known; it usually arises in the medullary cavity and extends outward to involve adjacent soft tissues. A similar appearing, very rare tumor arising from the chest wall has been separately categorized as a neuroepithelioma, or Askin's tumor. Ewing's sarcoma is extremely rare in blacks.

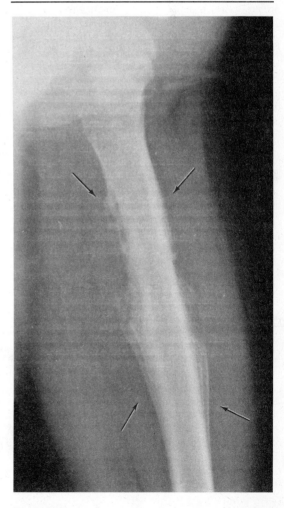

Figure 30–8. X-ray of the femur demonstrating a prominent diaphyseal destructive lesion (arrows) consistent with Ewing's sarcoma.

Clinical Findings

Ewing's sarcoma is either localized or metastatic at diagnosis. It most frequently involves the long bones rather than the flat bones. Long bone tumors usually originate in the diaphysis (Figure 30–8). The most common sites of metastasis are lung, other bones, bone marrow, and lymph nodes. The most frequent symptom is pain, which may precede diagnosis by as long as 6 months. Initially, the tumor may not be seen on x-ray but can be identified on bone scan. Consequently, a child with persistent bone pain and a negative x-ray should have a bone scan to rule out the possibility of tumor. The pain also may be referred, as is seen when knee pain is a presentation of a high femoral or pelvic lesion.

Treatment & Prognosis

Ewing's sarcoma of the extremities generally carries a better prognosis than pelvic or flat bone disease. Localized Ewing's sarcoma is a curable disease in two-thirds of patients. It is primarily treated with radiotherapy (> 4500 cGy) and chemotherapy (vincristine, dactinomycin, cyclophosphamide, and doxorubicin for 18 months). The 5-year disease-free survival for patients with metastatic disease is less than 20%.

In a few instances, amputation or removal of the involved bone may be considered. Tumor limited to the clavicle has an excellent prognosis if the clavicle is removed. Amputation may be considered in smaller prepubertal children if administration of radiation will result in significant limb disparity and morbidity as a result of growth retardation. Radiation is administered to the entire bone and may result in the appearance of second malignancies (ie, osteosarcoma and acute leukemia) and severe nonhealing fractures.

OSTEOSARCOMA

Clinical Findings

Osteosarcoma occurs most frequently in mid and late adolescence. It arises from bone and is pathologically characterized by production of malignant osteoid. The sites most frequently involved are the distal femur, proximal tibia, and proximal humerus. The presenting symptoms are pain and a palpable mass. The tumor characteristically arises as a lytic lesion in the metaphysis (Figure 30–9), in contrast to Ewing's sarcoma, which often arises in the diaphysis. Most patients have localized disease at diagnosis. Metastases most frequently are observed in the lungs and less frequently in other bones. Initial laboratory tests include a CT scan of the lungs, skeletal survey, and bone scan to rule out metastases.

Treatment & Prognosis

After the diagnosis is established by biopsy, amputation is generally the treatment of choice. In some

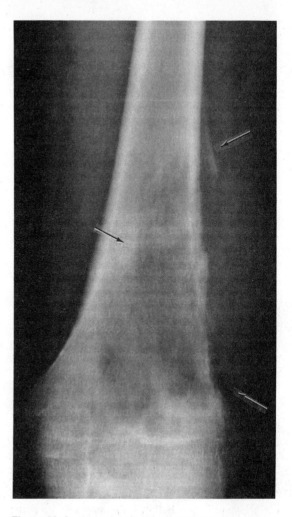

Figure 30–9. X-ray of the femur demonstrating a lytic metaphyseal lesion (arrows) in a patient with osteosarcoma.

instances, limb salvage operations may be performed. The tumor is considered radioresistant, and radiotherapy is reserved for palliation or preparation for some limb salvage procedures. Many oncologists believe that adjunctive chemotherapy significantly increases the cure rate by destroying micrometastasis and preventing pulmonary or bone recurrence, which historically occurs in 80–85% of patients with localized disease at diagnosis treated by amputation alone. Some pediatric oncologists advocate a course of chemotherapy prior to surgery to gauge tumor responsiveness and assess whether specific drugs will be useful for an individual patient. In general, the long-term disease-free survival for patients with localized osteosarcoma treated with surgical and chemotherapeutic modalities ranges from 50% to 70%. The prognosis is better for distant extremity tumors and poorer for more proximal tumors. Unresectable osteosarcoma is usually incurable.

Approximately 10–20% of patients with pulmonary metastatic disease either at diagnosis or after amputation may be salvaged with vigorous chemotherapy and often-repeated thoracotomy and metastasectomies. Bone metastases are not responsive to therapy, are salvage of these patients is not currently possible.

RETINOBLASTOMA

Retinoblastoma arises from neuronal elements in the retina and often is multicentric in origin. It is usually diagnosed in the first year of life and is an autosomal dominant familial disease in approximately 20% of cases. The disease is unilateral in 80% of cases and bilateral in 20%. Familial cases more frequently are bilateral and are usually diagnosed in younger infants.

Clinical Findings
The majority of patients will present with a "cat's eye," or white retinal reflex called leukokoria (Figure 30–10). Other symptoms may include strabismus, ocular inflammation, and poor vision. Initial laboratory evaluation includes a CT scan, skeletal survey, bone marrow aspirate, and cerebrospinal fluid evaluation to determine the extent of disease. Over 90% of children have disease limited to the orbit at diagnosis.

Treatment & Prognosis
Diagnosis is usually confirmed by therapeutic enucleation. In bilateral cases, this is done on the most involved eye. If there is no evidence of optic nerve involvement or extraocular extension, no further therapy is needed. If extraocular disease is suspected or documented, radiotherapy to the tumor bed and optic nerve are indicated. In bilateral disease, the remaining intraocular tumor may be successfully eradicated with radiotherapy, light coagulation, or cryo-

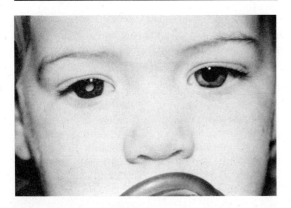

Figure 30–10. Cat's eye reflex, or leukokoria, seen in the right eye of a child with retinoblastoma.

therapy depending on its location and size. At present, no role for chemotherapy has been clearly documented in this disease. The cure rate for localized retinoblastoma is in excess of 85%, whereas metastatic disease is uniformly fatal.

If there is a family history of retinoblastoma or if the tumor is bilateral, then 50% of the patient's offspring may have retinoblastoma. The offspring of sporadic unilateral cases have a 15% chance of developing retinoblastoma. If there is no family history of retinoblastoma, the parents of a child with unilateral retinoblastoma have a less than 10% chance of having other children with retinoblastoma.

HISTIOCYTOSIS X

Histiocytosis X represents a varied group of clinical syndromes that have in common the pathologic proliferation of histiocytes. Usually, these histiocytes have Langerhans' granules demonstrable by electron microscopy. Whether this disorder can be considered a cancer remains controversial, since spontaneous resolution has been observed in some cases.

Disseminated Histiocytosis X
Also referred to as Letterer-Siwe disease, this disorder occurs predominantly in children under 1 year of age. Involved areas may include skin, liver, spleen, lung, and bones. The scaling dermatitis or macular papular rash is usually impressive and is usually associated with massive hepatosplenomegaly. The pulmonary involvement may resemble miliary tuberculosis and can result in significant respiratory distress. Treatment with vinblastine is frequently helpful. The overall mortality is 30–50%.

Hand-Schüller-Christian Disease
This histiocytosis syndrome has a peak incidence at 3 years of age, and there is usually more limited organ involvement. Characteristically there is involvement of the hypothalamus and pituitary with clinical diabetes insipidus. Frequently bony lytic lesions may be seen on radiologic evaluation. Therapy is usually successful and includes irradiation to the tumor and chemotherapy with vinblastine. The diabetes insipidus is usually not reversible, and vasopressin replacement therapy is required for life.

Eosinophilic Granuloma
This disorder may present at any age and usually involves one or more lytic bone lesions. They usually are noticed on routine x-ray or are associated with local pain or pathologic fracture. Vertebral involvement may result in sudden paralysis associated with pathologic fracture.

Treatment may consist of no more than surgical curettage. A minimal amount of local irradiation is used as curative therapy. This disorder rarely progresses to disseminated histiocytosis X.

PSYCHOSOCIAL IMPLICATIONS OF CANCER IN CHILDREN

Once diagnosed with cancer, the child and the child's family must be informed of the diagnosis, and appropriate psychosocial support should be provided. The work of the pediatrician is greatly facilitated in this effort in a pediatric cancer center setting in which pediatric oncology social workers, nurses, and psychologists participate and act as resources for the family. The emotional impact on the family and the dependent nature of the parent-child unit results in disruption of family life-style that is different from the disruption that occurs when an adult family member develops cancer. Specifically one or both parents must devote significant time and emotional support to the child. This often results in missed work or in unemployment, financial and marital difficulties, and frustration on the part of other siblings, who frequently do not understand what is happening or feel that they are being treated unequally. In addition, unrealistic guilt feelings arise in both parents and siblings, who may feel that they somehow contributed to or caused the cancer or perhaps delayed its diagnosis. Alternatively, the young patient may feel that he or she is being punished with this illness. Such concerns must be identified and addressed by the pediatric oncology team.

The physicians must also determine or provide guidelines about how much information the child should be given and whether consent or assent for therapy should be obtained from the child. Generally when a child is 6–8 years old, some explanation of the problem should be aimed at the child and assent should be sought. Adolescents generally should be asked to give informed consent, and the physician and treatment team need to be alert to specific patient fears and concerns particularly as they impact on appearance and disruption of peer interaction.

Decisions to stop therapy when unresponsive progressive disease occurs are even more complex. Frequently at this point in the disease the older child and adolescent has regressed emotionally and requires the special understanding found in a pediatric setting. Young children are most worried about separation from parents, but most psychologists believe that the finality of death can be understood by patients over 14 years of age. Once death has occurred, the support staff should continue to maintain contact with the family for several months or even years. Unresolved issues and guilt feelings regarding previous decisions frequently resurface and require clarification by the staff. These issues often can be addressed several months after death. Holidays, birthdays, and death anniversaries are particularly difficult times for family members, and availability and inquiries on the part of the pediatric oncology staff are often appreciated.

LATE SIDE EFFECTS OF CANCER THERAPY IN CHILDREN

With the improved prognosis of childhood cancer and the longer survival of these patients, late side effects of cancer therapy have been seen. They occur only in a minority of children but are of concern to oncologists. Children frequently tolerate chemotherapy and surgery better than adults. On the other hand, radiation therapy must be limited depending on the age of the child. The toxicity from radiation is often exaggerated by its deleterious effect on growth. Thus, arrest of bone or muscle growth in a child given radiotherapy may result in considerable morbidity later in life that is not seen in adult patients. A second complication is the increased incidence of a second malignancy. Overall, approximately 4% of children who are long-term survivors of cancer develop a second neoplasm. This is particularly true of children receiving large amounts of radiation or alkylating agents. For instance, patients with Hodgkin's disease treated with combined modality therapy have a 5–12% chance of developing a second cancer, usually myeloid leukemia, within 15 years of therapy given for Hodgkin's disease. Similarly, retinoblastoma patients given radiotherapy to the orbit have an increased incidence of osteosarcoma in the radiation field. Other examples of late side effects seen in less than 2–5% of children include heart disease in children given anthracyclines, restrictive lung disease in children given bleomycin, and aplastic anemia as a result of alkylating agents. Hemorrhagic cystitis and bladder cancer can occur after administration of cyclophosphamide. Cisplatin results in deafness and some renal dysfunction in approximately 10% of treated patients. Sterility may result from radiation and alkylating agents. Hormone deficiency can result from radiation therapy when organs such as the thyroid gland, testis, or hypothalamus are included in the radiation field. Similarly, therapy-related growth hormone deficiencies have been reported in children with ALL. Children undergoing extensive pelvic surgery for rhabdomyosarcoma have considerable morbidity related to removal of the bladder and sometimes the rectum. With the utilization of bone marrow transplantation for the treatment of leukemia and other malignancies, graft-versus-host disease is seen in approximately half these patients, with complications serious enough to cause fatalities in 5–10%. When total body irradiation is used in preparative regimens, growth retardation may be dramatic with development of short stature and sometimes hypoplastic lungs.

PEDIATRIC AIDS

In December 1991, approximately 5000 children in the USA were identified as having AIDS. Over 90% acquired human immunodeficiency virus (HIV) infection from the mother congenitally. This pediatric AIDS population is projected to increase dramatically. A smaller percentage of children (< 10%) acquired the infection through transfusion prior to screening of blood products (1985). However, this mode of acquisition has been virtually eliminated.

Clinical Findings

Clinical findings in pediatric AIDS patients may differ from those in adult AIDS patients in a variety of ways.

A. Growth failure is a prominent symptom in pediatric patients.

B. Neurologic involvement with significant delays in development eventually occurs in most children.

C. Lymphocytic interstitial pneumonia occurs almost exclusively in young pediatric patients with a mean age incidence of 15 months and must be distinguished from *Pneumocystis* pneumonia (usually by biopsy).

D. Parotid swelling is common in children but uncommon in adults.

E. Major bacterial infectious complications are more prominent in children, presumably as a result of damage to the B cell system by HIV.

F. Kaposi's sarcoma is rare in children, and lymphomas occur less frequently.

G. Cardiomyopathy is more frequent in pediatric patients.

In general, the CDC-specified diagnosis for establishment of AIDS are similar for adults and children except that recurrent invasive bacterial infections and lymphoid interstitial pneumonitis are unique to the pediatric population. Both pediatric and adult patients may experience opportunistic infections including invasive *Candida albicans, Cryptococcus* infection, *Cryptosporidium* diarrhea, cytomegalovirus retinitis or pneumonia, and *Pneumocystis* pneumonia. In addition, other complications, such as idiopathic thrombocytopenia purpura, recurrent fever, lymphoma, and wasting are common in both pediatric and adult HIV infection. Lymphadenopathy and hepatic and renal involvement also occurs in both groups.

Pediatric patients with HIV infection may have severe problems without the lymphopenia or extremely low helper lymphocyte counts as seen in adults. Unlike the case for adults, hypergammaglobulinemia is a common feature of pediatric HIV infection. Antibody production is usually nonspecific and polyclonal. B cell dysfunction is prominent, and consequently these children may not produce antibody after immunization.

HIV testing in children is less reliable than in adults. False-positive antibody tests (ELISA and Western blot) in infants can occur as a result of passive acquisition from a seropositive mother. The false-positive result may persist for as long as 1 year without apparent true infection. False-negative results also may occur as a result of B cell dysfunction in children and failure to produce specific antibody. The HIV antigen test is diagnostic of infection when positive; however, the majority of infected children have a negative test. Newer tests for HIV nucleic acids including in situ hybridization and the polymerase chain reaction for amplification of HIV DNA will facilitate the diagnosis of HIV infection in children.

Diagnosis & Prognosis

Current estimates suggest that more than 60% of HIV-infected children will develop AIDS (with a lower incidence in transfusion-acquired versus congenitally acquired infection). The disease may evolve rapidly in the first months of life or may occur insidiously over more than a 5-year period. The mother and frequently the father may also succumb to AIDS before or after the child's death, further confounding the tragedy.

Pediatric HIV infection is classified as indeterminate in asymptomatic perinatally exposed infants (< 15 months of age) who have only a positive antibody test. Diagnosis of asymptomatic HIV infection in this group requires the presence of a positive antigen test or the presence of abnormal immune studies in an HIV antibody–positive infant. Diagnosis of symptomatic HIV infection or AIDS is made with the appearance of fever or diarrhea of greater than 1 month duration, failure to thrive, wasting, progressive neurologic disease, lymphoid interstitial pneumonitis, opportunistic infection with a CDC-specified disease, two or more episodes of serious bacterial infection, or a CDC-specified secondary cancer (lymphoma, Kaposi's sarcoma). The inclusion of failure to thrive, lymphoid interstitial pneumonitis, and recurrent serious bacterial infection in the diagnosis of AIDS is unique to pediatrics.

Treatment

Children with HIV infection should be encouraged to participate in school and educational activities if possible. Infected children have the right to have the diagnosis withheld from teachers and caretakers if the children are in control of their body fluids. On the other hand, symptomatic children with obvious immunosuppression should avoid environmental contacts that could place them at risk for severe secondary infection. Live immunizations generally should not be given to HIV-infected children, but they should receive other routine vaccinations and killed poliomyelitis vaccine.

These children should be supported nutritionally, and hyperalimentation may be necessary as the disease progresses. Intravenous gammaglobulin (200–300 mg/kg) may be given every 2–3 weeks to compensate for B cell defects in some children. Zidovudine (AZT) should be considered when the disease progresses. Septra prophylaxis may be used to prevent *Pneumocystis* infection; however, it is often poorly tolerated in these patients, who demonstrate an increased incidence of myelosuppression and systemic reactions. Alternatively, aerosolized pentamidine may be considered in the older child. Amphotericin B and acyclovir may be necessary to manage fungal and viral complications. Curative therapy does not currently exist for pediatric AIDS patients, and treatment goals are limited to optimizing quality of life and minimizing inpatient hospitalization.

REFERENCES

Allegretta GJ, Weisman SJ, Altman AJ: Oncologic Emergencies I and II: Metabolic and space-occupying consequences of cancer and cancer treatment. *Pediatr Clin North Am* 1985;**32:**601.

Allen JC et al: Brain tumors in children: Current cooperative and institutional chemotherapy trials in newly diagnosed and recurrent disease. *Semin Oncol* 1986;**13:**110.

Brodeur GM et al: International criteria for diagnosis, staging, and response to treatment in patients with neuroblastoma. *J Clin Oncol* 1988;**6:**1874.

Burgert EO Jr et al: Multimodal therapy for the management of nonpelvic, localized Ewing's sarcoma of bone: Intergroup study IESS-II. *J Clin Oncol* 1990;**8:**1514.

Cavenee WK et al: Prediction of familial predisposition to retinoblastoma. *N Engl J Med* 1986;**314:**1201.

Crist WM et al: Prognosis in children with rhabdomyosarcoma: A report of the intergroup rhabdomyosarcoma studies I and I. *J Clin Oncol* 1990;**8:**443.

Finlay JL, Uteg R, Giese WL: Brain tumors in children. 2. Advances in neurosurgery and radiation oncology. *Am J Pediatr Hematol Oncol* 1987;**9:**256.

Gaynon PS et al: Modified BFM therapy for children with previously untreated acute lymphoblastic leukemia and unfavorable prognostic features: Report of Children's Cancer Study Group, study CCG-193P. *Am J Pediatr Hematol Oncol* 1988;**10:**42.

Glasser DB et al: Survival, prognosis, and therapeutic response in osteogenic sarcoma. *Cancer* 1992;**69:**698.

Grabowski EF, Abramson DH: Intraocular and extraocular retinoblastoma. *Hematol Oncol Clin North Am* 1987;**1:**721.

Hammond GD: The cure of childhood cancers. *Cancer* 1986;**58(Suppl 2):**407.

Health Guidelines for the attendance in day-care and foster care settings of children infected with human immunodeficiency virus. *Pediatrics* 1987;**79:**466.

King NMP, Cross AW: Children as decision makers: Guidelines for pediatricians. *J Pediatr* 1989;**115:**10.

Lampkin BC et al: Biologic characteristics and treatment of acute nonlymphocytic leukemia in children. *Pediatr Clin North Am* 1988;**35:**743.

Leikin S: A proposal concerning decisions to forgo life-sustaining treatment for young people. *J Pediatr* 1989;**115:**17.

Magrath IT: Malignant non-Hodgkin's lymphomas in children. *Hematol Oncol Clin North Am* 1987;**1:**577.

Maurer HM, Ruymann FB, Pochedly C: *Rhabdomyosarcoma and Related Tumors in Children and Adolescents.* CRC Press, 1991.

Miser JS, Pizzo PA: Soft tissue sarcomas in childhood. *Pediatr Clin North Am* 1985;**32:**779.

Osband ME: Histiocytosis X: Langerhans' cell histiocytosis. *Hematol Oncol Clin North Am* 1987;**1:**737.

Pao WJ, Kun LE: Hodgkin's disease in children. *Hematol Oncol Clin North Am* 1989;**3:**345.

Poplack DG, Reaman G: Acute lymphoblastic leukemia in childhood. *Pediatr Clin North Am* 1988;**35:**903.

Rowland RG: Testicular germ-cell neoplasms: Curative approaches. *Hematol Oncol Clin North Am* 1988;**2:**467.

Scott GB et al: Survival in children with perinatally acquired human immunodeficiency virus type I infection. *N Engl J Med* 1989;**321:**1791.

Trigg ME: Bone marrow transplantation for treatment of leukemia in children. **Pediatr Clin North Am** 1988;**35:**933.

Wilm's tumor: Status report, 1990. *J Clin Oncol* 1991;**9:**877.

Woods WG et al: Neuroblastoma represents distinct clinical-biologic entities: A review and perspective from the Quebec neuroblastoma screening project. *Pediatrics* 1992;**89:**114.

Yeager AM: Bone marrow transplantation in children. *Pediatr Ann* 1988;**17:**694.

AIDS-Related Malignancies

31

Geoffrey R. Weiss, MD, & Jeffrey A. Scott, MD

The acquired immunodeficiency syndrome (AIDS) emerged as a clinical entity in early 1981 with publications of reports of *Pneumocystis carinii* pneumonia and Kaposi's sarcoma in previously healthy young homosexual men. Definitions of the syndrome were quickly published by the Centers for Disease Control, recognizing the frequent occurrence of an otherwise rare malignancy as one hallmark of this condition. Over the past decade, AIDS has assumed epidemic proportions, and its clinical presentations, viral etiology, and epidemiologic behavior are now well established. Kaposi's sarcoma and a variety of other cancers are major contributors to morbidity and mortality of AIDS.

Evidence strongly supports the human immunodeficiency virus (HIV), a retrovirus identified in 1983, as the cause of AIDS. The virus has been isolated from blood, semen, bone marrow, tears, saliva, vaginal secretions, cerebrospinal fluid, urine, feces, and various other tissues. Because the mode of transmission of HIV is by blood-borne infection or by sexual transmission, major human risk groups for AIDS include homosexual or bisexual men, intravenous drug abusers, heterosexual contacts of infected individuals, infants born of infected mothers, and recipients of infected blood products. No risk factors can be identified for approximately 5% of AIDS patients. An estimated 1 million individuals in the USA have been infected by the virus; 5–7% of seropositive adults progress annually to symptomatic AIDS.

Fundamental to the clinical manifestations of AIDS are the immune abnormalities induced by the virus. Patients often present with an absolute lymphopenia, largely related to a decrease in T-helper (CD4+) lymphocytes. As the disease progresses to the frank syndrome, there is an inverted T-helper to T-suppressor ratio due mostly to a fall in the number of T-helper cells and a rise in the number of T-suppressor cells. Patients may be anergic to a battery of recall antigens and may exhibit a polyclonal hypergammaglobulinemia.

KAPOSI'S SARCOMA

In 1872, Kaposi first described an unusual tumor in the skin that he termed "idiopathic multiple pigmented sarcoma of the skin." Until the AIDS epidemic, Kaposi's sarcoma (KS) was a rare tumor, occurring with an incidence of 20–60 per 1 million population. In the AIDS population, KS is a manifestation of the syndrome in 30% of cases (epidemic variant).

Variants of KS

A. Classical KS: The majority of patients with classical KS are white men of eastern European or Mediterranean ancestry, most commonly of Italian or Jewish heritage. Classical non–AIDS-related KS occurs in a male-to-female ratio of 15:1. It is prevalent in the sixth through eighth decades of life. Patients with classical KS present with asymptomatic blue or brownish-red patches, plaques, or nodules of the skin that are confined predominantly to the lower extremities and feet. Despite their vascular appearance, the lesions do not bleed excessively when cut, and venous stasis or lymphedema may be the main symptomatic complaints. Over years' time, the lesions enlarge and coalesce, producing cosmetic problems and local invasion of bone and soft tissue. The clinical course of classical KS is indolent and relatively benign; visceral involvement rarely occurs. Median survival of patients with classical KS is 13 years, but more protracted courses are not unusual, and spontaneous regressions have been observed. One-third of classical KS patients develop a second malignancy, usually a lymphoreticular or lymphomatous condition.

B. African KS: KS is an endemic illness in equatorial Africa, constituting 3–9% of all malignancies. Unlike Burkitt's lymphoma, African KS is limited to the sub-Saharan continent. It occurs in children and in adults in the fourth through seventh decades. Males predominate in a ratio of 13:1 in adults and 3:1 in children. Children and young adults are most commonly afflicted with lymphadenopathic KS, which is characterized by massive lymph node infiltration and enlargement, frequent cutaneous involvement, and rapid progression to visceral involvement and prompt mortality. Nodular KS is the most common adult form of endemic disease. Plaquelike or nodular cutaneous lesions progress slowly and rarely become visceral in extent. Florid KS presents with more rapidly growing cutaneous lesions that become superficially eroded and may penetrate soft tissues and bone. Infiltrating KS is an aggressive form that more deeply penetrates soft tissues and often produces painful bone lesions.

C. Immunosuppression-related KS: Patients undergoing organ transplantation and requiring long-term immunosuppression are at risk of developing KS. Renal transplant recipients have a 400–500% greater incidence of KS than the general population; 0.4% of renal transplant recipients develop KS. The development of KS in this population is believed to be partially related to the use of immunosuppressive agents to prevent organ rejection. Males predominate, and the disease occurs at a mean age of 42 years. The clinical presentation may range from localized skin involvement to widespread visceral involvement. Clinical behavior may be indolent or rapidly progressive. Mucocutaneous disease may occasionally regress upon attenuation or withdrawal of immunosuppressive therapy. Death is more often related to infective complications of immunosuppression than to complications of KS except in individuals having visceral involvement.

D. Epidemic (HIV-related) KS: Epidemic KS occurs most often in HIV-infected homosexual males and less often in infected children and hemophiliacs. Cutaneous lesions begin as small, fleshy, reddish-purple plaques occurring singly, in small clusters, or in widely distributed groups. Typical sites of involvement include the tip of the nose, the forehead, the hard palate, or the alveolar ridge. With time, visceral involvement may follow the cutaneous disease, not uncommonly involving the gastrointestinal tract, the lymph nodes, or the lungs. When occurring as the sole manifestation of AIDS, epidemic KS may be slow-growing or rapidly progressive; the disease is especially lethal when associated with opportunistic infection. Occasional spontaneous regression of disease may be observed.

Pathology

There are three histopathologic variants of KS: anaplastic, spindle cell, and mixed cell. Each of these forms has been observed in the variants of KS. The mixed-cell form is the most common variant observed in HIV-related KS. Typically, this variant displays slitlike vascular structures lined by large atypical endothelial cells, surrounding spindle cells, and diffuse red cell extravasation. Few mitoses are observed, and numerous inflammatory cells may infiltrate the malignant tissue.

The cell of origin in KS remains a matter of controversy. Endothelial cells of lymphatic or vascular origin are the principal cells believed to give rise to KS lesions. A variety of etiologic agents have been proposed: infectious agents, chronic antigenic stimulation, and environmental or genetic causes. In HIV-related KS, cytomegalovirus (CMV) infection has been suggested as the cause because of the presence of CMV antibodies in patient sera, and CMV DNA sequences and antigens have been found in the KS lesions.

Staging & Clinical Findings

No staging system for HIV-related KS has provided useful information regarding prognosis or clinical management. The progression of the disease is variable, ranging from indolent to rapid progression, circumscribed to multicentric presentation, involvement of skin, lymph nodes, or viscera singly to simultaneously. The outlook seems to be better in those who present with a few geographically limited lesions. Those individuals without preceding or simultaneous infection, weight loss, fever, or night sweats ("B" symptoms or whose T-helper lymphocytes exceed 300/µL also fare better. Characteristic sites of involvement include the palate and oropharynx, tip of the nose, soles of the feet, penis, and eyelids. A "storm" of small or coalescent lesions may appear on the groin and thigh and progress centrifugally. Progression of the disease to lymph nodes had little prognostic impact, but visceral involvement, especially of the lung and gastrointestinal tract, is associated with adverse survival expectation.

KS lesions may appear in combinations of the following typical clinical pictures:

A. Cutaneous KS: Early lesions may initially appear as subcutaneous dark red or blue palpable tumor masses. These lesions may be isolated in clusters on any cutaneous site.

B. Plaque Stage and Nodular KS: KS lesions may present or evolve into large plaques commonly appearing on the soles of the feet, the lower extremities, and less commonly on the trunk or upper extremities. Exophytic lesions may occur in a similar distribution, may bleed, and may become painful. Unusually, deep invasion of the skin may produce lymphedema, nerve entrapment, or bone erosion.

C. Late-stage KS: Lymphedema of various body regions occurs with or without extensive superficial cutaneous involvement in the same distribution. The lower extremities, genitalia, and face are the most common sites of edema formation, which is clinically firm, woody in texture, and nonpitting. With sustained evidence of cutaneous or lymphatic KS, the development of visceral evidence of the disease becomes more likely. In patients with pulmonary infiltrates, pulmonary KS is a particularly ominous diagnostic development. KS may involve any portion of the gastrointestinal tract, from mouth to anus. KS lesions may reveal themselves to oropharyngeal or upper or lower gastrointestinal tract endoscopic evaluation. Other sites of visceral involvement may occur but are distinctly more unusual.

Treatment

The management of HIV-related KS is particularly challenging for the clinician, especially when confronted with existing immunosuppression and the need for effective anticancer therapy. Indeed, since most therapeutic interventions in the management of this disease are largely palliative, a strong case may be made for a period of observation in the individual whose health is not immediately threatened by the recent appearance of KS lesions. This strategy may spare the patient exposure to treatments that may be life-threatening until such risks are warranted. In addition, this approach permits the establishment of the pace of malignant growth and an estimation of the urgency of therapeutic need. The following therapies may be applied to the palliation of HIV-related KS.

A. Surgery: Surgical intervention in the management of HIV-related KS is limited to diagnostic biopsy and to excision of cosmetically troublesome or locally uncomfortable lesions. The latter approach is motivated by the presence of painful, protruding, or infected lesions. Skin healing is usually satisfactory. Further, bleeding or obstructive KS lesions in the gastrointestinal, pulmonary, or genitourinary tracts not amenable to relief by other measures may be managed surgically. However, surgery offers little in the way of curative potential or lasting control of visceral lesions.

B. Radiation Therapy: Radiation is one of the most effective palliative therapeutic tools in the control of epidemic KS. Doses as low as 3000 cGy and sometimes lower accomplish local regression of lesions. Symptomatic oropharyngel and palatine lesions may be relieved by the application of radiation therapy, particularly against a background of painful gum or mucosal lesions, malocclusion, dysphagia, or chronic mucosal infection. Therapy is likely to be accompanied by oral mucositis with secondary involvement by *Candida* sp. Maintenance of meticulous oral hygiene and analgesia will permit tolerance of such therapy.

Similarly, cutaneous lesions may be locally painful and less commonly locally invasive into nerve trunks or bone. Such lesions appearing at sites of frequent trauma, such as the soles of the feet and palms of the hands, may be particularly prone to pain, disruption, or infection. Orthovoltage or electron beam therapy may provide relief of symptoms but infrequently leads to loss of pigmentation. Deeper soft tissue involvement leading to facial or extremity lymphedema is also amenable to treatment with radiation therapy.

C. Chemotherapy: The aggressive use of chemotherapy in epidemic KS is tempered by the risk of additive immunosuppression accompanying such use. The impact of chemotherapy on the survival of KS-afflicted individuals is obscure owing to the multifold clinical conditions afflicting the AIDS patient. Careful use of the following agents may result in safe, gratifying, and prompt regression of more disseminated KS lesions.

The *Vinca* alkaloids (vinblastine, vincristine) may be used singly or in alternating combination. Vinblastine may be administered at a dosage of 0.1 mg/kg intravenously weekly, increasing the dosage as bone marrow tolerance permits. Each dose may be delivered if total granulocytes exceed 1000/mm^3 prior to each weekly dose. Toxicity of therapy is limited to leukopenia, occasional nausea and vomiting, and rare neurotoxicity and alopecia. Vincristine may be administered weekly in doses of 1.2–2 mg/m^2. This agent more commonly produces neuropathy. Both vincristine and vinblastine have produced objective antitumor responses in 20–40% of KS patients. The two agents may be utilized in these same doses on alternating weekly schedules. Such therapy seems capable of boosting the response rate to 45%. Doses of vincristine and vinblastine are reduced by 25% for disabling paresthesias or granulocyte counts below 1500/mm^3, respectively.

Doxorubicin is an active agent in epidemic KS, producing some benefit in 15–40% of treated patients. The drug may be safely administered at dosages of 15–20 mg/m^2 weekly or every other week. Leukopenia and mild alopecia may be the predominant toxicities.

Etoposide in dosages of 100–150 mg/m^2 orally or intravenously daily for 3 days every 28 days may produce responses in over 40% of patients. The drug is myelosuppressive and causes occasional nausea, vomiting, and alopecia.

Bleomycin is a minimally toxic drug that may have modest activity against KS, particularly when avoidance of myelosuppression or of immunosuppression is desired. Bleomycin may be administered on a weekly schedule in doses of 10–20 mg/m^2 intravenously. Its primary toxicities include hypersensitivity reactions, fever, and rarely pulmonary toxicity.

Combination chemotherapy for epidemic KS is rarely used, principally owing to the risk of immunosuppression and opportunistic infection. Such an approach is generally limited to individuals with rapidly progressive disease and few alternative therapeutic options.

D. Biologic Response Modifier: Alpha interferon possesses antiviral, anticancer, and immunostimulatory activity that may theoretically provide desired effects in the KS-afflicted AIDS patient. Alpha interferon is administered in dosages of 10–30 million units subcutaneously or intramuscularly daily, 5 days per week or 3 times per week. Twenty percent to 40% of treated patients may experience regression of KS. Adverse effects are frequent and may be disabling in the AIDS patient. They include fever, chills, fatigue, nausea, occasional vomiting, diarrhea, liver function abnormalities, leukopenia, thrombocytopenia, and anemia. If treatment is tolerated, it should be continued as long as the patient continues to experience some benefit in control of KS.

NON-HODGKIN'S LYMPHOMA

Various acquired or congenital immune deficiencies are associated with the development of an increased incidence of malignant lymphoma. Over the past 5 years, there has been a dramatic increase in the incidence of malignant lymphomas among HIV-infected individuals. In 1985, an epidemiologic survey conducted by the University of Southern California Surveillance Program, a cancer registry for Los Angeles County, demonstrated a significant increase in the incidence of B cell malignancies, immunoblastic lymphoma, and diffuse noncleaved small-cell lymphoma among never married males. The case definition for AIDS was revised in 1985 to include high-grade B cell lymphomas in patients with HIV-positive serology.

The cause of AIDS-related lymphoma is obscure, but a viral etiology remains an area of active investigation. Coexistent infections with HTLV-1, human B-lymphoma virus (HBLV), and Epstein-Barr virus (EBV) in patients with AIDS-related lymphoma have been reported. The role of these viruses in lymphoma causation is uncertain.

Epidemiology

Non-Hodgkin's lymphoma occurs in up to 10% of patients with AIDs. The majority are HIV-infected homosexual or bisexual men, followed in incidence by intravenous drug abusers. Thirty-one percent of lymphoma patients have had a preceding diagnosis of opportunistic infection and 18.5% a prior diagnosis of Kaposi's sarcoma. A prospective study of the natural history of persistent generalized lymphadenopathy in HIV-infected individuals disclosed a risk of B cell lymphoma exceeding 1000 times normal.

Pathology

The spectrum of non-Hodgkin's lymphoma occurring in HIV-infected patients differs from that seen in the general population. Essentially all lymphomas are of B cell origin and are high grade. In AIDS-related non-Hodgkin's lymphoma, 60–90% of patients develop high-grade lesions in contrast to a 10% incidence of high-grade lesions in the general population. Diffuse noncleaved small-cell lymphoma is first in frequency, followed by diffuse large-cell immunoblastic lymphoma. An increased incidence of intermediate-grade lymphoma, predominantly diffuse large-cell lymphoma, has recently been observed. The Centers for Disease Control has revised the definition of AIDS to include intermediate-grade lymphomas among the criteria for diagnosis. Although not included in the case definition for AIDS, chronic lymphocytic luekemia, multiple myeloma, and low-grade lymphoma are reported to be of higher incidence in HIV-infected individuals.

Staging

In most nonimmunosuppressed patients acquiring non-Hodgkin's lymphoma, the disease is characterized by lymph node involvement, and stage IE or stage IV disease occurs in only 39% of cases. In HIV-infected patients, extranodal presentation is observed in up to 85%. In comparison to the general population, non-Hodgkin's lymphoma in HIV-infected patients occurs more often in the central nervous system (CNS) and gastrointestinal tract. CNS presentation may be observed in a third of patients and may represent the sole site of disease in 15% of patients. It is noteworthy that 93% of patients with CNS lymphoma manifest bone marrow involvement by the lymphoma. "B" symptoms (fevers, night sweats, weight loss exceeding 10% of normal body weight) are common, and their presence is difficult to discriminate from similar symptoms in HIV-infected patients who contract opportunistic infection.

Treatment & Prognosis

The prototypical patient with AIDS and non-Hodgkin's lymphoma is younger than most patients with non-AIDS lymphoma, has a high-grade malignancy, presents with extranodal disease, and suffers rapidly progressive disease. Median survival is 6–10 months. CNS relapse has been reported in 25–40% of patients and is not prevented by the early and prophylactic use of chemotherapy agents intrathecally or by agents that cross the blood-brain barrier.

Patients with high-grade HIV-related non-Hodgkin's lymphoma present a difficult therapeutic challenge. The use of multiagent chemotherapy regimens at conventional dosage is accompanied by the hazard of deepening immunosuppression and the risk of accelerated mortality from opportunistic infection. Recent clinical trials suggest that the overall prognosis with systemic multiagent therapy of HIV-related non-Hodgkin's lymphoma is poorer than with systemic multiagent therapy of the same disease in the general population. Achievement of complete response is less reliable and maintenance of complete response is less durable in AIDS-related lymphoma. Furthermore, evidence suggests that multiagent chemotherapy regimens at attenuated dosage may more effectively induce durable responses without the attendant risk of mortality from opportunistic infection. Individuals with CD4+ (helper) lymphocyte counts exceeding 100 and with good performance status appear to tolerate therapy better and survive longer.

PRIMARY CNS LYMPHOMA

Lymphoma confined to the CNS represents 25% of HIV-related non-Hodgkin's lymphoma. Patients may present with a variety of nonspecific neurologic findings including headache, memory loss, somnolence, confusion, focal sensorimotor manifestations, seizures, and cranial nerve palsies. Single or multiple enhancing lesions may be observed on CT scan, and the primary differential diagnostic concern is intracranial toxoplasmosis (less commonly bacterial, fungal, or mycobacterial abscess). It is reasonable to initiate anti-*Toxoplasma* therapy and collect *Toxoplasma* serologic specimens upon detection of discrete intracranial lesions on CT scan or MRI of the brain. If the patient clinically improves after 2 weeks of observation and CT scan lesions regress in this interval, brain biopsy may be avoided. If serology is negative, the patient fails to respond to therapy, or scan findings do not regress, brain biopsy is indicated to ascertain the diagnosis.

Primary CNS lymphoma is routinely treated with whole-brain irradiation to doses of 3000–3500 cGy. Despite induction of CNS tumor regression or remission, the prognosis is poor. Mortality following whole-brain irradiation is usually a consequence of progressive CNS lymphoma or the onset of opportunistic infection.

HODGKIN'S DISEASE

Hodgkin's disease is observed in patients with AIDS but is not included at present as a case definition for AIDS. Although the incidence of Hodgkin's disease among AIDS patients is lower than that of non-Hodgkin's lymphoma, its occurrence cannot be solely attributed to its usual manifestation in this young age group. AIDS patients afflicted with Hodgkin's disease exhibit frequent extranodal involvement, poor response to therapy, and presentation at advanced stage. Mixed cellularity is the most common histologic feature. The prognosis is poor owing to a high incidence of opportunistic infection.

Although it is not clear that the incidence of Hodgkin's disease is increased in the AIDS population, the interaction of HIV infection and Hodgkin's disease does appear to affect the outcome of the disease adversely.

OTHER CANCERS

A variety of cancers unusual in the general population occur with increased frequency among the homosexual/bisexual population and secondarily in the HIV-infected population. Squamous cell carcinoma of the anus, squamous cell carcinoma of the head and neck and of the esophagus, mixed germ cell tumors of the testis, hepatocellular carcinoma, and malignant melanoma are observed in AIDS patients and may occur in unusual anatomic sites. The occurrence of these illnesses in young men was known before the emergence of AIDS.

CLINICAL TRIALS

Physicians should offer HIV-infected patients with cancer every opportunity to participate in clinical trials of new anticancer therapies. Such studies are often available through a national network of AIDS Clinical Trials Groups (ACTGs). Investigational trials permit access to potentially active new anticancer agents for treatment of this group of especially vexing cancers.

REFERENCES

Abrams D, Volberding P: Alpha interferon therapy of AIDS-associated Kaposi's sarcoma. *Semin Oncol* 1986;**13**:43.

Friedman-Klein A, Laubenstein L: Disseminated Kaposi's sarcoma in homosexual men. *Ann Intern Med* 1982;**96**:693.

Gelmann E, Longo D: Combination chemotherapy of disseminated Kaposi's sarcoma in patients with the acquired immune deficiency syndrome. *Am J Med* 1987;**82**:456.

Gill P, Levine A: AIDS-related malignant lymphoma: Results of prospective treatment trials. *J Clin Oncol* 1987;**5**:1322.

Groopman J: Neoplasms in the acquired immune deficiency syndrome: The multidisciplinary approach to treatment. *Semin Oncol* 1987;**14**:1.

Krown S: The role of interferon in the therapy of epidemic Kaposi's sarcoma. *Semin Oncol* 1987;**14**:27.

Laubenstein L, Krigel R: Treatment of epidemic Kaposi's sarcoma with etoposide or a combination of doxorubicin, bleomycin and vinblastine. *J Clin Oncol* 1984;**2**:1115.

Levine A, Gill P: Malignancies in the acquired immunodeficiency syndrome. *Curr Probl Oncol* 1987;**11**:211.

Levine A, Meyer P: Development of B-cell lymphoma in homosexual men. *Ann Intern Med* 1984;**100**:7.

Real F, Oettgen H: Kaposi's sarcoma and the acquired immunodeficiency syndrome: Treatment with high and low doses of recombinant leukocyte A interferon. *J Clin Oncol* 1986;**4**:544.

Rosenblum M, Levy R: Primary central nervous system lymphomas in patients with AIDS. *Ann Neurol* 1988;**23**:S13.

Volberding P, Conant M: Chemotherapy in advanced Kaposi's sarcoma. *Am J Med* 1983;**74**:652.

Volberding P, Abrams D: Vinblastine therapy for Kaposi's sarcoma in the acquired immunodeficiency syndrome. *Ann Intern Med* 1985;**103**:335.

Ziegler J, Beckstead J: Non-Hodgkin's lymphoma in 90 homosexual men: Relation to generalized lymphadenopathy and to the acquired immunodeficiency syndrome. *N Engl J Med* 1984;**311**:565.

Section VI.
Management of Treatment Toxicities

Nausea & Vomiting

32

Philip D. Hall, PharmD, & John G. Kuhn, PharmD

With the development of high-dose and aggressive dose-intensive chemotherapy, the management of treatment-related toxicities has become increasingly important. Nausea and vomiting can be a psychologically devastating and sometimes a life-threatening side effect of cancer chemotherapy. Twenty-five percent to 50% of patients undergoing chemotherapy will either refuse further treatment or delay a course of therapy because of uncontrolled nausea and vomiting. The potential consequences of uncontrolled nausea and vomiting include decreasing the chance for prolonged disease-free survival or cure and decreasing the patient's quality of life.

Physiology of Emesis

The three stages of emesis are nausea, retching, and vomiting. The stages do not always occur in this sequence, nor does one stage automatically lead to another stage. Nausea, an awareness of the urge to vomit, is associated with a loss of gastric tone and motility and with reflux of the duodenal contents into the stomach.

During retching, the gastric contents move forcibly upward owing to a positive abdominal pressure and a concomitant negative pressure in the thorax. The positive abdominal pressure results from a contraction of the abdominal wall musculature, while the negative intrathoracic pressure is generated by a strong inspiratory movement involving the diaphragm and chest wall muscles.

Vomiting is the coordinated expulsion of gastric contents. It involves coordination of diaphragmatic and abdominal musculature contractions along with opening of the gastric cardia.

Coordination of vomiting is under the control of the emetic center in the medulla oblongata. Areas adjacent to the emetic center include the respiratory center, vasomotor center, salivatory center, and cranial nerves VIII and X. The emetic center coordinates nausea and vomiting through these adjacent areas. The emetic center receives input from three areas: peripheral afferents, the chemoreceptor trigger zone, and the cortex. Vagal and sympathetic afferents from the periphery may activate the emetic center. Seroto-nin receptors are located in both the periphery and the chemoreceptor trigger zone. Most total body serotonin is located in the enterochromaffin cells in the gastrointestinal tract. Cisplatin can induce the release of serotonin by damaging the gastrointestinal tract. The serotonin released by the enterochromaffin cells stimulates the vagal and splanchnic nerve receptors that project into the emetic center. Increased urine concentrations of 5-hydroxyindoleacetic acid (5-HIAA), the main metabolite of serotonin, have been found in patients receiving cisplatin. The number of episodes of emesis increased as urinary concentrations of 5-HIAA increased. The chemoreceptor trigger zone, also located in the medulla oblongata, is able to detect toxins (drugs) in blood and cerebrospinal fluid. It is postulated that the chemoreceptor trigger zone signals the emetic center through certain transmitters: dopamine, histamine, enkephalins, serotonin, and prostaglandins. Histamine blockade inhibits only that vomiting due to vesticular causes. The stimulation of the emetic center by the cortex remains poorly understood. It is hypothesized that the cortex is responsible for anticipatory nausea and vomiting.

Clinical Findings

Nonspecific signs and symptoms include flushing, pallor, sweating, salivation, and tachycardia or bradycardia. All these findings are under control of the autonomic nervous system, whereas retching and vomiting are under control of the somatic nervous system.

Chemotherapy-induced nausea and vomiting has significant clinical importance. Uncontrolled nausea and vomiting can prompt dose reductions and delayed or even missed courses of chemotherapy. Uncontrolled nausea and vomiting reduces the patient's quality of life. In addition, it can cause nutrition disorders and electrolyte imbalances, including malnutrition (anorexia and malabsorption), electrolyte losses (Na^+, K^+, Cl^-, HCO_3^-, Mg^{2+}), systemic alkalosis, and dehydration. Other clinical consequences of uncontrolled nausea and vomiting include aspiration pneumonia, mucosal tears (Mallory-Weiss, Boerhaave's), and pathologic fractures.

In the cancer patient with nausea and vomiting, before these symptoms are attributed to chemotherapy, other common causes of nausea and vomiting should be ruled out (Table 32–1).

Certain patient characteristics help identify a patient's likelihood to have nausea and vomiting from a chemotherapeutic regimen. Elderly patients and patients with a history of heavy alcohol consumption have decreased nausea and vomiting with chemotherapy. Patients with susceptibility to motion sickness or with poor previous emetic control are at increased risk for chemotherapy-induced nausea and vomiting. Younger patients are at greater risk for anticipatory nausea and vomiting and have an increased incidence of dystonic reactions when receiving high-dose metoclopramide. Approximately 30% of patients younger than 30 years of age experience dystonic reactions as compared with 2% of patients over age 30.

A. Acute Nausea and Vomiting: Acute nausea and vomiting is the development of nausea or vomiting within 24 hours of chemotherapy treatment. Most clinical trials focus on the prevention of acute nausea and vomiting.

B. Anticipatory Nausea and Vomiting: Anticipatory nausea and vomiting is the development of nausea or vomiting prior to or in anticipation of chemotherapy. Risk factors are age below 50 years, treatment with agents with a high emetic potential, previous posttreatment nausea or vomiting, susceptibility to motion sickness, and prolonged treatment (> 4 months). The best treatment of anticipatory nausea and vomiting is prevention with a good antiemetic regimen. Behavioral therapy and drugs that are amnestic and anxiolytic (lorazepam, diazepam) can be effective in preventing or treating this condition.

C. Delayed Nausea and Vomiting: Delayed nausea and vomiting is the development of nausea or vomiting more than 24 hours after treatment. Cisplatin causes nausea or vomiting in 21–60% of patients 24–120 hours after therapy. Delayed nausea and vomiting is not as severe as the acute form. Patients receiving chemotherapy agents with delayed onset or long duration of nausea and vomiting should receive antiemetic prophylaxis.

Emetic Potential of Chemotherapeutic Agents

Three factors should be considered: dose, single agent or combination therapy, and onset and duration of nausea and vomiting caused by a chemotherapeutic agent (Table 32–2).

Treatment With Antiemetic Agents

Table 32–3 lists doses, schedules, and routes of administration of antiemetic agents. Figure 32–1 gives the proposed site of action.

Most clinical trials have focused on preventing acute nausea and vomiting with high-dose cisplatin regimens. These antiemetic regimens may be tried with other highly emetogenic agents or chemotherapy regimens (eg, CHOP, MOPP, ABVD; see Tables 29–4 and 29–10). Few trials have considered the less emetogenic regimens; therefore, dosing of antiemetics is generally based on the emetic potential of the chemotherapeutic agent and onset and duration of nausea and vomiting.

A. Phenothiazines: Phenothiazines are proposed to work by dopaminergic blockade in the chemoreceptor trigger zone. The piperazine derivatives (thiethylperazine, perphenazine, prochlorperazine) are more effective than aliphatic derivatives (chlorpromazine). Side effects include central nervous system depression, sedation, hypotension, and extrapyramidal effects (dystonic reactions, akathisia). High-dose prochlorperazine (0.2–1.2 mg/kg intravenously) is currently being investigated to prevent chemotherapy-induced nausea and vomiting. The dose-limiting toxicity (occurring at the 1.2 mg/kg dose level) is hypotension, which is reversed by a fluid load.

B. Butyrophonones: Butyrophonones (haloperidol, droperidol) are more potent inhibitors of dopamine in the chemoreceptor trigger zone than phenothiazines. Clinically, haloperidol and droperidol are highly effective antiemetics. Side effects include sedation, extrapyramidal effects, and hypotension.

C. Metoclopramide: Metoclopramide (a substituted benzamide) exerts its antiemetic effect at low doses by blocking dopamine receptors in the chemoreceptor trigger zone, blocking serotonin receptors at high doses, and increasing gastrointestinal motility. The antiemetic efficacy and toxicity of metoclopramide are dose-and route-related. Standard doses (10 mg orally or intravenously) of metoclopramide will not provide adequate protection against highly emetogenic agents such as cisplatin. Higher doses of metoclopramide (0.5–3 mg/kg intravenously) administered on a regular schedule before and after chemotherapy, reduces or eliminates nausea and vomiting in the majority of patients receiving even highly

Table 32–1. Common causes of nausea and vomiting in cancer patients.

Central nervous system
Drug-induced (narcotics, antifungals)
Increased intracranial pressure (primary tumor, metastasis)
Severe or chronic pain
Anticipatory nausea and vomiting

Gastrointestinal
Gastric outlet obstruction
Radiation enteritis
Hepatic metastasis
Uremia

Metabolic
Hypercalcemia
Hypoadrenalism

Table 32–2. Emetic potential of chemotherapeutic agents.

Incidence	Agent	Dose (mg/m^2)	Onset (hours)	Duration (hours)
Very high (>90%)	Cisplatin	≥75	1–6	24–120
	Dacarbazine (DTIC)	>500	1–3	1–12
	Melphalan (L-PAM)	180	3–6	6–12
	Nitrogen mustard	6	5–2	8–24
	Cytarabine	>1000	Related to rate of infusion	2–4
	Cyclophosphamide[1]	2200 (60 mg/kg)	4–12	12–24
	Carmustine (BCNU)	≥200	2–4	4–24
	Lomustine (CCNU)	≥60	2–6	4–6
	Streptozocin	>500	1–4	12–24
High (60–90%)	Cisplatin	60–75	1–6	24–120
	Dacarbazine	<500	1–3	1–12
	Cytarabine	250–1000	6–12	3–5
	Carmustine	<200	2–4	4–24
	Cyclophosphamide[1]	1000–2000	4–12	12–24
	Lomustine	<60	2–6	4–6
	Doxorubicin	75	4–6	6+
	Methotrexate	≥250	4–12	3–12
	Mitomycin	10	1–4	48–72
	Procarbazine	100	24–27	Variable
	Azacitidine	200	1–3	3–4
Moderate (30–60%)	Cisplatin	<60	1–6	24–120
	Cyclophosphamide	500–1000	4–12	12–24
	Methotrexate	≥100, <250	4–12	3–12
	Doxorubicin	>20, <75	4–6	6+
	Fluorouracil	≥1000	3–6	- - -
	Vinblastine	6	4–8	- - -
	Teniposide (VM-26)	60–170	3–8	- - -
	Asparaginase	>5000 U	1–3	- - -
	Busulfan	148 (4 mg/kg)	- - -	- - -
	Pentostatin	2–4	- - -	- - -
	Carboplatin	>120	6–12	24
	Ifosfamide	1200	1–2	- - -
	Etoposide (VP-16)[2]	>100	3–8	- - -
Low (10–30%)	Methotrexate	<100	4–12	3–12
	Fluorouracil	<1000	3–6	- - -
	Doxorubicin	≤20	4–6	6+
	Cytarabine	≤20	6–12	3–5
	Bleomycin	10 U	3–6	- - -
	Mercaptopurine	100	4–8	- - -
	Hydroxyurea	1000–6000	6–12	- - -
	Mitoxantrone	10–14	- - -	- - -
Very low (<10%)	Vincristine	1.4	4–8	- - -
	Chlorambucil	1–3	48–72	- - -
	Busulfan	2–6	- - -	- - -
	Thioguanine	100	4–8	- - -
	Cyclophosphamide (oral)	100	- - -	- - -
	Interferon (α, B, γ)[3]	Variable	- - -	- - -

[1]Aberrant taste (metallic or salty).
[2]Incidence is greater with oral preparation.
[3]Nausea and vomiting more frequent with α-interferon doses ≥10 million units.

emetogenic chemotherapy regimens. Side effects include diarrhea, sedation, and extrapyramidal effects (dystonic reactions, akathisia).

D. Serotonin Antagonists: Ondansetron is the only serotonin antagonist approved for use in the USA at this time. Serotonin antagonists selectively bind to the 5-hydroxytryptamine (5-HT$_3$, serotonin) receptors. Their mechanism of action is thought to be serotonin blockade in the periphery (vagus nerve) and the chemoreceptor trigger zone. Clinical trials have found these agents to be effective against high-

dose cisplatin and to lack extrapyramidal side effects. Side effects include headache, mild sedation, diarrhea, dry mouth, transient elevations in liver transaminases, and dizziness. Other serotonin antagonists under investigation are granisetron and ICS 205–930.

E. Corticosteroids: The mechanism of action of corticosteroids (dexamethasone, methylprednisolone) is unknown, but it is postulated that inhibition of prostaglandin synthesis may be responsible for its antiemetic activity. A corticosteroid in combination with metoclopramide, a phenothiazine, a butyro-

Table 32–3. Antiemetic drugs.

Agent	Dose/Schedule	Route of Administration	Side Effect
Phenothiazines			
Prochlorperazine (Compazine)	5–10 mg every 4–6 hours	PO, IM, IV	Extrapyramidal effects, sedation, hypotension
	25 mg every 6–8 hours	PR	
Thiethylperazine (Norzine, Torecan)	10 mg every 6–8 hours	PO, IM, IV, PR	
Perphenazine (Trilafon, others)	4–6 mg every 6 hours	PO, IM, IV	
Butyrophenones			
Haloperidol (Haldol, others)	1–3 mg every 2–8 hours	PO, IM, IV	Sedation, extrapyramidal effects, hypotension
Droperidol (Inapsine, Innovar, others)	10 mg, then 4 mg every 2 hours for 4 doses	IV	
Corticosteroids			
Dexamethasone (many preparations)	10–20 mg every 6–12 hours	IV	Insomnia, mood change, hyperglycemia
	8 mg twice daily for 2 days, then 4 mg twice daily for 2 days	PO	
Methylprednisolone (Medrol, others)	125–500 mg every 6 hours	IV	
Benzamides			
Metoclopramide (Reglan, others)	2 mg/kg every 2 hours for 5 doses	IV	Sedation, extrapyramidal effects, diarrhea, akathisia, bronchospastic reaction
	3 mg/kg every 2 hours for 2 doses	IV	
	3 mg/kg load, then 0.5 mg/kg/h for 12 hours	IV (continuous)	
	0.5–3 mg/kg every 2–6 hours	PO	
Serotonin antagonists			
Ondansetron (Zofran)	0.15 mg/kg every 4 hours for 3 doses	IV	Headache, hiccups, sedation, diarrhea, dizziness, transient increase in liver transaminases
	0.3 mg/kg pre- and 3.5 hours postchemotherapy	IV	
	8 mg IV load, then 1 mg/h for 24 hours	IV (continuous)	
	32 mg for 1 dose prechemotherapy	IV	
	8 mg every 8 hours for 2–3 days	PO	
Cannabinoids			
Dronabinol (Marinol)	5–10 mg/m^2 every 3–4 hours	PO	Sedation, euphoria, hypotension, memory loss, dysphoric reactions, dry mouth, ataxia
Others			
Lorazepam (Ativan, others)	1–2 mg/m2 every 4 hours (maximum dose, 3 mg)	PO, IV	Sedation, hypotension
Diphenhydramine (Benadryl, others)	25–50 mg every 4–6 hours	PO, IV	Sedation, anticholinergic effects
Benztropine (Cogentin, others)	1–2 mg every 8 hours	PO, IV	Anticholinergic effects
Combination therapy (for cisplatin-containing moderate to highly emetic regimens)			
Ondanstron[2]	0.15 mg/kg IV 30 minutes prechemotherapy, then every 4 hours for 3 doses		
Dexamethasone	20 mg IV 30 minutes prechemotherapy		
Metoclopramide[2,3]	2 mg/kg IV 30 minutes prechemotherapy, then every 2 hours for 3–4 doses		
Dexamethasone	20 mg IV 30 minutes prechemotherapy		
Lorazepam	1–2 mg IV 30 minutes prechemotherapy		
Diphenhydramine	25–50 mg IV 30 minutes prechemotherapy		

[1]PO = orally; IV = intravenously; IM = intramuscularly; PR = rectally.
[2]For other schedules, see individual drugs.
[3]Alternative choice is haloperidol or droperidol.

phonone, or ondansetron is more effective than any of these agents used alone. Side effects are generally minimal and well tolerated. They include mild euphoria, insomnia, lethargy, mood changes, hyperglycemia, and perianal itching associated with a rapid infusion.

F. Benzodiazepines: Benzodiazepines (lorazepam, diazepam) do not have a direct antiemetic ef-

fect. Their activity is mediated through their amnestic or anxiolytic effects. Lorazepam and diazepam may be useful in preventing akathesia but not dystonic reactions when used in combination with dopamine blockers. These agents are particularly useful in preventing and treating anticipatory nausea and vomiting. Side effects include sedation, drowsiness, urinary incontinence, and anterograde amnesia.

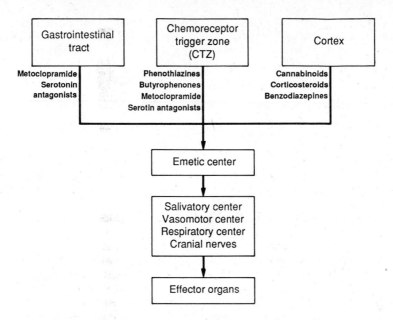

Figure 32–1. Physiology of nausea and vomiting and antiemetic sites of action.

G. Cannabinoids: The mechanism of action of cannabinoids (dronabinol, nabilone) is poorly understood. Interference with higher cortical input, inhibition of prostaglandin synthesis, or inhibition of cyclic AMP synthesis have been proposed for their antiemetic effects. Side effects include sedation, dry mouth, dizziness, confusion, ataxia, nervousness or anxiety, dysphoric reactions (hallucinations, fear, paranoia), and depressed mood. The presence of a "high" has been associated with the cannabinoid's antiemetic activity; however, the concomitant use of phenothiazines can block the "high" while maintaining antiemetic efficacy.

H. Antihistamines: Antihistamines (diphenhydramine) and anticholinergics (benztropine) are often used in antiemetic regimens to control extrapyramidal side effects of metoclopramide, phenothiazines, or butyrophenones. They may have activity in patients with a history of motion sickness but have little to no activity in chemotherapy-induced nausea and vomiting as single agents.

I. Antiemetic Combinations:

1. The addition of dexamethasone (10–20 mg orally or intravenously) and diphenhydramine (50 mg intravenously) improved the antiemetic control of metoclopramide (2 mg/kg intravenously for 5 doses) in patients receiving high-dose cisplatin. Short-course metoclopramide (3 mg/kg intravenously for 2 doses) with dexamethasone and diphenhydramine is equally effective. Short-course metoclopramide may be better suited for outpatient use, but it is associated with a higher incidence of delayed nausea and vomiting. A comparison of the addition of lorazepam (1.5 mg/m^2 for one dose intravenously, maximum

dose = 3 mg) or diphenhydramine (50 mg intravenously for one dose) to short-course metoclopramide and dexamethasone (20 mg intravenously for one dose) found no difference between the two regimens. Less akathisia and anxiety was observed in the lorazepam-treated group. A continuous infusion of metoclopramide (3 mg/kg intravenous bolus, then 0.5 mg/kg/h for 12 hours) is as effective as bolus-dose metoclopramide (2 mg/kg intravenously for 5 doses) in patients receiving high-dose cisplatin. This method of administration may be useful in bone marrow transplant recipients and inpatients.

2. A study comparing ondansetron (0.15 mg/kg intravenously every 4 hours for 3 doses) to metoclopramide (2 mg/kg intravenously every 2 hours for 3 doses, then every 3 hours for 3 doses) in patients receiving high-dose cisplatin ($\geq$ 100 mg/m^2) found that patients receiving ondansetron had a higher rate of complete response (40% versus 30%), a higher complete plus major response rate (65% versus 51%), and a lower median number of emetic episodes (one versus two) than did patients receiving metoclopramide. The addition of dexamethasone (20 mg intravenously before chemotherapy) to ondansetron (0.15 mg/kg for one dose before chemotherapy, then every 4 hours for 2 doses after chemotherapy) increased the complete protection from nausea and vomiting as compared to ondansetron alone in patients receiving cisplatin-based chemotherapy.

3. Haloperidol (3 mg intravenously for 5 doses) in an alternative to metoclopramide (2 mg/kg intravenously for 5 doses) in patients receiving cisplatin (>70 mg/m^2); however, metoclopramide demonstrates a small advantage in controlling nausea and vomiting. Droperidol has also been suggested as an alternative to metoclopramide. The addition of dexamethasone and lorazepam with or without diphenhydramine may improve the efficacy of haloperidol and droperidol. Dronabinol and nabilone have also been suggested as alternatives in patients with refractory chemotherapy-induced nausea and vomiting.

4. Of patients receiving high-dose cisplatin, 20–68% will experience delayed nausea and vomiting. The above regimens offer good protection for acute nausea and vomiting but offer no protection for delayed nausea and vomiting. The combination of oral metoclopramide (0.5 mg/kg 4 times daily for 4 days) plus oral dexamethasone (8 mg twice a day for 2 days, then 4 mg twice a day for 2 days) was more effective than oral dexamethasone alone or placebo in preventing delayed nausea and vomiting in patients receiving high-dose cisplatin. This regimen is begun 24 hours after the patient receives chemotherapy. Patients still require an appropriate antiemetic regimen to prevent the acute nausea and vomiting. Oral antiemetics can be effective in patients with delayed nausea and vomiting, and the use of other oral antiemetics (haloperidol, prochlorperazine) may also be considered to prevent delayed nausea and vomiting.

Treatment Recommendations

Antiemetics are more effective when administered prophylactically. They should begin 0.5–24 hours before chemotherapy and be given "around-the-clock" and *not* as needed. Posttreatment therapy should continue for 12–120 hours after therapy depending on prior patient response and the emetic potential (onset and duration) of the chemotherapeutic agents.

Supportive care measures may improve the response rate of antiemetics. Sympathetic personnel, avoidance of harsh colors and smells in the clinic, and a quiet and relaxing environment may improve the patient's antiemetic control. The use of hard candy to mask the metallic taste caused by such agents as cyclophosphamide may be beneficial. Patients should be instructed to avoid hot (spicy) and greasy foods for a few days following therapy and to eat lightly on the day of treatment. Patients should be cautioned to avoid their favorite foods on the day before and the day after treatment because food aversions can develop during therapy. Patients who receive sedative antiemetics in the clinic should be advised to arrange for transportation.

REFERENCES

Agostinucci WA et al: Continuous intravenous infusion versus multiple bolus doses of metoclopramide for prevention of cisplatin-induced emesis. *Clin Pharm* 1988;**7:** 454.

Cebeddu LX et al: Efficacy of ondansetron and the role of serotonin in cisplatin-induced nausea and vomiting. *N Engl J Med* 1990;**322:**810.

Craig JB, Powell BL: Management of nausea and vomiting in clinical oncology. (Review.) *Am J Med Sci* 1987;**293:** 34.

Gralla RJ et al: Antiemetic efficacy of high-dose metoclopramide: Randomized trials with placebo and prochlorperazine in patients with chemotherapy-induced nausea and vomiting. *N Engl J Med* 1981;**305:**905.

Grunberg SM et al: Comparison of antiemetic effect of high-dose intravenous metoclopramide and high-dose intravenous haloperidol in a randomized double-blind crossover study . *J Clin Oncol* 1984;**2:**782.

Hainsworth J et al: A single-blind comparison of intravenous ondansetron, a selective serotonin antagonist, with intravenous metoclopramide in the prevention of nausea and vomiting associated with high-dose cisplatin chemotherapy. *J Clin Oncol* 1991;**9:**721.

Kelley SL et al. Trial of droperidol as an antiemetic in cisplatin chemotherapy. *Cancer Treat Rep* 1986;**70:**469.

Kris MG et al: Controlling delayed vomiting: Double-blind, randomized trial comparing placebo, dexamethasone alone, and metoclopramide plus dexamethasone in patients receiving cisplatin. *J Clin Oncol* 1989;**7:**108.

Kris MG et al: Incidence, course, and severity of delayed nausea and vomiting following the administration of high-dose cisplatin. *J Clin Oncol* 1985;**3:**1379.

Lindley CM, Bernard S, Fields SM: Incidence and duration of chemotherapy-induced nausea and vomiting in the outpatient oncology population. *J Clin Oncol* 1989;**7:** 1142.

Morrow GR: Chemotherapy-related nausea and vomiting: Etiology and management. *CA* 1989;**39:**89.

Roila F et al: Prevention of cisplatin-induced emesis: A double-blind multicenter randomized crossover study comparing ondansetron and ondansetron plus dexamethasone. *J Clin Oncol* 1991;**9:**675.

Oral Complications of Cancer Therapy

33

Spencer W. Redding, DDS

COMPLICATIONS SECONDARY TO CHEMOTHERAPY

Rapidly dividing cancer cells are the primary target for cancer chemotherapy. Cells that are undergoing accelerated growth and division are more sensitive to the effects of chemotherapy. Normal cells that rapidly divide are also susceptible to cancer chemotherapy. These cells include bone marrow, gastrointestinal mucosa (including oral mucosa), reproductive cells, and hair. Disruption of cellular activity of the oral mucosa and the bone marrow leads to breakdown of selected oral tissues. As a result, odontogenic infection, oral hemorrhage, and oral mucositis can occur, and oral complications of chemotherapy are common. Approximately one-fourth of patients receiving cancer chemotherapy, or 250,000 patients in the USA, experience oral complications secondary to cancer chemotherapy each year.

Odontogenic Infection

Odontogenic infection (involving the teeth and their supporting structures) in the patient receiving cancer chemotherapy predisposes that patient to significant morbidity and even mortality. The neutropenia resulting from bone marrow suppression secondary to cancer chemotherapy can result in systemic spread of an oral infection that otherwise would be limited to the oral cavity in a healthy patient. These infections result from one of three causes: (**1**) periapical infection secondary to severe tooth decay involving a tooth pulp, (**2**) periodontal infection secondary to loss of supporting bone surrounding the teeth, or (**3**) pericoronal infection commonly associated with partially impacted third molar teeth (Figure 33–1). In a normal healthy individual, such infections would be limited to the oral cavity. In the patient receiving chemotherapy, oral organisms associated with these infections are a significant cause of septicemia. Since patients receiving cancer chemotherapy commonly become neutropenic approximately 7 days after chemotherapy is begun, potential sources of odontogenic infection should be eliminated prior to initiation of chemotherapy.

Diagnosis and elimination of sources of odontogenic infection prior to the initiation of cancer chemotherapy is the mainstay of management to prevent the serious sequelae of these infections. The patient requires a thorough intraoral evaluation, including x-rays, by dental personnel as soon as the determination for cancer chemotherapy is made. The periodontal status of all remaining teeth should also be evaluated. Potential sources of odontogenic infection must be eliminated by tooth extraction, root canal therapy, or oral prophylaxis. Since there is commonly little time before chemotherapy begins, dental diagnosis and treatment should be performed in an aggressive manner. If the patient is already neutropenic, the use of prophylactic antibiotics should be considered with any dental therapy. Because of a shift in oral flora toward more gram-negative organisms in patients receiving cancer chemotherapy, a broad-spectrum synthetic penicillin such as ticarcillin with clavulanic acid should be used (Table 33–1). Other therapies that should be performed prior to chemotherapy are the (**1**) restoration of any gross carious lesions in the remaining teeth, (**2**) elimination of any rough or sharp edges on the remaining teeth, and (**3**) institution of oral hygiene instruction and subsequent reinforcement during chemotherapy.

If aggressive prechemotherapy oral evaluation and treatment is performed, odontogenic infections during chemotherapy should be largely eliminated. If odontogenic infection does occur after chemotherapy has begun, treatment is more difficult. If the patient's neutrophil count is less than 500, the dental and medical personnel managing the patient must determine whether to treat the patient or wait until the neutropenia resolves. If the decision is made to treat the patient and if tooth extraction or periodontal scaling is necessary, the patient must have a platelet count of at least 50,000. With tooth extraction, local measures of hemostasis can be employed. An absorbable gelatin sponge (Gelfoam) or microfibrillar collagen powder (Avitene) soaked with thrombin may be placed in the extraction socket to speed hemostasis. (The patient should also receive prophylactic antibiotics when neutropenic.)

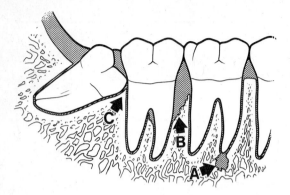

Figure 33–1. *A:* Periapical infection occurs at the root end of the tooth secondary to dental decay. *B:* Periodontal infection surrounds the tooth secondary to periodontal disease. *C:* Pericoronal infection occurs under a flap of gum tissue around a tooth that has inadequate space to erupt properly (usually a mandibular third molar).

Hemorrhage

Bone marrow toxicity secondary to chemotherapy results in a decreased production of megakaryocytes, which in turn can significantly reduce the number of circulating platelets (thrombocytopenia). The resulting thrombocytopenia can lead to significant complications whenever hemorrhage is present in the body. The structures of the oral cavity receive a rich blood supply, and bleeding is common with all types of oral manipulation. Oral bleeding can be a particular problem in patients who already have inflammation present as gingivitis or periodontal disease. The most common forms of oral bleeding in this patient population are gingival hemorrhage and hematoma formation (Figure 33–2). Postoperative bleeding secondary to any type of dental surgical procedure can be difficult to control. Therefore it is critical to eliminate potential sources of oral hemorrhage prior to initiation of cancer chemotherapy.

The mainstay of prevention of oral hemorrhage during cancer chemotherapy is the elimination of sources of oral inflammation prior to the initiation of chemotherapy. This is accomplished by tooth extraction, root canal therapy, or oral prophylaxis. If localized oral bleeding should occur, some local measures can be applied. Initially, digital pressure can be applied with moistened cotton gauze. This can be supplemented by applying topical thrombin to the gauze to act as a hemostatic agent. Avitene powder can be applied to localized areas of gingival bleeding. This will act as a matrix for clot formation in the area. If generalized gingival bleeding occurs, Avitene powder can be applied in 2 custom-made plastic oral carrier (Figure 33–3). If bleeding does not respond to the above local measures, the patient probably will need a platelet transfusion in order to raise the platelet count to achieve adequate hemostasis.

Oral Mucositis

Oral mucositis (inflammation of oral mucosal tissues commonly with ulceration) is often a serious complication of cancer chemotherapy. These areas of ulceration can be generalized or localized and often cause the patient severe discomfort. If severe enough, this oral pain will lead to a reduction in oral intake, thus compromising the patient's nutritional status at a time when adequate nutrition is essential. An often overlooked consequence of oral mucositis secondary to cancer chemotherapy is the potential for spread of oral organisms to the systemic circulation through ulcerated tissue. These ulcers can be the portal of entry for bacterial, fungal, and viral organisms.

A. Direct Toxicity–Induced Mucositis: Direct toxicity–induced oral mucositis is considered to be the result of a direct effect of the chemotherapeutic agents on oral epithelium. Oral epithelium is a rapidly dividing cell type and therefore very susceptible to the effect of cancer chemotherapy. The chemotherapeutic agent is toxic to the DNA of the basal cell layer of the oral epithelium. Surface layers of cells continue to exfoliate even though the basal layers are not being replaced, resulting in ulceration of the affected tissue. This process is characterized by an initial generalized tissue erythema followed by a white pseudomembrane formation. The pseudomembrane then sloughs off, leaving ulcerated tissue beneath (Figure 33–4). Direct toxicity–induced mucositis usually occurs within 7–10 days following the initiation of chemotherapy and heals subsequent to cessation of the treatment.

B. Indirect Toxicity-Induced Mucositis: Indirect toxicity–induced oral mucositis is believed to be a result of the effect of chemotherapy on the bone marrow, rendering the patient less able to fight infection. This leads to infection of oral tissue by opportunistic organisms, including normal oral bacteria, fungi (primarily *candida*), and viruses (primarily herpes virus).

1. Bacterial–Bacterial infection usually involves secondary infection of an area of existing chronic infection (eg, periodontal lesions) or secondary infection of an area of trauma (eg, from chewing or oral manipulation). Oral ulceration spreads from the initial area of tissue breakdown. These lesions progress during the period of the patient's neutropenia at the nadir of the neutrophil count, beginning approximately 12–16 days after the initiation of chemotherapy. These lesions usually heal or regress as the neutrophil count returns to normal.

2. Fungal–The most common fungal organism that initiates mucositis is *Candida albicans*. It commonly presents as a white curdlike covering on an oral soft tissue (Figure 33–5). Patients may complain of a burning sensation but often are unaware of the presence of infection. When the white areas are rubbed from the tissue, a red inflamed surface is exposed. Frank ulceration, however, is uncommon. Re-

Table 33–1. Drugs commonly used to treat oral complications of cancer therapy.

Drug	Dosage	Comment
Ticarcillin with clavulanic acid (Timentin)	3.1 g 1 hour before procedure, then 3.1 g 6 hours later.	Extend postoperative dosing if delayed wound healing is a concern. Amoxicillin with clavulanic acid (Augmentin), 500 mg every 8 hours, can be used postoperatively if an oral medication is desired.
Acyclovir (Zovirax) sterile powder	5 mg/kg every 8 hours for 7 days.	Prepare with sterile water. ***Caution:*** Transfuse over at least 1 hour to prevent renal tubular damage.
Acyclovir (Zovirax) capsules	200 mg orally 5 times per day for 7 days.	Prophylaxis: Patients who are seropositive for HSV prior to bone marrow transplantation should begin acyclovir therapy, 200 mg 3 times per day for 1 day, before their conditioning chemotherapy and continue for 6 weeks. If oral mucositis develops and oral intake is compromised, begin intravenous acyclovir, 5 mg/kg every 8 hours. Reinstitute oral acyclovir when oral intake resumes.
Nystatin (Mycostatin, others) oral suspension	Rinse with 4 mL for 2 minutes, and swallow, 4 times per day.	
Clotrimazole (Mycelex, others) troches	Dissolve 1 troche (10 mg) in mouth 5 times per day for 14 days.	
Ketoconazole (Nizoral) tablets	200 mg/d.	
Fluoconazole (Diflucan) tablets	100 mg/d.	
Lidocaine (Xylocaine, others) viscous solution	Rinse with 1 tablespoonful, and expectorate, every 2 hours.	
Dyclonine (Dyclone) 1% topical solution	Rinse with 1 teaspoonful, and expectorate, every 2 hours.	Prepare 50% mixture by volume with magnesium hydroxide (eg, Milk of Magnesia).
Carboxypropylcellulose tannic acid gel with benzocaine (Oratect)		Apply gel to areas of oral ulceration, and let dry. Reapply when previous application has sloughed.
Chlorhexidine (Peridex) oral rinse	Rinse with 15 mL vigorously for 30 seconds, and expectorate, 3 times per day after meals.	Continue during period of chemotherapy.
Stannous fluoride (Gel-Kam, others) gel 0.4%	Apply 8 drops in custom-made oral tray, and place in mouth 5 minutes per day.	
Fluocinonide (Lidex, others) gel 0.05%	Apply to ulcerated area 4 times per day with cotton swab.	

cent data suggest that oral candidiasis is a more common vector for systemic candidiasis in the cancer chemotherapy patient than was previously thought. Most patients who develop candidal fungemia while on chemotherapy will have had preexisting oral candidiasis. Multiple areas of tissue ulceration as a result of oral mucositis can be an entry source for *Candida* into the bloodstream.

3. Viral–Herpes simplex virus (HSV) appears to play a significant role in complicating oral mucositis. These infections reflect a reactivation of HSV, not primary infections. Patients who are significantly immunosuppressed, such as those receiving chemotherapy, commonly develop oral soft tissue lesions complicated by reactivation of the virus. These ulcerations differ in appearance and duration from those herpes simplex ulcers that occur in otherwise healthy patients. These ulcerations can appear in any

soft tissue area in the oral and circumoral region. The lesions are large, involve multiple areas, and are painful (Figure 33–6). Up to 40% of mucositis lesions that occur in patients on cancer chemotherapy are complicated by HSV reactivation.

C. Treatment: Health care personnel can have significant impact on reducing patient morbidity secondary to cancer therapy in the management and treatment of oral mucositis. Identifying the cause is critical. All lesions should be evaluated for HSV. The most reliable technique is viral culturing on each lesion. If viral culturing is not available, other techniques can be used such as exfoliative cytology and immunofluorescence staining using polyclonal and monoclonal antibodies. A high degree of suspicion for HSV should be maintained by treating personnel. All lesions should also be evaluated for this Candida by means of Gram's stain or a potassium hydroxide

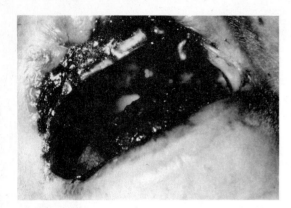

Figure 33–2. Severe intraoral bleeding in a patient who was thrombocytopenic secondary to cancer chemotherapy.

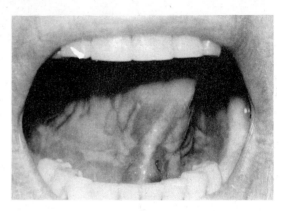

Figure 33–4. Generalized oral mucositis of the ventral surface of the tongue secondary to the direct effect of cancer chemotherapy.

wet preparation. Culture results of these lesions may be misleading, since many patients are oral carriers of *Candida albicans* but do not have clinical infection.

A patient who is positive for HSV should be treated with either intravenous or oral acyclovir (Table 33–1). In general, oral acyclovir is used for outpatients with less severe disease and intravenous acyclovir for inpatients with more severe disease. If a patient's lesion is positive for *Candida albicans,* the patient should be treated with nystatin oral suspension, clotrimazole troches, ketoconazole tablets, or fluconazole tablets (Table 33–1). For cost reasons, it is preferable to begin treatment with nystatin oral suspension. If this is not effective, the patient should be switched to clotrimazole troches; as a last treatment, the patient should be switched to ketoconazole or fluconazole. The patient's liver function should be monitored if ketoconazole or fluconazole is used.

The patient should be given a topical anesthetic for oral pain relief. Viscous lidocaine or dyclonine mixed with magnesium hydroxide (eg, Milk of Magnesia) can be utilized. A carboxypropylcellulose tannic acid gel combined with benzocaine (Oratect) can be used to treat large areas of oral ulceration. Acting as an oral bandage, this combination has been shown to provide significant pain relief for up to 3 hours (Table 33–1). If the patient's oral pain is severe, systemic pain medication should be utilized. The commonly available parenteral narcotics are drugs of choice.

Antimicrobial mouth rinses may help reduce oral complications of cancer chemotherapy. One such oral rinse, chlorhexidine, has been shown to decrease the severity of oral mucositis in patients receiving cancer chemotherapy. It is thought to exert this action by reducing the load of oral bacteria, thus lessening the secondary effect of oral bacteria in mucositis. Chlorhexidine has also been found to have antifungal properties and to be effective against *Candida al-*

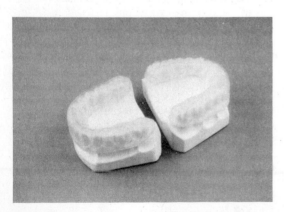

Figure 33–3. Custom-made plastic oral carriers that can be used for Avitene powder or daily fluoride treatments.

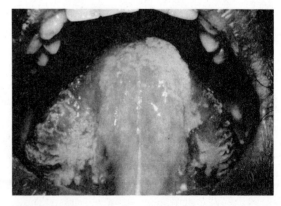

Figure 33–5. Candidiasis of the ventral surface of the tongue in a patient receiving cancer chemotherapy. (Courtesy of CS Miller, DDS.)

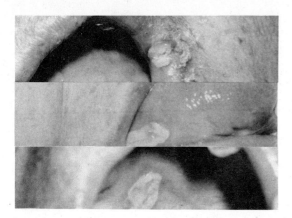

Figure 33–6. Herpes simplex virus infection of the oral commissure **(A)**, lateral border of the tongue **(B)**, and palate **(C)** in a patient receiving cancer chemotherapy.

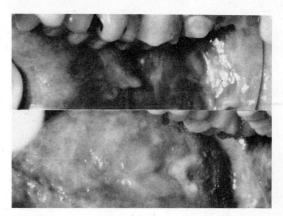

Figure 33–7. Oral mucositis secondary to graft-versus-host disease in an allogeneic bone marrow transplant patient. **A:** buccal mucosa. **B:** Lateral border of the tongue. Both are reverse views taken with oral mirrors (Courtesy of D Haslam, DDS.)

bicans. Chlorhexidine should be considered as a prophylactic oral rinse during chemotherapeutic regimens to cut down on secondary oral infection (Table 33–1).

Complications Specific to Bone Marrow Transplant Patients

Patients receiving bone marrow transplantation receive high doses of chemotherapy and often total body irradiation. As a result, oral complications are more severe. Oral mucositis tends to be more aggressive and lasts longer. HSV infection is more frequent; up to 60% of mucositis lesions have an HSV component that responds to acyclovir therapy.

Graft-versus-host disease (GVHD) is a common complication of allogeneic bone marrow transplantation. Oral involvement includes chronic oral mucositis and xerostomia. The mucositis can range from simple tissue erythema to frank ulceration, with patient discomfort directly related to the amount of tissue ulceration (Figure 33–7). Duration of mucositis may be short in acute GVHD or may remain a permanent complication of chronic GVHD.

Xerostomia results from the Sjögren's syndrome–like effects of GVHD on the salivary glands. Salivary flow can be greatly reduced, and salivary constituents are altered. Sodium and lysozyme levels are increased, whereas phosphate and IgA levels are decreased. These salivary changes make the patient prone to aggressive dental decay.

Diagnosis of GVHD can be aided by oral soft tissue biopsies. Labial mucosal and minor salivary gland biopsies can help grade the extent of GVHD. Treatment of GVHD-induced mucositis usually involves topical (eg, Lidex) and then systemic (eg, oral prednisone) corticosteroids (Table 33–1). Prevention of dental decay secondary to xerostomia is critical. Patients must practice scrupulous oral hygiene in-cluding brushing and flossing. Custom-made oral fluoride carriers should be used daily (Figure 33–3). Chlorhexidine oral rinses should be considered.

Acyclovir prophylaxis is a rational preventive therapy in bone marrow transplant patients who are seropositive for HSV prior to transplant.

COMPLICATIONS SECONDARY TO HEAD & NECK RADIOTHERAPY

Head and neck irradiation resulting in significant oral changes can mainly be confined to those tumors that involve the oral and perioral structures. More than 30,000 patients are diagnosed each year in the USA with oral cancer and nearly 50% receive head and neck irradiation as part of their therapy. Side effects of irradiation to oral structures, if not treated aggressively, can result in significant patient morbidity. It is common for head and neck radiotherapy to be curative but to leave the patient with a serious permanent oral side effect.

Radiation combines with water in cells to form free radicals that disrupt the nucleotide sequence in genetic material, causing cell death. Because of this action on the genetic level, cells that undergo rapid mitosis such as tumor cells are radiosensitive. Normal cells that undergo rapid cell division are sensitive to the effect of radiation as well. Commonly involved tissues in the oral cavity include epithelial cells, alveolar osteoblasts, and osteocytes. Glandular acinar ductal cells of salivary glands are radiosensitive as well. The side effects of radiation lead to the oral complications of mucositis, xerostomia, radiation caries, and osteoradionecrosis.

Oral Mucositis

Oral mucositis secondary to head and neck irradiation is a direct result of the effect of irradiation on the DNA of the basal cell layer of oral epithelium. Growth of these cells is diminished. Cells superficial to the basal cell layer continue to exfoliate in a normal pattern. Since the basal cell layer is not being replenished, the epithelium progressively thins and eventually ulcerates.

The presentation of oral mucositis begins with a reddening of the involved epithelium. A whitish membrane, which represents sloughing epithelial tissue, then forms and eventually exfoliates, leaving an ulcerated surface for the duration of the mucositis (Figure 33–8). This process usually begins approximately 2 weeks following the initiation of radiation therapy and lasts 2–3 weeks following the last treatment. Patients experience pain, burning, hoarseness, sensitivity to spicy foods, and difficulty speaking or swallowing.

Mucositis can be seen with total radiation doses of as low as 1000 cGy but is more common with doses of greater than 2000 cGy. Since most patients receive 6000–7000 cGy, oral mucositis is often severe. The most common opportunistic infection that develops is secondary to the organism *Candida albicans.* Such lesions should be evaluated by Gram's stain or a potassium hydroxide wet preparation.

Treatment is largely palliative. Numerous topical anesthetics have been suggested. Viscous lidocaine can be used as a rinse to lessen oral pain. A combination of dyclonine and magnesium hydroxide can also be used to make the patient more comfortable, especially during eating (Table 33–1). Patients should be advised to avoid spicy foods and ingest a bland diet. Over-the-counter mouth rinses containing alcohol should be avoided because of their astringent and irritating properties. Patients should be encouraged to continue to practice good oral hygiene using a soft toothbrush or a sponge-tipped swab. If infection due to *Candida albicans,* develops, the patient should be given nystatin oral suspension, clotrimazole troches, ketoconazole tablets, or fluconazole tablets (Table 33–1).

Xerostomia

If the patient's salivary glands, particularly the sublingual, submandibular, and parotid glands, lie within the port of head and neck irradiation, xerostomia is a common result. Head and neck irradiation induces inflammation and degenerative changes in the salivary gland acini and ducts. Edema and inflammatory infiltration of glands begins early in the course of radiotherapy. Eventually glandular fatty degeneration, necrosis, and small blood vessel fibrosis occur. Radiation tends to have more of an effect on the serous portion of the salivary glands than on the mucous component. Therefore, saliva becomes thicker and more difficult for the patient to manage (Figure 33–9). The pH of the saliva commonly decreases significantly, to as low as 4.0. There is a quantitative decrease in saliva production as well as a marked increase in salivary sodium, chloride, magnesium, and protein levels.

The diminished volume of saliva and the increased viscosity and tackiness decrease its lubricating and cleansing properties. Patients complain of extreme mouth dryness, coughing, loss of taste, and loss of appetite. Xerostomia begins during the first 2 weeks following initiation of radiation therapy. Signs and symptoms of xerostomia can occur with radiation doses as low as 1500 cGy. Irreversible salivary changes often require a dosage of 4000–6000 cGy. Since most patients receiving head and neck irradiation are given at least 6000 cGy, xerostomia is a common problem.

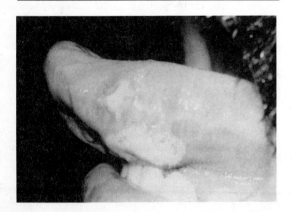

Figure 33–8. Oral mucositis of the lateral border of the tongue in a patient receiving ionizing irradiation for an oral tumor.

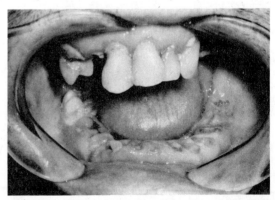

Figure 33–9. Xerostomia and severe generalized dental decay (radiation caries) in a patient who received head and neck radiation therapy 2 years previously for an oral tumor.

Treatment is largely palliative. Numerous saliva substitutes are available. These agents contain a combination of glycerine, electrolytes, and fluoride. They also include sodium carboxymethyl cellulose and sorbitol. These products are used to help improve overall mouth wetness, buffering capacity, and cariostatic support. Many patients find the saliva substitutes objectionable, and the cost can be prohibitive. These patients are encouraged to carry a container of water and to take frequent sips, especially at night and during eating. Some patients receive help from saliva stimulants, eg, sugar-free lemon drops or chewing gum. Patients with severe xerostomia can be given pilocarpine to stimulate salivary flow.

Radiation Caries

Because of the severe xerostomia developed by patients receiving head and neck radiation, the normal relationships of the oral microbiota are disrupted. This disruption leads to a rapid and aggressive form of dental caries (radiation caries). The cause is believed to be solely xerostomia secondary to head and neck irradiation. Once teeth are fully developed in the arch, head and neck irradiation will not have a deleterious effect on the teeth themselves. Teeth not in the direct radiation beam are also affected by radiation caries, since xerostomia can cause destruction of any tooth.

Salivary flow is reduced, and the quality and constituents of the saliva change. The pH of the saliva becomes more acidic, and there is a reduction in salivary immunoproteins. Secondary to these changes is a shift in the oral microbiota to more acidogenic and cariogenic forms, including *Streptococcus mutans, Lactobacillus* sp, and *Actinomyces* sp. With the lessening in the ability of the saliva to lubricate food, patients tend to shift to a diet that is high in refined carbohydrates. All these factors lead to an increase in the incidence of dental caries.

Radiation caries is characterized by a typical distribution of dental decay. The most commonly involved tooth surfaces are the cervical areas at the gum line and the cusp tips. Decay on the cusp tips of teeth is unusual in other types of decay and therefore is specific for radiation caries. The decay is rapidly progressive. As decay progresses, it eventually results in amputation of the tooth crown over a relatively short period of time ($\leq$ 1–2 years) (Figure 33–9). It is common for patients with radiation caries to lose complete function of their dentition. Severe reduction in mastication follows as well as problems secondary to odontogenic infection. Patients may regain some amount of salivary flow following head and neck radiation therapy; however, most experience reduction in salivary flow, and radiation caries can be a lifelong problem.

The critical factor in prevention of radiation caries is institution of scrupulous oral hygiene measures to reduce the load of oral bacteria. Patients must be taught meticulous techniques for oral hygiene and use them for the rest of their lives. Measures include toothbrushing and the use of dental floss. Patients should be followed for oral hygiene evaluation and therapy at brief intervals, probably no longer than 3 months. Patients should be encouraged to minimize intake of refined carbohydrates. Topical fluoride therapy is effective in reducing the incidence of radiation caries. It should be delivered in a plastic oral carrier that can be fabricated by the patient's dentist. Chlorhexidine has not been studied for this indication; however, its efficacy in other patient populations that are prone to high caries rates warrant its use as a prophylactic mouth rinse in patients susceptible to radiation caries.

Osteoradionecrosis

Osteoradionecrosis is the most serious side effect of head and neck irradiation. It is not an infectious disease but rather an area of devitalized bone. It can be defined as an area of exposed bone lying within a previous field of radiation that is present for at least 3 months. This denuded bone is a result of the effects of head and neck irradiation. Irradiation may produce periarteritis and endarteritis in the blood vessels of soft tissue and bone, which leads to vessel wall thickening and narrowing of the lumen of the vessels. The blood supply to the alveolus is compromised, and death of osteocytes and osteoblasts occurs. These cells are replaced in the marrow by connective tissue and fat, resulting in an alveolar bone that is hypovascular, hypocellular, and hypoxic with diminished repair and remodeling capability. When this bone becomes traumatized secondary to infection or surgical procedures, it cannot repair itself because of the reduced blood supply and "dead bone" is the result.

Osteoradionecrosis typically presents as an area of denuded bone following tooth extraction or soft tissue trauma in a patient who has received head and neck irradiation (Figure 33–10). The potential for osteoradionecrosis appears to increase with time following head and neck irradiation. Approximately 10–15% of patients who receive head and neck radiation therapy for oral tumors ultimately develop osteoradionecrosis. Over 90% of cases occur in the mandible, probably because of its greater bone density, which allows a higher absorption of the radiation dose, and also because of its poorer blood supply compared to that of the maxilla. Osteoradionecrosis most commonly occurs with total radiation doses greater than 6000 cGy and is infrequent at doses below this level. It is confined to the area of direct radiation and not to subsequent structures. Osteoradionecrosis is more common in patients who receive internal radiation with implants than in those who receive external radiation, probably because of the higher localized radiation dose delivered by internal source.

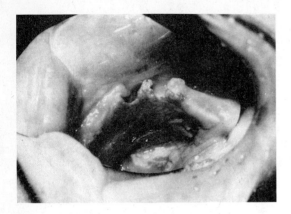

Figure 33–10. Osteoradionecrosis of the anterior mandible in a patient who received head and neck irradiation. Reverse view taken with an oral mirror. (Courtesy of JT McAnear, DDS.)

The most effective mode of treatment is prevention. Elimination of potential sources of oral infection prior to radiation therapy is critical. All teeth with a poor prognosis should be removed, including impacted teeth, teeth with moderate to severe periodontitis, teeth with extensive decay, and teeth with periapical lesions. Extraction of teeth and other therapies should be performed at least 14 days prior to the beginning of radiation therapy to allow for adequate healing. Full mouth extraction of teeth is indicated only if the patient is poorly compliant with therapy and will not implement meticulous oral hygiene and use of topical fluoride. If dental care requiring treatment of infection is necessary following radiation therapy, a conservative approach is appropriate. Root canal therapy is preferred over extractions. If extraction is necessary, hyperbaric oxygen therapy should be considered. Hyperbaric oxygen increases the vascularity of the affected bony areas, thus delivering more oxygen to the tissues. This therapy provides a better potential for healing. Once osteoradionecrosis occurs, the most successful therapy is hyperbaric oxygen treatment to stimulate healing plus debridement and antibiotic usage. Patients who do not respond to this therapy should receive alveolar resection following hyperbaric oxygen. Alveolar resection is indicated in patients who exhibit intractable pain, recurrent severe infections, or the potential for pathologic fracture. Because hyperbaric oxygen treatment is expensive and not available to all patients, aggressive preventive dental treatment before and after head and neck irradiation should be the rule.

REFERENCES

Ferretti GA et al: Chlorhexidine for prophylaxis against oral infections and associated complications in patients receiving bone marrow transplants. *Oral Surg Oral Med Oral Pathol* 1987;**114:**461.

Greenberg MS et al: The oral flora as a source of septicemia in patients with acute leukemia. *Oral Surg Oral Med Oral Pathol* 1982;**53:**32.

Greenberg MS et al: Oral herpes simplex infections in patients with leukemia. *J Am Dent Assoc* 1987;**114:**483.

Gold D, Corey L: Acyclovir prophylaxis for herpes simplex virus infection. *Antimicrob Agents Chemother* 1987;**31:**361.

Katz S: The use of fluoride and chlorhexidine for the prevention of radiation caries. *J Am Dent Assoc* 1982;**104:**164.

Marx RE, Johnson RP: Studies in the radiobiology of osteoradionecrosis and their clinical significance. *Oral Surg Oral Med Oral Pathol* 1987;**64:**379.

Meunier F et al: Fluconazole therapy of oropharyngeal candidiasis in cancer patients. Pages 169–174 in: *Recent Trends in the Discovery, Development and Evaluation of Antifungal Agents.* Fromtling RA (editor). Prous Science Publishers, 1987.

Montgomery MT: Head and neck radiation: Dental considerations. In: *Internal Medicine for Dentistry,* 2nd ed. Rose L, Kaye D (editors). Mosby Year Book, 1989.

Montgomery MT, Redding SW, LeMaistre CF: The incidence of oral herpes simplex virus infection in patients undergoing cancer chemotherapy. *Oral Surg Oral Med Oral Pathol* 1986;**61:**238.

Peterson DE, Elias EG, Sonis ST (editors): *Head and Neck Management of the Cancer Patient.* Martinus Nijhoff, 1986.

Redding SW: Oral considerations of cancer chemotherapy. In: *Internal Medicine for Dentistry,* 2nd ed. Rose L, Kaye D (editors). Mosby Year Book, 1989.

Redding SW, Rinaldi MG, Hicks JL: The relationship of oral *Candida tropicalis* infection to systemic candidiasis in a patient with leukemia. *Spec Care Dent* 1988;**8:**111.

Silverberg E, Lubera J: Cancer statistics, 1988. *CA* 1988;**38:**5.

Bone Marrow Suppression

34

E. Randolph Broun, MD

Bone marrow suppression is a common occurrence following the administration of cytotoxic therapy, either chemotherapy or radiotherapy. Most morbidity and mortality is secondary to infection or bleeding due to granulocytopenia or thrombocytopenia. A few antineoplastics and hormonal agents do not cause myelosuppression, eg, vincristine, bleomycin, asparaginase, efloxate (investigational), prednisone, and tamoxifen. Most commonly used chemotherapeutic agents cause reversible granulocytopenia and thrombocytopenia when given in standard doses.

Anemia

Many cancer patients have hemoglobin values around 10–11 g/dL as a result of the "anemia of chronic disease." This degree of anemia is usually well tolerated and does not require therapy.

Anemia in the setting of malignancy may be due to either accelerated loss or slowed production of red blood cells. Increased loss of red blood cells may result from hemorrhage (acute or chronic), splenic sequestration, or hemolysis. Causes of hemorrhage in cancer patients are surgery, disruption of vascular and mucosal integrity by cytotoxic therapy or malignant invasion, thrombocytopenia, and anticoagulation. The combination of mucositis and thrombocytopenia is commonly encountered and poses a particular risk of blood loss. Nutritional factors and marrow involvement with tumor often causes anemia in cancer patients.

Treatment, when indicated, is with packed red blood cells (PRBCs). Transfusion is not necessary until the patient is symptomatic; easy fatigability, shortness of breath, and headache are common symptoms. In general, patients with hemoglobin values of 7 g/dL or lower require transfusion; those with chronic anemia may tolerate a hemoglobin level of 7–8 g/dL without difficulty. However, older patients and those with underlying cardiac or pulmonary disease need a higher hemoglobin level, around 10–11 g/dL. Acute blood loss is less well tolerated, and transfusion is required when the hemoglobin value is 9–10 g/dL, especially in the face of orthostatic hypotension.

Three types of immediate transfusion reactions are associated with PRBC transfusions. Febrile reactions are the most common. They are not associated with signs or symptoms of hemolysis and are due to reactions to leukocyte or platelet antigens. They are treated with antipyretics. Allergic reactions manifested as urticaria and occasionally bronchospasm and anaphylaxis are thought to be caused by sensitivity to protein components in transfused plasma. These reactions are best managed with antihistamines and, if necessary, corticosteroids. The most serious type of reaction is a hemolytic transfusion reaction manifested by fever, low back and flank pain, nausea, and chest discomfort that is usually associated with ABO incompatibility and intravascular hemolysis. In the case of a hemolytic reaction, the goal is to maintain urine output at 100 mL/h by intravenous fluids and mannitol if necessary. The remaining blood in the unit should be returned to the blood bank for evaluation.

Leukocyte depletion of blood components is assuming increasing importance in transfusion support. While washing of PRBCs results in a residual leukocyte count of approximately 5×10^8, available filters (eg, PALL RC400, BF4) can provide a product with less than 2.5×10^5 residual leukocytes. Some transfusion-related problems including alloimmunization and the transmission of cytomegalovirus can be reduced or avoided by reducing the residual leukocytes to $\leq 10^6$. Other problems, such as febrile transfusion reactions, transfusion-related graft-versus-host disease, and immunomodulation, may also be helped by leukocyte depletion. Patients who should be considered candidates for leukocyte-depleted PRBCs and platelets are those who would be expected to receive a large number of transfusions, eg, in the setting of leukemic induction therapy or bone marrow transplantation, neonates, severely immunocompromised patients, and those in whom bone marrow transplantation is a possibility in the upcoming weeks or months.

Erythropoietin, which is normally produced in the kidney has been shown to improve the anemia due to chronic renal failure. Since patients with solid tumors have decreased levels of circulating erythropoietin, clinical trials are exploring the value of erythropoietin in patients with the anemia of malignancy. Patients with advanced, refractory cancer were treated with erythropoietin, 100–150 U/kg subcutaneously 3 times weekly, resulting in increases in hematocrit of 2.9–5.8%. Pretreatment erythropoietin levels were not predictive of response. Patients having prior treatment with cisplatin particularly benefited from such therapy.

Granulocytopenia

The most common serious side effect of cytotoxic therapy is bone marrow suppression. It occurs in a fairly predictable pattern depending on the agent and schedule utilized. For most standard dose regimens, the granulocyte and platelet nadir occurs at 10–14 days after the administration of chemotherapy and persists for 3–5 days. Uneventful rapid recovery is the rule. There are notable exceptions to this general statement. Non–cycle-specific agents such as nitrosoureas, melphalan, busulfan, and procarbazine are associated with a late nadir and prolonged recovery, necessitating dosing at 6-week or longer intervals instead of the usual 3–4 weeks. The reason for this variation lies in the marrow cell compartment primarily affected; those agents affecting only the pool of rapidly proliferating cells (phase- and cycle-specific agents) are associated with an early nadir and quick recovery, whereas those agents acting on the more slowly dividing stem cell pool produce a late nadir with a prolonged period of cytopenia.

Patients receiving radiation therapy may also experience myelosuppression. The problem increases as more of the axial skeleton (containing active bone marrow in adults) is included in the radiation port. Even patients receiving localized radiation therapy, however, may develop falling peripheral blood counts.

Therapy is primarily supportive. The risk of complications due to cytopenia is related to the degree of leukopenia or thrombocytopenia. Patients with an absolute granulocyte count (AGC) of less than 1000/μL are at increased risk for serious infection.

$$AGC = \frac{\text{Total white blood cell count} \times \frac{\%\text{ polymorphonuclear leukocytes}}{} + \%\text{ band forms}}{100}$$

The risk escalates rapidly as the AGC falls below 500/μL and is related to the duration of neutropenia. The use of empiric broad-spectrum antibiotics for febrile patients with neutropenia (AGC < 1000/μL or < 500/μL depending on the institution) that are directed against gram-negative infections has significantly decreased morbidity and mortality rates. Monotherapy with ceftazidime, 2 g every 8 hours, or imipenem-cilastatin may be adequate, particularly in patients with moderate neutropenia (AGC > 100) that is expected to be of brief duration, which is the usual case in patients receiving standard dose regimens for solid tumors. Patients receiving leukemic induction therapy or bone marrow transplant preparative regimens who are expected to have prolonged neutropenia may be better served by a two-agent regimen (eg, piperacillin, 4 g every 6 hours, plus amikacin or ceftazidime). Patients treated with these empiric regimens frequently develop gram-positive or fungal infections requiring specific therapy. For gram-positive infections, vancomycin (25–40 mg/kg/d in 2 divided doses) is commonly utilized. Amphotericin (0.5–1 mg/kg/d) is currently recommended for systemic fungal infections.

The use of granulocyte transfusions is controversial. There are reports of neutropenic patients with progressive infections despite the use of antibiotics who have benefited from this mode of therapy. More recent studies in patients treated aggressively with antibiotics have not shown a benefit for granulocyte transfusions. Since granulocyte transfusions have not been shown to be of value in controlled studies, they should not be used routinely. The toxic effects of granulocyte transfusion consist of fever and chills in most patients and pulmonary infiltrates in approximately 16%. Simultaneous administration of amphotericin B may be associated with an increased incidence of pulmonary complications. The potential for transmission of viral agents such as cytomegalovirus or human immunodeficiency virus (HIV) must also be considered. The usual dose of granulocytes is approximately 1×10^{10} cells per transfusion, and a minimum of four daily transfusions should be administered for gram-negative sepsis. If there is no improvement in the clinical picture, daily transfusions for a prolonged period of time (2–3 weeks) may be necessary.

A more promising mode of therapy is the use of colony-stimulating factors (CSFs). Granulocyte colony-stimulating factor (G-CSF) has been evaluated in several studies to prevent the neutropenia due to chemotherapy. A reduction in the number of days of neutropenia was noted, with patients who had not received prior cytotoxic therapy showing the best response. Studies are continuing to determine whether reduction in infections also occurs in this population. The recommended dose of G-CSF is 5 μg/kg/d subcutaneously.

Granulocyte-macrophage colony-stimulating factor (GM-CSF) has been the most extensively investigated CSF in clinical trials. It has been shown to improve peripheral white blood cell counts in several bone marrow failure states including aplastic anemia, myelodysplastic syndromes, and the acquired immunodeficiency syndrome (AIDS). One study reported a 31% decrease in the number of days of neutropenia with successive cycles of myelosuppressive chemotherapy compared to a single untreated cycle. The effect persisted with repeated administrations of GM-CSF with successive cycles of chemotherapy up to 5 cycles. The recommended dose of GM-CSF is 250 μg/m²/d subcutaneously or by prolonged intravenous infusion.

Thrombocytopenia

Thrombocytopenia is usually due to lack of production rather than consumption of platelets. However, a low platelet count in cancer patients should be thoroughly investigated because there are numerous possible causes. A bone marrow aspirate is particularly helpful in this regard; if megakaryocytes are present, it is unlikely that underproduction can account for thrombocytopenia.

In general, thrombocytopenic patients who are not bleeding do not need to be transfused until the platelet count falls below $20,000/\mu L$. Mild-to-moderate thrombocytopenia is well tolerated and, in the absence of bleeding, requires no replacement therapy. In the presence of bleeding, platelet counts greater than $50,000/\mu L$ do not need replacement; however, levels below $50,000/\mu L$ should probably be transfused up to a level of $50,000/\mu L$. Platelet counts less than $20,000/\mu L$ are associated with an increased instance of spontaneous bleeding, and platelet transfusions are of value in preventing and controlling bleeding and so enhancing survival in thrombocytopenic patients.

Platelet transfusions, while effective, have several drawbacks. Under normal circumstances, platelets circulate for only 9–10 days, and so the duration of benefit from a transfusion is limited. Because platelets are not routinely cross-matched, immunocompetent recipients develop antibodies to surface antigens (such as HLA antigens) and become alloimmunized, rendering them refractory to further platelet transfusions. Since 40–50% of leukemic patients become alloimmunized, this phenomenon is independent of the number of units transfused. Leukocyte depletion of blood products decreases the incidence of alloimmunization. Patients refractory to random donor platelets can usually be maintained with HLA-identical platelets, although this approach is costly and time-consuming.

Patients with platelet counts of $20,000–30,000/\mu L$ who are expected to regain marrow function should be given prophylactic platelet transfusions. This is usually accomplished with 6–8 units given 2–3 times weekly; however, it is not unusual for daily transfusions to be required. The platelet count is the guide and should be maintained at approximately $25,000/\mu L$. Occasionally, patients refractory to transfusions may require daily or several times daily transfusions to maintain an adequate platelet count. Continuous infusion of platelets (0.5–1 unit/h) has been used but not in a controlled fashion.

A unit of platelets is defined as the number of platelets routinely harvested from a unit of fresh whole blood. The yield is about 7×10^{10} platelets per unit. The theoretically expected increment in platelet count from the transfusion of a unit of platelets of $10,000–12,000/\mu L$ is not usually seen owing to accelerated consumption secondary to fever, sepsis, bleeding, or alloimmunization.

Bone Marrow Transplantation

The most extreme example of bone marrow suppression secondary to therapy is seen following conditioning for bone marrow transplantation. These patients are typically treated with high-dose combination chemotherapy or chemoradiotherapy with myeloablative intent. Bone marrow that was either harvested from the patient (autologous) or from a donor (allogeneic) is infused following the preparative regimen. Nadir blood counts typically occur around the time of marrow reinfusion, and absolute neutropenia persists for 7–10 days. With the routine use of either G-CSF (5 µg/kg/d) or GM-CSF (250 µg/m^2/d), patients typically require 14–16 days to achieve an absolute granulocyte count of 0.5×10^9/L. Since neither of these factors speeds platelet recovery, platelet transfusions are necessary until approximately 21 days following marrow infusion. These patients require aggressive blood product support in conjunction with broad-spectrum antibiotics, hyperalimentation, and frequently analgesics.

Recent studies with peripheral blood stem cell harvests have demonstrated their effectiveness at reconstituting hematopoietic function. Peripheral stem cells are harvested by multiple leukaphereses (8–10) usually performed 10–14 days after cytotoxic chemotherapy plus GM-CSF to enhance the yield. The advantage of peripheral stem cell transplants is somewhat earlier engraftment of white cells, which is thought to be secondary to the infusion of circulating committed progenitors. Peripheral blood stem cells are used in place of autologous bone marrow.

REFERENCES

Anderson KC: Who should receive leukodepleted blood components? *Transfus Sci* 1992;**13**:107.

Bodey GP et al: Quantitative relationships between circulating leukocytes and infection in patients with acute leukemia. *Ann Intern Med* 1966;**64**:328.

Deversaux S et al: GM-CSF accelerates neutrophil recovery after autologous bone marrow transplantation for Hodgkin's disease. *Bone Marrow Transplant* 1989;**4**:49.

Dutcher JP et al: Alloimmunization following platelet transfusion: The absence of a dose response relationship. *Blood* 1980;**57**:395.

Gabrilove J et al: A phase I/II study of rhG-CSF in cancer patients at risk for chemotherapy-induced neutropenia. *Proc Am Soc Hematol* 1987;**394**:135a.

Gaydos LS, Freireich EJ, Mantel N: The quantitative relation between platelet count and hemorrhage in patients with acute leukemia. *N Engl J Med* 1962;**266:**905.

Henderson ES: The granulocytopenic effects of cancer chemotherapeutic agents. Pages 207–221 in: *Drugs and Hematologic Reactions.* Dimitrov NV, Nodine JH (editors). Grune & Stratton, 1974.

Higby EJ et al: The prophylactic treatment of thrombocytopenic leukemia patients with platelets: A double blind study. *Transfusion* 1974;**14:**440.

Karp DD et al: Pulmonary complications during granulocyte transfusions: Incidence and clinical features. *Vox Sang* 1982;**42:**57.

Morstyn G et al: Effect of granulocyte colony stimulating factor on neutropenia induced by cytotoxic chemotherapy. *Lancet* 1988;**2:**667.

Platanias LC et al: Treatment of chemotherapy-induced anemia with recombinant human erythropoietin in cancer patients. *J Clin Oncol* 1991;**9:**2021.

Pizzo PA et al: A randomized trial comparing ceftazidime alone with combination antibiotic therapy in cancer patients with fever and neutropenia. *N Engl J Med* 1986;**315:**552.

Schimpff SC et al: Empiric therapy with carbenicillin and gentamicin for febrile patients with cancer and granulocytopenia. *N Engl J Med* 1971;**284:**1061.

Winston DJ, Ho WG, Gale RP: Therapeutic granulocyte transfusions for documented infections. *Ann Intern Med* 1982;**97:**509.

Cardiac Toxicity

35

Daniel D. Von Hoff, MD

When a patient with cancer presents with a cardiac problem, the differential diagnosis is large. Included is involvement of the heart by the tumor itself (eg, invasion of the myocardium by solid tumor or leukemic infiltrates), nonbacterial thrombotic endocarditis, and side effects of prior treatment (radiotherapy, chemotherapy, or both).

COMPLICATIONS SECONDARY TO RADIATION THERAPY

Radiation therapy is associated with several cardiac side effects including electrocardiographic changes, late-onset atherosclerotic cardiovascular disease, and pericarditis with or without effusions and with or without constriction. The incidence of clinically apparent irradiation-induced disease is dose related. Shielding of the heart (for total doses of ≤ 3000 cGy) has decreased the incidence of irradiation-induced cardiac toxicity.

With a greater percentage of patients being cured of their cancer, whether or not they would prematurely develop irradiation-related coronary artery disease became an important question. Most reported instances of premature coronary artery disease were from a time span when radiotherapy techniques were not optimal (eg, no shielding). More recent studies have observed no excessive risk of irradiation-related ischemic heart disease.

Pericarditis secondary to radiation therapy can be noted within a year after completion of therapy or many years later. The effusion that may accompany the pericarditis may cause cardiac tamponade, necessitating pericardiocentesis or placement of a cardiac window. A constrictive pericarditis can also occur. This complication can be treated by pericardiectomy.

COMPLICATIONS SECONDARY TO CHEMOTHERAPY

Doxorubicin

Doxorubicin (Adriamycin, Rubex, others) is one of the most widely used antineoplastic agents. Its cardiac effects include acute electrocardiographic changes and a cumulative, drug-induced cardiomyopathy.

A. Electrocardiographic Changes: A large variety have been noted in association with administration of doxorubicin, but in general they are of little clinical consequence. The most common is ectopy (premature ventricular contractions). However, sudden death, presumably due to an arrhythmia, has been reported. Acute myocardial infarctions have also been reported.

B. Drug-Induced Cardiomyopathy: Doxorubicin-induced cardiomyopathy is more serious and is associated with significant morbidity and mortality (28–61%). The overall incidence of doxorubicin-induced cardiomyopathy ranges from 0.4% to 9% and is related to total cumulative dose.

It is impossible to distinguish doxorubicin-induced congestive heart failure (CHF) from other types of cardiomyopathies. The first signs may include tachycardia and a nonproductive cough. After this initial period, the usual symptoms and signs of CHF become evidence (dyspnea, orthopnea, engorgement of neck veins, gallop rhythm, hepatomegaly, ankle edema, cardiomegaly, and pleural effusion. The time of onset of CHF after the last dose of doxorubicin ranges from 0 days to 7 years (mean of 33 days and median of 23 days). The possibility of very late (> 10 years) onset of doxorubicin-induced CHF should always be kept in mind when evaluating a patient who has received that agent.

The most important risk factor is cumulative dose of doxorubicin administered. In initial studies, adult patients who received more than 550 mg/m^2 of doxorubicin had a significant increase in doxorubicin-induced CHF. Based on that information, it is recommended that doxorubicin be stopped when the total dose of 550 mg/m^2 is reached. However, in a retrospective study, the author and colleagues noted that there is not an absolute level above which drug-induced CHF occurs but rather a continuum of increasing incidence of CHF with increasing total doses of doxorubicin (Figure 35–1). Thus, if a patient's tumor is responding to treatment with doxorubicin and the patient has reached a total dose of 550 mg/m^2, some objective measurement of cardiac function, such as cardiac biopsy or another noninvasive method,

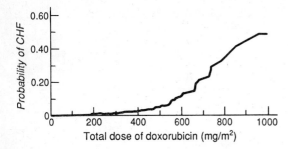

Figure 35–1. Cumulative probability of developing doxorubicin-induced congestive heart failure (CHF) versus total cumulative dose of doxorubicin (3941 patients, with 88 cases of CHF). (Reproduced, with permission, from Von Hoff DD et al: Risk factors for doxorubicin-induced congestive heart failure. *Ann Intern Med* 1979;**91**:712.)

should be considered to help determine whether to continue the drug.

Another risk factor for development for doxorubicin-induced CHF is schedule of drug administration. Earlier studies indicated that doxorubicin administered as a weekly dose or given daily for 3 days every 21 days was less cardiotoxic than a single dose given every 21 days. Another important study showed that doxorubicin given as a continuous infusion is less likely to produce CHF.

Other risk factors include increased patient age, preexisting cardiac disease, prior mediastinal radiation, and concomitant administration of other cytotoxic agents. Only the latter two have been definitely shown to be risk factors. Most investigators feel that patients who have had prior mediastinal radiation should have cumulative doses of doxorubicin limited to 400 mg/m². The same recommendation is made for patients who are receiving concomitant cyclophosphamide. However, these recommendations are based on little clinical trial information.

The standard for monitoring cardiac damage has been the endomyocardial biopsy as described by Billingham et al. Since now all institutions have the necessary experience to monitor patients with that technique, other noninvasive methods including serial ECGs to look for decreased voltage of the QRS complex, cardiac ejection fractions measured with radionuclide techniques, echocardiography, and the QRS-Korotkoff interval have been tried. Only radionuclide cineangiography has survived as a trusted method, despite some evidence of a poor correlation between cardiac biopsy findings and ejection fractions measured by that technique. A baseline study is usually performed before the first dose of doxorubicin is administered. If the baseline ejection fraction measured by this technique is abnormal, other nonanthracycline chemotherapy should be considered. Patients are then followed with serial ejection fractions. If there is a significant deterioration in

the ejection fraction, therapy with doxorubicin should be discontinued. A recently reported method for evaluating for the early onset of doxorubicin-induced CHF is the elevation in blood levels of atrial natriuretic peptide in patients who eventually developed CHF.

The treatment for doxorubicin-induced CHF is the same as for other types of CHF, including salt restriction, diuresis, and digitalis. Discontinuation of doxorubicin is essential. Aggressive medical therapy is important because of increasing evidence that the cardiomyopathy may be reversible.

Several agents have been proposed to prevent doxorubicin-induced cardiac damage, including coenzyme Q10, alpha-tocopherol, prenylamine, and ICRF 187. Only ICRF 187 shows convincing evidence of modulating the onset of doxorubicin-induced CHF (eg, it allows larger doses of doxorubicin to be administered without development of CHF).

C. Other Factors: CHF also is being noted in patients undergoing surgery and in women in childbirth, when those patients have had prior doxorubicin. This result may be due to fluid retention or fluid administration during those procedures. Patients with a prior history of doxorubicin administration require careful perioperative management of fluids.

Daunorubicin

Daunorubicin (Cerubidine) has a more limited spectrum of antitumor activity and is most commonly used in treatment regimens for patients with acute leukemia. Cardiac toxicity includes acute electrocardiographic changes and daunorubicin-induced CHF.

A. Electrocardiographic Changes: The most common electrocardiographic findings are low voltage of the QRS complex and nonspecific ST-T wave changes. These changes are reversible and are not predictive for the onset of CHF.

B. Drug-Induced Cardiomyopathy: Daunorubicin-induced CHF is, like doxorubicin-induced CHF, related to total dose of drug administered (Figure 35–2). The time from the last dose of daunorubicin to the onset of cardiomyopathy ranges from 2 to 280 days (mean of 80 days, median of 60 days). To date, there is little information whether schedule of drug administration makes difference in terms of cardiomyopathy, but some investigators note that patients who receive high total doses of daunorubicin over short periods of time develop cardiomyopathy more readily than those who receive daunorubicin over longer periods of time. No systematic studies of other risk factors (eg, prior mediastinal radiation, concomitant chemotherapy) have been undertaken.

Treatment is the same as for doxorubicin-induced CHF, namely, supportive care. In several series, the deaths of more than 70% of patients with this complication were secondary to the CHF.

There have been no systematic studies of methods

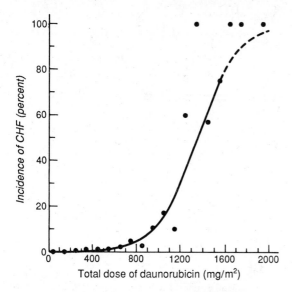

Figure 35–2. Percent incidence of congestive heart failure (CHF) in patients receiving daunorubicin (5613 patients, with 65 cases of CHF). (Reproduced, with permission, from Von Hoff DD et al: Daunomycin-induced cardiotoxicity in children and adults: A review of 110 cases. *Am J Med* 1977;**62**:200.)

to predict the development of daunorubicin-induced CHF. For routine patient management, the use of radionuclide cineangiography appears reasonable. At present, there is no known method to protect against the development of daunorubicin-induced cardiomyopathy.

Other Anthracyclines

A large number of other anthracyclines are undergoing clinical trials including epirubicin, detorubicin, idarubicin hydrochloride, esorubicin hydrochloride, and other compounds. Epirubicin appears to be slightly less cardiotoxic than doxorubicin and has recently been approved for use in the USA. It is too early to determine whether the other agents will have less cardiotoxicity than does either doxorubicin or daunorubicin.

Cyclophosphamide

Hemorrhagic cardiac necrosis has been noted only with very high doses (120–240 mg/kg given over 1–4 days) of cyclophosphamide (Cytoxan, Neosar, others). This uncommon toxicity may become more common with the increasing number of patients being treated with the agent owing to bone marrow transplantation. The presenting signs of this toxicity are tachycardia and refractory CHF. The cardiac necrosis is fatal in almost all instances. The use of cyclophosphamide in combination with other agents (eg, carmustine plus cytarabine plus thioguanine) may be more cardiotoxic than cyclophosphamide alone.

Mitoxantrone

Mitoxantrone (Novantrone) is an anthracene derivative used for treatment of patients with acute leukemia. The agent also has antitumor activity against breast cancer and lymphoma. Mitoxantrone has been associated with transient electrocardiographic changes as well as decreased ejection fractions and congestive heart failure. Electrocardiographic changes include nonspecific ST-T wave changes.

However, drug-induced CHF is rare (1.5% in one study of 601 patients). Most patients who developed CHF had cumulative doses of mitoxantrone greater than 100 mg/m². Those patients who also had had prior doxorubicin had a higher incidence of CHF. Prospective studies using radionuclide scans to evaluate left ventricular function to evaluate the myocardial toxicity of mitoxantrone have shown a small but definite decrement in left ventricular ejection fraction. Endomyocardial biopsy studies have shown that mitoxantrone is cardiotoxic but to a minor degree at the total doses used in that study.

Caution is needed when cumulative doses of mitoxantrone greater than 100 mg/m² are used. Serial cardiac ejection fractions appear to be the best way to follow potential cardiac damage.

Fluorouracil

This frequently used pyrimidine analog is rarely associated with cardiac side effects. The one most consistently reported is angina pectoris. This angina usually occurs several hours after injection. Echocardiograms performed in patients showing signs of myocardial ischemia thought to be secondary to fluorouracil indicate left ventricular dysfunction. Pretreatment with nitrates and calcium channel blockers fails to prevent the signs and symptoms of myocardial ischemia. Myocardial infarctions have also been reported in association with infusion of fluorouracil.

Diethylstilbestrol

Diethylstilbestrol (DES) is used extensively to treat patients with prostate cancer. Studies by the Veterans Administration Cooperative Urological Research Group indicate that a dose of 5 mg/d is associated with cardiovascular deaths. This incidence is lower if a dose of 1 mg of DES is utilized.

Cisplatin

Although rare, there are case reports of myocardial ischemia associated with administration of combinations containing cisplatinum (Platinol) in patients with or without prior mediastinal radiation therapy. In addition, cisplatin-induced bradycardia and paroxysmal supraventricular tachycardia have been reported.

Interleukin-2

A few patients administered interleukin-2 (IL-2) have developed supraventricular arrhythmias, myocardial ischemia (angina), and rarely myocardial infarctions resulting in death.

Homoharringtonine

Homoharringtonine HHT is a new agent with documented activity in patients with acute leukemia. Its main side effects are tachycardia and arrhythmias. Characterization of these side effects requires additional clinical trials.

Amsacrine

Amsacrine (AMSA) is a new agent with documented activity in patients with acute non-lymphocytic leukemia. The compound has been reported to cause electrocardiographic changes, atrial and ventricular arrhythmias (hypokalemia predisposes to them) resulting in sudden death, congestive heart failure, and myocardial necrosis. There appears to be no cumulative dose effect.

REFERENCES

Alexander J et al: Serial assessment of doxorubicin cardiotoxicity with quantitative radionuclide angiocardiography. *N Engl J Med* 1979;**300**:278.

Billingham M et al: Endomyocardial biopsy findings in Adriamycin-treated patients. *Proc Am Assoc Cancer Res* 1976;**17**:281.

Collins, C, Weiden PL: Cardiotoxicity of 5-fluorouracil. *Cancer Treat Rep* 1987;**71**:733.

Corn BW, Trock BJ, Goodman RL: Irradiation-related ischemic heart disease. *J Clin Oncol* 1990;**8**:741.

Goldberg BA et al: Cyclophosphamide cardiotoxicity: An analysis of dosing as a risk factor. *Blood* 1986;**68**:1114.

Legha SS et al: Reduction of doxorubicin cardiotoxicity by prolonged continuous intravenous infusion. *Ann Intern Med* 1982;**96**:133.

Muggia F et al: Protective effect of the bispiperazinedione ICRF-187 against doxorubicin-induced cardiac toxicity in women with advanced breast cancer. *N Engl J Med* 1988;**319**:745.

Perez DJ et al: A randomized comparison of single-agent doxorubicin and epirubicin as first-line cytotoxic therapy in advanced breast cancer. *J Clin Oncol* 1991;**9**:2148.

Shenkenberg TD, Von Hoff DD: Mitoxantrone: A new anti-cancer drug with significant clinical activity. *Ann Intern Med* 1986;**105**:67.

Steinherz LJ et al: Cardiac toxicity 4 to 20 years after completing anthracycline therapy. *JAMA* 1991;**266**:1672.

Talcott JA, Herman TJ: Acute ischemia vascular events and cisplatin. *Ann Intern Med* 1987;**107**:121.

Weiss RB et al: Amsacrine-associated cardiotoxicity: An analysis of 82 cases. *J Clin Oncol* 1986;**4**:918.

Pulmonary Toxicity

36

Jay Peters, MD

Approximately 75% of immunocompromised hosts having impaired antibody formation, defective cell-mediated immunity, or reduced granulocyte function will develop pulmonary complications of cancer therapy. About three-quarters of these patients will have an infectious process, and one-third will have two or more causes of their pulmonary symptoms, eg, infection plus drug-induced lung disease or recurrent malignancy plus radiation pneumonitis. The pulmonary toxicity of chemotherapeutic agents and irradiation presents a dilemma because the chest x-ray is not diagnostic of a specific entity and the clinical presentation may mimic an infectious process. The four causes of pulmonary disease in cancer patients presenting with an abnormal chest x-ray are (**1**) extension of the malignancy to the lung, (**2**) an opportunistic infection, (**3**) a new, unrelated disease process, and (**4**) a pulmonary reaction to either chemotherapeutic agents or irradiation. Invasive diagnostic tests such as bronchoscopy with transbronchial biopsy or open-lung biopsy are often required to establish the diagnosis.

COMPLICATIONS SECONDARY TO RADIATION THERAPY

Irradiation to the thorax can produce changes in the lung (Table 36–1), heart, pericardium, esophagus, and spinal cord. The incidence of radiation pneumonitis is difficult to assess, since some authors consider radiographic changes as diagnostic for radiation pneumonitis whereas others denote it as a clinical syndrome. Symptoms develop in only 5–15% of patients; however, an appreciable number will die of radiation pneumonitis. Irradiation to the thorax is mainly used in the treatment of cancers of the breast, lymphoma, and lung.

In breast cancer, the incidence of radiologic evidence of pneumonitis is 30–70% (mean of 40%). Only 8–15% of these patients develop symptoms of respiratory failure due to radiation pneumonitis, and clinically significant radiation pneumonitis is extremely rare in patients with breast cancer. Late radiologic findings of radiation fibrosis occur in 50–60% of patients but are rarely associated with symptoms.

In the largest series reported on lymphoma, clinical radiation pneumonitis occurred in 6.4% of patients who received irradiation to the mediastinum alone, 15% of patients who were reirradiated to the mediastinum, and 33% of patients who received irradiation to the mediastinum and lung (with a 5.8% mortality). More recently, technical improvements have reduced this incidence of radiation pneumonitis in patients with lymphoma.

In lung cancer, the incidence of radiographic changes varies from 10% to 100%. Symptoms develop in 15–45% of patients and may be a contributing cause of death in as many as one-third of patients with symptomatic radiation pneumonitis.

The incidence and severity of radiation pneumonitis is related to technical factors such as the volume of lung irradiated, the amount of irradiation, and the rate of delivery. The volume of lung irradiated is considered the limiting factor in lung tolerance. As an example, 3000 cGy delivered to a quarter of the lung volume rarely produces symptomatic pneumonitis; however, the same quantity delivered to the entire volume of both lungs will likely result in death. The second most important factor appears to be the rate of delivery or fractionation. As little as 1500 cGy has proved fatal when given as a single dose, yet this same dose given in 8–10 fractions would not be expected to cause any adverse effects. The amount of lung damage is less a function of total dose than rate of delivery, since fractionation permits time for injured tissue to undergo repair.

Pathophysiology & Histopathology

Absorption of x-rays by tissues accelerates electrons, generating highly reactive free radicals that may break chemical bonds. In the presence of oxygen, the free radicals produce organic peroxides, leading to irreversible chemical lesions and significantly more tissue damage. Irradiation damages two types of cells: nongenetic material, eg, proteins or polysaccharides, and genetic material, eg, DNA.

Damage to nongenetic material causes immediate damage including increased permeability of membranes and connective tissue fragmentation. These effects rarely lead to clinically detectable lesions. Damage to genetic material occurs only when the cell enters mitosis, in which phase chromosomal damage

Table 36–1. Characteristics of radiation injury to the lung.

	Radiation Pneumonitis	Radiation Fibrosis
Onset after therapy	6–12 weeks	6–12 months
Symptoms	Dyspnea, cough, fever	Progressive dyspnea
X-ray features	Reticulonodular infiltrate	Linear streaks radiating from prior pneumonitis
Response to corticosteroids	Common	Rare

leads to inability of the cell to reproduce. Irradiation-induced chromosomal damage affects those cells with the highest mitotic rates—capillary endothelial cells, type II pneumonocytes, and bronchial epithelial cells.

Histopathologic changes occur in two phases: an early phase, which begins about 2 months after irradiation, and a late phase, which occurs 6 or more months after irradiation. In the early phase, an interstitial edema with a lymphocyte infiltrate occurs and is associated with the formation of hyaline membranes (an organized proteinaceous exudate) in the alveolar space. The capillary endothelium becomes hyperplastic and protrudes into the lumen of the blood vessel. Later fibrinoid necrosis and thrombosis develop. Changes in the bronchial wall occur, including bronchial wall necrosis, squamous metaplasia, and bronchiectasis. These histopathologic changes in the bronchial wall account for the signs and symptoms such as the nonproductive cough experienced by these patients.

In the late phase, the histologic appearance is dominated by dense fibrosis and thickening of the alveolar wall. This fibrosis is associated with minimal inflammation but occurs in the setting of sclerotic obliteration of small muscular pulmonary arteries. Vascular calcification is common and sometimes extensive. These histopathologic changes account for the progressive dyspnea associated with the increased work of breathing and also for the lack of response to anti-inflammatory drugs when used at this stage.

Clinical Findings

The clinical features have two distinct phases: an early phase known as acute radiation pneumonitis, which occurs 6–12 weeks after radiation therapy, and a late phase known as radiation fibrosis, which occurs 6–12 months after completion of therapy. As a general rule, patients entering the late phase have progressed from acute radiation pneumonitis and either failed to seek medical attention or failed to respond to treatment. A small proportion of patients will develop radiation fibrosis without prior symptoms of acute pneumonitis.

A. Radiation Pneumonitis: The cardinal symptom of radiation pneumonitis is dyspnea, often associated with a persistent cough. The cough is initially nonproductive but later progresses to produce small quantities of either white or slightly blood-tinged sputum. Frank hemoptysis is uncommon and should be attributed to another cause. Fever and constitutional symptoms are frequently noted and may be marked. Pleuritic pain is uncommon.

Physical examination of the chest initially reveals inspiratory crackles with progression of pneumonitis. A pleural friction rub or evidence of a pleural effusion may be detected. In severe cases, signs of respiratory failure—cyanosis, tachypnea, and tachycardia—may appear. Left untreated, acute cor pulmonale may develop and is associated with a high mortality.

Laboratory tests may reveal moderate leukocytosis and elevated erythrocyte sedimentation rate. Arterial blood gas measurements frequently show hypoxemia, but hypercapnia is unusual unless there is a significant history of underlying lung disease.

Radiologic abnormalities are invariable in radiation pneumonitis. Initially there may be an interstitial infiltrate. This type of infiltrate is often referred to as reticulonodular, since it consists of "lines" and "dots." A patchy alveolar infiltrate suggests a bacterial pneumonia.

Differentiating features of radiation pneumonitis are the relatively sharp borders and limitation of the infiltrate to the margins of the port (Figure 36–1). One of the most characteristic features of radiation pneumonitis is that the infiltrate does not conform to anatomic segments of the lung. Pleural effusions occur in approximately 10% of cases, but they are generally small and remain stable over long periods of time.

Radiation pneumonitis may last several weeks and subside without sequelae or may last several months and slowly regress. The course is variable and in severe cases may progress from mild dyspnea to respiratory failure in a matter of days.

B. Radiation Fibrosis: Most patients develop radiation fibrosis following an episode of symptomatic radiation pneumonitis; however, a small percentage of patients develop symptoms only during the stage of fibrosis. Progressive dyspnea is the only uniform symptom. Fever and sputum production should suggest an infectious complication or secondary bronchiectasis. When the area of fibrosis is small, many patients will be asymptomatic. In a few patients with either extensive fibrosis or significant preexisting lung disease, chronic respiratory failure develops. This syndrome is characterized by reduced exercise tolerance, exertional dyspnea, orthopnea, and cyanosis that can progress to chronic cor pulmonale.

Pulmonary function tests reveal a restrictive defect with diminished forced expiratory volume (FEV_1) and forced vital capacity (FVC) while the ratio of FEV_1 to FVC remains normal. Total lung capacity and diffusion capacity are both reduced.

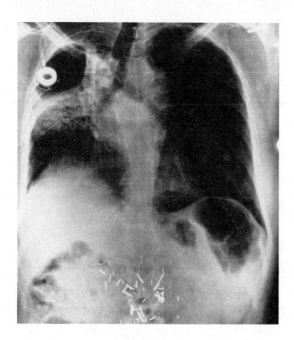

Figure 36–1. Chest x-ray demonstrating the sharply delineated borders of the radiation port in a 59-year-old patient presenting with radiation fibrosis.

Chest x-rays reveal linear streaks radiating from prior areas of pneumonitis. Contraction of these lesions leads to volume loss with shifts of the trachea, mediastinum, and diaphragm. Fibrosis may also lead to scoliosis with the spine concave toward the area of fibrosis. Occasionally, contraction of densely fibrotic lung tissue leads to hyperinflation in adjacent areas ("cicatricial emphysema"). In the upper lobes, this can resemble active tuberculosis.

Risk Factors

The most important factors that can potentiate the detrimental effects of radiation are prior irradiation, chemotherapeutic agents, and withdrawal from corticosteroids. Reirradiation of the mediastinum in Hodgkin's disease is associated with a threefold increase in the frequency of radiation pneumonitis. In these cases, severe pneumonitis usually presented earlier. Thus, when patients undergo re-treatment, special care should be taken in planning the radiotherapy regimen to reduce the incidence of radiation pneumonitis.

Many chemotherapeutic agents have been shown to potentiate the effects of irradiation in animal models. Since both chemotherapy and radiotherapy produce reactive oxygen molecules, marked synergistic toxicity is theoretically possible. However, only busulfan, bleomycin, and mitomycin have been shown in clinical studies to potentiate to pulmonary toxicity of radiotherapy.

Withdrawal from corticosteroids may precipitate or unmask radiation pneumonitis. This is important in patients with lymphoma who may receive combination chemotherapy that includes prednisone. Such regimens should include gradual tapering of corticosteroids in patients who have undergone recent radiotherapy.

Treatment

Three modalities of therapy have been used in the treatment of radiation pneumonitis: anticoagulants, antibiotics, and corticosteroids. Anticoagulants and antibiotics have not proved beneficial. Although no controlled clinical trials have been performed to confirm the beneficial effects of corticosteroids, there are sufficient animal data and clinical experience to support the use of corticosteroids in acute radiation pneumonitis.

In most centers, corticosteroids are initiated as soon as the diagnosis is considered reasonably certain. Prednisone, 60–100 mg/d, is usually sufficient to produce a satisfactory clinical response. Once a clinical response is obtained, the dose is maintained at 20–40 mg/d for several weeks and then slowly tapered. The prophylactic use of corticosteroids to prevent radiation pneumonitis has largely been abandoned.

There is no clinical evidence that radiation fibrosis responds to corticosteroids. Since clinically it may be difficult to distinguish when pneumonitis resolves and the phase of fibrosis begins, many patients are given a short course of corticosteroids and are rapidly tapered if there is no physiologic and clinical response.

COMPLICATIONS SECONDARY TO CHEMOTHERAPY

Chemotherapy-induced pulmonary disease was first recognized in 1961 in association with busulfan. Bleomycin, methotrexate, and cyclophosphamide have become increasingly associated with drug-induced pulmonary disease. Difficulties for the oncologist stem from the facts that drug-induced injury **(1)** mimics other pulmonary diseases, **(2)** can be fatal, and **(3)** may occur after the drug has been discontinued. The diagnosis of drug-induced lung disease is made by a history of exposure to the drug, histologic evidence consistent with drug-induced injury, and exclusion of other causes of lung injury.

Three typical patterns of injury have emerged (Table 36–2). The most acute form is hypersensitivity lung disease. This disorder has been associated with bleomycin, methotrexate, and procarbazine. Patients present with an acute syndrome of dyspnea, nonproductive cough, and fever that progresses over several hours to days. Pulmonary or peripheral eosinophilia in combination with an acute pulmonary infiltrate is

Table 36–2. Types of cytotoxic lung injury.

Pattern of Injury	Associated Drugs	Clinical Features
Hypersensitivity	Bleomycin, methotrexate, procarbazine	Progressive dyspnea, cough, and fever over days to weeks
Chronic pneumonitis	All categories of drugs	Chronic dyspnea and dry cough over weeks to months
Pulmonary edema	Cytarabine, cyclophosphamide, teniposide, and methotrexate	Signs and symptoms of heart failure

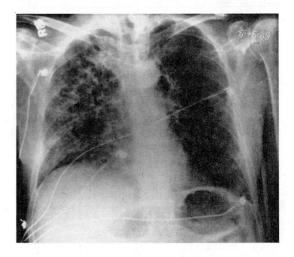

Figure 36–2. Chest x-ray of a patient with progressive dyspnea and low-grade fever. Autopsy revealed that the patient died of cytotoxic lung injury secondary to use of mitomycin.

the hallmark of this syndrome. Laboratory studies may reveal 10–20% of the white blood cell count to be eosinophils; however, this finding is not invariable and often the eosinophils are confined to the lung. In general, this form of cytotoxic lung injury has a good prognosis with discontinuation of the drug, use of corticosteroids, or both.

The second syndrome is chronic pneumonitis and fibrosis secondary to cytotoxic injury. This pattern of injury is the most common syndrome associated with chemotherapy. Chronic pneumonitis with fibrosis occurs with essentially all categories of cytotoxic drugs. The typical presentation includes progressive dyspnea on exertion, fatigue, a nonproductive cough, and occasionally fever that develops over several weeks to months. Auscultation of the lung reveals rales. This syndrome is often misinterpreted as an infectious disease, congestive heart failure, or idiopathic pulmonary fibrosis. Clubbing, which occurs in three-fourths of patients with idiopathic fibrosis, is not reported to be a feature of cytotoxic drug–induced lung disease. The chest x-ray usually shows an interstitial pattern but may reveal a mixed alveolar-interstitial pattern. Pulmonary function tests are abnormal in essentially all patients with cytotoxic lung injury. The carbon monoxide diffusing capacity may be diminished prior to a fall in lung volumes. For this reason, serial diffusion capacity studies are used to detect early pulmonary toxicity in order to discontinue treatment before the onset of clinical symptoms. Treatment usually includes discontinuation of the drug and a trial of corticosteroids. Response to corticosteroids is variable and anecdotal except with mitomycin-induced lung injury, where it is usually favorable and often dramatic.

The final form of cytotoxic lung injury is drug-induced noncardiogenic pulmonary edema, which is a rare reaction occasionally seen with cytarabine, methotrexate, teniposide, and cyclophosphamide. Signs and symptoms are identical to those seen in heart failure except that they occur in the face of a normal left ventricular pressure. The presumed cause is a capillary leak syndrome, and the prognosis is variable and relates to extent of injury.

Pathogenesis & Histopathology

The mechanism of cytotoxic lung injury is not known, but it is postulated to be a direct toxic reaction. Accumulation of drug within cells can cause fragmentation of DNA. Oxygen-mediated injury may also play an important role. Several cytotoxic agents generate toxic oxygen-derived substances such as superoxide anion (O_2^-), hydrogen peroxide (H_2O_2), and hydroxyl radicals ($OH^·$). The toxic effect of these agents reflects participation of these molecules in oxidation-reduction reactions in which fatty acid oxidation may lead to membrane instability. Cytotoxic drugs may induce pulmonary injury through alterations in the normal balance between oxidants and antioxidants.

The pathologic changes induced by chemotherapeutic agents are similar in appearance but differ in degree. These changes consist of alveolar cell dysplasia and an interstitial lymphocyte infiltration. The presence of eosinophils lends support to the diagnosis of a drug reaction. Fibrosis is a function of the duration of therapy. Even in the fibrotic stage, dysplastic cells may be noted.

Cytopathologic changes, consisting of dysplastic cells with enlarged hyperchromatic nuclei and congealed chromatin, are characteristic of chemotherapy-induced lung injury.

Risk Factors

Predisposing factors for the development of pulmonary toxicity from chemotherapeutic agents include cumulative dose, radiation therapy, oxygen therapy, and age. Although some pulmonary toxicity appears to be idiosyncratic, bleomycin, busulfan, and carmustine show enhanced toxicity with increasing dose. With busulfan, pulmonary damage occurs above the critical dose of 500 mg. In contrast, bleomycin and carmustine may occasionally produce pulmonary damage at low doses. Bleomycin-induced pulmonary toxicity usually occurs after a total dose of 450–500 mg. Carmustine, on the other hand, shows a linear relationship between cumulative dose and toxic effects to the lung.

Since both irradiation and chemotherapy are thought to produce injury through the production of reactive oxygen metabolites, synergistic toxicity seems likely. However, busulfan, bleomycin, and mitomycin are the only cytotoxic drugs for which clinical data support such synergy. Similarly, oxygen therapy might be expected to result in higher concentrations of oxygen metabolites and increase the injury caused by these agents. Yet only bleomycin and cyclophosphamide have been shown to exacerbate oxygen-induced pulmonary damage.

Increasing age may be associated with a decrease in the antioxidant defense system. This implies that pulmonary toxic effects would be increased in older patients. Such a correlation has been identified only with bleomycin. Better markers are needed to identify which patients are at risk for developing pulmonary toxicity from chemotherapeutic agents.

Cytotoxic Agents

A. Antibiotics:

1. Bleomycin–Bleomycin is used primarily in the treatment of squamous cell carcinoma, lymphoma, and testicular tumors. Skin and pulmonary toxicities limit the dosage tolerated in many patients. In humans, bleomycin-induced injury is predominately confined to the alveoli in the periphery of the lung. Ultrastructure studies show that the drug induces a vascular lesion with secondary edema and also produces necrosis of type I pneumonocytes. This leads to pulmonary fibrosis, which can be severe and debilitating.

Some degree of pulmonary injury develops in 4–10% of patients treated with bleomycin, and 1–2% die of drug-induced pulmonary disease. The critical dose above which pulmonary injury increases dramatically appears to be 450–500 units. Doses as low as 100 units have produced significant toxicities.

Two types of radiation injury are also reported with bleomycin. The first is due to its radiosensitizing properties, and the pulmonary injury is not limited to the port but extends to the surrounding lung. The second is radio-recall, a phenomenon by which previously irradiated lung develops injury associated with the administration of the drug.

In addition, high inspired concentrations of oxygen (average $FIO_2 = 4$) during bleomycin administration may enhance the development of pulmonary fibrosis. This phenomenon is not usually noted in studies 1–2 months after bleomycin administration; however, it seems prudent to use the lowest FIO_2 necessary to adequately oxygenate the patient.

The best treatment for bleomycin-induced lung injury is early withdrawal of the agent. Therefore, many clinicians follow the diffusion capacity of carbon monoxide and withdraw the drug if there is a 20% reduction in this value. Corticosteroids have been used with some success and should probably be initiated when pulmonary toxicity is suspected.

2. Mitomycin–Mitomycin is an alkylating antibiotic used primarily in the treatment of gastrointestinal malignancies and also of breast and lung cancers. The incidence of pulmonary toxicity is reported to be 3–12%, but the effect of this drug is difficult to estimate, since most of these patients receive multiple chemotherapeutic agents. Pulmonary damage is not thought to relate to age, dose regimen, or total dose. Irradiation and oxygen therapy may increase the risk of injury. The mortality of mitomycin-associated lung injury is estimated to be 50% but can be decreased by early withdrawal of the drug and administration of corticosteroids.

B. Alkylating Agents:

1. Busulfan–Busulfan is used primarily in the treatment of myeloproliferative disorders, especially chronic myelogenous leukemia. Subclinical pulmonary toxicity is estimated to be 40–45% and about 4% of patients develop symptomatic lung disease. The pulmonary fibrosis seen with busulfan can develop as early as 2 months into therapy but on average occurs after 3 years of therapy. This delay is significantly longer than with most cytotoxic agents. No patient treated with less than 500 mg of busulfan has developed clinical lung toxicity.

No therapy has been defined for busulfan-induced lung injury. Initially, the agent should be discontinued. Since this disorder carries a high mortality secondary to progressive fibrosis, a trial of corticosteroids is usually attempted. The mean survival after diagnosis of pulmonary fibrosis is only 5 months.

2. Cyclophosphamide–Cyclophosphamide is effective against a wide range of cancers and inflammatory disorders. Pulmonary toxicities have occurred in patients with both malignant and nonmalignant disorders with a frequency of less than 1%. Pulmonary toxicity does not appear to be related to age, underlying disease, duration, or dose of the drug or to radiotherapy. While one animal study showed increased toxicity when associated with oxygen exposure, no clear relationship has been noted in humans. The clinical course is similar to that for other cytotoxic agents except that fever is noted in over half the cases. The prognosis is variable, and about 60% recover with cessation of the drug alone or in combination with corticosteroids.

3. Chlorambucil–Chlorambucil is used primarily in the treatment of hematologic cancer. Eleven well-documented cases of chlorambucil-induced pulmonary toxicity have been reported. The pattern of toxicity resembles that seen with cyclophosphamide. Half the patients die of respiratory failure despite the initiation of corticosteroids. The value of any specific therapy is unclear.

C. Antimetabolites:

1. Methotrexate–Methotrexate is a folate antagonist used in the treatment of malignant and nonmalignant disorders including leukemia, choriocarcinoma, osteogenic sarcoma, and psoriasis. The exact incidence of pulmonary toxicity is not known but is estimated at 4–8%.

This drug can be administered orally, intramuscularly, or intravenously. Pulmonary toxicity appears to relate to frequency of administration and not to route of administration. Patients receiving the drug either daily or weekly are more likely to develop lung damage. Age, total dose, and duration of therapy do not relate to the frequency of pulmonary toxicity.

Many patients develop findings consistent with a hypersensitivity pneumonitis including fever and eosinophilia, granulomatous changes on some lung biopsies, and the development of disease despite very low doses of the drug. Clinically, the presentation may be subacute or chronic. The subacute form is associated with fever, pleuritic pain, and a peripheral blood eosinophilia in 40% of patients. Skin eruptions occur in 20%. The prognosis is very good, with a mortality of around 1%. Some reports have noted clearing of infiltrates despite continuation of the drug; however, discontinuation of the drug and initiation of corticosteroids are thought to induce a dramatic resolution in most patients.

2. Azathioprine and mercaptopurine–Acute drug-induced pneumonitis has occurred in three pa-tients taking azathioprine and one patient taking mercaptopurine. Initiation of corticosteroids and cessation of the drug led to improvement in each case.

D. Other Cytotoxic Drugs:

1. Carmustine (BCNU)–Carmustine is a nitrosourea used in the treatment of intracranial malignancies, lymphoma, and myeloma. When carmustine is the only agent used to treat intracranial cancer, pulmonary toxicity develops in 20–30% of the cases. Overall, carmustine is thought to induce symptomatic pulmonary lesions in 5% of patients. Younger patients are more likely to develop pulmonary toxicity, but this may be related to the longer duration of therapy and larger total dose given to younger patients. A unique feature of carmustine-induced lung disease is the occurrence of fibrosis in the absence of inflammatory cell infiltration. The lung injury can be so severe that respiratory failure and death occurs within several days; however, most cases progress over several months. Many patients develop pulmonary fibrosis while receiving corticosteroids for intracranial malignancy, making the use of corticosteroids in this disorder questionable.

2. Procarbazine–Procarbazine is used primarily in the treatment of lymphoma. This agent has been associated with a hypersensitivity pneumonitis that on biopsy reveals mononuclear cell infiltration with foci of eosinophils. The clinical manifestations are almost identical to those seen with methotrexate. Treatment consists only of stopping the drug, yet corticosteroid use would seem reasonable.

3. *Vinca* alkaloids–Vinblastine and vindesine have been reported to cause diffuse interstitial infiltrates and respiratory failure in 11 patients. Each of these patients was receiving mitomycin concomitantly. The role of mitomycin is unknown, but unlike in other cases of cytotoxic drug–induced lung injury, bronchospasm and obstruction on pulmonary function testing were noted. Lung biopsy revealed a nonspecific inflammatory reaction with dysplasia of the alveolar lining cells and fibrosis.

REFERENCES

Radiation Therapy

Ellis F: Dose, time, and fractionation: A clinical hypothesis. *Clin Radiol* 1969;**30**:1.

Gross NJ: Pulmonary effects of radiation therapy. *Ann Intern Med* 1977;**86**:81.

Libshitz HL, Southard ME: Complication of radiation therapy: The thorax. *Semin Roentgenol* 1974;**9**:41.

Smith JC: Radiation pneumonitis. *Am Rev Respir Dis* 1963;**87**:647.

Chemotherapy

Gockerman JP: Drug-induced interstitial lung diseases. *Clin Chest Med* 1982;**3**:521.

Green MR: Pulmonary toxicity of antineoplastic agents. *West J Med* 1977;**127**:292.

Bleomycin

Holoye PY et al: Bleomycin hypersensitivity pneumonitis. *Ann Intern Med* 1978;**88**:47.

· Yagoda A et al: Bleomycin, an antitumor antibiotic: Clinical experience in 274 patients. *Ann Intern Med* 1972;**77**:861.

Mitomycin

Andrews AT et al: Mitomycin and interstitial pneumonitis. *Ann Intern Med* 1979;**90**:127.

Gunstream SR et al: Mitomycin-associated lung disease. *Cancer Treat Rep* 1983;**67**:301.

Busulfan

Burns WA, McFarland W, Matthews MJ: Busulfan-induced pulmonary disease: Report of a case and review of the literature. *Am Rev Respir Dis* 1970;**101**:408.

Oliner H et al: Interstitial pulmonary fibrosis following busulfan therapy. *Am J Med* 1961;**31**:134.

Cyclophosphamide

Patel AR et al: Cyclophosphamide pneumonitis. *Thorax* 1978;**33**:89.

Topilow AA, Rothenberg SP, Cottrell TS: Interstitial pneumonia after prolonged treatment with cyclophosphamide. *Am Rev Respir Dis* 1973;**108**:114.

Chlorambucil

Cole SR, Myers TJ, Klatsky AU: Pulmonary disease with chlorambucil therapy. *Cancer* 1978;**41**:455.

Methotrexate

Sostman HD, Matthay RA, Putman CE: Methotrexate-induced pneumonitis. *Medicine* 1976;**55**:371.

Lascari AD et al: Methotrexate-induced sudden fatal pulmonary reaction. *Cancer* 1977;**40**:1393.

BCNU

Durant JR et al: Pulmonary toxicity associated with bischloroethylnitrosourea (BCNU). *Ann Intern Med* 1979;**90**:191.

Procarbazine

Jones SE et al: Hypersensitivity to procarbazine (Matulane) manifested by fever and pleuropulmonary reaction. *Cancer* 1972;**29**:498.

Vinca Alkaloids

Kris MG et al: Dyspnea following vinblastine or vindesine administration in patients receiving mitomycin plus *Vinca* alkaloid combination therapy. *Cancer Treat Rep* 1984;**68**:1029.

Luedke D et al: Mitomycin C and vindesine associated pulmonary toxicity with variable clinical expression. *Cancer* 1985;**55**:542.

37

Renal Toxicity

T. Dwight McKinney, MD

Patients with cancer are subject to a variety of different types of renal, fluid and electrolyte disorders (Table 37–1). Some result from direct effects of neoplasia, such as urinary tract obstruction by tumor, or from indirect effects, such as hypercalcemic nephropathy. Others, eg, glomerulonephritis and nephrotic syndrome, are due to immunologic reactions associated with neoplasia. Immunosuppressed patients may develop severe infections, and acute renal failure may result from some of these infections, eg, gram-negative bacteremia with septic shock and disseminated intravascular coagulation. Treatment of infections, particularly with aminoglycoside antibiotics or amphotericin B, is often complicated by acute renal failure. Finally, renal injury may be a consequence of therapy directed to the patient's neoplasm. Often, renal injury represents the dose-limiting factor in these therapies. The most frequent forms of renal injury that may result from antineoplastic therapy are discussed below.

COMPLICATIONS SECONDARY TO CHEMOTHERAPY

Cisplatin

Cisplatin is a compound frequently used in therapy of several solid tumors. The drug may produce a variety of renal abnormalities, and nephrotoxicity limits the dose (Table 37–2). Renal excretion represents the primary mode of disposition of cisplatin. The initial half-life of cisplatin is 1 hour or less, followed by a late half-life of 24–60 hours or more. Although up to half an administered dose may undergo urinary excretion within 24 hours, the drug may be detected in urine for up to 30 days following a single dose. Urinary excretion is due to glomerular filtration and tubular secretion. Studies suggest that the secretory component may involve both organic cation and organic anion transport pathways. The highest tissue levels of cisplatin are found in the kidneys, liver, and spleen.

The most important form of cisplatin nephrotoxicity is acute renal failure associated with necrosis of the renal tubules. Decreased renal function is unusual with a single dose below 50 mg/m^2 but progressively increases with higher doses and is correlated with peak plasma levels of ultrafilterable platinum. Typically, azotemia appears within 2–4 days of therapy and becomes maximal within 6–10 days. Recovery of renal function occurs within 2–3 weeks if damage is not severe. Irreversible renal damage, largely manifested by chronic tubulointerstitial disease, may occur with repeated courses of cisplatin or with initially severe injury. Concomitant exposure to other nephrotoxins, particularly the aminoglycoside antibiotics alone or in combination with cephalosporins, is associated with greater nephrotoxicity. Other potential nephrotoxins, especially aminoglycosides, should be avoided if possible in patients who have received cisplatin within the past several days. Additionally, the drug should be administered with caution in individuals with underlying renal insufficiency, regardless of cause.

The pathophysiologic mechanisms responsible for cisplatin nephrotoxicity remain uncertain. As in many other forms of acute toxic renal disease, renal vascular resistance is increased and renal blood flow is reduced in the early stage of experimental cisplatin-induced renal injury. In the experimental setting, renal hemodynamics may be improved (but not restored to normal) in cisplatin-treated animals with extracellular fluid volume expansion. Some evidence suggests that the renal vasoconstriction occurring soon after cisplatin administration is not due to activation of the renin-angiotensin system.

Clinically, the most important factor identified to provide protection against cisplatin nephrotoxicity is maintenance of a high urine flow rate with intravenous saline, possibly combined with furosemide or mannitol. Use of isotonic or hypertonic saline as the vehicle for administering cisplatin appears to reduce nephrotoxicity without decreasing its antitumor activity. This effect may be due to lesser aquation of the parent compound; the aquated form of the drug may be more nephrotoxic. Administration of cisplatin as a slow continuous infusion over several hours may also decrease nephrotoxicity.

Several agents are being investigated for their ability to ameliorate cisplatin nephrotoxicity, among them, probenecid, sulfur-containing nucleophiles and sulfhydryl protective agents, the organic thiophosphate WR-2721 [S-2-(3-aminopropylamino)ethyl phosphorothioic acid], sodium thiosulfate, diethyl-

Table 37–1. Categories and examples of renal and electrolyte disorders in patients with neoplasia.

Disorders due to underlying malignancy
  Direct effects
    Urinary tract obstruction by neoplastic cells
    Infiltration of kidneys by neoplastic cells
    Lactic acidosis
    Hyperuricemia
  Indirect effects
    Hypercalcemia and hypercalcemic nephropathy
    Uric acid nephropathy
    Glomerulonephritis
    Myeloma of kidney
    Syndrome of inappropriate antidiuretic hormone secretion (SIADH)
    Hypokalemia from Cushing's syndrome due to ectopic ACTH
Disorders due to antineoplastic therapy
  Nephrotoxic effects of drugs or radiation therapy
  Tumor lysis syndrome
Disorders due to associated therapy or diagnostic agents
  Drug-induced acute renal failure
    Acute tubular necrosis, eg, resulting from aminoglycoside antibiotics, amphotericin B, or radiographic contrast medium
    Drug-induced acute allergic interstitial nephritis, eg, resulting from penicillin, sulfonamide, or allopurinol therapy
Other disorders
  Acute renal failure associated with sepsis
  Prerenal azotemia resulting from poor oral intake and vomiting

dithiocarbamate, glutathione, adenosine antagonists, calcium channel blockers and selenium.

Another common nephrotoxic effect of cisplatin therapy is renal magnesium wasting. This may cause symptomatic hypomagnesemia and resulting complications including hypocalcemia, tetany, and hypokalemia. Hypomagnesemia may occur in as many of 50% of patients receiving cisplatin and may persist for several weeks following administration of the drug. Thus, serum magnesium levels should be measured at regular intervals and replacement therapy begun if needed. The renal tubular defect responsible for magnesium wasting is not certain.

Other renal complications of cisplatin therapy include renal sodium wasting occurring several weeks

Table 37–2. Renal and electrolyte complications of cisplatin therapy.

Acute renal insufficiency associated with acute tubular necrosis
Chronic renal insufficiency associated with chronic tubulointerstitial disease
Renal magnesium wasting with magnesium deficiency with or without hypomagnesemia
  Hypocalcemia resulting from magnesium deficiency
  Renal potassium wasting resulting from magnesium deficiency
Renal sodium wasting resulting in extracellular volume depletion or hyponatremia
Renal concentrating defect resulting in polyuria

after therapy is begun. This has been associated with decreased activity of the renin-angiotensin-aldosterone system and may be accompanied by hyponatremia and signs of extracellular volume depletion including orthostatic hypotension. Polyuria, evidently resulting initially from impaired release of antidiuretic hormone and later from decreased interstitial tonicity of the renal medulla, may also occur following cisplatin therapy.

Initial studies suggest that carboplatin, an analog of cisplatin, may be a useful antineoplastic agent having significantly less nephrotoxitiy than cisplatin.

Nitrosoureas

Progressive renal damage has been documented in some patients receiving the nitrosoureas carmustine and lomustine, generally when given as part of the therapy for malignant brain tumors or malignant melanoma. Renal damage seems to be more frequent in children. In one report, six of six children receiving a total dose of lomustine greater than 1500 mg/m^2 developed renal damage. In adults receiving similar doses, the incidence of renal damage was 26%. Nephrotoxicity is manifested by the insidious development of azotemia and, particularly in children, a progressive decrease in renal size. Renal damage becomes evident during repeated courses of chemotherapy but more frequently develops months after therapy is completed. Once present, renal damage tends to be progressive and may continue to end-stage disease requiring chronic dialysis therapy. Chronic renal insufficiency is not accompanied or preceded by abnormalities of the urinary sediment, proteinuria, hypertension, or an episode of acute renal failure. Renal pathologic changes in nitrosourea-induced renal injury consist predominantly of interstitial fibrosis and glomerular sclerosis with wrinkling, thickening, and duplication of the glomerular capillary basement membrane. Immunofluorescence and electron microscopic examinations rarely reveal findings consistent with immune-mediated renal injury.

The pathogenesis of nitrosourea nephrotoxicity is uncertain. These compounds are rapidly metabolized, and most of the metabolites are excreted in the urine within several hours of administration of the drugs. It is generally believed that renal injury results from direct toxic effects of the drugs or their metabolites. Although the renal pathology in this setting is in many respects similar to that observed in chronic radiation nephritis, hypertension and proteinuria, which are common in the latter disorder, are not observed.

Since the development of nephrotoxicity is dose-related and no factors predict the development of renal failure, renal damage can be best avoided by limiting the cumulative dose of the nitrosoureas to less than 1400–1500 mg/m^2. Furthermore, if an otherwise unexplained increase in the blood urea nitrogen or serum creatinine concentration is observed during therapy with the nitrosoureas, the drugs should be discontinued.

Streptozocin

Streptozocin is a glucosamine-nitrosourea most frequently used in therapy of pancreatic islet cell tumors. Its dose-limiting adverse effect is nephrotoxicity. The parent compound is rapidly metabolized after administration, with some of the metabolites having more alkalyating activity than the parent compound. Streptozocin is most concentrated in the kidney and liver, and urinary excretion of metabolites represents the major mode of disposition of the drug. Nephrotoxicity occurs in 28–73% of patients. Pathologic changes in the glomeruli and interstitial inflammation have been described with streptozocin nephrotoxicity. Both glomerular and tubular functional abnormalities and acute and chronic renal insufficiency may occur. Proteinuria is often the first manifestation of renal damage. This is usually mild, and only rarely is proteinuria present in nephrotic quantities (> 3.5 g/d). Multiple abnormalities of proximal tubular function, either alone or in combination (Fanconi's syndrome), are also frequent. These include phosphaturia (with hypophosphatemia), type II (proximal) renal tubular acidosis (with bicarbonaturia and hyperchloremic metabolic acidosis), uricosuria (with hypouricemia), kaliuresis (with hypokalemia), glycosuria (with normal serum glucose concentration), and aminoaciduria. Although renal abnormalities may occur after only one or a few doses, more commonly they are observed after repeated doses. No predictive factors for the development of streptozocin-induced nephrotoxicity or measures to prevent it have been identified. If administration of streptozocin is stopped when only mild renal abnormalities are present, they may disappear.

Methotrexate

Methotrexate is a folic acid antagonist used in the treatment of a variety of hematologic malignancies and solid tumors. Urinary excretion of the parent drug, primarily by glomerular filtration and, to a lesser extent by secretion utilizing organic anion pathways, represents the principal mode of disposition. Greater than 50% of an administered dose is excreted within 12 hours of administration. Methotrexate is concentrated in urine to levels severalfold higher than those in plasma. Because of this and because the solubility of the drug is less in acidic fluid, when given in high doses (> 500 mg/m^2) methotrexate may precipitate in the lumen of distal nephron segments and result in intrarenal obstruction and acute renal failure. Although unusual with low-dose therapy, acute renal failure has been an important cause of morbidity and mortality with high-dose methotrexate therapy. In addition to tubular obstruction, tubular necrosis may result from direct toxic effects of methotrexate. Development of renal failure

prolongs the half-life of the drug and may result in other toxic manifestations, particularly myelosuppression. This is especially true if leucovorin (given to protect normal tissues from the drug) is not utilized concomitantly and not continued until blood levels of methotrexate fall.

Several measures may be used to lessen the incidence of methotrexate nephrotoxicity. First, the concentration of the drug in urine can be decreased by maintaining extracellular fluid volume expansion and a high urine flow rate (> 100 mL/h) with intravenous fluids. Second, since the solubility of methotrexate in urine is increased tenfold by elevation of urine pH from 5.7 to 6.9, urine should be alkalinized to a pH of 7.0 or more by means of intravenous fluids that contain sodium bicarbonate prior to administration of the drug. A high flow of alkaline urine should also be maintained for the first day following high-dose methotrexate. Third, methotrexate should be given with caution to individuals with underlying renal insufficiency. Finally, drugs that may inhibit renal proximal tubular organic anion secretory pathways, eg, salicylates (and several other nonsteroidal anti-inflammatory drugs), should not be prescribed during methotrexate therapy. Both renal function and methotrexate blood levels should be measured 24–48 hours following administration of the drug, and if leucovorin therapy is being given, this should be continued if blood levels are greater than 9×10^{-7} mol/L at 48 hours. A concentration less than this predicts that the level at 72 hours will likely be in the safe range and leucovorin may be discontinued. It should be noted that leucovorin does not prevent intrarenal precipitation of methotrexate. Determining the clearance of a small dose of methotrexate is useful in calculating the amount of drug to be given in a high-dose regimen. Although hemodialysis, peritoneal dialysis, and charcoal hemoperfusion may cause a transient fall in the plasma concentration of methotrexate, because of the rapid rebound in plasma levels soon after these treatments are discontinued, they are not useful therapies in patients with toxic plasma concentrations of the drug.

Mitomycin

Fifteen percent to 40% of patients receiving mitomycin, usually in combination with other agents for treatment of a variety of solid tumors, develop manifestations of renal disease. These include azotemia, mild proteinuria, and hematuria, which generally occur several months after therapy with mitomycin is instituted. In some cases, acute renal failure occurs in association with microangiopathic hemolytic anemia, thrombocytopenia, and hemoglobinuria, a constellation of findings resembling the hemolytic uremic syndrome. Renal disease may be accompanied by severe hypertension. Most patients with renal abnormalities have received multiple courses of mitomycin resulting in a cumulative dose of 90 mg or more.

Renal pathologic changes include mesangial disruption, nuclear atypia of renal tubular cells, and, in those with microangiopathic hemolytic anemia, fibrin thrombi and fibrinoid necrosis of the glomerular capillary loops. The pathogenetic basis for mitomycin nephrotoxicity is not known. In some patients, blood transfusions appear to exacerbate the microangiopathic process. Except for supportive measures, there is no established therapy for mitomycin nephrotoxicity. Plasmapheresis has been reported to be useful in isolated cases. Mitomycin should be discontinued if renal disease becomes apparent.

Interleukin-2

Recombinant interleukin-2 (IL-2), generally in combination with lymphokine-activated killer cells, has been administered on an experimental basis to some patients with advanced cancer. A host of findings, including hypotension necessitating administration of large volumes of intravenous fluids, oliguria with low urinary sodium excretion, azotemia, and massive fluid retention typically occurs. Although the responsible mechanisms are not known, these findings are most consistent with marked prerenal azotemia. In addition to IL-2, most patients receive other drugs, particularly the nonsteroidal anti-inflammatory agent indomethacin, possibly indicating a role for decreased prostaglandin production. Typically, abnormalities develop shortly after IL-2 therapy begins and generally resolve within several days after its discontinuation. The most severe impairment in renal function tends to occur in individuals with underlying renal insufficiency.

COMPLICATIONS SECONDARY TO RADIATION THERAPY

Radiation Nephritis

Exposure of the kidneys to fractionated radiation in excess of 2000–3000 cGy may result in delayed renal damage that may take one of several forms. Acute radiation nephritis develops 6–12 months following renal irradiation. Clinical features include hypertension, salt retention with edema, proteinuria, microscopic hematuria, pyuria, anemia, and azotemia. Patients may be left with varying degrees of chronic renal insufficiency, or acute radiation nephritis may progress to end-stage renal failure. Chronic radiation nephritis may follow acute radiation nephritis or may develop by itself after a latent interval as long as several years following renal irradiation. Clinical features are similar to those observed in acute radiation nephritis. Progression to end-stage renal failure may occur. Both benign and malignant hypertension may develop from 2 to several years following renal irradiation. Finally, isolated proteinuria may occur, usually several years after renal irradiation.

The pathogenesis and progression of irradiation-induced renal injury is incompletely understood. It is not clear whether the initial injury is to the renal tubules or to vascular components. Renal pathologic changes include mesangial and glomerular sclerosis and chronic interstitial nephritis. The small renal arteries and arterioles typically show collagenous intimal thickening. Fibrinoid necrosis of the small renal arteries and glomeruli may be observed, particularly in the setting of malignant hypertension.

There is no specific treatment for radiation nephritis. Adequate control of blood pressure should diminish the rate of renal functional impairment. The most important feature of treatment is prevention by limiting exposure of the kidneys to total irradiation of 2000 cGy or less delivered in fractionated doses over several days. Decline in renal function following irradiation to the kidneys may be related as much to the amount of renal tissue exposed as to the dose of irradiation, and doses higher than 2000 cGy may be tolerated with acceptable levels of renal toxicity if the field of exposure is limited to 50% or less of the kidney. Since unilateral radiation nephritis may represent a surgically correctable cause (ie, by nephrectomy) of severe hypertension associated with activation of the renin-angiotensin system, this should be kept in mind in individuals with a unilaterally small kidney who have received previous radiation therapy.

TUMOR LYSIS SYNDROME

Patients with certain hematologic malignancies, particularly acute leukemia and undifferentiated (including Burkitt's and non-Burkitt's forms) and lymphoblastic lymphoma, may develop spontaneous acute renal failure due to overproduction of uric acid and precipitation of uric acid in the lumen of the renal tubules resulting in intrarenal obstruction (acute uric acid nephropathy). More frequently, however, acute renal failure in these patients follows massive cytoreductive chemotherapy or radiation therapy. With massive cell lysis, in addition to release of uric acid and its purine precursors, other cellular constituents, particularly phosphates and potassium, enter the extracellular fluid. Even though blood levels of these substances may not be elevated, increased urinary excretion of phosphate and potassium are frequent. As a result of the release of cellular constituents, a constellation of abnormalities, termed tumor lysis syndrome, may be seen. It may include acute renal failure, hyperuricemia, hyperphosphatemia (with hypocalcemia secondary to the calcium phosphate solubility product in blood being exceeded), and hyperkalemia. Patients with baseline renal insufficiency are more likely to develop worsening renal function in this setting. Although acute uric acid nephropathy may follow massive cytoreductive therapy, since most of these patients receive allopurinol prior to chemotherapy and generally do not subsequently develop severe hyperuricemia, acute uric acid nephropathy alone is a less likely cause of their acute renal failure. It has been suggested that precipitation of phosphate salts in the tubule lumen is a major contributor to renal failure.

The chance of developing acute renal failure due to tumor lysis syndrome can be minimized by the following guidelines. If possible, allopurinol should be given in a dose of 300–400 mg/m^2 for 3–4 days prior to administration of cancer therapy. Thereafter, the dose should be reduced to one-half this amount, since a rare complication of high-dose allopurinol administration is xanthine nephrolithiasis. Sodium bicarbonate may be administered to alkalinize the urine and increase uric acid excretion. However, since phosphate salts are less soluble in alkaline solutions, alkali therapy should be discontinued prior to administration of cancer therapy. Patients should be well hydrated, and a high urine flow rate ($\geq$2–3 L/d) should be established prior to administration of cancer therapy, generally, by intravenous administration of fluids. Strong consideration should be given to performing dialysis in patients with baseline renal insufficiency before beginning cancer therapy. Acute dialysis (generally hemodialysis) is indicated not only in patients with acute renal failure but also in those who develop significant hyperuricemia or hyperphosphatemia after cancer therapy in the absence of azotemia in an attempt to prevent acute renal failure. Hemodialysis is effective in removing uric acid and, to a lesser extent, phosphate. It is also an effective treatment for hyperkalemia. In patients with acute renal failure occurring in this setting, renal function generally returns to baseline in 1–3 weeks. In addition to acute uric acid nephropathy and tumor lysis syndrome, other causes of renal failure should be excluded in these patients, including that due to ureteral obstruction from tumor and other nephrotoxic sources, especially drugs such as aminoglycoside antibiotics and radiographic contrast medium.

OTHER CAUSES OF NEPHROTOXICITY

Other pharmacologic and immunologic agents used in treatment of malignancies occasionally cause nephrotoxicity. Recombinant leukocyte alpha and gamma interferon has been associated with acute interstitial nephritis, acute tubular necrosis, proteinuria, and nephrotic syndrome. Both reversible azotemia and renal tubular abnormalities, including bicarbonate, sodium, glucose, and phosphorus wasting and polyuria, have been reported after azacytidine therapy. Nephrotoxicity has also been reported as an unusual complication in patients treated with daunorubicin, doxorubincin, ifosfamide, mithramycin, and dacarbazine.

REFERENCES

Bennett WM, Elzinga LW, Porter GA: Tubulointerstitial disease and toxic nephropathy. Pages 1430–1496 in: *The Kidney.* Brenner BM, Rector FC Jr (editors). Saunders, 1991.

Christiansen, NP et al: Nephrotoxicity of continuous intravenous infusion of recombinant interleukin-2. *Am J Med* 1988;**84:**1072.

Giroux L, Better P, Giroux L: Mitomycin-C nephrotoxicity: A clinico-pathologic study of 17 cases. *Am J Kidney Dis* 1985;**6:**28.

Groth S et al: Acute and long-term nephrotoxicity of cisplatinum in man. *Cancer Chemother Pharmacol* 1986;**17:**191.

Krochak RJ, Baker DG: Radiation nephritis: Clinical manifestations and pathophysiologic mechanisms. *Urology* 1986;**27:**389.

McCroskey RD et al: Acute tumor lysis syndrome and treatment response in patients treated for refractory chronic lymphocytic leukemia with short-course, high-dose cytosine arabinoside, cisplatin, and etoposide. *Cancer* 1990;**66:**246.

McKinney TD: *Renal Complications of Neoplasia.* Praeger, 1986.

McKinney TD: Tubulointerstitial diseases and toxic nephropathies. Pages 568–579 in: *Cecil Textbook of Medicine.* Wyngaarden JB, Smith LH Jr, Bennett JC (editors). Saunders, 1992.

Narins RG et al. The nephrotoxicity of chemotherapeutic agents. *Semin Nephrol* 1990:**10:**556.

Quesada JR et al: Clinical toxicity of interferons in cancer patients: A review. *J Clin Oncol* 1986;**4:**234.

Ries F, Klastersky J: Nephrotoxicity induced by cancer chemotherapy with special emphasis on cisplatin toxicity. *Am J Kidney Dis* 1986;**5:**368.

Rieselbach RE, Garnick MB: Renal disease induced by antineoplastic agents. Pages 1275–1299 in: *Diseases of the Kidney.* Schrier RW, Gottschalk CW (editors). Little, Brown, 1988.

Saferstein R et al: Cisplatin nephrotoxicity. *Am J Kidney Dis* 1986;**8:**356.

Schacht RG et al: Nephrotoxicity of nitrosoureas. *Cancer* 1981;**48:**1328.

Shalmi CL et al: Acute renal dysfunction during interleukin-2 treatment: Suggestion of an intrinsic renal lesion. *J Clin Oncol* 1990;**8:**1839.

Skinner R et al: Assessment of chemotherapy-associated nephrotoxicity in children with cancer. *Cancer Chemother Pharmacol* 1991;**28:**81.

Weiss RB: Streptozocin: A review of its pharmacology, efficacy, and toxicity. *Cancer Treat Rep* 1982;**66:**427.

Section VII.
Oncologic Emergencies

Infection in the Neutropenic or Immunocompromised Patient

38

Rebecca Johnson Irvin, PharmD, & Jim M. Koeller, MS

An immunocompromised host has a substantial and prolonged dysfunction of cellular and humoral immunity secondary to specific immunosuppressive therapy or disease process. Immunocompromised patients are subject to a host of bacterial, fungal, viral, and other opportunistic infections. A neutropenic patient has an abnormally small number of neutrophils in the circulating blood and is more susceptible to bacterial and fungal infections. Leukemics having an absolute neutrophil count (ANC) less than 1000 cells/mm^3 and patients with solid tumors having an ANC less than 500 cells/mm^3 are at significant risk for developing infections. ANCs less than 500 cells/mm^3 are associated with over 70% of septic episodes and 90% of disseminated fungal infections in the neutropenic or immunocompromised host. Fatality rates range from 30% to 70% depending on the degree and duration of neutropenia. While the basic medical evaluation in the two populations is the same, the underlying cause of infection is often different (Table 38–1).

Reasons for Immunodeficiency
A. Neutrophil Count: Neutropenia is usually defined as an absolute neutrophil count (ANC) of 500 cells/mm^3 or less in patients with solid tumors or 1000 cells/mm^3 or less in leukemic patients. The ANC is the sum of the percent of neutrophils and band forms, multiplied by the total number of white blood cells (WBCs). As an example,

WBCs = 1000 Differential = **55 segmented neutrophils**
5 band forms
30 lymphocytes
10 monocytes
ANC = (0.55 + 0.05) × 1000 = 600 cells/mm^3

The neutrophil count and duration of neutropenia are probably the most significant factors determining the risk of infection. As the neutrophil count decreases and the duration of neutropenia increases, the risk of infection by bacteria, fungi, and opportunistic organisms increases substantially. Patients who have re-

ceived prior chemotherapy or radiotherapy are particularly vulnerable to infectious processes secondary to defects in neutrophil function and decreased bone marrow reserve.

B. Defects in Cell-Mediated and Humoral Immunity: Cell-mediated immunity is conferred by T lymphocytes and executed by lymphocytes and macrophages. Pathogens susceptible to lymphocytes and macrophages include certain bacteria, viruses, fungi, protozoa, helminths, *Chlamydia, Rickettsia,* and *Treponema pallidum.* Irradiation, cytotoxic drugs (eg, cyclophosphamide), and corticosteroids are agents responsible for altering cell-mediated immunity. Dysfunctional cellular immunity is an integral part of some disease processes, eg, Hodgkin's disease and the acquired immunodeficiency syndrome (AIDS).

The humoral immune response produces opsonizing and bactericidal antibodies against organisms such as *Streptococcus pneumoniae, Haemophilus influenzae, Neisseria meningitidis, Pneumocystis carinii,* and *Giardia.* Patients with multiple myeloma, chronic lymphocytic leukemia, or splenectomy are vulnerable to the above organisms owing to altered humoral immunity. Hypogammaglobulinemia does not appear to predispose patients to fungal or viral infections when cellular immunity remains intact.

C. Alterations in Physical Barriers: Disturbance of physical barriers, such as the skin, gastrointestinal tract, urinary tract, and respiratory mucosa, during chemotherapy or invasive procedures provides a portal of entry for invasive organisms. Indwelling intravenous or urinary catheters, intubation devices, venipuncture sites, bone marrow aspirations, drug extravasations, and surgery disrupt protective barriers, and their use should be approached cautiously in neutropenic and immunocompromised patients.

D. Nutritional Status: Good nutritional status is important in maintaining cell-mediated immunity, since decreased phagocytic and lymphocytic function, as well as impaired healing of skin and mucosal

Table 38–1. Risk factors for infection in neutropenic or immunocompromised patients.

Defect	Underlying Disease
Neutropenia	Leukemia, bone marrow transplant (early) cancer chemotherapy
Defects in cellular and humoral immunity	Hodgkin's disease, bone marrow transplant, AIDS, multiple myeloma, chronic lymphocytic leukemia
Alterations in physical barriers	
Decreased nutritional status	
Obstruction due to tumor or surgery	Lung cancer, gynecologic cancer
Central nervous system dysfunction	
Alterations in microbacterial flora	

barriers, has been reported in nutritionally depleted patients. Although nutritional support has not been shown to have an impact on survival in cancer patients, it may be of benefit in bone marrow transplant recipients and patients being treated with curative intent.

E. Obstruction: Pulmonary obstruction due to the primary malignancy can increase the risk of anaerobic infections such as *Bacteroides* sp, *Fusobacterium nucleatum*, and *Peptococcus*. *Pseudomonas aeruginosa* and *Klebsiella pneumoniae* are common pathogens associated with urinary tract obstructions. Neutropenic and immunocompromised patients, should be evaluated for infectious causes secondary to obstructive processes.

F. Central Nervous System Dysfunction: Central nervous dysfunction due to the primary malignancy or to metastasis may adversely affect protective mechanisms, leading to increased risk of infection. Loss of the gag reflex may predispose a patient to aspiration pneumonia, while impaired micturition secondary to neurologic dysfunction may lead to urinary tract infections.

G. Alterations in Bacterial Flora: Since 80% of documented infections are caused by the patient's own bacterial flora, colonization of the respiratory and gastrointestinal tract with virulent organisms is a primary concern. Colonization is dependent on exposure of the neutropenic host to organisms that attach to mucosal or epithelial tissues. Two important determinants of colonization are extensive antibiotic use and the type of bacteria and fungi inhabiting a particular medical center. Intensive care units and cancer wards are particularly noted for harboring virulent strains of bacteria or fungi that can establish residence in a neutropenic or immunocompromised host. Broad-spectrum antibiotic use alters gut anaerobic flora, increasing the susceptibility of the host to colo-

nization by more virulent organisms such as *P aeruginosa*.

BACTERIAL INFECTIONS

Bacterial infections account for up to 75% of all infections in the neutropenic or immunocompromised patient (Table 38–2). Gram-negative organisms account for 60–70% of bacterial infections. Rates of gram-positive infections as high as 60% have been reported at some institutions. *Staphylococcus epidermidis* is being recognized with increased frequency as a true pathogen primarily owing to the use of central venous catheters. Documented anaerobic organisms account for less than 5% of bacterial infections in these patients, probably because of poor culturing techniques for anaerobes.

Clinical Findings

Fifty-five percent of neutropenic or immunocompromised patients with proved bacteremia have no physical signs of infection, eg, abscesses lack pus formation, pyuria is absent from urinary tract infections, cough is without purulent sputum, and pharyngitis is without exudate or adenopathy. Fever is usually the only indication of an infectious process, and fever that persists for more than 2 hours unassociated with administration of blood products is considered due to an infectious process in these patients until proved otherwise. Fever is defined as three oral temperature readings above 38 °C in a 24-hour period or a single oral temperature of 38.5 °C. Noninfectious causes of fever include blood products, amphotericin B, graft rejection, lymphoma, leukemia, tumor fever, and tumor necrosis. Antipyretics and corticosteroids should be avoided if possible, since they can mask fever. Respiratory changes such as dyspnea, hemoptysis, nonproductive cough, and pleuritic chest pain may represent early signs of sepsis. Hyperventilation and respiratory alkalosis may be seen alone or with hypoxemia. Confusion, disorientation, changes in consciousness, headache, and nausea and vomiting are signs of central nervous system infection or sepsis. Skin lesions should also be evaluated. *P aeruginosa, Staphylococcus aureus, Salmonella typhosa,* and *H influenzae* are examples of bacteria that produce skin lesions which may aid in diagnosis. Septic shock with hypotension can be seen in up to

Table 38–2. Common bacterial organisms causing infection in neutropenic or immunocompromised patients.

Gram-positive	Gram-negative
Staphylococcus aureus	Pseudomonas aeruginosa
Staphylococcus epidermidis	Escherichia coli
Streptococcus sp	Klebsiella pneumoniae

40% of patients with septicemia, predominately with gram-negative infections.

Diagnosis

Diagnosis begins with physical and neurologic examination. Common sites of infection are the periodontium, sinuses, pharynx, skin, esophagus, lungs, urinary tract, colon, and anus. Digital examination of the rectum should not be undertaken, since it can lead to transient seeding of blood by bacteria colonized in the rectum. If erythemia, tenderness, or swelling is found around an intravenous catheter site and the patient is otherwise clinically stable, the catheter should be removed by changing it over a guide wire, and the catheter tip and site should be cultured. In a few cases, it may be necessary to remove the catheter and place a new line on the opposite side. Skin lesions should be cultured or biopsied if possible. Two sets of blood cultures should be obtained: one from a peripheral vein and one from the central venous catheter, if present. Urine, sputum, mouth swab, and stool samples should be procured and sent for culture and Gram staining. With multiple fever spikes, cultures need only be obtained daily.

Chest x-ray should be obtained; however, as many as 60% of patients will have an abnormal chest x-ray but only half of these abnormal x-rays will reveal an infectious cause. Pneumococcal infection, *Klebsiella* infection, and pulmonary hemorrhage may present as a dense air space consolidation associated with air bronchograms. Pneumocystis pneumonia, viral infections, leukoagglutinin reactions, and drug-induced disease can demonstrate an interstitial pattern on the chest x-ray. Cavitating lesions are suggestive of fungal, tubercular, or nocardial infection. Sinus films may be helpful, particularly in diagnosing bacterial or fungal infections in patients with tender mastoid sinuses. Signs of central nervous system infection, eg, confusion, disorientation, and changes in consciousness, should be evaluated promptly by means of lumbar puncture. Bone marrow aspiration may yield a positive diagnosis of bacterial or fungal infection.

While bronchoalveolar lavage yields a specific diagnosis of opportunistic infection in one-third of the immunocompromised population, the complications of exacerbated respiratory failure and bleeding, especially in a thrombocytopenic patients, limit its utility. Open lung biopsy is considered a last resort in most institutions for obtaining a specific diagnosis in suspected pulmonary infections, since most immunocompromised patients are poor surgical candidates.

Treatment

A. General Considerations: Empiric therapy is instituted in the neutropenic patient prior to organism indentification owing to the low microbacterial yield from cultures and high mortality rate if left untreated.

Antibiotics should cover common bacterial organisms, possess synergistic properties, have low toxicity, bear bactericidal properties, and be cost effective.

The most important aspect of antimicrobial selection is to know which organisms commonly occur in the hospital in question and their antibiotic sensitivity and resistance patterns. Antibiotics selected for empiric therapy must be bactericidal for the commonly isolated organisms in that institution. Resistance to aminoglycosides, antipseudomonal penicillins, cephalosporins, and methicillin should be taken into consideration.

The empiric use of a single antimicrobial agent for the neutropenic patient is an alternative to combination therapy. Clinical trials with ceftazidime or imipenem have demonstrated efficacy during the first 72 hours of therapy. Ciprofloxacin has also been evaluated for use as empiric monotherapy. However, questions regarding the appropriate dose of ciprofloxacin, the higher incidence of superimposed infections when compared to ceftazidime, and the problem of increased ciprofloxacin resistance by microorganisms have yet to be resolved, and caution should be exercised if ciprofloxacin is used as monotherapy. Monotherapy should not be used in the following situations: institutions without continued microbiologic monitoring procedures, institutions with resistance problems to gram-negative infections, when treating profoundly neutropenic patients for prolonged periods (patients should be reevaluated within 48–72 hours after starting empiric therapy), and institutions without adequate monitoring personnel.

B. Gram-negative Organisms: Empiric therapy consists of a combination of an aminoglycoside and an antipseudomonal pencillin, ceftazidime, or imipenem (Table 38–3). The dose of aminoglycoside is based on ideal body weight, and renal function determines the scheduling interval. Usually a loading dose of gentamicin or tobramycin, 2 mg/kg, amikacin, 7.5 mg/kg, is given with the maintenance dose calculated based on published nomograms (such as that provided by Hull and Sarubbi). Aminoglycoside serum concentrations should be obtained after the third dose with desired peak concentrations of 6–10 μg/mL for gentamicin or tobramycin or of 20–30 μg/mL for amikacin. Higher peak concentrations (gentamicin or tobramycin, 8–10 μg/mL, or amikacin, 25–35 μg/mL) are necessary to obtain adequate aminoglycoside penetration in lung tissue for patients with pneumonia. Nephrotoxicity and ototoxicity are associated with aminoglycoside use and are frequently observed in dehydrated, geriatric, or renally compromised individuals. Use of multiple nephrotoxic and ototoxic drugs increases the risk of toxicity.

Antipseudomonal penicillins are used in combination with aminoglycosides as initial empiric therapy. Common adverse effects of these drugs include hypersensitivity reactions, gastrointestinal reactions,

Table 38–3. Antibiotics used to treat neutropenic patients.

Drug	Dose
Aminoglycosides	
Gentamicin	2 mg/kg loading dose, then per nomogram
Tobramycin	2 mg/kg loading dose, then per nomogram
Amikacin	7.5 mg/kg loading dose, then per nomogram
Antipseudomonal penicillins	
Azlocillin[1]	3 g every 4 hours or 4 g every 6 hours by slow intravenous infusion
Mezlocillin[1]	3 g every 4 hours or 4 g every 6 hours by slow intravenous infusion
Piperacillin[1]	3 g every 4 hours or 4 g every 6 hours by slow intravenous infusion
Ticarcillin[1]	3 g every 4 hours by slow intravenous infusion
Ticarcillin/clavulanate[1]	3.1 g every 4 hours by slow intravenous infusion
Miscellaneous	
Aztreonam[1]	2 g every 6–8 hours by slow intravenous infusion
Ceftazidime[1]	1 g every 8 hours by slow intravenous infusion
Imipenem-cilastatin	500 mg every 6 hours by slow intravenous infusion
Ciprofloxacin	300–400 mg intravenously every 12 hours
Gram-positive coverage	
Vancomycin[1]	1 g every 12 hours by slow intravenous infusion
Anaerobic coverage	
Clindamycin	600–900 mg every 6–8 hours by slow intravenous infusion
Metronidazole[2]	500 mg every 6 hours by slow intravenous infusion

[1] Adjust dose for creatinine clearance <50 mL/min.
[2] Adjust dose for hepatic dysfunction.

skin rash, phlebitis, platelet dysfunction, and electrolyte imbalance of sodium and potassium.

Ceftazidime is the only third-generation cephalosporin with reliable activity against *P aeruginosa*. Ceftazidime is generally well tolerated with common adverse effects limited to hypersensitivity reactions, gastrointestinal effects, and superinfection (especially with gram-positive organisms). Because resistant strains of *P aeruginosa* and *Enterobacter* have developed during therapy with single-agent ceftazidime, observation is mandatory.

Imipenem is a carbapenem that has good activity against gram-negative, gram-positive, and anaerobic organisms. Adverse effects include hypersensitivity reactions, gastrointestinal side effects, eosinophilia, seizures (in patients with renal failure or underlying seizure disorders), transient increases in hepatic enzymes, and superinfection. Its use as monotherapy has been associated with reports of resistant strains of *Pseudomonas* sp; therefore, addition of an aminoglycoside may be necessary for patients failing to respond to imipenem alone.

Ciprofloxacin, a broad-spectrum fluoroquinolone, is an alternative empiric antibiotic for beta-lactam–allergic neutropenic patients. The drug is well tolerated. Ciprofloxaxin as empiric monotherapy should be approached with caution owing to increasing antimicrobial resistance and superinfections with gram-positive organisms.

Aztreonam, a monobactam antibiotic with a narrow spectrum of activity against gram-negative organisms, can replace the antipseudomonal penicillin or cephalosporin in allergic patients. Since the drug is not effective against gram-positive or anaerobic organisms, it should never be used singly in a neutropenic patient. Alternative antibiotic regimens for patients with renal failure for whom an aminoglycoside may be contraindicated include a double beta-lactam (ceftazidime/piperacillin) or beta-bactam/monobactam (ceftazidime/aztreonam) combination.

C. Gram-positive Organisms: A documented gram-positive infection or significant clinical sign is required to initiate vancomycin therapy. If a patient continues to have fever after 48–72 hours of initial empiric coverage and has an indwelling intravenous catheter, vancomycin (1 g intravenously every 12 hours) should be added. Patients with decreased renal function (≤50 mL/min) should receive 1 g intravenously every 24–48 hours depending on the creatinine clearance. Vancomycin levels should be obtained after the third dose to document adequate peak serum concentrations of 20–40 µg/mL and trough (nadir blood level) concentrations of less than 10 µg/mL. Adverse effects of vancomycin include "red man's syndrome" (flushing of the neck and upper chest secondary to a rapid infusion rate), ototoxicity, nephrotoxicity, and hypersensitivity reactions. Vancomycin infusion times greater than 1 hour decrease the incidence of red man's syndrome.

Teicoplanin, a new glycopeptide antibiotic, has comparable activity to vancomycin in febrile neutropenic patients.

D. Anaerobic Infections: Anaerobic infections account for less than 5% of documented infections in neutropenic patients. A high index of suspicion for an anaerobic abscess or bacteremia must be present prior to initiating metronidazole or clindamycin therapy. Metronidazole or clindamycin should be added to empiric regimens lacking anaerobic coverage. Metronidazole is bactericidal, amebicidal, and trichomonacidal. Adverse effects include gastrointestinal reactions, peripheral neuropathy, hypersensitivity reactions, and superinfection. Clindamycin is bacteriostatic or bactericidal depending on the drug concentration at the site of the infection and the susceptibility of the organism. The drug is generally active against most gram-positive cocci and anaerobic bacteria. Adverse effects include gastrointestinal reactions, pseudomembranous colitis, local reactions, and transient increases in liver function tests.

FUNGAL INFECTIONS

Fungal infections are difficult to treat in the neutropenic or immunocompromised host, since functioning granulocytes are necessary for resolution of infection. Neutropenic patients remaining febrile for 4–7 days with broad-spectrum antimicrobial coverage are generally started on empiric intravenous amphotericin therapy to prevent fungal overgrowth, treat "subclinical" infections, and decrease mortality secondary to mycotic disease.

ASPERGILLOSIS

Aspergillosis is caused by *Aspergillus fumigatus* in one-half to two-thirds of infected patients and *Aspergillus flavus* in the remainder. Infection occurs when spores are aerosolized in the environment and colonized in the nasal sinuses, palate, epiglottis, and lungs.

Clinical Findings
Presenting symptoms for pulmonary invasion include dyspnea, tachypnea, nonproductive cough, pleuritic chest pain, hemoptysis, fever, and chills. Headache, local tenderness, infarction, and hemor-

rhage may be present in paranasal sinus invasion. Skin invasion by *A flavus* appears as an erythematous or violet-colored edematous indurated plague that progresses to a necrotic ulcer with a black eschar. Only one-fourth to one-half of disseminated cases are diagnosed early. A mycetoma (noninvasive fungal ball within a preexisting cavity) presents clinically with a potentially life-threatening hemorrhage.

Diagnosis
Culturing of throat, nasal, and tracheal secretions, and blood are necessary but usually provide little information, since the diagnosis will be missed in up to 75% of cultured patients. Chest x-ray may reveal a necrotizing bronchopneumonia, hemorrhagic pulmonary infarction, or both. Early diagnosis by aggressive biopsy technique is essential for effective treatment.

Treatment
Amphotericin B is the antifungal agent of choice for invasive aspergillosis (Table 38–4). Amphotericin B toxicity (Table 38–5) includes decreased glomerular filtration rate, renal tubular acidosis, hypokalemia, hypomagnesemia, thrombophlebitis, fever, shaking chills, and nausea and vomiting. Pretreatment with acetaminophen and diphenhydramine may prevent fever and histaminic effects, and chills can generally be alleviated with 50 mg of intravenous meperidine. Nephrotoxicity is generally seen within a few weeks of therapy and is usually reversible with total amphotericin doses less than 4 g. If the serum creatinine rises above 3 mg/dL, toxicity may be reduced by using an every-other-day schedule or decreasing the daily or total dose. Surgical excision is the treatment of choice for patients with mycetoma, but inhaled amphotericin therapy may be useful if the patient is not a surgical candidate.

CANDIDIASIS

Candida albicans and *Candida tropicalis* possess a strong affinity for host tissues and prosthetic devices, making these the most virulent *Candida* sp. *Candida*

Table 38–4. Protocol for amphotericin B administration.

Day 1	A 1-mg test dose in 100–250 mL of 5% dextrose in water is infused over 2–4 hours. Pulse, respiration rate, temperature, and blood pressure are monitored closely. If no anaphylactic reaction occurs 1 hour after infusion, the patient may receive 0.25 mg/kg over 2–4 hours. Premedication with diphenhydramine and acetaminophen may prevent adverse effects. Chills can be eliminated with 50 mg of meperidine.
	or
Day 1	The initial test dose can be given as part of the first maintenance dose by infusing the equivalent of 1 mg from the intravenous fluid containing 0.25 mg/kg. If no anaphylactic reaction occurs, the rest of the maintenance dose can be given.
Day 2 and beyond	Patients should receive 0.5 mg/kg/d in 5% dextrose in water (incompatible with normal saline) over 2–4 hours until the ANC is above 500 cells/mm³ or the total dose necessary to treat infection is reached. Some patients with documented fungemia may require 1–1.5 mg/kg/d.

Table 38–5. Adverse effects of amphotericin B.

Adverse Effect	Preventive Measure
Nephrotoxicity	? Use sodium loading.
Hypokalemia	Monitor and supplement K^+.
Hypomagnesemia	Monitor and supplement Mg^{2+}.
Thrombophlebitis[1]	Add heparin (1200–1600 units) to each bag of amphotericin B
Fever, chills	Give corticosteroids[2], meperidine, diphenhydramine, acetaminophen.
Anaphylactic reaction	Discontinue drug.

[1]Peripheral administration of amphotericin B.
[2]Corticosteroids may enhance potassium wasting.

sp are considered normal flora in the oropharyngeal and gastrointestinal tracts, skin, and vagina in 50%, 5%, and 20–30%, respectively, of the normal population. Clinical disease is propagated by candidal overgrowth at normal colonization sites and by invasion of mucocutaneous surfaces and the bloodstream.

Clinical Findings

The mucosal surfaces of the oropharynx, gastrointestinal tract, and vagina are common overgrowth sites for *Candida* in the neutropenic or immunocompromised patient. Discrete, raised white plaques on an erythematous base in the oropharynx may be associated with pain. Patients presenting with severe retrosternal pain and dysphagia should be evaluated for esophogeal candidiasis. *Candida*-induced endocarditis is observed in heroin addicts, cancer chemotherapy recipients, prosthetic valve implant recipients, and patients with prolonged intravenous catheter use or with superimposed bacterial endocarditis. The presentation is variable and may include fever, murmur, embolic phenomena (brain, kidney, and spleen), and skin manifestations. Pulmonary infections secondary to *Candida* rarely manifest themselves clinically, but when present, the symptoms are similar to those of *Aspergillus* sp. Patients with chronic indwelling urinary catheters are susceptible to urinary tract candidiasis and may present with benign to severe symptoms of cystitis. Disseminated candidiasis is more common in patients receiving parenteral hyperalimentation, having surgery in sites of *Candida* overgrowth, or receiving immunosuppressive therapy.

Diagnosis

Microscopic examination of mucocutaneous plaques from involved sites leads to the diagnosis of oropharyngeal candidiasis. Candidal endophthalmitis, a common metastatic finding, is characterized by a white cottonball-like area of chorioretinitis extending out into the vitreous. *Candida* sp frequently colonize the tracheobronchial tree of immunocompromised patients, so positive findings from sputum or bronchial secretions are not helpful. Histologic confirmation of *Candida* invasion of lung tissue is required for definitive diagnosis. Echocardiography may be beneficial in detecting the large vegetations seen in candidal endocarditis. Intravenous and urinary catheters should be inspected for signs of candidiasis, and urine and blood cultures should be obtained, although blood cultures are often negative or latently positive in 50% of cases. Serologic tests are not consistently useful.

Treatment

Neutropenic or immunocompromised patients should be started on empiric topical antifungal therapy with nystatin pastilles or suspension or clotrimazole troches to suppress oral candidal overgrowth (Table 38–6). An oral solution of amphotericin B (50 mg in 1 L of sterile water) is an alternative to nystatin or clotrimazole therapy, but clinical trials are lacking. Fluconazole, a synthetic triazole derivative, is effective in the treatment of oropharyngeal candidiasis in neutropenic patients. Drugs that interact with fluconazole include warfarin, cyclosporine, phenytoin, rifampin, sulfonylurea antidiabetic agents, and thiazide diuretics. Oral ketoconazole can be given. An acid environment is necessary to promote ketoconazole absorption, so concomitant use of H_2 antagonists and antacids is ill-advised. Other drugs that interact with ketoconazole include hepatotoxic drugs, phenytoin, antitubercular agents, warfarin anticoagulants, and cyclosporine. Candidal esophagitis is treated with nystatin suspension, clotrimazole troches, low-dose amphotericin B (10–355 mg over 4–18 days), miconazole, or ketoconazole. Fluconazole is considered the drug of choice for esophageal candidiasis in many hospitals. Disseminated or pulmonary candidiasis requires

Table 38–6. Antifungal dosing regimens.

Drug	Dose	Side Effect/Comment
Nystatin suspension	5–10 mL swish and swallow 4 times daily	Bitter taste, irritation
Clotrimazole troches	10 mg dissolved 5 times daily	Abnormal liver function tests
Amphotericin B solution	15 mL orally 4–5 times daily	Taste, ?efficacy
Ketoconazole	200 mg orally daily	Hepatotoxicity, gastrointestinal effects (nausea and vomiting), gynecomastia in men
Fluconazole	200 mg orally on day 1, then 100 mg daily	Rash, gastrointestinal effects, transient increases in aspartate aminotransferase, alanine aminotransferase, alkaline phosphatase, gamma glutamyl transferase, and bilirubin

treatment with amphotericin B to a total dose of 2 g. Amphotericin B with concomitant flucytosine may be required in patients with disseminated candidasis. Intravenous fluconazole has been successfully used for systemic candidiasis in amphotericin B–intolerant patients.

CRYPTOCOCCUS

Cryptococcus neoformans is the yeastlike organism mainly found in pigeon or chicken excreta that is responsible for cryptococcal disease in humans. Infection is presumed to be acquired by inhalation of organism-laden particles. The major clinical impact is in the central nervous system.

Clinical Findings
Pulmonary manifestations of cryptococcosis include cough, chest pain, fever, hemoptysis, dyspnea, and night sweats. In immunocompromised patients, pulmonary *C neoformans* infection can lead to dissemination or meningeal infection. Meningeal cryptococcal infection usually has an acute or subacute onset, with headache, fever, dizziness, ataxia, impaired mentation, irritability, decreased visual acuity, and rarely seizures. Space-occupying lesions of the brain and spinal cord are responsible for neurologic findings such as papilledema and cranial nerve palsies.

Diagnosis
A segmental consolidation or coin lesion, occasionally with cavitation, is the typical chest x-ray finding for pulmonary cryptococcosis. Multiple nodules or diffuse disease, an interstitial or miliary pattern, hilar adenopathy, or pleural effusion may also be found. Sputum cultures positive for *C neoformans* do not provide causation for infection, since the organism may be colonizing the tracheobronchial tree. Space-occupying lesions of the brain can be visualized by CT scan, which can localize mass cryptococcal lesions. Cerebrospinal fluid (CSF) evaluation for cryptococcal meningitis demonstrates an elevated opening pressure, increased protein level, depressed glucose level, and low white blood cell count that is primarily lymphocytic. India ink preparation of the CSF smear demonstrates cryptococci in 60% of infected patients. The latex agglutination test for cryptococcal antigen is the most useful serologic test for cryptococcosis and is positive in the CSF in over 90% of cases.

Treatment
Cryptococcal meningitis is universally fatal if left untreated. Treatment is limited to amphotericin (0.6–1 mg/kg/d) or amphotericin B (0.3 mg/kg/d) plus flucytosine (150 mg/kg/d). Side effects of flucyosine include gastrointestinal effects, which can be severe,

elevated liver enzymes, and of greatest concern in the neutropenic patient, hypoplasia of bone marrow. Flucytosine is renally eliminated, and nephrotoxicity from concomitant amphotericin B therapy can lead to elevated flucytosine concentrations and enhanced toxicity. Monitoring of renal, hepatic, and hematologic measurements is mandatory. Fluconazole has been used with some success in AIDS-related cryptococcal meningitis, but clinical trials in the neutropenic or immunocompromised cancer patient are lacking.

MUCORMYCOSIS

Infectious complications due to Mucoraceae, including *Rhizopus, Mucor,* and *Absidia* sp, are most commonly found in patients with lymphoma, diabetes, and leukemia, and in patients who are chronically immunocompromised or receiving corticosteroids. Mucormycosis clinically resembles invasive aspergillosis. The organisms are ubiquitous, growing on decaying vegetation and other organic matter. Infection is initiated by direct inoculation onto unaccustomed surfaces or by lodging in the lower respiratory tract or paranasal sinuses.

Clinical Findings
Rhinocerebral mucormycosis begins in the nasal sinus, extends to the paranasal sinus, and either progresses through the cribriform plate and into the frontal lobe or progresses into the retro-orbital region and through the apex of the orbit into the brain. Symptoms include fever, headache, lethargy, loss of vision, facial swelling, and proptosis. Cavernous sinus thrombosis due to early retinal artery involvement or internal carotid artery thrombosis is a frequent complications. The second, third, fourth, and sixth cranial nerves are often affected with progressive invasion. Obtundation and neurologic syndromes are seen with metastatic spread to the brain.

Pulmonary mucormycosis is manifested by pulmonary infarction and hemorrhage. Symptoms include cough, hemoptysis, fever, pleurisy, and varying degrees of dyspnea.

Cutaneous mucormycosis has been associated with contaminated elastic adhesive tape used for operative wounds or intravenous sites in immunocompromised patients. Lesions associated with vessel infarctions may be nonspecific or resemble ecthyma gangrenosum.

Disseminated mucormycosis can involve the spleen, kidney, liver, heart, duodenum, pancreas, stomach, and omentum and is characterized by vessel infarction of surrounding parenchyma. Symptoms are usually nonspecific.

Diagnosis
Biopsy demonstrating the presence of invasive or-

ganisms is the only reliable method for definitive diagnosis. Sinus films may demonstrate nodular thickening of the mucosa of multiple sinuses, cloudy sinus without fluid levels, and destruction of bony walls of multiple sinuses. Chest x-ray findings include a patchy, nonhomogeneous infiltrate, consolidation, cavity formation, and rarely pleural effusion. Bronchoscopy may aid in diagnosis, and lung perfusion scans and CT scans may define the extent of disease. CSF findings are nonspecific and may include elevated CSF pressure, slight pleocytosis, and mild protein elevation. Cultures from blood, CSF, urine, or sputum rarely harbor the organism. Biopsy or scraping of any suspicious lesion for histopathologic examination and culture should be done.

Treatment

Successful treatment depends on early diagnosis, systemic antifungal therapy, surgical debridement, and control of the underlying disease. Aggressive surgical debridement of necrotic and devitalized tissue early in the diagnosis with concomitant amphotericin B therapy offers the best chance for cure. High daily doses of amphotericin B, 0.7–1.5 mg/kg/d, are probably necessary to provide adequate antifungal concentrations. Synergy between amphotericin B and rifampin, flucytosine, and tetracycline analogs has been suggested, but clinical trials are lacking. The total cumulative dose of amphotericin B required for treatment is not known, but 2–4 g has been utilized in most studies.

VIRAL INFECTIONS

Viral infections in immunocompromised hosts are the result of disrupted mucocutaneous membranes of the respiratory, gastrointestinal, and genitourinary tracts and lack of normally functioning lymphocytes, plasma cells, and macrophages that prevent viral shedding. Viruses most likely to infect this popula-

tion include cytomegolovirus, herpes simplex, herpes zoster, and varicella-zoster (Table 38–7).

CYTOMEGALOVIRUS

Cytomegalovirus (CMV) is a herpesvirus. It is ubiquitous and can be associated with severe disease in immunocompromised hosts (eg, leukemics and bone marrow transplant recipients). The virus can cause a primary infection—first infection in a seronegative patient—or more commonly a secondary infection—reactivation of a latent infection or reinfection in a seropositive patient. Complications include hepatitis, Guillain-Barré syndrome, meningoencephalitis, myocarditis, thrombocytopenia, hemolytic anemia, gastroenteritis, esophagitis, retinitis, and interstitial pneumonia.

Clinical Findings

Interstitial pneumonitis is a common manifestation of CMV infection. Two types of pneumonitis are seen clinically: (1) Miliary CMV pneumonitis presents with sudden tachypnea with severe respiratory distress and hypoxemia, and most patients require a respirator or die within 3 days. (2) Diffuse CMV pneumonitis follows an indolent course of fever, nonproductive cough, and respiratory complaints that can lead to respiratory failure. Risk factors for CMV pneumonitis include acute graft-versus-host disease, total body irradiation with lung doses greater than 600 cGy, increased age, pretransplant seropositive patients, and Caucasian race. CMV infection of the liver clinically presents with increased serum aminotransferase and bilirubin levels and is usually clinically indistinguishable from other causes of viral hepatitis. Gastrointestinal presentation of CMV infection ranges from asymptomatic to ulceration, bleeding, and perforation of the esophagus, stomach, small intestine, or colon and may be confused with gastrointestinal graft-versus-host disease in the bone marrow transplant patient. CMV retinitis usually occurs 6 months or more after transplantation, and patients usually present with nonspecific complaints of scotoma, blurred vision, and decreased visual acuity. The ocular lesion appears as a white granular necrotic patch with patches of flame-shaped intraretinal hemorrhages superimposed.

Table 38–7. Viral infections.

Virus	Treatment	Prevention/Attenuation
Cytomegalovirus	Ganciclovir, intravenous immune globulin, ?foscarnet	?Ganciclovir Seronegative blood products
Herpes simplex	Acyclovir	?Intravenous immune globulin
Varicella-zoster	Acyclovir	Acyclovir Varicella-zoster immune globulin or intravenous immune globulin
Herpes zoster	Acyclovir	?Acyclovir

Diagnosis

Definitive diagnosis is obtained by identification of CMV in affected tissue culture. Infection with CMV in the urine or saliva is common after bone marrow transplantation and is usually not life-threatening. Cultures are useful in most symptomatic patients (pneumonitis or hepatitis) who will be excreting virus into the saliva and urine, making negative culture results useful in excluding the diagnosis of disseminated CMV infection. Serologic tests (detection of IgG antibody against CMV) in immunocompromised hosts can give false-negative results secondary to a dysfunctional immune system, delaying the diagnosis or causing it to be missed in patients who fail to mount a response. Chest x-ray shows a localized interstitial infiltrate that progresses to bilateral involvement in days to weeks. Tissue biopsy or bronchoalveolar lavage is helpful in establishing the diagnosis.

Treatment

Therapy of established CMV pneumonitis, the most devastating of CMV infections in transplant recipients, with acyclovir, vidarabine, or trifluorothymidine has been unsuccessful. The combination of ganciclovir (2.5 mg/kg intravenously every 8 hours for 14–20 days) and CMV hyperimmune globulin (400 mg/kg on days 1, 2, and 7 and 200 mg/kg on day 14) or high-dose immune globulin (500 mg/kg intravenously every other day for 10 doses) has been successful in a few studies. Side effects of ganciclovir include neutropenia, thrombocytopenia, and increased bilirubin, alkaline phosphatase, and serum creatinine levels. A dose adjustment is required in patients with impaired renal function. Larger control led trials are needed, but the combination of ganciclovir and immune globulin appears promising.

Foscarnet is a pyrophosphate analog with good activity against CMV. It is an alternative for ganciclovir-intolerant patients, and clinical improvement has been demonstrated in transplant patients with CMV infection. Adverse effects include renal toxicity, phlebitis at infusion site, lower back pain, hypocalcemia, hyperphosphatemia, and decreased hemoglobin concentration.

HERPES SIMPLEX VIRUS

Reactivation of herpes simplex virus (HSV) in seropositive (>1:8 or 1:16) bone marrow transplant patients usually occurs at a median of 17 days after initiation of chemotherapy with or without total body irradiation. Primary infection with HSV is very rare.

Clinical Findings

Mucocutaneous manifestations are seen in 85% of HSV infections, while genital infections occur in only 15%. Mucocutaneous lesions are exudative or ulcerative and may involve the hard and soft palate, gingiva, tongue, lip, buccal mucosa, or facial area. Infection in mucosal and deep cutaneous layers results in friability, necrosis, bleeding, severe pain, and inability to eat or drink. Concomitant HSV and *Candida* infections are frequently seen.

HSV esophagitis may be an extension of an oral lesion or reactivation that has spread to the esophagus via the vagus nerve. Presenting symptoms include odynophagia, dysphagia, substernal pain, and weight loss. HSV pneumonitis is uncommon (6–8% of biopsy proved cases of pneumonitis) in bone marrow transplant recipients and presents as a focal necrotizing or bilateral interstitial pneumonitis. Liver involvement, which presents with fever, leukopenia, and abrupt elevations of serum transaminases and bilirubin, is rare and carries a grave prognosis. The hallmark of herpes encephalitis is fever, headache, focal neurologic symptoms (especially of the temporal lobe), and changes in personality or sensorium. Lesions of the genital tract may be vesicles, pustules, or painful erythematous ulcers that are widely spaced with a bilateral distribution on the external genitalia. Perianal herpetic lesions in immunocompromised hosts are probably spread by autoinoculation from HSV-infected saliva or finger lesions. Symptoms can include anorectal pain, anorectal discharge, tenesmus, and constipation.

Diagnosis

Staining of scrapings from the base of the lesions with Wright's, Giemsa, or Papanicolaou's stain should demonstrate giant cells or intranuclear inclusions of a herpesvirus infection. Isolation of HSV in tissue culture confirms the diagnosis.

Differentiation between HSV-1 and HSV-2 is accomplished by restriction endonuclease analysis of viral DNA. Serologic assays are not helpful for diagnosing acute infections, but are useful in determining seropositive patients who may need prophylactic acyclovir therapy during bone marrow transplantation.

Prevention

Acyclovir prophylaxis should be used in seropositive patients with a high incidence of clinically significant HSV infection who are undergoing bone marrow transplantation or intensive chemotherapy for leukemia. An intravenous dose of 250 mg/m^2 every 8 hours or oral dose of 200–400 mg 5 times daily has been effective.

Treatment

Intravenous acyclovir, 5 mg/kg every 8 hours for 7–10 days, is the drug of choice for HSV infections. Higher intravenous doses, 10 mg/kg every 8 hours for 10 days, are required for treatment of HSV encephalitis.

Side effects include local reactions at the injection site, headaches, transient increases in blood urea nitrogen and serum creatinine levels, especially with rapid infusion, and nausea, vomiting, and diarrhea with oral therapy.

VARICELLA-ZOSTER VIRUS

1. VARICELLA

Varicella-zoster virus (VZV) is responsible for two different clinical entities: varicella, or chickenpox, and herpes zoster, or shingles. The primary infection with VZV is extremely contagious and is likely to be transmitted by the respiratory route, followed by localized replication, seeding of the reticuloendothelial system, and viremia.

Clinical Findings

The primary infection with VZV consists of fever and malaise followed by lesions on the face, scalp, mucous membranes, neck, trunk, and extremities. The characteristic lesion is a superficial vesicle surrounded by a halo of erythema accompanied by intense pruritus. If the immunocompromised host is left untreated, new vessels will continue to form for as long as 2 weeks from the onset of infection. Immunocompromised children often have a difficult clinical course including cutaneous bacterial superinfection, otitis media, meningoencephalitis, and pneumonia. Secondary bacterial superinfection of the skin with *Staphylococcus* or *Streptococcus* sp results from excoriation of skin lesions following scratching. Central nervous system involvement in children usually appears 20 days after rash onset and presents with cerebellar ataxia and meningeal irritation.

Elevated protein levels and lymphocytes are found in the CSF. Pneumonitis usually appears 3–5 days into the illness and presents with cough, dyspnea, tachypnea, and fever. Physical findings include cyanosis, pleuritic chest pain, and hemoptysis. Chest x-ray reveals nodular infiltrates and interstitial pneumonitis. Hepatitis, with increased serum transaminases, is usually asymptomatic, although a few patients experience nausea and vomiting.

Diagnosis

Lesions should be cultured for virus by aspirating 3–4 vesicles with a tuberculin syringe attached to a 25-gauge needle. The base of the lesion should be rubbed with the bevel of the needle during aspiration to obtain VZV-laden epithelial cells. Inoculation of the specimen into tubes containing human foreskin fibroblast cells should occur as soon as possible. If culture is not available, the base of the lesion can be scraped and the cellular material examined for the presence of multinucleated giant cells (Tzanck test). Demonstration of seroconversion or a fourfold or greater antibody rise when comparing acute and convalescent samples (by serologic detection of antibodies to VZV) may confirm the diagnosis.

Prophylaxis

Passive immunization for the immunocompromised child who is at significant risk for developing progressive varicella is accomplished by using varicella-zoster immune globulin (VZIG) (Table 38–8). The immunoglobulin should be given within 96 but preferably 48 hours of exposure. Postexposure administration of VZIG may only ameliorate rather than prevent varicella-zoster infection in previously uninfected immunocompromised children. Since VZIG may prolong the incubation period of varicella infections from 15 days in normal patients to 31 days in VZIG-treated patients, most cases of varicella infection in VZIG treated patients occur 28 days after virus exposure. Immunocompromised children with a prior history of varicella infection are considered to have immunity and do not require VZIG administration unless they subsequently received a bone marrow transplantation. Recipients of bone marrow transplants are considered susceptible to VZV and should receive postexposure VZIG prophylaxis when indicated.

Dosing recommendations for adults do not exist; 625 units is probably sufficient to ameliorate or prevent varicella infection in healthy adults, with higher doses probably needed in immunocompromised adults. The drug is administered intramuscularly and should not be given intravenously. In individuals with thrombocytopenia or a bleeding disorder, the benefit of VZIG administration should outweigh the possible risks of bleeding. If VZIG is not available or advisable, intravenous immune globulin (IVIG), 200–300 mg/kg, results in antibody titers similar to those of VZIG.

Treatment

The treatment of choice for varicella infections is intravenous acyclovir, 10 mg/kg 3 times per day for 5–10 days depending on clinical improvement. The dose is adjusted for renal function. The use of VZIG for treatment of varicella-zoster infections is currently not recommended. The patient should be isolated, preferably in a room with negative pressure

Table 38–8. Dose recommendations for VZIG administration in children.

Weight (kg)	VZIG dose
≤10	125 units (1 vial)
10.1–20	250 units (2 vials)
20.1–30	375 units (3 vials)
30.1–40	500 units (4 vials)
>40	625 units (5 vials)

ventilation, to prevent nosocomial spread of the virus.

2. HERPES ZOSTER

Herpes zoster, or shingles, is the common manifestation of the reactivation of VZV from the dorsal root ganglia of the spinal cord or the ganglion of a cranial nerve. The probability of developing herpes zoster increases with age, underlying disease, and emotional or physical stress. VZV infection occurs in approximately 50% of bone marrow transplant patients, with a median onset of 4–5 months.

Clinical Findings

Shingles usually begins with unilateral pain that is described as deep, searing, knifelike, or burning and precedes the rash by several days to a week. The closely cropped vesicles usually erupt within the thoracic dermatomes but may also occur within the cranial nerves. An ophthalomology consultation is required for patients with fifth cranial nerve involvement to evaluate corneal scarring. Disseminated zoster generally occurs 2–11 days after the onset of dermatomal cutaneous lesions and can involve distal cutaneous sites, the lung, liver, central nervous system, or gastrointestinal tract. Cutaneous dissemination occurs in one-third of immunocompromised hosts and is associated with a 5–10% increased risk of pneumonitis, meningoencephalitis, hepatitis, and other serious complications. Headache, fever, photophobia and meninigitis are symptoms of meningoencephalitis.

Postherpetic neuralgia is probably the most debilitating complication of herpes zoster. This syndrome is defined as pain persisting for at least 1 month after onset of acute herpes zoster and may persist for years. The exact incidence of postherpetic neuralgia is not known but is probably around 17%. Pain management is difficult. Common treatment modalities include amitriptyline, carbamazepine, capsaicin, phenytoin, and transcutaneous electrical nerve stimulation (TENS).

Diagnosis

The lesions are usually characteristic, but confusion may arise when sacral zoster mimics recurrent herpes simplex. The diagnosis is made by culture.

Treatment

Immunocompromised patients who have systemic clinical manifestations of herpes zoster should be treated with acyclovir. Therapy should begin immediately but is probably of benefit as long as new lesions are still forming. Acyclovir, 10 mg/kg every 8 hours for 7–10 days, has been shown to retard the spread of cutaneous lesions, reduce the frequency of visceral zoster development, decrease acute pain, and promote resolution of rash. The dose is adjusted for patients with renal failure. Side effects include local tissue irritation, transient increases in hepatic enzymes, decreased renal function, and central nervous system toxicity.

Prophylaxis

Prophylactic oral acyclovir has been shown to decrease the incidence of herpes zoster in bone marrow transplant patients; however, after acyclovir cessation the rate of VZV infection increases to that of the normal population. Currently, prophylactic acyclovir cannot be universally recommended to prevent VZV dissemination, especially since patients can receive intravenous acyclovir at the earliest sign of infection and achieve equally satisfying results.

MISCELLANEOUS VIRUSES

Adenovirus can cause life-threatening interstitial pneumonia, hepatitis, gastroenteritis, hemorrhagic cystitis, and meningoencephalitis. Patients present with malaise, fever, lethargy, fatigue, night sweats, and gastrointestinal symptoms. Respiratory symptoms include nonproductive or slightly productive cough, tachypnea, and dyspnea. Laboratory findings include elevated hepatic enzyme levels. Chest x-ray may show bilateral diffuse pulmonary infiltrates or alveolar infiltrates. Serologic studies may not indicate the cause of illness. Diagnosis is often made postmortem when the virus is isolated from infected tissues.

Respiratory syncytial virus is a rare cause of severe diffuse pneumonitis in immunocompromised patients. Fever, productive or nonproductive cough, rhinorrhea, sore throat, and shortness of breath are some clinical symptoms. Physical examination reveals increased respiratory rate, rales or rhonchi, and wheezing. Sinusitis can be documented by radiographs, and bilateral interstitial infiltrates are present on chest x-ray. Blood gas determinations usually reveal hypoxemia. Diagnosis can be made by isolating the virus or viral antigen from throat, sputum, bronchoalveolar lavage, lung tissue, or sinus aspirate. Treatment includes supplemental oxygen, assisted ventilation, and possibly aerosolized ribavirin therapy. Ribavirin, 6 g/d diluted in 300 mL of sterile water, is given over 12–18 h/d by a small-particle aerosol generator. The drug should be given for at least 3 days and not more than 7 days; however, some clinicians feel that prolonged therapy may be necessary in these patients.

Epstein-Barr virus (EBV) may be responsible for the increasing numbers of donor B cell lymphomas noted after bone marrow transplantation. Acyclovir may be able to prevent these EBV-induced lymphoproliferative disorders, but more clinical trials are necessary.

PROTOZAL INFECTIONS

PNEUMOCYSTIS PNEUMONIA

P carinii is the major protozoal pathogen in immunosuppressed patients. Impaired cellular immunity with reactivation by latent infection is thought to be the most important factor in the development of pneumocystis pneumonia. Patients who have been treated with cytotoxic drugs or corticosteroids for long periods are particularly susceptible to *P carinii*.

Clinical Findings
The onset of infection is usually insidious with patients typically complaining of fever, nonproductive cough, and dyspnea. Tachypnea, tachycardia, and cyanosis can be found on physical examination, but lung auscultation is usually normal. Hypoxemia, increased alveolar arterial oxygen gradient, and respiratory alkalosis can be demonstrated by arterial blood gas measurement. Chest x-ray classically consists of bilateral diffuse infiltrates with air bronchograms developing over time.

Diagnosis
Pneumocystis pneumonia is diagnosed by finding the organism in body fluids or tissues. The cyst form can be demonstrated with methenamine silver stain, while the trophozoite form is best seen with Wright's stain. Invasive procedures are usually necessary to obtain the diagnosis, since the organism is rarely found in the sputum or by transtracheal aspiration. Transbronchial biopsy, with or without bronchoalveolar lavage, gives a lower diagnostic yield than open lung biopsy but is an alternative in unstable patients. Open lung biopsy provides the best specimen for diagnosis and generally is performed when bronchoscopy is nondiagnostic. Serologic diagnosis is currently not useful.

Prevention
Low-dose trimethoprim-sulfamethoxazole (trimethoprim, 150 mg/m^2) on 3 consecutive days of the week has been used in children with acute lymphocytic leukemia for prevention of *P carinii* pneumonitis. Bone marrow transplant patients are currently given trimethoprim-sulfamethoxazole (trimethoprim, 5–10 mg/kg/d; sulfamethoxazole, 25–50 mg/kg/d) 10 days prior to transplantation and then daily or twice a week during days 30–50 after transplantation. The drug is also given for the duration of chronic graft-versus-host disease. For trimethoprim-sulfamethoxazole–intolerant patients, inhaled pentamidine, dapsone-trimethoprim, or dapsone alone can be used for *P carinii* prophylaxis.

Treatment
High-dose trimethoprim-sulfamethoxazole (trimethoprim, 20 mg/kg/d; sulfamethoxazole 100 mg/kg/d) for 14 days is required for treatment of *P carinii* pneumonia. Adverse reactions include allergic reactions, agranulocytosis, thrombocytopenia, leukopenia, nausea, Stevens-Johnson syndrome, and diarrhea. Pentamidine isethionate, 4 mg/kg/d intramuscularly or intravenously for 14 days, is alternative therapy when trimethoprim-sulfamethoxazole fails or is contraindicated. The many adverse effects of pentamidine include hypotension, tachycardia, nausea and vomiting, facial flushing, pleurisy, local irritation, hypoglycemia, azotemia, bone marrow suppression, and sterile abscess formation at the injection site.

TOXOPLASMOSIS

Toxoplasma gondii is the causative agent. A few cases of devastating neurologic or disseminated disease, probably due to reactivation of latent infection as a result of defective cell-mediated immunity, in bone marrow transplant recipients have been reported. Seronegative recipients of organs transplanted from seropositive donors are at particular risk as are patients with hairy cell leukemia. Patients appear to be at highest risk between days 20 and 100 after transplantation.

Clinical Findings
CNS involvement is seen in half the cases of toxoplasmosis in immunocompromised patients. Three clinical pictures have evolved: (1) diffuse encephalopathy with or without seizures, (2) meningoencephalitis, and (3) singular or multiple enlarging mass lesions. Predominant symptoms are usually nonspecific and include headache, drowsiness, and disorientation. Fever and dyspnea are manifestations of pneumonitis, which may occur in up to one-third of immunosuppressed patients with toxoplasmosis. Disseminated toxoplasmosis may be manifested as myocarditis, pericarditis, and lymphadenitis.

Diagnosis
CSF abnormalities are nonspecific and include mild lymphocytic pleocytosis, normal or slightly elevated protein levels and normal glucose levels. In *Toxoplasma* pneumonitis, chest x-ray reveals a diffuse bilateral pulmonary infiltrate. Organisms in the bronchoalveolar lavage fluid occasionally provide the diagnosis. Serologic studies do not play an important role in diagnosis in immunocompromised pa-

tients, since the humoral immune system is usually depressed. The diagnosis is established by isolation of the trophozoite form of *T gondii* from tissue (brain, lymph node, or lung) or bodily fluids.

Treatment

The combination of pyrimethamine and sulfadiazine is the treatment of choice. An oral loading dose of pyrimethamine, 100 mg/d for 1–2 days, followed by 25 mg every other day is usually adequate. In the immunodeficient patient with severe disease, the dose can be increased to 50 mg/d for the first few weeks of therapy. Adverse effects include bone marrow suppression, gastrointestinal effects, headache and dysgeusia. Folinic acid, 10 mg orally with each pyrimethamine dose, may decrease the incidence of bone marrow suppression. An oral loading dose of sulfadiazine, 75 mg/kg (up to 4 g), is given, followed by 100 mg/kg/d (up to 8 g) in two divided doses. Spiramycin, clindamycin, and trimethoprim-sulfamethoxazole are second-line treatment.

CRYPTOSPORIDIOSIS

Cryptosporidium is a rare cause of diarrhea in the immunodeficient patient or bone marrow transplant recipient. Infection is caused by ingestion of viable cysts. Patients present with abdominal pain and profuse, watery, nonbloody diarrhea, usually without fever, nausea, or vomiting. Diagnosis is established by culturing oocysts from the stool. There is no effective pharmacologic treatment, and patients should be supported with fluid and electrolyte therapy.

MISCELLANEOUS INFECTIONS

CHLAMYDIAL INFECTIONS

Chlamydial infections are rare in bone marrow transplant patients with interstitial pneumonia. In the few cases that have been described, infection occurred 4–13 weeks after transplantation, and patients showed an interstitial infiltrate on chest x-ray. *Chlamydia trachomatis* has been noted in bone marrow transplant recipients by serologic evidence and sputum culture. Intravenous erythromycin (2 g/d) is the drug of choice for serious infections.

MYCOBACTERIAL INFECTIONS

Mycobacterial infections (*Mycobacterium tuberculosis, Mycobacterium fortuitum, Mycobacterium kansasii* and, *Mycobacturium avium-intracellulare*) occur in 1% of bone marrow transplant recipients. Patients usually have constitutional symptoms of fever, chills, fatigue, anorexia, night sweats, and cough. Chest x-ray may show an apical or subapical patchy infiltrate in early chronic tuberculosis. A bilateral upper lobe infiltrate with patchy, soft, scattered infiltrates with or without cavitation is especially suggestive. Diagnosis is made from positive sputum, bronchoscopy specimen, or open lung biopsy, Treatment depends on the type of mycobacterium isolated. High-risk patients include those with well-established histories of inadequately treated tuberculosis, known family contacts, recent skin test conversion, past skin test positivity, and previous bacillus Calmette-Guérin (BCG) immunotherapy. These patients should be screened by skin test prior to organ transplantation or induction chemotherapy, and prophylactic oral isoniazid (300 mg/d) should be considered in those who test positive.

LEGIONELLA

A few cases of infection due to *Legionella bozemanii* and *Legionella pneumophila* in immunocompromised hosts have been reported. These individuals present with fever, nonproductive cough, dyspnea, and multilobar infiltrates on chest x-ray. Sputum or bronchoalveolar lavage culture provides the diagnosis. Erythromycin, 3–4 g/d intravenously for 1 week, followed by 2 g/d orally for 2 weeks is the treatment of choice. Rifampin (600 mg/d) is adjunctive treatment to erythromycin in severely ill patients or patients not adequately responding to erythromycin therapy.

DURATION OF THERAPY

The duration of therapy in neutropenic patients depends on the documentation of infection, ANC, incidence of febrile episodes. Following is a guide for duration of empiric therapy in patients who are neutropenic, febrile, and taking antibiotics.

(1) If defervescence occurs, the culture is negative, and the ANC is greater than 500 cells/mm^3, discontinue antibiotics.

(2) If defervescence occurs, the culture is positive, and the ANC is greater than 500 cells/mm^3, a 14-day course of antibiotics or appropriate total dose of antifungal therapy according to culture and sensitivity should be completed.

(3) If the patient is afebrile but remains neutropenic (ANC < 500 cells/mm^3), continue therapy until

the ANC is greater than 500 cells/mm^3. Some groups advocate stopping therapy sooner if the patient is clinically well, the culture is negative, and the patient has completed 7–14 days of therapy. The patient is followed closely and, if fever recurs, is placed back on antibiotics. Patients with profound neutropenia (ANC < 100) should be continued on antimicrobial agents.

(4) If the patient continues to be febrile, reevaluate by physical examination, cultures, and other appropriate procedures. Therapy generally is continued if infectious causes of fever cannot be ruled out.

AUGMENTATION OF HOST DEFENSE

GRANULOCYTE TRANSFUSION

The use of granulocyte transfusions in neutropenic patients is controversial. Current evidence suggests that the benefits of newer empiric therapy (antibiotics and colony-stimulating factors) outweigh the risks of granulocyte transfusions, and they cannot be recommended for neutropenic patients. These transfusions can produce interstitial-alveolar pulmonary infiltrates, transmission of CMV to seronegative patients, sensitization, fever, and chills. Some authors report an increased incidence of pulmonary complications with concomitant administration of amphotericin B and granulocytes. Therefore, concurrent administration of these therapeutic modalities should be employed judiciously.

PROPHYLACTIC ANTIBIOTICS FOR GUT DECONTAMINATION

"Gut decontamination" is proposed to rid the gastrointestinal tract of potentially invasive gram-negative bacilli that can lead to infection in the neutropenic host. Antibiotics with selective activity against gram-negative aerobic bacilli are preferred, since they leave the more innocuous anaerobic flora intact. Many oral antibiotic regimens have been designed to accomplish this goal, but study design, side effect profile, and questions of efficacy limit their overall utility. Trimethoprim-sulfamethoxazole has been the most consistently studied drug, but with results are conflicting. Concerns about high incidence of side effects, possible myelosuppressive activity, fungal superinfection, and selection of resistant gram-negative organisms have limited the drug's overall acceptability. Norfloxacin and ciprofloxacin have been evaluated in trials for infection prophylaxis in patients with acute leukemia. These drugs are better tolerated and have better activity against *Pseudomonas* sp than trimethoprim-sulfamethoxasole. Although studies have shown a decrease in gram-negative infections with the oral fluoroquinolones, no reduction in infection-related mortality rates has been reported and there has been an increase in gram-positive infections.

INTRAVENOUS IMMUNE GLOBULIN

Intravenous immune globulin (IGIV) has shown some benefit in allogeneic bone marrow transplant recipients. Patients receiving weekly (IGIV 500 mg/kg) showed decreased gram-negative septicemia, interstitial pneumonitis, and acute graft-versus-host disease and required a decreased number of platelet transfusions. Survival and risk of relapse were unaltered.

Patients with chronic lymphocytic leukemia receiving IVIG, 400 mg/kg every 3 weeks, had decreased incidence of moderate infections (requiring oral antibiotics) and remained free of serious bacterial infection for a longer period. The high cost of administering routine prophylaxis to all patients with chronic lymphocytic leukemia may outweigh the benefit in patients whose infections may be controlled by oral antibiotics. More trials documenting efficacy are needed.

COLONY-STIMULATING FACTORS

Colony-stimulating factors (CSFs) are a family of glycoproteins that promote stem cell proliferation, hematopoietic differentiation, and functional activity of mature granulocytes and macrophages. CSFs have been used to stimulate bone marrow recovery in patients with aplastic anemia, neutropenia due to chemotherapy and ablative therapy with subsequent bone marrow transplantation, and AIDS. The exact mechanism of action is not known. The role of CSFs in treating or preventing infection in neutropenic patients is currently not well defined. (See also Chapter 34.)

MONOCLONAL ANTIBODIES

HA-1A is a monoclonal IgM antibody that binds specifically to many endotoxins as well as a broad range of clinical isolates of gram-negative bacteria. In a large multicenter trial of septic patients, HA-1A was compared to placebo. Overall mortality was unchanged. The subset population of HA-1A patients with gram-negative bacteremia and septic shock had a decreased mortality. Studies in neutropenic patients are lacking.

REFERENCES

Anaissie E et al: Fluconazole therapy for chronic disseminated candidiasis in patients with leukemia and prior amphotericin B therapy. *Am J Med* 1991;**91**:142.

Bodey GP et al: Quantitative relationships between circulating leukocytes and infection in patients with acute leukemia. *Ann Intern Med* 1966;**64**:328.

Feldman S, Lott L: Varicella in children with cancer: Impact of antiviral therapy and prophylaxis. *Pediatrics* 1987;**80**:465.

Hathorn JW, Rubin M, Pizzo PA: Empirical antibiotic therapy in the febrile neutropenic cancer patient: Clinical efficacy and impact of monotherapy. *Antimicrob Agents Chemother* 1987;**31**:971.

Hughes WT et al: Guidelines for the use of antimicrobial agents in neutropenic patients with unexplained fever. *J Infect Dis* 1990;**161**:381.

Klastersky J: Concept of empiric therapy with antibiotic combinations: Indications and limits. *Am J Med* 1986; **80**:2.

Klastersky J: Empiric treatment of infection during granulocytopenia. *Ann Oncol* 1990;**1**:255.

Liany R et al: Ceftazidime versus imipenem-cilastatin as initial monotherapy for febrile neutropenic patients. *Antimicrob Agents Chemother* 1990;**34**:1336.

Maddux MS, Barriere SL: A review of complications of amphotericin B therapy: Recommendations for prevention and management. *Drug Intell Clin Pharm* 1980; **14**:177.

McCabe RE: Diagnosis of pulmonary infections in immunocompromised patients. *Med Clin North Am* 1988; **72**:1067.

Mertelsmann R et al: Hematopoietic growth factors in bone marrow transplantation. *Bone Marrow Transplant* 1990;**6**:73.

Pennington JE: Newer uses of intravenous immunoglobulins as anti-infective agents. *Antimicrob Agents Chemother* 1990;**34**:1463.

Pizzo PA et al: Approaching the controversies in antibacterial management of cancer patients. *Am J Med* 1984; **76**:436.

Pizzo PA et al: The child with cancer and infection: Empiric therapy for fever and neutropenia, and preventive strategies. *J Pediatr* 1991;**119**:679.

Pizzo PA et al: The child with cancer and infection: Nonbacterial infections. *J Pediatr* 1991;**119**:845.

Rubin M et al: Gram-positive infections and the use of vancomycin in 550 episodes of fever and neutropenia. *Ann Intern Med* 1988;**108**:30.

Saral R, Burns WH, Prentice HG: Herpes virus infections: Clinical manifestations and therapeutic strategies in immunocompromised patients. *Clin Haematol* 1984;**13**: 645.

Schmidt GM et al: A randomized, controlled trial of prophylactic ganciclovir for cytomegalovirus pulmonary infection in recipients of allogeneic bone marrow transplants. *N Engl J Med* 1991;**324**:1005.

Sullivan KM et al: Immunomodulatory and antimicrobial efficacy of intravenous immunoglobulin in bone marrow transplantation. *N Engl J Med* 1990;**323**:705.

Ziegler EJ et al: Treatment of gram-negative bacteremia and septic shock with HA-1A human monoclonal antibody against endotoxin. *N Engl J Med* 1991;**324**:429.

39 Superior Vena Cava Syndrome

Arlene J. Zaloznik, MD

Essentials of Diagnosis
- Shortness of breath, chest pain, cough.
- Venous distention of neck and thorax.
- Facial edema.
- Tachypnea.

Obstruction of the superior vena cava (SVC) can present as an acute, subacute, or chronic process. The symptom complex and characteristic physical findings occur most frequently in the setting of an intrathoracic neoplasm.

Etiology
Historically, SVC syndrome was associated with benign causes (aortic aneurysm, usually syphilitic, and chronic mediastinitis). Currently, over 90% of cases of SVC obstruction are due to some form of malignant process. Lung cancer accounts for 67–82% of cases, with small-cell cancers making up the majority of lung cancers. Lymphomas are second in frequency, causing 5–15% of cases. Thymomas and germ cell tumors are other primary mediastinal malignancies that may cause SVC syndrome. Metastatic disease is responsible for 3–20% of cases, with breast cancer being the most common.

Benign causes of SVC syndrome include fibrous mediastinitis from granulomatous disease (usually histoplasmosis) and substernal goiter. The increasing use of central indwelling catheters and resultant thrombotic potential may create an additional risk factor for the development of SVC syndrome in the cancer patient.

Pathophysiology
The SVC is the major vessel for drainage of venous blood from the head, neck, upper extremities, and upper thorax. It is located in the middle mediastinum, surrounded by the trachea, right bronchus, aorta, pulmonary artery, and the perihilar and paratracheal lymph nodes. Because of its compliance and easy compressibility, this vessel is vulnerable to space-occupying lesions in its vicinity.

Extensive venous collateral circulation usually involving the azygous and hemiazygous systems may develop when there is obstruction of the SVC. Other collateral channels include the internal mammary veins, lateral thoracic veins, paraspinous veins, and the esophageal venous network. Engorgement of the subcutaneous veins of the neck and thorax is a typical physical finding in SVC syndrome.

Obstruction of the SVC may be due to extrinsic compression, direct invasion by disease process, or thrombosis. Extrinsic compression generally occurs in a gradual manner, so venous collateral channels have time to develop. The obstruction is well tolerated, and the patient has few symptoms. When the obstruction is due to a rapidly expanding malignancy, it occurs quickly without the development of collateral channels. It is less well tolerated and is often associated with more severe symptoms.

The extent and severity of the primary disease do not always correlate with the severity of the SVC syndrome.

Clinical Findings
A. Symptoms and Signs: Patients with superior vena cava obstruction complain of face, neck, and arm swelling; shortness of breath; orthopnea; and cough. The skin of the face may appear flushed. Other symptoms include hoarseness, stridor, tongue swelling, nasal congestion, epistaxis, dysphagia, headache, dizziness, syncope, lethargy, and chest pain. Symptoms are aggravated by bending forward, stooping, or lying down.

The most common signs are dilatation and tortuosity of the veins of the upper body; swelling of the face, neck, or arms; and plethora or cyanosis of the face. Other signs include proptosis, glossal edema, rhinorrhea, laryngeal edema, mentation changes, and elevation of the venous and cerebrospinal fluid pressures.

Signs and symptoms of prognostic importance include headache, vertigo, visual disturbances, decreased mentation, stupor, somnolence, and convulsions indicating cerebral edema; or hoarseness and stridor suggesting upper airway obstruction.

B. Diagnostic Studies: The SVC syndrome was once considered a life-threatening emergency, and patients were often treated without histologic confirmation of malignancy. Diagnostic procedures were avoided because they were considered hazardous. However, every effort must be made to confirm a diagnosis of cancer before antineoplastic therapies are instituted. The clinical diagnosis is usually apparent without extensive diagnostic tests. The chest x-ray will show a mass in most patients. Other common radiologic abnormalities include superior mediastinal widening and pleural effusion. A CT scan of the thorax will further define the anatomy of intrathoracic structures and pathologic lesions. The importance of contrast venography remains controversial. Its greatest value is for those patients in whom surgical bypass is being considered for an obstructed vena cava. Since more than half the patients with SVC syndrome will not have a primary diagnosis, the remainder of the diagnostic studies involve obtaining tissue. Sputum cytology, fine needle aspiration cytology, bronchoscopy, thoracentesis, lymph node biopsy, bone marrow biopsy, and mediastinoscopy can be used in the attempt to identify the underlying cancer. Thoracotomy is diagnostic when all other procedures have failed. However, care should be taken to avoid the more invasive diagnostic options because of the patient's propensity for brisk venous bleeding at or above the level of obstruction.

Treatment

The goals of therapy are to relieve the symptoms and to cure, if possible, the underlying cancer. Small-cell cancer of the lung, non-Hodgkin's lymphoma, and germ cell tumors are potentially curable.

A. Emergency Measures: Patients with life-threatening cerebral or laryngeal edema may require immediate radiation therapy without a firm diagnosis.

B. Specific Measures: Radiation therapy is the primary treatment. Irradiation is directed to the gross tumor plus a 2-cm margin surrounding the tumor and to the mediastinal, hilar, and supraclavicular nodes to a total dose of 30–50 cGy. The total dose is dependent on patient condition, extent of disease, response of the disease to treatment, and histology of the tumor. Chemotherapy alone may be beneficial for patients with chemosensitive tumors such as small-cell lung cancer, non-Hodgkin's lymphoma, and germ cell tumors. Relief from signs and symptoms usually occurs with 7–14 days with evidence of benefit 24 hours after onset of treatment in some cases.

C. General Measures: Rest in bed with the head elevated relieves some symptoms. Diuretics and reduced sodium intake help reduce upper extremity edema. Corticosteroids may be of some benefit in reducing cerebral edema and in reducing the inflammatory reactions associated with tumors and radiation therapy although their value has not been proved. Anticoagulant and thrombolytic therapy have limited usefulness.

D. Surgical Measures: Surgery to remove thrombi or to bypass obstruction of the SVC has not been widely applied but represents a measure that may be utilized when more conservative therapy (chemotherapy or radiation) fails. Venographic procedures are being evaluated whereby the obstruction may be relieved by placement of an expansile stent in the lumen of the compressed vessel.

Course & Prognosis

Most patients with SVC syndrome respond to radiation treatment. After 3–4 days of therapy, 77% of patients are subjectively better, and by day 7, 91% are subjectively better. Objective relief of signs occurs more slowly, with 89% of patients showing objective relief in 14 days. The failure rate of radiation therapy is 10–20%. The relapse rate may be as high as 50%. Failure of radiation therapy appears to be related to the presence of a thrombus in the SVC. The mean survival of patients with SVC syndrome caused by malignant disease is 6–7 months. Approximately 10% of patients with lung cancer and 45% of patients with lymphoma are alive at 30 months.

REFERENCES

Ahmann FR: A reassessment of the clinical implications of the superior vena cava syndrome. *J Clin Oncol* 1984;**2**:961.

Nieto AF, Doty DB: Superior vena cava obstruction: Clinical syndrome, etiology, and treatment. *Curr Probl Cancer* 1986;**10**:442.

Schraufnagel DE et al: Superior vena caval obstruction: Is it a medical emergency? *Am J Med* 1981;**70**:1169.

Yahalom J: Superior vena cava syndrome. Chapter 58 in: *Cancer: Principles & Practice of Oncology*, 3rd ed. DeVita VT Jr, Hellman S, Rosenberg SA (editors). Lippincott, 1989.

Central Nervous System Emergencies

Pamela Zyman New, MD

BRAIN METASTASES

Brain metastasis is one of the most common complications of cancer, possibly second only to metabolic encephalopathy. Autopsy studies have verified an incidence of 25% in patients who died of cancer. As patients survive their primary tumors longer owing to improved therapy, the incidence of brain metastases will likely increase. Metastases make up 15–30% of all intracranial lesions.

Pathogenesis

Most metastases reach the brain by hematogenous spread. The majority of these patients will have tumor involving the lung, either as the primary (60%) or as another step in the metastatic process for a primary located elsewhere (Table 40–1). A chest x-ray is often helpful in diagnosing the source, and if no lesion is identified, CT scan or MRI of the lung may reveal small metastases. In the few patients for whom this mechanism of spread is not identified, the pathogenesis may involve (1) spread through Batson's venous plexus, (2) tumor embolus through a patent foramen ovale, or (3) tumor filtered through lungs with only local or microscopic growth.

Brain metastases occur anywhere within the brain, but the distribution in general follows the proportionate blood flow to specific areas of the brain. Most occur within the hemispheres including gray and white matter (80%), about 15% occur in the cerebellum, and less than 5% present in the brain stem. Multiple metastases occur in 50% of patients; the tumor types responsible most often are melanoma and lung cancer (Table 40–2). Metastases from breast, colon, and renal cell carcinoma are more often single. Primary tumors originating from the pelvis more often produce posterior fossa metastases.

Clinical Findings

A. Symptoms and Signs: The most common history obtained is one of headache evolving over days to weeks followed by progressive focal neurologic symptoms, such as hemiparesis. Headache is more common in the patient with multiple metastases or with a metastasis involving the posterior fossa.

The classic early morning headache, which is thought to be associated with raised intracranial pressure, occurs in only about 40% of patients who have headache. Papilledema occurs in only 25% of patients with brain metastases. Seizures may be a presenting sign of metastasis and occur in about 15%. An additional 5–10% present with acute neurologic deficits because of hemorrhage into a metastasis or sudden growth and swelling surrounding the lesion. A nonfocal encephalopathy may be the initial sign in 1–2% of patients.

B. Diagnostic Tests: Diagnosis is based on imaging, either CT scan or MRI. Accuracy of the CT scan can be improved by performing multiple thin sections or infusing the patient with double-dose intravenous contrast material. For a specific tissue diagnosis, biopsy may be necessary if the primary is not known. The differential diagnosis includes primary brain tumor, brain abscess, stroke, and hemorrhage in some cases. In the case of a brain lesion with an appearance suggestive of metastasis on CT scan or MRI (ie, ring enhancing, surrounding edema) in a patient with no history of cancer, evaluation should begin with the lung. If the patient's history and a careful physical examination do not suggest a source (including chemistries, complete blood count, and urinalysis), consideration may be given to abdominal-pelvic CT scan. Further evaluation is seldom fruitful.

Treatment

Management must be individualized on the basis of such factors as the patient's neurologic status, the extent of systemic disease, as well as the number and site of the metastases. The standard treatment consists of corticosteroids followed by radiation therapy. All patients should be started on corticosteroids at the time of diagnosis. The usual initial dose is dexamethasone, 4 mg/d orally in 4 divided doses. Whole-brain irradiation is an important part of therapy, and the course is shorter than for the patient with a primary brain tumor. Doses per fraction may range from 150 to 400 cGy per day over 5–10 days, for a total of 3000–5000 cGy. Dexamethasone should be continued throughout the course of radiation therapy and gradually tapered at its completion. Most patients

Table 40–1. Cell types or primaries of solid tumor brain metastases.

Type	Frequency (%)
Lung	60–65
Breast	15–20
Kidney and urinary tract	6–10
Gastrointestinal tract	5–8
Melanoma	5–7

thus treated will experience adequate palliation. Large retrospective studies have shown that death is usually due to progressive systemic cancer rather than to brain metastases. The patient population defined here most often are those patients who have either multiple metastatic lesions or a large burden of tumor elsewhere in the body.

For the subgroup of patients whose only metastasis is to the brain and whose primary disease is fairly well controlled, the cause of death may well be related to the metastatic lesion, which certainly warrants more aggressive management in an effort to prolong survival. Data available from a well-controlled prospective study support an improved survival for patients with a single brain metastasis who are also good surgical candidates and have minimal tumor outside the brain or whose systemic cancer is responding well to therapy and who then undergo surgical excision of the metastasis followed by radiation therapy.

Prognosis

Regardless of the type of therapy, the occurrence of brain metastasis is associated with a poor prognosis. Those who receive no treatment at all have a median survival of 1 month. With the addition of corticosteroid treatment, survival can be increased to 2 months. Most of these patients die as a result of their brain tumor. The addition of whole-brain irradiation increases the median survival to 3–6 months. Data from retrospective studies show that over half these patients die of progressive systemic cancer and not as a result of their brain metastasis. Recently published

Table 40–2. Solid neoplasms with the highest tendencies toward central nervous system metastasis.

Type	Frequency (%)
Melanoma	40–50
Germ cell tumor	50–60
Bronchopulmonary cancer	40–50
Small cell	48
Undifferentiated forms	17
Squamous cell	17
Breast	40–50
Renal	20
Head and neck	20–25
Gastrointestinal, including liver and pancreas	2–15

prospective studies have further shown that in the case of single brain metastasis and minimal systemic disease, overall survival is significantly longer in the patients who have had surgery plus whole-brain radiation therapy (median of 10 months) versus those who have had only whole-brain radiation therapy (median of 4 months). Quality of life was also significantly better in the group receiving surgical resection and whole-brain radiation therapy.

Chemotherapy may also effect the regression of brain metastases in certain situations. Reports are becoming available that suggest favorable results in patients who have brain metastases from chemosensitive tumors, have had no prior systemic therapy or brain irradiation, have minimal systemic disease, and have a good performance status.

SPINAL CORD COMPRESSION

Incidence

Spinal cord compression occurs in approximately 5% of cancer patients. Its occurrence as the presenting sign of malignancy ranges in various series from 5% to 40%. The majority of cases occur in the thoracic spine (60–70%).

Every type of neoplasm has been reported to spread to the spine. However, roughly half of all cord-compressive lesions result from either breast or lung cancer (Table 40–3).

Pathophysiology

Approximately 90% of cord-compressive lesions arise by extension of vertebral lesions into the peridural space. The cord is then damaged by direct compression, with demyelination and axonal damage, as well as by secondary vascular compromise leading to ischemia, edema, and ultimately infarction of the cord. Some tumors, however, such as lymphoma and neuroblastoma, can spread to paravertebral nodes and directly enter the epidural space through the intervertebral foramina, without involving the vertebrae. Pelvic tumors can spread through Batson's venous plexus to the epidural space. Most tumors remain in the epidural space. Only 3–5% of cord-compressive lesions are intramedullary. These arise by hematogenous spread.

Table 40–3. Types of neoplasm causing spinal cord compression.

Primary Neoplasm	Frequency of Epidural Metastasis (%)
Lung	12–33
Breast	16–28
Lymphoma/leukemia	6–16
Prostate	4–9
Myeloma	3–7
Renal	3–7
Unknown primary	2–14

Other factors that may cause spinal cord compression as an indirect result of a metastatic tumor are pathologic vertebral fracture, kyphosis, and spinal instability. Most epidural metastases occur over one or two spinal segments, but they may be even more extensive. One or more noncontiguous epidural lesions may also be present at the time of diagnosis (10–30% of patients), and these may or may not be symptomatic. This situation occurs most often in breast cancer, prostate cancer, and multiple myeloma.

Clinical Findings

A. Symptoms and Signs: Ninety percent of patients have pain, usually localized to the involved spinal segments, as their initial complaint. Fifty percent to 75% may develop redicular pain. The local pain is either midline or off to one side. It usually is a dull, constant ache that increases when lying supine and is relieved by sitting or standing. When the pain is radicular, it is usually unilateral. This presentation is more common in the cervical and lumbar regions. After pain, other neurologic signs and symptoms develop, including weakness, sensory changes, and bladder and bowel dysfunction. At this point, progression can be rapid. Paraplegia can develop in hours to days. Approximately two-thirds of patients will have sensory loss or weakness by the time that the diagnosis of cord compression is made, and half will have in addition bladder and possibly bowel sphincter loss. The proportion of patients not ambulatory at the time of diagnosis ranges in various studies from 15% to 50%. Rarely, these neurologic signs and symptoms may develop without pain. Half the patients who are paraplegic at diagnosis have deteriorated rapidly over 24–48 hours after a variable period of pain with or without minor neurologic symptoms.

Less common presentations of cord compression include gait ataxia without weakness, herpes zoster along the dermatomes of compressed nerve roots, Brown-Séquard syndrome (usually secondary to a pathologic fracture or dislocation), and a conus medullaris syndrome of acute urinary retention and constipation without motor or sensory signs.

B. Diagnostic Tests: Evaluation usually begins with plain films of the spine, 80–90% of which will be positive in patients with carcinoma. Abnormalities include erosion of pedicles, vertebral collapse, and a paravertebral mass. Plain films of the spine are revealing in only 30–40% of cord compressions secondary to lymphoma because of the potential for lymphoma to spread through the intervertebral foramina without involving bone. Radionuclide bone scans are as sensitive as plain films but have a higher incidence of false positives from non-neoplastic disease.

Following plain film evaluation, myelography followed by CT scan is performed, or an MRI of the cord may be obtained. Controversy exists over which study is ultimately more sensitive. Benefits of panmyelography followed by CT scan include easy visualization of the entire cord in 1–2 hours plus the provision of cerebrospinal fluid (CSF) for examination. MRI is less invasive, on the other hand, and may yield multiplanar images. The quality of the MRI equipment available for spinal cord evaluation is of great importance.

Indications for myelography or MRI in cancer patients are the signs and symptoms of nerve root or spinal cord impingement described above. Any patient in this population with myelopathy should be considered a medical emergency requiring immediate myelography. Other patients with suspected lesions should be evaluated expeditiously, with the realization that sudden deterioration may occur. Myelography or MRI is recommended for cancer patients with unexplained back pain (even if plain films are normal), multiple vertebral metastases and pain, or paravertebral tumors.

Differential Diagnosis

Consider epidural abscess, epidural hematoma, herniated disk, and radiation myelopathy (if the spinal cord had previously been in a field of radiation, whether for epidural tumor involvement or for treatment of the systemic cancer).

Treatment

When a diagnosis of spinal cord compression is suspected, a definitive evaluation should be initiated immediately and treatment begun as soon as possible in an attempt to halt progression and minimize neurologic loss. Once the diagnosis of spinal cord compression is made, treatment with corticosteroids must begin. A 100-mg intravenous bolus of dexamethasone is given to patients with myelopathy or a complete block on the myelogram (or both). It may be given even before the myelogram is performed if a high-grade block is suspected. The initial dose of dexamethasone is followed by 24 mg every 6 hours orally and is tapered through the course of irradiation. The dose may be increased if the patient again deteriorates during radiation treatment. Patients with a partial block may begin with a smaller dose of dexamethasone, 5 mg every 6 hours orally. Almost 85% of patients will experience pain relief from corticosteroids alone.

Radiation therapy should then follow emergently, the optimal dose being 2000–4000 cGy in 10–14 fractions, spanning two normal vertebral levels above and below the myelographic lesion.

The traditional surgical approach has been laminectomy to "decompress" the neural elements. No prospective studies show that this increases the benefits of radiation therapy. Perioperative mortality may be as high as 10%, and morbidity is of the order of 10–50%. The latter consists of poor wound healing and the risk of wound infection in a patient receiving corticosteroids and ultimately irradiation to the involved operative field. Other morbidity includes hematomas, CSF leak, meningitis, and spinal instability with neurologic deterioration.

Definitive indications for surgery include the occasional patient with tumor located predominantly posterior to the cord, which is fairly easy to decompress as opposed to the normal situation where the tumor arises anteriorly from the vertebral body itself. The patient who presents with myelopathy and evidence by myelogram or MRI of an epidural mass but who does not carry a diagnosis of cancer requires at least a tissue diagnosis for proper management.

New surgical procedures have also been designed to fit the pathophysiology involved in cord compression. These include anterior surgical approaches and resection of involved vertebral bodies, both of which result in better tumor debulking and neural decompression than are offered by the posterior approach. Another advantage of surgery is due to the fact that radiation cannot correct the pain and neurologic deficits from angulation deformities or collapsed vertebrae. A diseased vertebral body can be replaced by methyl methacrylate, and the spine can be stabilized by metal pins, rods, or bone grafts. The ideal candidate to undergo vertebral resection is a young patient with a single site of spinal metastasis who has normal neurologic examination, a minimal systemic tumor burden, and an anticipated long duration of survival.

Prognosis

Pain relief after treatment with irradiation and corticosteroids (with or without surgery) occurs in 70–80% of patients and is less satisfactory in patients with kyphosis or spinal instability. The decrease in pain does not always correlate with neurologic improvement, which depends mainly on the patient's pretreatment neurologic status. Approximately 80% of patients who are fully ambulatory prior to treatment remain ambulatory, but less than 5% of paraplegic patients ever walk again. Given the same pretreatment neurologic condition, patients who have spinal epidural metastatic disease of prostate or breast cancer, myeloma, or lymphoma tend to have a better response to treatment than patients with lung cancer or other tumors. Patients with more radioresistant tumors tend to do more poorly.

CARCINOMATOUS MENINGITIS

Carcinomatous meningitis or leptomeningeal metastasis involves the spread of malignant cells to the subarachnoid spaces, producing free-floating tumor cells in the CSF. The incidence of this form of metastasis has become more recognized as a cause of morbidity and mortality especially as survival improves for the various tumor types involved.

Incidence

The occurrence of carcinomatous meningitis is the highest among the adenocarcinomas (about 75% will have this type of solid tumor) (Table 40–4). Most lung tumors are adenocarcinomas and small-cell carcinomas. Melanoma is also a frequent primary. Many patients with carcinomatous meningitis from the latter two sources also have parenchymal brain metastasis.

Of the hematologic malignancies, meningeal spread in acute lymphocytic leukemia is well recognized. Prophylaxis with craniospinal irradiation and intrathecal chemotherapy has dramatically changed the course of this once uniformly fatal illness in children. The incidence in acute nonlymphocytic leukemia is also significant especially in patients with a large tumor burden as manifested by elevated LDH level, elevated count of abnormal peripheral white blood cells, and extramedullary leukemia infiltration. Of patients diagnosed with acute undifferentiated leukemia, those most at risk for carcinomatous meningitis have myelomonocytic or monocytic subtypes. A high proportion of patients with acute myelomonocytic leukemia (AMML) and leptomeningeal spread also have a specific chromosome abnormality: an inversion of chromosome 16. The presentation of AMML and chromosome 16 inversion carries a 33% higher risk of developing leptomeningeal carcinomatosis than does the diagnosis of any other acute nonlymphocytic leukemia.

Patients with non-Hodgkin's lymphoma develop leptomeningeal disease usually at a time when their illness is progressing and no longer responding to treatment. The most common subtypes for this complication to occur are Burkitt's, diffuse large cell, lymphoblastic, and undifferentiated lymphomas. Carcinomatous meningitis is also reported to occur in Hodgkin's disease.

In addition, a number of primary central nervous system CNS neoplasms invade the leptomeningeal space. Among those most commonly involved is the medulloblastoma; again, the prophylactic use of craniospinal irradiation is a mandatory part of therapy for these patients. Other tumors with a propensity to seed the CSF pathways include ependymoma and germ cell tumors. Oligodendroglioma and glioblastoma are also capable of spreading in this fashion but less commonly than the above tumors. (See also Chapter 19.)

Table 40–4. Occurrence of tumor types in carcinomatous meningitis.

Type	Frequency (%)	Mean (%)
Breast	22–64	45
Lung	10–41	24
Melanoma	10–19	14
Gastrointestinal tract	1–6	
Genitourinary tract	1–4	

Pathogenesis

The route by which systemic malignant cells reach the subarachnoid spaces is thought to involve hematogenous spread via the arachnoid veins. This pathway has been documented for the leukemias and most likely is the route for most solid tumors as well. Tumor cells can also reach the meninges by direct extension as in the case of metastases to the dura, superficial brain cortex, ventricular ependymal lining, or choroid plexus. Tumor cells can also spread along perineural sheaths of the cranial nerves or spinal nerve roots and gain entry into the subarachnoid space.

Once malignant cells have gained access to the CSF space, they tend to settle in areas of stasis, normally at the base of the brain and along the cauda equina. Autopsy data support the assumption that the cells then multiply in either a linear fashion or from nodules on the surface of the brain or nerve roots. Infiltration of cranial or spinal nerves (or both) can also occur, as well as extension of tumor cells into the Virchow-Robin spaces and invasion of brain or spinal cord parenchyma. Approximately half the patients will have communicating hydrocephalus as a result of tumor cells infiltrating the arachnoid granulations and preventing CSF resorption. Noncommunicating hydrocephalus can occur from obstruction of the cerebral aqueduct by tumor cells preventing outflow of CSF. Leptomeninges may become fibrotic, and nerve roots often become matted together. The ultimate response of the nerve root is to undergo axonal destruction with wallerian degeneration.

Clinical Findings

A. Symptoms and Signs: The clinical hallmark of carcinomatous meningitis is the combination of signs and symptoms that verity multifocal involvement of the brain, cranial nerves, or spinal nerve roots. There is no specific clinical feature for any underlying tumor type. The initial complaint is most often an alteration of cognitive function, which may be related either to diffuse infiltration of the surface of the brain by tumor or to increased intracranial pressure secondary to hydrocephalus. Almost one-half of patients with carcinomatous meningitis will present with headache, vomiting, and altered mental status. Focal seizures and focal cerebral dysfunction, either transient or permanent, can also occur. The ischemic basis for the latter symptoms has been verified by the arteriographic demonstration of beading of cerebral vessels in patients with leptomeningeal disease.

Cranial nerve findings are listed in Table 40–5 in the order of their occurrence. Cauda equina involvement is represented by multiple root signs including radicular pain, dermatomal sensory loss, weakness, reflex asymmetry, and bowel and bladder symptoms. Myelopathy occurs rarely as a result of direct cord in-

Table 40–5. Cranial nerve involvement in leptomeningeal carcinomatosis.

Finding	Cranial Nerve Involved
Ocular motor paresis	III, IV, V
Facial weakness	VII
Hearing loss, tinnitus	VIII
Visual loss	II
Facial numbness, pain	V
Hoarseness, dysphagia	IX, X

vasion by tumor cells or extrinsic compression by a tumor nodule.

B. Diagnostic Tests: The definitive diagnosis of carcinomatous meningitis is the demonstration of malignant cells in the CSF. Repeated taps are frequently necessary. The chance of obtaining a positive cytologic specimen on the first lumbar puncture has been reported as 50%, whereas three spinal fluid analyses increase the sensitivity of cytologic examination to about 85%. Between 5% and 10% of patients with autopsy-proved leptomeningeal disease have persistently negative CSF cytology. False-negative and false-positive results can occur in patients with lymphoma.

CSF is, however, abnormal in almost all patients with carcinomatous meningitis (0–3% of patients in several series had completely normal CSF on the first tap). Characteristic but nonspecific abnormalities on initial lumbar puncture are shown in Table 40–6.

The composition of CSF obtained from the ventricle may be significantly different from that obtained from the lumbar region, even when obstruction to the CSF pathways is not present. Fluid obtained from the respective area of involvement determined by the predominant clinical abnormalities produces the greatest diagnostic yield and is also the most useful in following the response to treatment.

Radiologic studies can assist in the diagnosis of carcinomatous meningitis. MRI, particularly with gadolinium infusion, may reveal enhancing deposits along the walls of the ventricles or the cortical sulci. The same abnormalities are occasionally detected by contrast CT scan. Communicating and noncommunicating hydrocephalus can be seen on either CT scan or MRI, and 35–70% of patients' abnormalities can be detected by CT scan alone.

Myelopathy followed by CT scan can be helpful when CSF is nonspecific and clinical symptoms are

Table 40–6. CSF abnormalities in carcinomatous meningitis.

Finding	Frequency (%)
Protein >50 mg/dL	70–80
White cells >5/mm³	50–70
Pressure >160 mm	50–54
Glucose <40 mg/dL	30–75

equivocal. Abnormal myelograms have been reported in 25–40% of patients with carcinomatous meningitis. Characteristic findings include thickened nerve roots, single or multiple nodules along the nerve roots, and occasionally an intradural block.

Biochemical markers in the CSF (Table 40–7) may be of help in the diagnosis when malignant cells are not present in the CSF, and they may contribute to the monitoring of therapy and early detection of recurrence of carcinomatous meningitis. β-Glucuronidase is also elevated in lung, breast, and CNS infections. Carcinoembryonic antigen (CEA), however, is least likely to show a false-positive elevation in CNS infection. $β_2$-Microglobulin is actually a portion of the HLA antigen complex and is restricted to myeloproliferative and lymphoproliferative disorders. Helpful CSF markers for the embryonal carcinomas are the well known alpha-fetoprotein and human chorionic gonadotropin (hCG). The assays used in detecting the above-mentioned markers may still have a significant percentage of false negatives; therefore, they should not be used as criteria to rule out carcinomatous meningitis. Nor should they be used as the sole criterion of diagnosis in the face of persistently negative CSF cytologic specimens. The markers are most useful in following the response to treatment; serial measurements revealing a decline are associated with successful therapy, whereas a rising level heralds a relapse of disease.

In the forefront of diagnostic technology lies the use of monoclonal antibodies to detect specific antigens and tumor cells in the CSF, combined with flow cytometry to detect abnormal DNA content in the tumor cells and thus diagnose carcinomatous meningitis from among a variety of systemic cancers.

Differential Diagnosis

Infectious meningitis with a subacute infection, such as tuberculosis or a fungal process, may present with findings similar to those of carcinomatous meningitis. The clinical features of increased intracranial pressure, altered mental status, and headache can also be seen in brain metastasis, stroke, or cerebral abscess. Other processes that can cause the spinal and root symptoms include epidural cord compression, brachial or lumbar plexopathy, intramedullary metastases, and radiation myelopathy.

Table 40–7. Biochemical markers and their relative frequency of occurrence in CSF of patients with leptomeningeal disease.

Tumor Type	CEA	$β_2$-Microglobulin	LDH-5 Isoenzyme
Breast	+		+++
Lung	+++		++
Melanoma	+		++
Lymphoma	–	++	+/–
CNS infection	+/–	+	+

Treatment

Untreated carcinomatous meningitis, especially related to solid tumors, results in death due to neurologic dysfunction within several months. Options for treatment include combinations of radiotherapy, intrathecal chemotherapy, and systemic chemotherapy.

Radiation therapy was the original method of treatment for leptomeningeal carcinomatosis. Total craniospinal axis radiation is no longer recommended, except in the case of meningeal leukemia, because of the risk of myelosuppression, which then limits chemotherapy for both the systemic and meningeal tumor. Myelosuppression is a particular risk in these cases because the vertebral column provides much of the functional bone marrow in adults. Irradiation is administered to areas of major clinical involvement at doses of 2000–3000 cGy in 10–15 fractions. In the case of radicular symptoms, the area most often involved is the region of the cauda equina. Radiation therapy is also useful for the treatment of ventricular outflow obstruction in the case of noncommunicating hydrocephalus, the relief of which is essential for the safe installation of chemotherapy into the ventricles. A field involving the base of the skull will also provide relief when cranial nerve palsies are a prominent finding.

The predominant mode of therapy for carcinomatous meningitis is intrathecal chemotherapy, since most chemotherapeutic agents do not cross the blood-brain barrier when administered systemically to achieve sufficient tumoricidal levels in CSF. The recommended method for delivery of intrathecal chemotherapy is through an intraventricular (Ommaya) reservoir, which requires a surgical procedure for placement but spares the patient the discomfort of repeated lumbar punctures. The reservoir can also be used to obtain an [111]indium DTPA (diethylene-triaminepentacetic acid) ventriculogram to verify that ventricular outflow is not obstructed. It is generally thought that intraventricular injections yield a better distribution of drug throughout the CSF compartment with more constant levels, but recent data from animal models suggest that at times a combination of lumbar and ventricular injections may be best for achieving adequate drug concentrations. Ventricular injections provide a high concentration of drug in the CSF surrounding the brain, but levels are much lower in the spinal cord region. The reverse is true with lumbar injections, so a combination of both may be optimal. Repeated lumbar punctures, on the other hand, may lead to local scar formation, making access into the CSF difficult. Radiotracer studies have shown that 10–15% of lumbar injections may end up in the epidural space or in subcutaneous fat. Another benefit of the Ommaya reservoir is to allow more frequent repetitive injections of low-dose drugs, resulting in less neurotoxicity from the agents instilled. Complications of the reservoir itself include obstruction, CSF leak, and most importantly infection, which can occur in 6–13% of patients. Most of these infections can be treated without removal of the reservoir.

The most commonly used drug for intrathecal injection is methotrexate, not only because of its efficacy but also because it seems to be better tolerated than most other agents. It is generally more effective for lymphomas, leukemias, and breast cancer than for other tumors. The standard intrathecal dose is 12–20 mg of methotrexate given twice weekly until the CSF improves, followed by the same dose at successively longer intervals. After each injection, patients are given oral doses of leucovorin to protect against myelosuppression caused by prolonged release of methotrexate into the circulation.

Other cytotoxic drugs that can be administered intrathecally include cytarabine and thiotepa. The former drug is useful mainly in lymphomas and leukemias and is given at a dose of 30–100 mg either in addition to or as a substitute for methotrexate. Cytarabine is much less active against solid tumors, but occasional responses are seen. Thiotepa, an alkylating agent, has been used with some success as a second-line drug in solid tumor carcinomatous meningitis, particularly that of breast and lung cancer origin. The standard dose is 10 mg per injection.

Prognosis & Complications

With radiation therapy and intrathecal chemotherapy, 75–80% of leukemia and lymphoma patients will have a CSF and clinical response; a large portion of these patients may attain a central nervous system remission. The prognosis is graver for solid tumors. Patients with breast cancer seem to have the best outcome, with a 40–80% response rate, a median survival of 6–7 months, and as many as 25% one-year survivors. The response rate of lung tumors is 25–40%, with the small-cell tumor response being at least 50% and the non–small cell tumor response much worse (rate of 20% and median survival of about 4 months). Patients with malignant melanoma have the worst outcome, with fewer than 20% responding to therapy and a very short median survival time (3.6 months). In addition to the type of tumor, the extent of neurologic dysfunction at the time of diagnosis contributes to duration of survival.

A major complication of the therapy for carcinomatous meningitis is the development of leukoencephalopathy, which generally begins weeks to months after beginning treatment. The onset is insidious with behavior or cognitive changes followed by dementia, spastic quadriparesis, and somnolence. Patients may stabilize or improve with the discontinuation of methotrexate, but few recover completely. The majority are left with serious sequelae. CT scans will reveal symmetric hypodensity of the deep hemispheric white matter. (MRI likewise confirms the presence of white matter change.) At autopsy foci of white matter necrosis and axonal swelling are seen. A similar situation can arise in patients receiving intrathecal or high-dose intravenous cytarabine. Overall incidence of leukoencephalopathy is about 10%, but many patients do not survive long enough to develop it. The incidence among 12-month survivors is thought to be as high as 40%. A synergistic effect occurs with the addition of cranial irradiation, especially if it is given prior to or during methotrexate treatment, and some authors feel that almost all patients who survive 1 year will develop leukoencephalopathy. The risk is further increased as the cumulative dose of methotrexate rises and in the presence of impaired CSF flow, with consequent delayed clearance of methotrexate from the central nervous system.

The more acute forms of toxicity in the treatment of carcinomatous meningitis involve the use of methotrexate itself, the most common syndrome being an acute sterile meningitis, which occurs in 5–40% of patients. Symptoms include headache, stiff neck, vomiting, fever, occasional seizures, altered mental status, and CSF pleocytosis beginning within several hours of treatment with intrathecal methotrexate or occasionally cytarabine. The entire syndrome resolves over 24–72 hours. CSF peak levels of methotrexate may be abnormally elevated in some patients, but this correlation is not always seen. A reversible subacute encephalopathy or myelopathy may develop several days to weeks into the treatment course, generally when infusions are closely spaced. A prolonged rate of clearance of methotrexate from the CSF is incriminated as the cause of this syndrome. Monitoring of CSF methotrexate levels should serve as a guide to the dosing of the drug and to minimizing toxicity.

REFERENCES

Brain Metastasis

Jellinger K: Pages 377–379 in· Therapy of Malignant Brain Tumors. Springer-Verlag, 1987.

LeChevalier T et al: Sites of primary malignancies in patients presenting with cerebral metastasis: A review of 120 cases. Cancer 1985;56:880.

Patchell RA: Brain metastasis. Pages 228–231 in: Current Therapy in Neurologic Disease 3. Johnson RT (editor). BC Decker, 1990.

Patchell RA: A randomized trial of surgery in the treatment of single brain metastasis. N Engl J Med 1990;322:496.

Spinal Cord Compression

Byrne T, Waxman S (editors): *Spinal Cord Compression*. FA Ramis, 1990.

Carmody RF et al: Spinal cord compression due to metastatic disease: Prognosis with MR imaging versus myelography. *Radiology* 1989;**173:**225.

Moore AJ, Uttley D: Anterior decompression and stabilization of the spine in malignant disease. *Neurosurgery* 1989;**25:**713.

Portenay RK et al: Back pain in the cancer patient: An algorithm for evaluation and management. *Neurology* 1987;**37:**134.

Posner JB: Back pain and epidural spinal cord compression. *Med Clin North Am* 1987;**71:**185.

Carcinomatous Meningitis

Gilbert M: Epidural spinal cord compression and carcinomatous meningitis. Pages 234–236 in: *Current Therapy of Neurologic Disease–3*. Johnson RT (editor). BC Decker, 1990.

Sculier JP: Treatment of meningeal carcinomatosis. *Cancer Treat Rev* 1985;**12:**95.

Wasserstrom WR, Glass JP, Posner JB: Diagnosis and treatment of leptomeningeal metastases: Experience with 90 patients. *Cancer* 1987;**49:**759.

Hypercalcemia of Malignancy

Gregory R. Mundy, MD

Hypercalcemia occurs commonly in patients with cancer and is responsible for morbidity and considerable mortality. Its prevalence depends on the setting. In the general population, cancer is the second most common cause of hypercalcemia, responsible for about one-third of cases. Only primary hyperparathyroidism is a more common cause, and these two diseases account for 90% of all cases. In the hospital setting, cancer becomes a relatively more common cause, since most patients with primary hyperparathyroidism are asymptomatic at the time of discovery. Hypercalcemia often is found when routine electrolyte measurements are performed. In many patients, hypercalcemia is an unexpected finding.

Hypercalcemia occurs most often in patients with the commonest malignancies, ie, carcinomas of the lung and breast (Table 41–1). It is also frequently seen in patients with squamous cell carcinomas of the head and neck, larynx, and oropharynx. It also occurs commonly in patients with carcinomas of the pancreas, kidney, and ovary. It is rare in patients with cancers of the female genitalia (except for squamous cell carcinomas) and extremely rare in patients with colon cancer. Some unusual cancers are associated with hypercalcemia. These include cholangiocarcinoma and VIPomas. In Japan, hypercalcemia often occurs in association with leukocytosis, particularly in patients with squamous cell carcinomas of the head and neck and the lung.

Pathophysiology

The mechanisms responsible for causing hypercalcemia in patients with cancer are heterogeneous and multiple (Figure 41–1). No single mechanism explains hypercalcemia in all types of cancer. Moreover, there is no clearly described situation in which the pathophysiology of hypercalcemia mimics that of primary hyperparathyroidism. In most patients with cancer, hypercalcemia appears to be due to a combination of increased bone resorption and decreased renal calcium excretion (Figure 41–2). In most cases increased absorption of calcium from the gut is not a cause of hypercalcemia, since gut absorption of calcium is decreased in the majority of patients. However, there are a few clearly described cases of lymphomas where gut absorption of calcium

is enhanced and hypercalcemia is associated with increased 1,25-dihydroxyvitamin D production by tumor cells.

Considerable evidence suggest that cancer patients have enhanced renal tubular calcium reabsorption. Its extent is probably similar to that which occurs in primary hyperparathyroidism.

Identification of factors produced by tumors that could influence calcium homeostasis has been an area of research for the past decade. As these factors have been characterized, it has become apparent that some tumors produce multiple factors that could increase bone resorption and potentially increase renal tubular calcium reabsorption.

A. Transforming Growth Factor Alpha (TGFα): is a polypeptide stimulator of cell growth and replication that is produced by many tumor cells in vitro and may be responsible for maintaining the transformed phenotype in target cells. It is a powerful stimulator of bone resorption in vitro, increasing the formation of new osteoclasts from precursors. It also increases plasma calcium when injected in vivo. It is responsible for the increased bone resorption that occurs in some animal models of hypercalcemia and probably plays an important role in the bone destruction associated with some human malignancies.

B. Parathyroid Hormone (PTH)–related Peptides: Many tumors associated with the humoral hypercalcemia syndrome (ie, the syndrome of hypercalcemia associated with a systemic mediator) produce a factor that binds to the PTH receptor and activates it. This tumor-associated protein has been identified and the gene cloned. It comprises 141 amino acids and has some amino acid sequence homology with PTH in the first portion of the aminoterminal end of the molecule (the portion of PTH that binds to the PTH receptor). This PTH-related protein stimulates bone resorption in vitro and vivo, increases renal tubular calcium reabsorption, and increases the plasma calcium in vivo.

C. Interleukin-1 Alpha (IL-1α): Both IL-1α and IL-1β are powerful bone resorbing factors. They stimulate osteoclastic bone resorption by causing proliferation of osteoclast progenitors and also act on mature preformed osteoclasts to stimulate bone resorption. IL-1α is associated with several human tu-

Table 41–1. Relative frequency of causes of hypercalcemia.

	No. of Patients	Percent of Cases
Primary hyperparathyroidism	111	54
Cancer	72	25
Lung	25	35
Breast	18	25
Hematologic (myeloma, lymphoma, etc)	10	14
Head and neck	4	8
Renal	2	3
Prostate	2	3
Unknown primary	5	7
Others	8	8

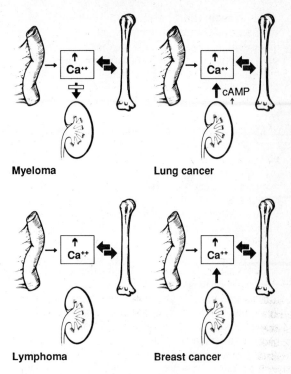

Myeloma   **Lung cancer**

Lymphoma   **Breast cancer**

Figure 41–2. Patterns of abnormalities in calcium homeostasis in patients with different types of cancer. In all cases, there is an increased in bone resorption. In patients with myeloma, there is decreased renal calcium excretion because of impaired glomerular filtration. In patients with lung cancer and breast cancer, there is impaired renal calcium excretion because of increased renal tubular calcium reabsorption. In some patients with lymphoma, absorption of calcium from the gut may be increased. (Reproduced, with permission, from Mundy GR: *Calcium Homeostasis: Hypercalcemia and Hypocalcemia,* 2nd ed. Martin Dunitz, 1990.)

mors associated with hypercalcemia, and it also may be produced by normal immune cells in response to the presence of a tumor as part of the host response.

D. Tumor Necrosis Factor (TNF): TNF is a cytokine produced by macrophages that shares many biologic properties with IL-1α. It stimulates osteoclastic bone resorption by causing proliferation of osteoclast progenitors and acting on mature osteoclasts to stimulate the formation of resorption lacunas. There are two closely related TNF molecules: TNFα and TNFβ (also called lymphotoxin). Lymphotoxin is produced by normal activated lymphocytes. Human myeloma cells produce lymphotoxin, and this may be the major mediator of bone destruction in myeloma. Moreover, infusions of lymphotoxin in mice cause hypercalcemia in vivo.

E. 1,25-Dihydroxyvitamin D: In most patients with hypercalcemia of malignancy, serum 1,25-dihydroxyvitamin D concentrations are suppressed. However, a few cases of T and B cell lymphomas and Hodgkin's disease have been associated with in-

creased circulating 1,25-dihydroxyvitamin D concentrations. Cells infected with the human T cell lymphotropic virus (HTLV) type 1, which causes one variety of adult T cell lymphoma, constitutively produce 1,25-dihydroxyvitamin D, indicating that extrarenal synthesis of 1,25-dihydroxyvitamin D occurs in this disease state and implicating this factor as a mediator of hypercalcemia in this situation.

Clinical Findings

A. Presentation with Hypercalcemia: Occasionally, a patient who presents with hypercalcemia without any obvious evidence of malignant disease is found to have an occult cancer on further investigation. Although relatively uncommon, occult malignancy as a cause of hypercalcemia may be more frequent in children that in adults. Certain tumor types may be associated with an occult malignancy, particularly carcinomas of the kidney or ovary. Rarely, it occurs with carcinoma of the lung and is extremely uncommon with carcinoma of the breast.

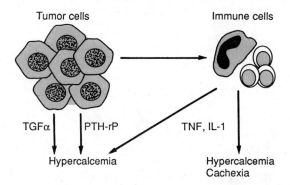

Tumor cells   Immune cells

TGFα   PTH-rP   TNF, IL-1

Hypercalcemia   Hypercalcemia Cachexia

Figure 41–1. Proposed mechanism for the pathophysiology of hypercalcemia in patients with solid tumors without metastases. The tumor (in this case, carcinoma of the lung) produces factors that stimulate bone resorption and renal tubular calcium reabsorption. The consequence is an increase in the serum calcium. (Reproduced, with permission, from Mundy GR: *Calcium Homeostasis: Hypercalcemia and Hypocalcemia,* 2nd ed. Martin Dunitz, 1990.)

B. Presentation with Hypercalcemia and Widespread Cancer: Hypercalcemia usually occurs in the setting of widespread bone metastases in a patient with disease that is metastatic not only to bone but also to other major organs such as liver and lungs. The commonest example is in the patient with breast cancer. Rarely do patients with breast cancer develop hypercalcemia unless they are in the last 3–6 months of life and have widespread bone disease. The symptoms and signs may be confused with those due to other causes, eg, cytotoxic drugs, advancing disease, or radiation therapy. This is particularly likely to occur in a patient who develops nausea and vomiting as a consequence of hypercalcemia or who is confused and disoriented. It is important to recognize hypercalcemia as the cause, since it is reversible in the majority of patients.

It is unusual for a patient with malignant disease to have a serum calcium level greater than 18 mg/dL, whereas occasional patients with primary hyperparathyroidism present with a serum calcium greater than 20 mg/dL. On the other hand, most patients with cancer and primary hyperparathyroidism have a serum calcium of less than 13 mg/dL.

Many patients with hypercalcemia are asymptomatic, particularly if the hypercalcemia is mild and has not developed rapidly. Symptoms are more prominent in those patients who have a rapid increase in the serum calcium. Symptoms are frequently related to the gastrointestinal tract, neurologic system, cardiovascular system, and kidney. The commonest gastrointestinal symptoms are nausea and vomiting. Anorexia and constipation are also occasionally found. Disorientation and confusion, frequently preceded by lethargy and loss of interest in the surroundings, are frequent features. Occasionally patients complain of headaches, and some become anxious or irritable. Insomnia and intractable nightmares occasionally occur and cease when hypercalcemia is relieved. A few patients show generalized muscle weakness. With severe hypercalcemia, confusion and disorientation are progressive and may lead to profound lethargy and coma. The comatose state is an ominous prognostic sign.

C. Laboratory Findings: Hypercalcemia in a patient with malignant disease is recognized most frequently when measurements of the serum calcium are performed routinely. The serum calcium should either be corrected for abnormalities in protein concentration or ionized calcium should be measured. Ideally, measurements of ionized calcium in the serum or whole blood are used. If ionized calcium measurements are unavailable, a correction formula for total serum calcium can be applied to account for abnormalities in the serum proteins. The usual correction formula is to allow 0.8 mg/dL of calcium for every gram of albumin that the serum albumin is less than 4 g/dL. Many patients, particularly those with advanced cancer, will be hypoalbuminemic, and

hypercalcemia will not be recognized if only the total cerumen calcium is considered.

Other important measurements include levels of the serum phosphorus, urinary or nephrogenous adenosine monophosphate (AMP), serum chloride, urinary calcium excretion, serum bone γ-carboxyglutamic acid, serum alkaline phosphatase, and serum creatinine. The serum phosphorus is frequently decreased in patients with humoral hypercalcemia, probably because tumor factors cause phosphate wasting. However, in patients with impaired renal function, it may be increased. It may also be increased in patients with increased serum 1,25-dihydroxyvitamin D concentrations, since this vitamin D metabolite increases phosphate absorption from the gut. Urinary and nephrogenous cyclic AMP are increased in patients with solid tumors who produce PTH-like peptides. The cyclic AMP is generated in the renal tubule cells, probably by activation of the PTH receptor by a tumor peptide. It is not a particularly useful diagnostic tool because it is also increased in patients with primary hyperparathyroidism. The serum chloride may be more useful in this regard. Most patients with primary hyperparathyroidism have a serum chloride greater than 103 meq/L. This occurs because PTH impairs bicarbonate reabsorption and leads to a mild form of renal tubular acidosis, accompanied by hyperchloremia. In contrast, most patients with the hypercalcemia of malignancy have a serum chloride less than 100 meq/L. Measurements of calcium excretion corrected for glomerular filtration or even for urinary creatinine are not useful in the differential diagnosis of hypercalcemia. Most patients with cancer have impaired calcium excretion for the level of serum calcium, similar to that seen in primary hyperparathyroidism.

The serum bone γ-carboxyglutamic acid protein has recently been measured as an index of bone turnover. It is not particularly useful in the differential diagnosis. It is usually decreased in patients with widespread metastatic bone disease. Serum alkaline phosphatase, in contrast, is usually increased and probably reflects a relative increase in bone formation occurring as a consequence of bone destruction. Alkaline phosphatase is often not increased in patients with myeloma because bone formation is not increased in this situation.

Renal function is normal in most patients with malignancy and hypercalcemia unless the serum calcium is greater than 13 mg/dL. Under these circumstances, the patient may become dehydrated and polyuric and may develop reversible renal failure. In the patient with cancer and fixed impairment of renal function, the most likely diagnosis is myeloma or lymphoma. In patients with myeloma, renal failure may be due to a combination of Bence Jones proteinuria, uric acid nephropathy, infection, or occasionally amyloidosis. In patients with lymphoma and fixed renal failure, consider ureteral obstruction due to enlarged retroperitoneal lymph nodes.

Treatment

All patients with hypercalcemia of malignancy, no matter how slight the increase in the serum calcium, should be actively treated. In malignant disease, hypercalcemia is usually progressive and should be reversed as soon as possible. Observation is reasonable only when the patient can be carefully followed.

The first principle of treatment is to treat the underlying cause. Unfortunately, in the majority of patients, this is not possible, since the disease is widespread at the time of diagnosis and only palliative therapy is possible. Nevertheless, chemotherapy or palliative therapy that reduces tumor bulk may be valuable in the treatment of hypercalcemia. For patients with myeloma who present with hypercalcemia, successful treatment of the malignant disease may also alleviate hypercalcemia.

A. Normal Saline: Rehydration with normal saline is the first treatment option. Many patients will have lost 5–10 L of extracellular fluid volume. Moreover, promotion of sodium diuresis always increases calcium excretion, thus improving the situation in which increased renal tubular calcium reabsorption is an important component of the hypercalcemia. However, this is not a useful form of maintenance therapy, and in many patients the lowering of the serum calcium is only of short-term benefit. The patient will rapidly become hypercalcemic again without further therapy.

A reasonable regimen is to administer 5–10 L by intravenous infusion in the first 24 hours (provided renal and cardiac function are normal, and depending on estimated fluid deficits) and then to give 2–3 L/d over the following days. Occasionally, patients become hypernatremic when infused with normal saline. Under these circumstances, hypotonic saline should be alternated with normal saline to maintain the serum sodium concentration in the normal range.

B. Bisphosphonates: The preferred form of therapy is to use a bisphosphonates. In the USA, the only bisphosphonates currently available are etidronate and pamidronate. Most patients will respond to etidronate given in doses of 7.5 mg/kg of body weight/d by intravenous infusion for 5–7 days in association with 2–3 L or normal saline per day, followed by oral administration. Etidronate probably should not be used in the patient with renal failure, particularly if the serum creatinine is greater than 3 mg/dL. Etidronate may cause a minor elevation in the serum phosphorus in patients with normal renal function. Pamidronate has recently been released by the FDA for use in the hypercalcemia of malignancy. This drug is preferable to etidronate. Nearly all patients will respond to pamidronate given in doses of 60–90 mg by intravenous infusion over 24 hours. Pamidronate should be used with caution in patients

with renal failure, particularly if the serum creatinine level is greater than 3 mg/dL.

C. Calcitonin and Corticosteroids: Calcitonin and corticosteroids used in combination are effective in lowering the serum calcium. They probably are not as effective as the bisphosphonates but have the advantage of a rapid mode of action and almost no toxicity when used in the short-term. They are useful for patients with major organ failure, especially renal failure, and particularly for patients with hypercalcemia due to hematologic cancer. Salmon calcitonin should be given in doses of 200 IU every 12 hours subcutaneously, and glucocorticoids can be given as hydrocortisone, 100 mg every 6 hours intravenously, or prednisone, 40 mg/d orally.

D. Plicamycin (Mithramycin): Plicamycin is effective in about 80% of patients. However, its toxicity has probably been underappreciated and its mode of administration is so clumsy that bisphosphonates or calcitonin and corticosteroids are preferred for acute management. It is nephrotoxic and should not be used in patients with renal failure. The dose is 15–25 mg/kg of body weight given by slow infusion over 4 hours. This should be repeated when the patient becomes hypercalcemic again. Responses may last from 5 days to 2 weeks.

E. Glucocorticoids: Glucocorticoids alone are usually not effective, particularly in hypercalcemia associated with solid tumors. They may be effective in patients with myeloma in doses equivalent to 40 mg of prednisone daily. However, they rarely reduce the serum calcium into the normal range.

F. Oral Phosphate: Oral phosphate is useful for patients who are ambulatory and require oral therapy. Oral phosphate may not be tolerated because of diarrhea, which occurs in a considerable proportion of patients It can be used in doses up to 2 g/d given in 3–4 divided doses. It is useful only in patients having a serum phosphorus less than 3.8 mg/dL and should not be used in patients with impaired renal function.

G. Gallium Nitrate: Gallium nitrate has recently become available in the USA for use in the hypercalcemia of malignancy. It is a very effective drug. It may be less toxic than plicamycin and should be used in those rare patients in whom pamidronate fails. There is less experience with this drug than with pamidronate.

Emergency Management

Patients who have a serum calcium greater than 13 mg/dL or who are symptomatic require urgent medical treatment. Serum calcium in this range may rise progressively and lead to rapid deterioration and death. Patients should be treated vigorously with normal saline intravenously to ensure normal extracellular fluid volume and to promote calcium diuresis. If possible, at least 3–5 L of normal saline should be given within the first 24 hours. In some patients, this may require simultaneous administration of loop diuretics such as furosemide, 40 mg by bolus injection every 6 hours, to prevent fluid overload. Larger doses of furosemide have been suggested to promote urinary calcium excretion, but the danger in an underhydrated patient probably outweighs the benefit. The author recommends immediate institution of salmon calcitonin 200 IU every 12 hours (or equivalent dose of human calcitonin). If the patient has a serum creatinine less than 2 mg/dL, intravenous etidronate by infusion 7.5 mg/kg of body weight/d should be commenced. If the serum calcium is greater than 2 mg/dL, hydrocortisone hemisuccinate, 100 mg every 6 hours, should be given by intravenous injection or infusion. Either treatment should lower the serum calcium into an acceptable range within 24 hours so that maintenance therapy can be used. For patients treated with etidronate, calcitonin can be withdrawn after 72 hours and the patient continued on etidronate infusions for a further 48 hours and then changed to oral etidronate treatment. For patients with compromised renal function who have responded well to the combination of calcitonin and glucocorticoids, this combination should be continued until the serum calcium is less than 12 mg/dL, and then the intravenous glucocorticoids should be changed to oral prednisone and gradually tapered over 1 week to the lowest dose possible to keep the serum calcium in the normal range. A dose equivalent to prednisone, 10 mg/d, is desirable. In the meantime, treatment for the underlying disease should be considered and instituted when feasible.

REFERENCES

Garrett IR et al: Production of the bone resorbing cytokine lymphotoxin by cultured human myeloma cells. *N Engl J Med* 1987;**317:**526.

Mosely JM et al: Parathyroid hormone–related protein purified form a human lung cancer cell line. *Proc Natl Acad Sci USA* 1987;**84:**5048.

Mundy GR: *Calcium Homeostasis: Hypercalcemia and Hypocalcemia,* 2nd ed. Martin Dunitz, 1990.

Mundy GR: Hypercalcemia of malignancy. *Kidney Int* 1987;**31:**142.

Mundy GR: The hypercalcemia of malignancy revisited. *J Clin Invest* 1988;**82:**1.

Mundy GR: Martin TJ: The hypercalcemia of malignancy: Pathogenesis and management. *Metabolism* 1982; **31:**1247.

Mundy GR, Wilkinson R, Heath DA: Comparative study of available medical therapy for hypercalcemia of malignancy. *Am J Med* 1983;**74:**421.

Stewart AF et al: Biochemical evaluation of patients with cancer-associated hypercalcemia: Evidence for humoral and nonhumoral groups. *N Engl J Med* 1980;**303:**1377.

Suva LJ et al: A parathyroid hormone–related protein implicated in malignant hypercalcemia: Cloning and expression. *Science* 1987;**237:**893.

Valentin A et al: Estrogens and anti-estrogens stimulate release of bone resorbing activity by cultured human breast cancer cells. *J Clin Invest* 1985;**75:**726.

Warrell RP et al: Gallium nitrate inhibits calcium resorption from bone and is effective treatment for cancer-related hypercalcemia. *J Clin Invest* 1984;**73:**1487.

Yates AJP et al: Effects of a synthetic peptide of a parathyroid hormone–related protein on calcium homeostasis, renal tubular calcium reabsorption, and bone metabolism. *J Clin Invest* 1988;**81:**932.

Malignant Effusions

42

Steven P. Kalter, MD

Malignant effusions represent abnormal accumulations of fluid exuded into a body cavity of limited capacity. This limited capacity may produce clinical sequelae that may occasionally be life threatening.

PLEURAL EFFUSION

Essentials of Diagnosis

- Persistent cough.
- Progressive shortness of breath.
- Chest x-ray findings of fluid in pleural cavity.
- Exudative pleural effusion with malignant cells seen on cytologic preparation.

General Considerations

Malignant pleural effusions are seen most often in patients who have lung cancer, breast cancer, or lymphoma.

Pathogenesis

In malignant effusions, a proteinaceous fluid is produced by malignant cells lining either the visceral or parietal pleura. This fluid production may be copious, or the malignant cells may line the visceral pleural cavity and "clog up" the visceral lymphatics, preventing fluid absorption. Hence, by either mechanism, fluid can accumulate in the pleural cavity, decrease effective lung volume, and cause clinical symptoms and signs.

Etiology

A malignant pleural effusion occurs only after malignant cells have invaded the parietal or visceral pleura or both. Invasion may be due to direct extension of tumor, eg, tumor from within the lung itself into the pleural cavity, or to hematogenous or lymphatic metastases preventing normal absorption of pleural fluid.

Pathology

By direct extension or metastasis, lung cancers are the most common tumors to create malignant effusions. Breast cancers usually metastasize to the lymphatics and cause effusions by lymphatic obstruction, often on the same side of the primary tumor. Lymphomas may cause lymphatic obstruction particularly in the mediastinum. When the thoracic duct is obstructed, a chylous effusion may result.

Histopathologic analysis of fluid often yields a specific diagnosis. When a patient has a known malignancy, thoracentesis can yield metastatic cytologic specimens. A pleural biopsy is necessary in the undiagnosed patient. Newer pathologic techniques are available that may better discriminate among the cytopathologic possibilities. Immunoperoxidase stains using monoclonal antibodies may differentiate among tumor types. The epithelial membrane antigen (EMA) stains positively for carcinomas. The common leukocyte antigen (CLA) stains positively for most lymphomas. Melanomas stain with S-100, whereas carcinomas do not. Sometimes it is difficult to differentiate between adenocarcinomas and mesothelioma in the pleural cavity. The adenocarcinomas will often stain for carcinoembryonic antigen (CEA) as well as EMA, where as the mesothelioma will not. Electron microscopy may even be necessary for diagnosis. Occasionally, the cytologic or pleural biopsy specimens remain negative, and a definitive open biopsy or thoracoscopic biopsy may be necessary.

Pathologic Physiology

The progressive accumulation of fluid in the pleural space will inevitably produce signs and symptoms. In most cases, several hundred milliliters of fluid will accumulate before the patient becomes symptomatic. Other patients may not become dyspneic until tension is produced on the contralateral hemithorax. The underlying functional status of the patient plays an important role; eg, the patient with chronic obstructive pulmonary disease and limited lung reserve will not be able to compensate for pleural fluid accumulation and will become symptomatic faster than a patient with a normal lung reserve.

Clinical Findings

A. Symptoms and Signs: Progressive fatigue, dyspnea, and pain are the usual presenting symptoms of a malignant pleural effusion. The patient may report a smothering sensation or heaviness in the chest. Usually there is orthopnea and progressive dyspnea on exertion, progressing to dyspnea at rest. The pain may suggest myocardial ischemia but typically worsens with a deep breath (pleuritic) but not with exertion (angina). There may be point tenderness, particularly if there is concomitant ipsilateral rib involvement.

Tachypnea and tachycardia usually accompany the dyspnea. A nonproductive cough may be present as well. The cough is usually worse upon reclining at night, and the patient may not be able to sleep supine owing to the cough and worsening dyspnea.

Tachycardia and fever are nonspecific and may or may not be present.

B. Laboratory Findings: Laboratory findings may be nonspecific; arterial blood gas measurements may show arterial hypoxemia in room air associated with hypocarbia and respiratory alkalosis as the hyperventilating patient attempts to compensate for hypoxemia. The pleural fluid almost always fulfills Light's criteria for an exudate: (1) lactic dehydrogenase (LDH) level >200, (2) ratio of fluid LDH to serum LDH >0.6, (3) protein level in fluid >3 g/dL, and (4) ratio of fluid protein to serum protein >0.5. Malignant cells are usually identified. Elevated CEA in the pleural fluid may indicate an adenocarcinoma. Electron microscopy may be useful in identifying specific features of carcinomas versus other malignancies (eg, mesothelioma). Differentiating malignant cells from clumps of benign reactive mesothelial cells may be difficult; definitive cytologic features of malignancy must be present before a diagnosis is rendered (this is especially relevant to lymphoma).

C. Imaging Findings: Standard chest x-ray usually identifies the pleural effusion. Typical features are blunting of the costophrenic angle and loss of the ipsilateral diaphragmatic surface (Figure 42–1). Small effusions on x-ray may be deceptive, since even the smallest effusion seen on x-ray contains 200–300 mL of fluid. CT scan of the chest will pick up smaller effusions, and the radiologist will help determine if the fluid is loculated. Ultrasound guidance can identify the best site for thoracentesis. In Meig's syndrome, the radiologist can often identify not only pleural effusion but also ascites and ovarian tumor by CT scan or ultrasound.

Differential Diagnosis

In the evaluation of malignant effusion, the key is to establish a diagnosis of malignancy. Rule out other possible explanations for the exudative effusion (Table 42–1). Benign effusions are usually transudates. Postinfectious parapneumonic effusion may be particularly difficult to distinguish from malignancy but should disappear with effective treatment of the pneumonia.

Complications & Sequelae

The most dreaded complication of malignant pleural effusion is respiratory failure as the effusion

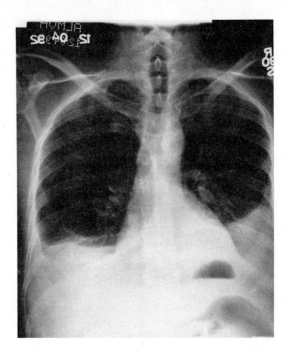

Figure 42–1. Bilateral pleural effusions in a patient with colon cancer.

grows and compresses lung parenchyma. Since many patients present with a pleural effusion of unknown cause, thoracentesis is often both diagnostic and therapeutic. A complication of thoracentesis is pneumothorax, and a chest x-ray should be ordered after each attempt. Delayed pneumothoraces occasionally

Table 42–1. Causes of pleural fluid transudates and exudates.[1]

Transudates	Exudates
Congestive heart failure	Parapneumonic effusion
Cirrhosis with ascites	Cancer
Nephrotic syndrome	Pulmonary embolism
Peritoneal dialysis	Empyema
Myxedema	Tuberculosis
Acute atelectasis	Connective tissue disease
Constrictive pericarditis	Viral infection
Superior vena cava obstruction	Fungal infection
Pulmonary embolism	Rickettsial infection
	Parasitic infection
	Asbestos pleural effusion
	Meigs' syndrome
	Pancreatic disease
	Uremia
	Chronic atelectasis
	Trapped lung
	Chylothorax
	Sarcoidosis
	Drug reaction
	Postmyocardial infarction syndrome

[1]Reproduced, with permission, from Stauffer JL: Pulmonary diseases. Chapter 7 in: *Current Medical Diagnosis & Treatment 1992.* Appleton & Lange, 1992.

occur. Progressive dyspnea for several hours or days after the thoracentesis should prompt chest x-ray evaluation. Sometimes fibrous scars form within the pleural cavity, leading to a loculated effusion. Loculated effusions can become a chronic problem and may never be successfully drained. A malignant pleural effusion may recur despite all therapeutic efforts. It may become infected, or bronchopleural fistulas may form, requiring chronic chest tube drainage and antibiotic therapy.

If all these treatments are unsuccessful, chemical pleurodesis is the next step. A chest tube is placed in the lowest possible anterior location in the thoracic cavity, and suction drainage is accomplished until all obvious fluid has been removed. A sclerosing agent is introduced into the pleural space, and the chest tube is clamped. Sclerosing agents include nitrogen mustard, bleomycin, quinacrine, tetracycline, and concentrated dextrose solutions. Recent evidence suggests that 60–90 units of bleomycin in 50 mL of sterile saline or dextrose solution is more effective than the other commonly used agents (tetracycline or doxycycline). After the admixture is introduced, the tube is clamped, and the patient changes position frequently so as to accomplish pleural symphysis. After 6–12 hours, suction is reapplied and continued until less than 100 mL of fluid is removed over 24 hours. The chest tube can be removed at that time. If this fails, the same technique using 500 mg–1 g of tetracycline should be attempted. Open pleurodesis with talc is a last resort if the above fails and the status of the patient allows it.

PERICARDIAL EFFUSION

Essentials of Diagnosis
- Shortness of breath.
- Chest pain.
- Elevated neck veins (jugular venous distension).
- Pulsus paradoxus.
- Electrical alternans.
- "Water bottle" heart seen on chest x-ray.
- Pericardial fluid seen on echocardiogram.

General Considerations
Development of a pericardial effusion in the cancer patient is not uncommon. As many as 21% of cancer patients develop some pericardial fluid at some time during the natural history of the disease. If accumulation of fluid is gradual, it may remain asymptomatic. On the other hand, rapid accumulation of fluid or accumulation of enough fluid to produce tamponade is a true oncologic emergency.

Pathogenesis
There is normally 5–10 mL of fluid in the pericardium. In malignant pericardial effusion, malignant cells usually invade the pericardium and produce an exudate. These tumors have spread to the pericardium either by direct extension or by hematogenous or lymphatic spread. Occasionally radiation therapy administered to the left chest or mediastinum can produce enough irritation to the pericardium to produce a pericardial effusion.

Etiology
Rarely, benign tumors of the chest or mediastinum (teratoma, fibroma, angioma) impinge on the pericardium and produce a "sympathetic" effusion. Primary malignant tumors of the pericardium (sarcoma, mesothelioma) accumulate hemorrhagic pericardiac fluid rapidly, leading to tamponade in most cases. Metastatic disease to the pericardium can result from almost any neoplasm but is most commonly due to lung or breast cancer, Hodgkin's and non-Hodgkin's lymphomas, melanomas, and gastrointestinal malignancies.

Postradiation pericarditis and consequent pericardial effusion usually occur within a few weeks (acute form) or within 12 months of the chest irradiation. Postradiation pericardial fibrosis can occur years after irradiation. This tends to be a more constrictive type of pericarditis and produces less pericardial fluid; it may be equally dangerous because the thickened pericardium is significantly less distensible and results in earlier breakdown of the heart's compensatory mechanisms.

Pathologic Physiology
Normally the heart beats smoothly in the few milliliters of pericardial fluid that serve as a lubricant. When enough pericardial fluid is present to decrease diastolic filling of the right ventricle and to decrease stroke volume, compensatory mechanisms attempt to maintain cardiac output. Contractility and heart rate increase. Peripheral vasoconstriction labors to increase venous return and ventricular filling pressure. Eventually the compensatory mechanisms are unable to compensate for the falling stroke volume. The consequent fall in cardiac output without corrective intervention eventually leads to circulatory collapse and death. How much fluid is required to produce circulatory collapse depends on the rate of accumulation of the fluid and the distensibility of the pericardium. If the pericardium distends slowly and some of the pericardial fluid is absorbed, a steady state may be reached and no clinical symptoms may develop.

Clinical Findings
A. Symptoms and Signs: The patient may experience no symptoms with a pericardial effusion until tamponade occurs. At this point there is usually apprehension or a feeling of doom. There may be a smothering feeling or chest pain. The patient may have dyspnea.

The heart tones are muffled and often distant. The patient may have a narrowed pulse pressure, often with systolic blood pressure below 100 mm Hg. There may be tachycardia. The systolic blood pressure may drop with inspiration (pulsus paradoxus), and if this drop exceeds 10 mm Hg, it is suggestive of pericardial tamponade.

B. Diagnostic Studies: Insertion of a right-sided heart catheter shows equalization of diastolic pressures in tamponade (pulmonary capillary wedge pressure, pulmonary artery end-diastolic pressure, right ventricular end-diastolic pressure, and right atrial pressure are within 5 mm Hg of each other). Chest x-ray shows cardiac enlargement often with a "water-bottle" configuration of the heart (Figure 42–2). The electrocardiogram shows reduced QRS voltage. Electrical alternans is almost pathognomonic of neoplastic cardiac tamponade. This variation in the size of the QRS complex is due to variation in heart position at the time of electrical depolarization, which in turn is due to the swinging motion of the heart when the pericardium is filled with a large volume of fluid. The echocardiogram is the most sensitive technique for diagnosing the presence of pericardial fluid. In the supine position, pericardial fluid collects posteriorly. As the pericardial effusion enlarges, fluid is seen both anteriorly and posteriorly.

Differential Diagnosis

Pulsus paradoxus may be seen in various types of cardiomyopathies, constrictive pericarditis, hypovolemic shock, and severe obstructive lung disease.

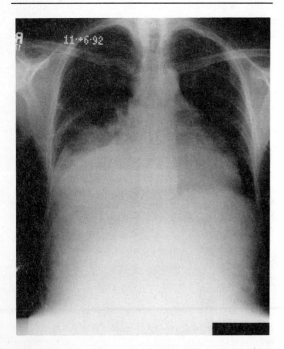

Figure 42–2. Typical "water bottle"–shaped heart of pericardial effusion in a patient with AIDS and Kaposi's sarcoma.

Pleural effusions on the echocardiogram can confuse the inexperienced interpreter. Pericardial masses or tumors should have increased density compared to free fluid. Irradiation-induced pericarditis may be difficult to differentiate from neoplastic involvement of the pericardium. Irradiation-induced pericarditis tends to occur 4–12 months after treatment. Half the patients who develop postradiation pericarditis are asymptomatic, and effusion is diagnosed only by echocardiogram. This type of effusion will resolve in 1–1.5 years. The other 50% of patients will have persistent, progressive pericardial effusions usually associated with chest pain and fatigue. Pericardiocentesis with cytologic analysis is indicated, but the specimen may be negative for malignant cells or uninterpretable, particularly in the case of well-differentiated lymphocytic lymphomas. Thoracotomy may be necessary to ascertain the diagnosis and to provide adequate pericardial drainage. For acute, symptomatic irradiation-induced pericarditis, a short course of systemic corticosteroids is probably indicated.

Complications & Sequelae

The most dreaded complication of a neoplastic pericardial effusion is pericardial tamponade. This is a medical emergency requiring emergent action in the acute setting. The patient with tamponade is usually anxious, diaphoretic, hypotensive, and tachycardic. Neck veins are elevated, and there is a pulsus paradoxus of greater than 10 mm Hg. Heart tones are distant. The echocardiogram shows a large pericardial effusion, and the electrocardiogram shows electrical alternans.

The patient with a neoplastic pericardial effusion or irradiation-induced pericarditis can develop constrictive pericarditis with jugular venous distention, hepatomegaly, and ascites. At the time of pericardiectomy, a patient who develops constrictive pericarditis should have the pericardium carefully inspected for tumor.

Treatment

If the patient is in shock owing to pericardial tamponade, intravenous normal saline should be given to maximize venous return and maintain blood pressure. If this alone does not stabilize the patient, emergent pericardiocentesis should be performed. A subxiphoid approach is preferred. A 2- to 3-inch, 18-gauge needle and 50-mL syringe are inserted just to the right of and below the xiphoid process with the tip of the needle aimed at the left shoulder. Often removal of 20–50 mL of fluid is adequate to reestablish an effective stroke volume. The two techniques used most frequently to provide durable relief of malignant pericardial effusion are creation of a pleuropericardial window and pericardiotomy. The pleuropericardial window is almost always effective but requires general anesthesia, which may be poorly tolerated by a debilitated cancer patient. Subxiphoid pericardiotomy is quick and can be performed under local anesthesia. Its efficacy is probably equal to that of the pleuropericardial window. Furthermore, a drainage catheter may be left in the pericardium for use with a sclerosing agent.

Intermittent pericardiocentesis has been used in the chronic situation for removal of reaccumulating pericardial fluid, but the use of intrapericardial sclerosing agents now obviates the need for repeated pericardiocentesis. The sclerosing agents used most frequently are tetracycline and bleomycin. The technique of intrapericardial sclerotherapy involves the instillation of a pericardial catheter into the pericardial space under continuous electrocardiographic monitoring. The fluid is allowed to drain for 12–24 hours and is cytopathologically and biochemically studied in the laboratory to confirm the diagnosis. Protein content, cell count, and bacterial, fungal, and acid-fast bacilli cultures are obtained. Once the malignant nature of the process has been confirmed, intrapericardial instillation begins. Lidocaine hydrochloride, 100 mg, is followed by tetracycline hydrochloride, 500 mg in 20 mL of normal saline. The catheter is clamped for 1–2 hours and then reopened. This procedure is repeated daily until the net drainage is less than 25 mL in 24 hours. Those few patients who do not respond can be treated with 5 units of bleomycin dissolved in 20 mL of sterile water. Both agents can cause fever but are otherwise well tolerated.

External beam radiation therapy can be used following failure of the aforementioned approaches. This technique is most useful in neoplasms having the greatest radiosensitivity, eg, lymphomas or leukemias, and is less successful in solid tumor effusions. External beam radiation therapy is adjunctive treatment when there is evidence of mediastinal involvement in addition to pericardial disease. The experimental technique of intrapericardial instillation of radioactive chromic phosphate ^{32}P showed a success rate of about two-thirds in one study.

MALIGNANT ASCITES

Essentials of Diagnosis
- Increased abdominal girth.
- Bloated feeling.
- Diffuse abdominal pain.
- Fluid wave on abdominal examination.
- Increased dullness to percussion of abdomen.
- Free peritoneal fluid seen in abdominal cavity on ultrasonography or CT scan.

General Considerations
Malignant ascites is often the initial presentation in patients with ovarian cancer. Other cancers may also produce ascites either initially or when recurrent.

Pathogenesis
The mechanism for fluid accumulation may involve either overproduction or under-reabsorption. Overproduction of ascitic fluid may be due to exudation of increased amounts of fluid accompanying increased permeability of the peritoneal membrane. Decreased reabsorption can result from either occluded diaphragmatic lymphatics or venous obstruction by tumor masses.

Etiology
Tumor deposits within the peritoneal cavity may produce ascites by overproduction of exuded fluid. This is seen most often in ovarian cancer and in malignant carcinomatosis due to pancreatic, colon, or breast cancers or lymphoma disseminated throughout the peritoneum. Metastatic disease in the liver may so impair hepatic function as to produce ascites due to liver failure. Hepatic involvement may produce obstruction at the level of the inferior vena cava and produce ascites (Budd-Chiari syndrome). In both latter examples, the ascites is transudative and cytologic specimens are usually negative.

Clinical Findings
A. Symptoms and Signs: The patient will usually note increased abdominal girth by increased size of the waistline and a feeling of increased abdominal fullness, bloating, or pain. Despite the fact that the patient has not been feeling well and has not been eating well, there is no significant weight loss; in fact, there may be a weight gain. Increased abdominal girth is measured by taking the abdominal circumference at the level of the umbilicus. A fluid wave is obtainable, and there is dullness to percussion. It may be possible to feel an abdominal or pelvic mass or "omental cake."

B. Laboratory Findings: The ascitic fluid is usually exudative. The cytologic specimen is positive in no more than half the patients with malignant ascites. Ascitic CEA levels are elevated in only 50% of patients with malignant ascites. Ascitic alpha-fetoprotein may be elevated in hepatoma patients. The ascitic CA-125 is not a specific tumor marker for ovarian cancer, since it may be elevated in patients with cirrhosis or hepatoma. When found in association with ovarian cancer, its value may increase or decrease depending on the progress of the cancer. Ascitic cholesterol levels of greater than 48 mg/dL are associated with cancer, whereas lower values are associated with benign conditions.

C. Special Studies: CT scan of the abdomen and pelvis may reveal an "omental cake" of tumor or show other signs of abdominal carcinomatosis. "Skinny" needle biopsy of tumor deposits under CT scan guidance may allow a diagnosis without resorting to exploratory laparotomy. If this technique does not provide adequate tissue for histologic and cytologic review, a larger needle can be used (eg, Trucut). Special stains for EMA, CEA, CLA, S-100, and alpha-lactalbumin (positive in breast cancer) can help provide diagnostic clues if the primary cancer is not known.

Cytology is most useful in confirming the diagnosis of a malignant effusion. To improve the yield, it is best to stain the smears (with the Papanicolaou and Giemsa stains) within 2 hours of aspiration. A stainable sediment is obtained by centrifuging 10- to 20-mL samples at 3000 revolutions per minute for 10 minutes.

Complications & Sequelae

The appearance of ascites in malignancy need not be a dire prognostic sign. It may be a sign at presentation, particularly in ovarian cancer, and may be amenable to treatment. Ascites per se may be little more than a cosmetic problem, since patients can well tolerate fluid accumulation within the peritoneum. Nonetheless, after more than 2–3 L of fluid accumulates, pressure symptoms may require treatment. Metastatic disease to the liver producing ascites as a consequence of liver failure is associated with a very short survival.

Treatment

The initial paracentesis for diagnostic purposes can also be an occasion to remove a large quantity of fluid (1–2 L) and reduce discomfort. If the patient has a treatable cancer, eg, ovarian or breast cancer or lymphoma, the response to intravenous or intraperitoneal chemotherapy may be manifested as a decrease in ascites. A diuretic such as spironolactone or spironolactone plus a thiazide may help decrease the quantity of ascitic fluid and produce symptomatic relief while awaiting a response from systemic therapy.

Should this approach not produce a complete remission, a Port-a-Cath (buried-subcutaneous) or Tenckhoff (transcutaneous) type catheter may be placed into the peritoneum for direct instillation of chemotherapy or for therapeutic paracentesis. Rarely does intraperitoneal chemotherapy produce a significant response if large intraperitoneal tumor masses are still present. If these measures prove inadequate and ascites is still a problem, consider insertion of a peritoneovenous shunt (Denver or LeVeen). This will allow reutilization of the proteins that would otherwise be evacuated and lost at time of paracentesis. The Denver shunt will consistently relieve ascites pressure problems 60–70% of the time. Complications include blocking of the catheter, infection, disseminated intravascular coagulation, and tumor embolism into the lung. Shunting is not recommended for patients with advanced metastatic liver disease.

Surgical Oncologic Emergencies

43

Michael P. Kahky, MD, Harold V. Gaskill III, MD, & Carey P. Page, MD

HEMORRHAGE

Hemorrhagic complications may result from any mucosal lesion in the gastrointestinal tract, from tumor necrosis, from erosion of major vessels, or from coagulation abnormalities imposed by the cancer (eg, leukemia) or by its treatment (surgery, radiotherapy, chemotherapy). Bleeding may occur into the lumen of the gut, into the tumor itself, into the organ of origin, into a body cavity, or into the retroperitoneum.

Upper Gastrointestinal Hemorrhage

Gastrointestinal tract hemorrhage is a common complication in the cancer patient because of mucosal involvement by tumors of the gastrointestinal tract, thrombocytopenia due to aggressive chemotherapy, and stress ulceration of the gut. Most episodes of upper gastrointestinal hemorrhage, however, are of nonmalignant origin. The decision to operate is based more on the rate and duration of bleeding than on the specific cause. Most bleeding episodes can be controlled nonoperatively.

Bleeding from sources proximal to the ligament of Treitz result in either "coffee-ground" vomitus or hematemesis. Begin resuscitation efforts immediately: secure intravenous access; draw blood for coagulation studies, blood count, and typing and crossmatching; and expand blood volume. Crystalloids are given intravenously to restore hemodynamic stability. If blood loss is estimated to be greater than 1000 mL, blood should be transfused immediately. Correction of coagulation abnormalities, platelet transfusions, and administration of antacids and H_2 blockers should be instituted. A Foley catheter is inserted to monitor urinary output and as an index of the adequacy of resuscitation and vital organ perfusion. A nasogastric tube or Ewald tube is inserted and the stomach is washed out with iced saline until the effluent clears. Nasogastric decompression reduces antral distention with a consequent release of gastrin, and it also allows clots to be removed from the stomach in preparation for endoscopy.

Flexible endoscopy is the first-line diagnostic procedure in patients with upper gastrointestinal bleeding to localize the site of bleeding. Though early endoscopy does not reduce mortality due to upper gastrointestinal bleeding, it will identify the bleeding site in 80–90% of patients, and sometimes is therapeutic as well as diagnostic.

A. Esophageal Bleeding: Bleeding from tumors of esophageal origin is usually manifested by hypochromic, microcytic anemia due to occult blood loss. Since these tumors rarely bleed massively, they rarely result in a surgical emergency because of bleeding. Patients on chemotherapy who have severe, sustained retching and vomiting can also bleed from Mallory-Weiss tears at the gastroesophageal junction. Candidal esophagitis, commonly seen in immunosuppressed cancer patients, can cause longitudinal esophageal ulceration and bleeding. Primary hepatic tumors, liver metastases, and liver involvement with myeloproliferative disorders can result in sufficient obstruction to portal blood flow to cause portal hypertension and esophageal varices, which can bleed massively.

Esophageal bleeding is usually self-limited and does not require an operation. Bleeding from esophageal tumors can usually be controlled by endoscopic coagulation. Mallory-Weiss tears often stop bleeding spontaneously. Patients who continue to bleed should undergo angiography. Intra-arterial vasopressin infusion or embolization of the left gastric artery can then be performed to control the bleeding. Candidal esophagitis can be diagnosed by its endoscopic appearance, and microscopic examination of esophageal washings can confirm the diagnosis. Oral nystatin or ketoconazole are effective treatment.

Bleeding from esophageal varices can be controlled in most instances by administration of intravenous vasopressin and, if necessary, tamponade with a Sengstaken-Blakemore tube. After bleeding is controlled, endoscopic sclerotherapy is particularly useful in obliterating varices, especially in patients in whom operation is to be avoided. Failure of response to these measures mandates surgical control of bleeding. A central portacaval shunt is the most effective surgical method of controlling bleeding esophageal varices.

B. Gastric and Duodenal Bleeding: Bleeding from the stomach and duodenum can result from both benign and malignant disorders. Stress gastritis with multiple mucosal erosions can result from ingested irritants, such as aspirin and corticosteroids, and can occur in the setting of sepsis and multiple system organ failure as a result of impaired mucosal blood flow. Stress gastritis has also been described as a complication of continuous hepatic artery infusion with floxuridine. The routine use of H_2 blocking agents and aggressive antacid therapy with monitoring of gastric pH in critically ill patients has made this complication less common than in the past. Benign gastric and duodenal ulcers can account for significant gastrointestinal bleeding in up to 25% of cancer patients. Corticosteroid therapy, thrombocytopenia, and sepsis can often aggravate preexisting ulcers and cause hemorrhage.

A variety of malignant conditions can cause bleeding from the stomach. Though blood loss from gastric adenocarcinoma is often occult, massive bleeding from tumor necrosis or arterial erosion can occur and may necessitate emergency operation. Gastric lymphomas frequently bleed during aggressive chemotherapy. As the tumor responds to drug treatment and undergoes necrosis, massive upper gastrointestinal hemorrhage can occur. Advanced lesions should be resected prior to chemotherapy, since the incidence of bleeding from necrotic tumors is high and may delay or prevent the completion of chemotherapy. Leiomyosarcoma of the stomach, gastric, carcinoids, and metastatic melanoma, though less common, can also cause massive upper gastrointestinal bleeding.

C. Bleeding from Ulcers: Bleeding from gastric ulcers or gastric cancers that fail to respond to medical management can occasionally be controlled by direct laser coagulation. If surgical resection is necessary, the location and extent of the ulcer determine the choice of operative procedure. Distal, lesser curvature ulcers can be adequately treated by vagotomy and antrectomy. More proximal ulcers require a more extensive resection. Bleeding gastric cancers, if not widely spread, should be resected for cure, and a wide subtotal gastrectomy is the procedure of choice. Bleeding peptic duodenal ulcer in the cancer patient is best treated by vagotomy, pyloroplasty, and oversewing of the bleeding point. In this situation, control of hemorrhage is the major concern, and amelioration of the ulcer disease is of secondary importance.

Lower Gastrointestinal Hemorrhage

Bleeding from a source distal to the ligament of Treitz generally manifests itself as blood passed per rectum, as either melenic stool or hematochezia.

Hemorrhage from the small intestine can cause melena or hematochezia and is very difficult to localize. Massive bleeding from either primary or metastatic tumors in the small intestine is rare but must be considered in the differential diagnosis of acute lower gastrointestinal bleeding. Radiation enteritis is an uncommon cause of small bowel bleeding. Cytomegalovirus enteritis has been described as a cause of small bowel hemorrhage in the immunosuppressed cancer patient.

Benign disease is often responsible for hemorrhage from the colon and rectum in the cancer patient. Diverticulosis, angiodysplasia, and ischemic colitis can all occur in this patient population. Major bleeding from colonic or rectal tumors is unusual and seldom requires emergent surgical intervention. Radiation proctitis can occur in patients treated for pelvic malignancies, but hemorrhage due to this condition is generally not life-threatening.

After resuscitative measures have been instituted, the first step in the evaluation of a patient with lower gastrointestinal bleeding is to exclude a source proximal to the ligament of Treitz. The presence of blood in the stomach on nasogastric aspiration indicates an upper gastrointestinal hemorrhage, and upper endoscopy is the next diagnostic procedure. If the nasogastric aspirate is clear, rigid proctosigmoidoscopy is then done to identify bleeding in the rectum and lower sigmoid colon. Colonoscopy then follows but is difficult to perform in the patient who is actively bleeding. Selective mesenteric angiography is the most accurate method for localizing lower gastrointestinal bleeding. After the bleeding point is localized, intra-arterial vasopressin will stop the bleeding in about half the cases. A rate of blood loss of 0.5–1 mL/min is necessary for arteriographic localization. Technetium scan may detect rates of blood loss as low as 0.1 mL/min. Less vigorous or intermittent bleeding can usually be detected by a radionuclide scan using technetium Tc 99m–labeled autologous red blood cells. This test can detect bleeding rates as low as 0.1 mL/min and is especially helpful in patients who are not continuously bleeding, since the labeled red cells remain in the blood pool for up to 24 hours. Labeled autologous blood scans are highly technique dependent and must be performed while the patient is bleeding.

Since colonic bleeding is usually not massive, emergent operations are not usually required. Segmental colectomy is the procedure of choice once the location of bleeding has been identified. Total abdominal colectomy is reserved for patients in whom the bleeding site has not been localized. If proctosigmoidoscopy has excluded a distal source of bleeding, then the distal bowel can be converted to a mucous fistula. If the status of the distal colon is unknown, the colon should be excised to the peritoneal reflection and Hartmann's pouch constructed. Anastomoses are generally not performed in patients in shock.

In frail patients with ongoing blood loss from rectal tumors, transanal fulguration of the tumor is often successful and avoids operation. Patients bleeding from radiation proctitis that does not respond to local measures (corticosteroid retention enemas, stool softeners) may require proximal diverting colostomy.

Small intestinal bleeding should be treated by segmental resection of the involved small bowel. The bleeding point in the small bowel is very difficult to localize preoperatively. At exploration, identification of the source of small bowel bleeding from tumor involvement is usually easy. Less certain, however, is localization of a small ulcerative or angiodysplastic lesion in the presence of a blood-filled small intestine. In actively bleeding patients, it is helpful to isolate multiple segments of the bowel with atraumatic clamps and then excise the segments that continue to fill with blood. Small bowel continuity is usually established with primary anastomosis.

INTESTINAL OBSTRUCTION

Cancer patients can develop intestinal obstruction due to either benign or malignant causes. In the absence of external hernias and in patients with previous operations and radiotherapy, the three primary considerations are adhesions, radiation fibrosis, and cancer.

Adhesions are the most common cause of intestinal obstruction. The small bowel is most often involved, and involvement usually is well distal to the ligament of Treitz. Small bowel obstruction has also been described as a complication of intraperitoneal chemotherapy. Small bowel obstruction secondary to malignancy is usually due to peritoneal carcinomatosis, although primary small bowel malignancies may initially present as intestinal obstruction. Carcinoma of the descending and sigmoid colon can cause intestinal obstruction, but in these instances the colonic distention is much more impressive, particularly with a competent ileocecal valve. Though malignant causes are more likely in patients with a prior history of colorectal cancer, known metastases, or advanced disease, benign causes of intestinal obstruction are still common. It should never be assumed that intestinal obstruction in the cancer patient is secondary to recurrent disease without some other confirmation eg, CT scan findings, palpable abdominal tumor mass, known carcinomatosis, histopathology.

Nausea, vomiting, abdominal distention, cramping abdominal pain, and obstipation are the classic symptoms of intestinal obstruction. On physical examination, the patient may demonstrate abdominal distention if the obstructive lesion is some distance distal to the ligament of Treitz. High small bowel obstruction may cause a deceptively flat abdomen. Auscultation of the abdomen may disclose high-pitched bowel sounds with rushes and tinkles if ileus has not supervened. Abdominal tenderness is usually mild and diffuse. Supine and upright films of the abdomen show air-filled loops of small bowel with differential air-fluid levels. Air may also be present in the colon if (1) the films are obtained early in the course, (2) the obstruction is incomplete, or (3) the patient has "treated" the bowel obstruction with enemas. Very high complete small bowel obstruction may result in an essentially "gasless" abdomen.

Distinguishing between mechanical intestinal obstruction and paralytic ileus is often difficult, particularly in the cancer patient. Patients receiving chemotherapy who are vomiting may have uncorrected losses of potassium, and hypokalemia drastically reduces gut motility. Narcotics can also impair bowel motility. Patients receiving *Vinca* alkaloids are particularly prone to paralytic ileus because of the neurotoxic effects of these drugs. Cisplatin may cause excessive renal losses of magnesium, which will reduce bowel motility.

Patients with intestinal obstruction generally are dehydrated owing to vomiting, lack of oral intake, and fluid loss into the bowel lumen and have some degree of metabolic derangement and acid-base imbalance. Resuscitation should begin with infusion of isotonic saline solution, and serial electrolyte and arterial blood gas values should be employed as guides to therapy. Passage of a nasogastric tube will relieve vomiting and decompress the stomach.

If the clinical presentation and x-ray findings are consistent with a colon obstruction, a limited barium enema should be performed. No preparation is necessary, since the study is done only to identify an obstructing lesion in the colon and not to define mucosal detail.

Whether the obstruction is partial or complete is the next determination. Incomplete obstruction sometimes responds to nasogastric or nasointestinal intubation, obviating the need for surgery. Patients with complete obstruction usually should be explored. Distinguishing simple from strangulated obstruction preoperatively is difficult, and there are no truly reliable physical signs or laboratory tests. Patients with incomplete obstruction, particularly if it is thought to be secondary to radiation enteritis or peritoneal carcinomatosis, may resolve with transnasal decompression alone. Whether nasointestinal intubation affords any advantage over nasogastric intubation is controversial, and most surgeons will use the method of decompression with which they have had the most success. Clinical signs must be followed carefully during this period of nonoperative therapy. Most patients who respond to decompression alone will do so within 72 hours.

Complete obstruction is treated by prompt surgical intervention once the patient is resuscitated and electrolyte abnormalities are corrected. If the patient is found to have a benign cause, standard surgical principles should be followed (adhesions lysed, internal hernias reduced, and so on). Complete obstruction due to carcinomatosis or radiation enteritis should be treated by side-to-side enteroenterosomy to bypass the obstructed segments. Aggressive attempts to dissect involved bowel loops increase the risk of entering the bowel lumen with the subsequent formation of enterocutaneous fistulas. This is a serious and avoidable complication in a critically ill patient. Postoperatively patients should receive parenteral nutritional support and prolonged tube decompression.

Colonic obstruction from carcinoma is managed according to the site of obstruction. Ascending colon lesions can be safely managed by resection and primary anastomosis. The conservative approach to obstructing left colon lesions is to perform a primary resection of the tumor and leave the patient with a temporary colostomy. This addresses the acute problem and allows time for endoscopic evaluation of the entire colon for synchronous lesions and for adequate bowel preparation for reanastomosis at a second operation. An alternative procedure is proximal decompression at the first operation and resection and anastomosis at a second operation.

INFLAMMATION

The extent and severity of suspected inflammatory lesions in cancer patients are often underestimated owing to their immunocompromised state and relative inability to manifest the usual components of an inflammatory response. Cancer patients are subject to the same types of inflammatory lesions seen in other patients of their age. Acute cholecystitis, pancreatitis, and diverticulitis are all seen in the oncology patient population. Two additional processes deserve comment: (**1**) anorectal inflammation, because it mandates different treatment in neutropenic patients, and (**2**) neutropenic enteritis, because it is peculiar to the cancer patient.

Acalculous Cholecystitis

A high index of suspicion is necessary to recognize acalculous cholecystitis, which generally occurs in an already ill and debilitated patient. Fever and localized upper right quadrant pain and tenderness are frequently seen but may be absent in the patient in whom the site of inflammation cannot be localized. Abnormal liver enzymes are almost always present. Leukocytosis may not occur. Suspicion, ultrasonography, and isotopic biliary tract imaging are the keys to diagnosis. A dilated gallbladder with a thickened wall and pericholecystic fluid are seen on sonography, which can be performed at the bedside if necessary. Findings of either delayed or nonvisualization of the gallbladder on the hepatobiliary scan support the diagnosis.

Cholecystectomy is the preferred treatment, but both operative cholecystostomy under local anesthesia and percutaneous, transhepatic cholecystostomy represent alternatives in the gravely ill patient. Mortality due to acalculous cholecystitis is about 6% mainly because it usually is not diagnosed until late in its course and because the patient in whom it occurs is usually gravely ill.

Pancreatitis

Acute pancreatitis may occur as a complication of chemotherapy. Asparaginase displays notable pancreatic toxicity, with an incidence of 15–16% in treated patients, and adverse effects can occur as late as 16 weeks after treatment. Acute pancreatitis has also been reported in patients receiving cytarabine, corticosteroids, and combination therapy with vincristine, methotrexate, mitomycin-C, fluorouracil, doxorubicin, and cyclophosphamide.

Nausea, vomiting, and midepigastric abdominal pain, often radiating posteriorly, are common symptoms. Physical findings of poorly localized upper abdominal tenderness, absent bowel sounds, and abdominal distention are products of generalized ileus secondary to retroperitoneal inflammation. Hemodynamic instability, massive fluid requirements, and oliguria are indicative of a more severe inflammatory process. The appearance of flank (Turner's sign) or periumbilical (Cullen's sign) ecchymoses are late signs of hemorrhagic pancreatitis.

The diagnosis of pancreatitis is made on the basis of the clinical presentation with laboratory evidence of pancreatic injury (elevated serum amylase or lipase, elevated urine amylase: creatinine ratio). CT scan may be helpful in imaging the inflammatory process and in providing a baseline for follow-up. Sonography is generally unrewarding in the presence of ileus.

Surgical intervention is reserved for the complications of pancreatitis (hemorrhage, abscess, persistent pseudocyst). Supportive therapy, however, is necessary in all cases of pancreatitis. Restoration of intravascular volume, correction of electrolyte imbalance, and nasogastric suction are the hallmarks of appropriate management. Nutritional support should be initiated after resuscitation because of the indeterminate duration of the process. Careful monitoring of hemodynamic status, electrolyte balance, glucose metabolism, coagulation status, and ventilation and oxygenation is essential.

Neutropenic Enteropathy

Neutropenic enteropathy is a syndrome of abdominal pain, distention, tenderness, and blood diarrhea seen in patients who are severely neutropenic from chemotherapy. The neutropenic state allows invasion of the gut mucosa by enteric pathogens with hemorrhage, ulceration, and in severe cases, perforation. Though generally a diffuse process, a predilection for the proximal colon has been seen ("neutropenic typhlitis" or "ileocecal syndrome").

Patients present with pain, diffuse abdominal tenderness, and diarrhea when their neutrophil count is lowest (<1000/mm^3). Gentle endoscopic examination of the colon can aid in determining the diagnosis. It is important to differentiate this process from pseudomembranous colitis, so stool should be assayed for *Clostridium difficile.*

Treatment is supportive with intravenous fluids, antibiotics to cover gut organisms, and possibly granulocyte transfusions. As the granulocyte count moves back toward normal and the patient's defenses recover, the process usually resolves. Continued hemorrhage, localized abdominal tenderness, perforation, or localized pneumatosis of the bowel wall signal the need for operation, usually resection. Mortality is high. (See also Chapter 38.)

Anorectal Inflammation

Anorectal infections are a potential source of morbidity and mortality in immunocompromised patients with cancer. Most frequently seen in patients with lymphoproliferative disorders and certain solid tumors, these infections typically occur during the induction phase of chemotherapy when the neutrophil count is lowest. An antecedent history of perianal problems (hemorrhoids, anal fissures, fistula in ano) often exists, allowing bacteria access to the local soft tissues.

Rectal pain is the cardinal symptom of the inflammatory process. Fever, erythema, and induration are often present, but the relative lack of neutrophils inhibits localization of the process and the formation of pus.

A history of anorectal irregularities should alert the clinician to the possibility of a necrotizing perianal infection. Such patients should have a rectal examination prior to the institution of chemotherapy, and rectal examination or instrumentation should be avoided during treatment. Sitz baths and stool softeners may help correct underlying irregularities.

Initial treatment of patients in whom anorectal infection is suspected is immediate, aggressive intravenous antibiotic therapy ensuring coverage of both aerobic and anaerobic organisms. Sitz baths and moist local heat afford symptomatic relief. Increasing numbers of neutrophils signal the return of host defenses and localization of the inflammatory process followed either by resolution, spontaneous drainage, or operative drainage.

When a fluctuant perirectal lesion does not improve with antibiotics and local measures, incision and drainage should be done. Local debridement may be necessary, but more extensive procedures do not seem to offer any advantage. Although radiation therapy has been advocated in the treatment of these infections in patients with leukemia, prospective randomized trials have not demonstrated any benefit.

VASCULAR ACCESS ESTABLISHMENT

Patients receiving intermittent chemotherapy for a short to intermediate period of time should have a central venous catheter placed percutaneously at the time of chemotherapy administration. This method provides reliable vascular access with minimal risk of central venous puncture if performed by an experienced physician. At the end of the course of chemotherapy, the catheter is removed and the patient discharged.

Patients requiring long-term vascular access for intermittent chemotherapy should have a subcutaneous infusion port placed early in their course. The subcutaneous port should be used only for the administration of chemotherapy and intravenous fluids. Early placement will preserve peripheral veins for subsequent blood sampling and administration of blood products or antibiotics.

Patients who will receive continuous chemotherapy for a short to intermediate period of time and in whom significant bone marrow toxicity is anticipated should have single or multilumen catheters placed percutaneously. Multilumen catheters provide two or three ports for the administration of intravenous fluids, antibiotics, and blood products in these potentially gravely ill patients. If the issue of catheter sepsis arises during therapy, it is easily addressed by exchanging catheters over a guide wire.

On occasion the surgeon is asked to provide vascular access in a desperately ill patient who is neutropenic and thrombocytopenic. In such instances, avoid percutaneous subclavian or internal jugular venous puncture, since the potential complications of hemothorax, pneumothorax, and cervical hematoma formation with airway compromise can be life-threatening. The external jugular vein is an excellent site for intravenous access in these patients. Its superficial position renders it accessible by either a percutaneous approach or a small cutdown. A flexible-tip guide wire can frequently be advanced to the central venous system. Hemostasis is easily obtained by direct pressure or, if the vein has been surgically exposed, by electrocautery and ligation of the vein proximal and distal to the venotomy. These procedures should be performed under local anesthesia in the operating room, and strict aseptic technique should be employed. Skin incisions should be closed with an absorbable subcuticular suture. Radiographic control is invaluable in facilitating correct placement of the catheter and essential in identifying the correct position of the catheter tip.

REFERENCES

General

Kemeny MM, Brennan MF: Surgical complications of chemotherapy in the cancer patient. *Curr Probl Surg* 1987;**24**:10.

Turnbull AD: *Surgical Emergencies in the Cancer Patient.* Year Book, 1987.

Turnbull AD: The surgical oncologist's role in the intensive care unit. Chapter 17, pp 318–338, in: *Critical Care of the Cancer Patient.* Howland W, Carlon GC (editors). Year Book, 1985.

Wilson RE: Surgical emergencies. Chapter 58, pages 2003–2015 in: *Cancer: Principles and Practice of Oncology,* 3rd ed. De Vita VT Jr, Hellman S, Rosenberg SA (editors). Lippincott, 1989.

Upper Gastrointestinal Bleeding

Cukingnan RA, Carey JS: Carcinoma of the esophagus. *Ann Thorac Surg* 1978;**26**:274.

Hubert JP Jr et al: The surgical management of bleeding stress ulcers. *Ann Surg* 1980;**191**:672.

Levine BA, Gaskill HV III, Sirinek KR: Portasytemic shunting remains the procedure of choice for control of variceal hemorrhage. *Arch Surg* 1985;**120**:296.

Pingleton SK: Recognition and management of upper gastrointestinal hemorrhage. *Am J Med* 1987;**83 (Suppl 6A)**:41.

Shiu MH et al: Management of primary gastric lymphoma. *Ann Surg* 1982;**195**:196.

Stothert JC Jr et al: Randomized prospective evaluation of cimetidine and antacid control of gastric pH in the critically ill. *Ann Surg* 1980;**192**:169.

Sugawa C, Benishek D, Walt A: Mallory-Weiss syndrome: A study of 224 patients. *Am J Surg* 1983;**145**:30.

Lower Gastrointestinal Bleeding

Beart R, Farnell M: Lower gastrointestinal bleeding. Pages 162–163 in: *Surgical Decision Making.* Norton LW, Eiseman B (editors). Saunders, 1988.

Buchman TG, Bulkley GB: Current management of patients with lower gastrointestinal bleeding. *Surg Clin North Am* 1987;**67**:651.

Intestinal Obstruction

Brolin RE: Partial small bowel obstruction. *Surgery* 1984;**95**:145.

Lillemoe KD et al: Surgical management of small bowel radiation enteritis. *Arch Surg* 1983;**118**:905.

Osteen RT et al: Malignant intestinal obstruction. *Surgery* 1980;**87**:611.

Sarr MG, Bulkley GB, Zuidema GD: Preoperative recognition of intestinal strangulation obstruction: Prospective evaluation of diagnostic capability. *Am J Surg* 1983;**145**:176.

Inflammation

Glenn J: Anorectal infections in immunocompromised patients with cancer. *Probl Gen Surg* 1985;**2**:333.

Howard RJ: Acute acalculous cholecytitis. *Am J Surg* 1981;**141**:194.

Savino JA, Scalea TM, Del Guercio LR: Factors encouraging laparotomy in acalculous cholecystitis. *Crit Care Med* 1985;**13**:377.

Vascular Access

Brothers TE et al: Experience with subcutaneous infusion ports in 300 patients. *Surg Gynecol Obstet* 1988;**166**:295.

Raaf JH: Results from use of 826 vascular access devices in cancer patients. *Cancer* 1985;**55**:1312.

Index

AAF. *See* 2-Acetylaminofluorene
Absolute neutrophil count, 355
Acalculous cholecystitis, 394
Accuracy, of screening tests, 35
Acetaminophen, in pain management, 132*t*
2-Acetylaminofluorene
  carcinogenicity of, 13*t*
  metabolism of, 13–14
N-Acetyltransferase, activity, and carcinogenesis, 12
Achlorhydria, 176
Acid phosphatase, in acute leukemia, 275
Acquired immune deficiency syndrome
  cancers related to, 315–319. *See also* Kaposi's sarcoma; Lymphoma(s), primary, of brain
  gastrointestinal, 177–178
  in children, 313–314
    clinical findings with, 313
    diagnosis of, 313
    incidence of, 313–314
    prognosis for, 313
    treatment of, 313–314
  and clinical trials, 319
  etiology of, 315
  GM-CSF therapy in, 123
  and hospice care, 66
  immune abnormalities in, 315
  lymphoma in, 297
  risk factors for, 315
Actinic keratosis, 218
Actinomycin, as radiosensitizer, 80
Actinomycin D. *See* Dactinomycin
Activity, in pain management, 135
Acupressure, in pain management, 135
Acute lymphocytic leukemia, 272. *See also* Leukemia(s), acute
  B cell, 274
  carcinomatous meningitis with, 375
  central nervous system prophylaxis, 277
  chemotherapy for, 105*t*, 277–278, 278*f*
    in children, 301–302
  in children, 299–302
    bone marrow transplantation for, 301–302
    clinical findings with, 300–301
    differential diagnosis, 301
    epidemiology of, 300*t*
    incidence of, 299–300

laboratory findings in, 300*f*, 300–301
  prognosis for, 302
  treatment of, 301–302
common ALL antigen-positive, 274
FAB classification of, 274, 275*t*
null, 274
pathogenesis of, 273–274
postremission therapy, 277
prognosis for, 279
remission induction, 277
T cell, 274
Acute myelogenous leukemia, 272. *See also* Leukemia(s), acute
  chemotherapy for, 277
    central nervous system prophylaxis, 277
    consolidation, 277
    intensification, 277
    maintenance, 277
  chromosomal abnormalities in, 274–275
  FAB classification of, 274, 275*t*
  pathogenesis of, 274
  postremission therapy, 277
  prognosis for, 277, 279
  remission induction, 277
Acute renal failure, in tumor lysis syndrome, 353–354
Acyclovir, 329*t*, 330–331
  for neutropenic or immunocompromised host, 363–366
Adenoacanthoma, endometrial, 200
Adenocarcinoma
  of bladder, 185
  cervical, 202, 204–205, 205*t*
  endometrial, 200–201
  of lung, 238, 239*t*
  vaginal, 208
  vulvar, 206
Adenoma(s), colonic, and colorectal cancer, 174
Adenosine deaminase, in acute leukemia, 275
Adenosquamous carcinoma
  endometrial, 200
  vulvar, 206
Adenovirus infection, in neutropenic or immunocompromised host, 365
Adjuvant therapy
  benefits of, 32, 33*t*, 33
  need for, evaluation of, 33

for osteosarcoma, 269, 270*t*
  for soft-tissue sarcoma, 269
Adnexal tumors, of head and neck, 218
Adoptive immunotherapy, 124
Adrenal cortex, cancer of, chemotherapy for, 104*t*
Adriamycin. *See* Doxorubicin
Adult T cell lymphoma-leukemia, 297
Aflatoxin, carcinogenicity of, 11, 42, 44, 44*t*
Agent Orange, carcinogenicity of, 264
AHH. *See* Aryl hydrocarbon hydroxylase
Ah polymorphism, 12
AIDS. *See* Acquired immune deficiency syndrome
Air pollution, 23
Alcohol
  as cocarcinogen, 23, 44, 44*t*
  and laryngeal cancer, 233, 235
  and oral cancer, 227–228
  and oropharyngeal/hypopharyngeal cancer, 230
Alkeran. *See* Melphalan
Alkylating agents, 106. *See also* specific agent
  as leukemogens, 273
  pulmonary toxicity of, 347–348
ALL. *See* Acute lymphocytic leukemia
Alpha-fetoprotein
  in cerebrospinal fluid, with leptomeningeal disease, 377
  with ovarian germ cell tumors, 198, 199*t*
  with testicular cancer, 187
Amikacin, for neutropenic patient, 358*t*
4-Aminobiphenyl, carcinogenicity of, 182
Aminoglutethimide, 115
  for breast cancer, 143
  in cancer treatment, 191
  side effects of, 115, 117*t*
  structure of, 111*f*
Aminoglycosides, for neutropenic patient, 357, 358*t*
Amitriptyline, in pain management, 132*t*
AML. *See* Acute myelogenous leukemia
Amphotericin B
  adverse effects of, 359, 360*t*
  dosage and administration, 359, 359*t*
  for neutropenic or immunocompromised host, 360*t*, 360–362

Note: An *f* following a page number refers to an illustration; a *t* refers to a table.

LANGE
medical books

LANGE medical books
are available at your local
health science bookstore
or by calling
Appleton & Lange
toll-free
1-800-423-1359
(in CT 838-4400).

See reverse side for a complete listing of LANGE titles.

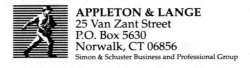

a smart investment in your medical career

Basic Science Textbooks

Color Atlas of Basic Histology
Berman
1993, ISBN 0-8385-0445-0, A0445-5
Jawetz, Melnick & Adelberg's
Medical Microbiology, 19/e
Brooks, Butel & Ornston
1991, ISBN 0-8385-6241-8, A6241-2
Concise Pathology
Chandrasoma & Taylor
1991, ISBN 0-8385-1320-4, A1320-9
Correlative Neuroanatomy, 21/e
deGroot & Chusid
1991, ISBN 0-8385-1332-8, A1332-4
Review of Medical Physiology, 16/e
Ganong
1993, ISBN 0-8385-8426-8, A8426-7
Basic Histology, 7/e
Junqueira, Carniero & Kelly
1992, ISBN 0-8385-0576-7, A0576-7
Basic & Clinical Pharmacology, 5/e
Katzung
1992, ISBN 0-8385-0562-7, A0562-7
Pharmacology
Examination & Review, 3/e
Katzung & Trevor
1993, ISBN 0-8385-7807-1, A7807-9
Medical Microbiology & Immunology
Examination & Board Review, 2/e
Levinson & Jawetz
1992, ISBN 0-8385-6262-0, A6262-8
Harper's Biochemistry, 23/e
Murray, et al.
1993, ISBN 0-8385-3562-3, A3562-4
Basic Histology
Examination & Board Review, 2/e
Paulsen
1993, ISBN 0-8385-0569-4, A0569-2
Basic & Clinical Immunology, 7/e
Stites & Terr
1991, ISBN 0-8385-0544-9, A0544-5
Basic Human Immunology
Stites & Terr
1991, ISBN 0-8385-0543-0, A0543-7

Clinical Science Textbooks

Clinical Cardiology, 6/e
Cheitlin & Sokolow
1993, ISBN 0-8385-1093-0, A1093-2
Fluid & Electrolytes
Physiology & Pathophysiology
Cogan
1991, ISBN 0-8385-2546-6, A2546-8
Basic and Clinical Biostatistics
Dawson-Saunders & Trapp
1990, ISBN 0-8385-6200-0, A6200-8
Basic Gynecology and Obstetrics
Gant & Cunningham
1993, ISBN 0-8385-9633-9, A9633-7
Review of General Psychiatry, 3/e
Goldman
1992, ISBN 0-8385-8428-4, A8428-3

Principles of Clinical Electrocardiography, 13/e
Goldschlager & Goldman
1989, ISBN 0-8385-7951-5, A7951-5
Medical Epidemiology
Greenberg
1993, ISBN 0-8385-6204-3, A6204-0
Clinical Neurology, 2/e
Greenberg, Aminoff & Simon
1993, ISBN 0-8385-1311-5, A1311-8
Basic and Clinical Endocrinology, 3/e
Greenspan
1991, ISBN 0-8385-0545-7, A0545-2
Occupational Medicine
LaDou
1990, ISBN 0-8385-7207-3, A7207-2
Clinical Anatomy
Lindner
1989, ISBN 0-8385-1259-3, A1259-9
Clinical Anesthesiology
Morgan & Mikhail
1992, ISBN 0-8385-1324-7, A1324-1
Dermatology
Orkin, Maibach & Dahl
1991, ISBN 0-8385-1288-7, A1288-8
Clinical Thinking in Surgery
Sterns
1988, ISBN 0-8385-5686-8, A5686-9
Smith's General Urology, 13/e
Tanagho & McAninch
1992, ISBN 0-8385-8608-2, A8608-0
General Ophthalmology, 13/e
Vaughan, Asbury & Riordan-Eva
1992, ISBN 0-8385-3115-6, A3115-1

CURRENT Clinical References

CURRENT Pediatric Diagnosis & Treatment, 11/e
Hathaway, et al.
1993, ISBN 0-8385-1440-5, A1440-5
CURRENT Obstetric & Gynecologic Diagnosis & Treatment, 7/e
Pernoll
1991, ISBN 0-8385-1424-3, A1424-9
CURRENT Emergency Diagnosis & Treatment, 4/e
Saunders & Ho
1992, ISBN 0-8385-1347-6, A1347-2
CURRENT Medical Diagnosis & Treatment 1993
Tierney, et al.
1993, ISBN 0-8385-1350-6, A1350-6
CURRENT Surgical Diagnosis & Treatment, 9/e
Way
1991, ISBN 0-8385-1426-X, A1426-4

LANGE Clinical Manuals

Dermatology
Diagnosis and Therapy
Bondi, Jegasothy & Lazarus
1991, ISBN 0-8385-1274-7, A1274-8
Office & Bedside Procedures
Chesnutt, Dewar & Locksley
1992, ISBN 0-8385-1095-7, A1095-7
Psychiatry
Diagnosis & Treatment, 2/e
Flaherty, Davis & Janicak
1993, ISBN 0-8385-1267-4, A1267-2
Neonatology
Management, Procedures, On-Call Problems, Diseases, Drugs, 2/e
Gomella
1992, ISBN 0-8385-1284-4, A1284-7
Drug Therapy, 2/e
Katzung
1991, ISBN 0-8385-1312-3, A1312-6
Ambulatory Medicine
The Primary Care of Families
Mengel & Schwiebert
1993, ISBN 0-8385-1294-1, A1294-6
Poisoning & Drug Overdose
Olson
1990, ISBN 0-8385-1297-6, A1297-9
Internal Medicine
Diagnosis and Therapy, 3/e
Stein
1993, ISBN 0-8385-1112-0, A1112-0
Surgery
Diagnosis & Therapy
Stillman
1989, ISBN 0-8385-1283-6, A1283-9
Medical Perioperative Management
Wolfsthal
1989, ISBN 0-8385-1298-4, A1298-7

LANGE Handbooks

Handbook of Gynecology & Obstetrics
Brown & Crombleholme
1993, ISBN 0-8385-3608-5, A3608-5
Pocket Guide to Diagnostic Tests
Detmer, et al.
1992, ISBN 0-8385-8020-3, A8020-8
Handbook of Poisoning
Prevention, Diagnosis, and Treatment
Dreisbach & Robertson
1987, ISBN 0-8385-3643-3, A3643-2
Handbook of Clinical Endocrinology, 2/e
Fitzgerald
1992, ISBN 0-8385-3615-8, A3615-0
Pocket Guide to Commonly Prescribed Drugs
Levine
1993, ISBN 0-8385-8023-8, A8023-2
Silver, Kempe, Bruyn & Fulginiti's
Handbook of Pediatrics, 16/e
Merenstein, Kaplan & Rosenberg
1991, ISBN 0-8385-3639-5, A3639-0